Nunn's Applied Respiratory Physiology

Commissioning Editors: Paul Fam/Natasha Andjelkovic
Project Development Manager: Tim Kimber
Project Manager: Kathryn Mason
Design Managers: Stewart Larkin/Jayne Jones
Illustration Manager: Mick Ruddy
Illustrators: Tim Loughhead/Robin Dean
Marketing Managers (UK/USA): Brant Emery/Emily M. Christie

Nunn's Applied Respiratory Physiology

Sixth Edition

Andrew B Lumb MB BS FRCA
Consultant Anaesthetist
St James's University Hospital;
Senior Clinical Lecturer
University of Leeds
Leeds, UK

Foreword by
Ronald G Pearl MD PhD
Professor and Chair
Department of Anesthesia
Stanford University
Stanford, CA, USA

ELSEVIER
BUTTERWORTH
HEINEMANN

ELSEVIER
BUTTERWORTH
HEINEMANN
An imprint of Elsevier Limited

First published 2005
First edition 1969
Second edition 1977
Third edition 1987
Fourth edition 1993
Fifth edition 2000

ISBN 0 7506 8791 6

British Library Cataloguing in Publication Data
A catalogue record for this book is available from the British Library

Library of Congress Cataloging in Publication Data
A catalog record for this book is available from the Library of Congress

Notice
Medical knowledge is constantly changing. Standard safety precautions must be followed, but as new research and clinical experience broaden our knowledge, changes in treatment and drug therapy may become necessary or appropriate. Readers are advised to check the most current product information provided by the manufacturer of each drug to be administered to verify the recommended dose, the method and duration of administration, and contraindications. It is the responsibility of the practitioner, relying on experience and knowledge of the patient, to determine dosages and the best treatment for each individual patient. Neither the Publisher nor the author assumes any liability for any injury and/or damage to persons or property arising from this publication.

The Publisher

Printed in Italy
Last digit is the print number: 9 8 7 6 5 4 3 2 1

Contents

Contents

Foreword to the Sixth Edition

I am honored to provide a foreword to this, the sixth edition of *Nunn's Applied Respiratory Physiology*. When the first edition of this work published in 1969, it instantly became the classic text on the subject. The teaching of respiratory physiology is interspersed throughout medical training, and the book fulfilled the needs of both the beginning student learning the essentials of respiratory physiology and the experienced clinician needing to learn more about a specific topic. Over the years, the subject of respiratory physiology has grown and evolved, and the book has kept pace. There have been major advances in our understanding of respiratory physiology on the organ, tissue, cellular, biochemical, and molecular levels. By the third edition of the book, it became necessary to create two parts to the book in order to separately emphasize basic principles and the applications of respiratory physiology. The fifth edition of the book, published in 2000 following Dr Nunn's retirement, was edited by Andrew Lumb and markedly increased the emphasis on clinical topics by adding a third section on physiology of pulmonary disease. In order to continue the goal of having a single yet comprehensive volume, the fifth edition included a major revision with removal of older literature and topics. This process parallels the process of curriculum revision that is occurring in medical schools throughout the world.

This sixth edition maintains the tradition of presenting respiratory physiology in a manner that can be understood by students, clinicians, and investigators. The book continues the three-pronged approach adopted in the fifth edition. The first part on basic principles covers anatomy, mechanics, control of breathing, ventilation, circulation, ventilation-perfusion matching, diffusion, carbon dioxide and oxygen, and non-respiratory functions of the lung. The second part on applied physiology discusses the effects of pregnancy, exercise, sleep, altitude, pressure, drowning, smoking, anesthesia, hypocapnia, hypercarbia, hypoxia, hyperoxia, and anemia. The third part on physiology of pulmonary disease discusses both specific clinical disorders (ventilatory failure, airways disease, pulmonary vascular disease, parenchymal lung disease, acute lung injury) and therapies (artificial ventilation, extrapulmonary gas exchange, and lung transplantation). Although the topics covered in the book are similar to the prior edition, the chapters have been fully updated and serve as a current reference. Visually, the book has been modernized with new illustrations, improved layout, and the addition of color. Key points and key references have been added to the chapters. The new edition has markedly expanded the coverage of molecular physiology and clinical pharmacology relevant to the lung, but with the format changes the book is now even shorter than before.

For more than three decades, *Nunn's Applied Respiratory Physiology* has been the standard book for understanding this important subject. This sixth edition will take a place on my bookshelf next to my well-used copy of the first edition. I anticipate that this new edition will soon be equally used and congratulate Dr Lumb on an outstanding update of this classic text.

Ronald G Pearl

Preface to the Sixth Edition

Over the past 36 years *Nunn's Applied Respiratory Physiology* has developed into a renowned textbook on respiration, providing both physiologists and clinicians with a unique fusion of underlying principles and their applications. With Dr John Nunn's retirement in 1991, a new author was required, and, as Dr Nunn's final research fellow in the Clinical Research Centre in Harrow, I was honoured to be chosen as his successor. As a practising clinician with an interest in medical education, changes to the sixth edition have again focused on combining a clear, logical and comprehensive account of basic respiratory physiology with a wide range of applications, both physiological and clinical. This approach acknowledges the popularity of the book amongst doctors from many medical specialities and will hopefully provide readers with a scientific background even greater insight into the applications of respiratory physiology. Clinical chapters in Part 3 of the book are not intended to be comprehensive reviews of the pulmonary diseases considered, but in each case they provide a detailed description of the physiological changes that occur, accompanied by a brief account of the clinical features and treatment of the disease.

For the sixth edition, the most noticeable change relates to the book's format, which has allowed better linkage between the text and tables/figures. Key references have been identified by an asterisk in the reference list following each chapter. These references are highlighted because they either provide outstanding recent reviews of their subject or describe research that has had a major impact on the topic under consideration.

The history of respiratory physiology (Chapter 13) is new for the sixth edition. Snippets of information on history had crept into many sections of previous editions, and I embarked on collating these into a single chapter. However, once research into this area began, it became clear that the evolution of our understanding of how and why we breathe travelled much farther back into history than I had anticipated. The story is fascinating, and peppered with starkly erroneous concepts, some of which persisted for many centuries, and vehement academic controversies.

In several chapters of this edition new information has been included about drugs that affect the respiratory system. Potential therapeutic use of drugs acting on pulmonary receptors has been the driving force for indepth research into the physiological mechanisms underlying receptor activity. For example, the molecular mechanisms of the β-adrenoreceptor in airway smooth muscle are now elucidated in enormous depth in the search for more efficacious agonists.

Advances in respiratory physiology since the last edition are too numerous to mention individually, but continue to focus on better understanding of physiological processes at the cellular and molecular levels. Understanding of several proteins involved in respiratory physiology has advanced rapidly in recent years. A fascinating example is pulmonary α_1-antitrypsin, which is now known to act like a mousetrap, offering an amino acid bait to protease enzymes which, when cleaved, causes the entire molecule to flip closed, trapping the protease within the α_1-antitrypsin molecule. Other examples include recently discovered molecular mechanisms for the actions of haemoglobin, carbonic anhydrase and band 3, the protein responsible for the exchange of chloride and bicarbonate ions across the red blood cell membrane.

I wish to personally thank the many people who have helped with the preparation of the book, including the numerous colleagues who have encouraged and assisted my acquisition of knowledge in subjects not so close to my own areas of interest. I am also indebted to Professor Pearl for his kind words in the Foreword, and to Professor Walker for providing the figure of the lung fibroblast guiding a neutrophil into the lung interstitium. I wish to thank the staff of the Leeds University Library Special Collections and the Wellcome Library, London, for their expertise concerning the historical documents used for researching and illustrating Chapter 13. I remain especially indebted to Dr Nunn for his continued support of the book and its author, and would like to thank him for once again providing an excellent Chapter 1 on the origins of Earth's atmosphere. Last, but by no means least, I would like to thank Lorraine, Emma and Jenny for tolerating a pre-occupied and reclusive husband/father for so long. Jenny, when aged 5, often enquired about my activities in the study, until one evening she nicely summarized my years of work by confidently informing me that 'if you don't breathe, you die'. So what were the other 471 pages about?

Andrew B Lumb

Preface to the First Edition

Clinicians in many branches of medicine find that their work demands an extensive knowledge of respiratory physiology. This applies particularly to anaesthetists working in the operating theatre or in the intensive care unit. It is unfortunately common experience that respiratory physiology learned in the preclinical years proves to be an incomplete preparation for the clinical field. Indeed, the emphasis of the preclinical course seems, in many cases, to be out of tune with the practical problems to be faced after qualification and specialization. Much that is taught does not apply to man in the clinical environment while, on the other hand, a great many physiological problems highly relevant to the survival of patients find no place in the curriculum. It is to be hoped that new approaches to the teaching of medicine may overcome this dichotomy and that, in particular, much will be gained from the integration of physiology with clinical teaching.

This book is designed to bridge the gap between pure respiratory physiology and the treatment of patients. It is neither a primer of respiratory physiology nor a practical manual for use in the wards and operating theatres. It has two aims. First, I have tried to explain those aspects of respiratory physiology that seem most relevant to patient care, particularly in the field of anaesthesia. Secondly, I have brought together in review those studies that seem to me to be most relevant to clinical work. Inevitably there has been a preference for studies of man and particular stress has been laid on those functions in which man appears to differ from laboratory animals. There is an unashamed emphasis on anaesthesia because I am an anesthetist. However, the work in this specialty spreads freely into the territory of our neighbours.

References have been a problem. It is clearly impracticable to quote every work that deserves mention. In general I have cited the most informative and the most accessible works, but this rule has been broken on numerous occasions when the distinction of prior discovery calls for recognition. Reviews are freely cited because a book of this length can include only a fraction of the relevant material. I must apologize to the writers of multi-author papers. No one likes to be cited as a colleague, but considerations of space have precluded naming more than three authors for any paper.

Chapters are designed to be read separately and this has required some repetition. There are also frequent cross-references between the chapters. The principles of methods of measurement are considered together at the end of each chapter or section.

In spite of optimistic hopes, the book has taken six years to write. Its form, however, has evolved over the last twelve years from a series of lectures and tutorials given at the Royal College of Surgeons, the Royal Postgraduate Medical School, the University of Leeds and in numerous institutions in Europe and the USA that I have been privileged to visit. Blackboard sketches have gradually taken the form of the figures that appear in this book.

The greater part of this book is distilled from the work of teachers and colleagues. Professor W Melville Arnott and Professor KW Donald introduced me to the study of clinical respiratory physiology and I worked under the late Professor Ronald Woolmer for a further six years. My debt to them is very great. I have also had the good fortune to work in close contact with many gifted colleagues who have not hesitated to share the fruits of their experience. The list of references will indicate how much I have learned from Dr John Severinghaus, Professor Moran Campbell, Dr John Butler and Dr John West. For my own studies, I acknowledge with gratitude the part played by a long series of research fellows and assistants. Some fifteen are cited herein and they come from eleven different countries. Figures 2, 3, 6, 11 and 15 [Figure 5.3 in the fourth edition, and Figures 3.4 and 3.1 in the fifth edition] which are clearly not my blackboard sketches, were drawn by Mr H Grayshon Lumby. I have had unstinted help from librarians, Miss MP Russell, Mr WR LeFanu and Miss EM Reed. Numerous colleagues have given invaluable help in reading and criticizing the manuscript.

Finally, I must thank my wife who has not only borne the inevitable preoccupation of a husband writing a book but has also carried the burden of the paperwork and prepared the manuscript.

John F Nunn

Part: One

Basic principles

Dr John F Nunn

KEY POINTS

- The mass of the Earth and its distance from the sun provide optimal conditions of gravity and temperature for long-term liquid surface water and the retention in its atmosphere of oxygen, nitrogen and carbon dioxide.
- Primitive life forms generated energy by photosynthetic reactions, which produced oxygen as a waste product, and by doing so they facilitated the development of an oxygen-containing atmosphere and aerobic organisms.
- Carbon dioxide was initially the main component of the Earth's atmosphere, but by 300 million years ago rock weathering and photosynthesis had reduced its concentration to current low levels.
- There is now an acceptance that burning of fossil fuels and deforestation are causing an increase in atmospheric carbon dioxide, unprecedented in the last 40 million years. However, there is no immediate likelihood of a physiologically significant reduction in oxygen concentration.

The atmosphere of Earth is radically different from that of any other planet in the solar system (Table 1.1). This is because of two main reasons. First, temperature has permitted the existence of liquid surface water for at least 4000 million years (Ma), and this has resulted in weathering of silicate rocks, reducing the concentration of carbon dioxide far below the levels still pertaining on the rocky planets Venus and Mars. Second, the existence of liquid surface water enabled living organisms to appear at a very early stage: life forms then evolved to undertake oxygenic photosynthesis. When oxygen sinks were saturated, oxygen appeared in the atmosphere and some organisms began to utilise highly efficient oxidative metabolic pathways. An atmosphere containing oxygen is in inorganic chemical disequilibrium and is an indication of the existence of life.

EVOLUTION OF THE ATMOSPHERE

Formation of Earth and the prebiotic atmosphere

The earth was formed by a relatively short-lived but intense gravitational accretion of rather large planetesimals, orbiting the newly formed sun some 4560 Ma ago. The kinetic energy of the impacting bodies was sufficient to raise the temperature to a few thousand degrees Celsius. This would have melted the entire Earth, resulting in loss of the primary atmosphere.

Earth cooled rapidly by radiation when the initial bombardment abated and the very high temperature (Hadean) phase is not thought to have lasted longer than a few hundred Ma. The crust solidified but massive outgassing continued, resulting in an atmosphere mainly comprising carbon dioxide and steam (Table 1.2), as probably occurred on Venus and Mars.[1,2] In the case of Earth, the water vapour condensed to surface water and there is good evidence that oceans existed about 3800 Ma ago and perhaps even earlier.[3] Once Earth's crust was cool and surface water was in existence, it was possible for comets and meteorites to leave a secondary veneer of their contents, including water and a wide range of organic compounds.[4]

Important physicochemical changes occurred in the early secondary atmosphere. Helium and hydrogen tended to be lost from the Earth's gravitational field. Ammonia dissociated to nitrogen and hydrogen, the former retained and the latter lost from the atmosphere. Some carbon dioxide might have been reduced by hydrogen to form traces of methane, but very large quantities slowly reacted with surface silicates to become trapped as carbonates, while forming silica (weathering). Traces of water vapour underwent photodissociation to hydrogen and oxygen. However, oxygen from this source was present in only minimal quantities. The early atmosphere is no longer thought to have been as strongly reducing as was formerly believed.[6]

Table 1.1 Composition of the atmosphere of Earth and the nearer planets

Planet	Atmosphere			
Mercury	Extremely tenuous			
Venus	Carbon dioxide	96.5%	+ Traces: argon, helium, neon,	
	Nitrogen	3.5%	krypton (all <20 ppmv)	
Earth	Nitrogen	78.08%	Water vapour – variable	
	Oxygen	20.95%	Neon	18.2 ppmv
	Argon	0.93%	Helium	5.2 ppmv
	Carbon dioxide	0.037%	Methane	1.8 ppmv
Mars	Carbon dioxide	95.3%	Oxygen	0.13%
	Nitrogen	2.7%	Carbon monoxide	0.27%
	Argon	1.6%	+ Traces: neon, krypton, xenon	
Jupiter	Hydrogen	89%	Methane	1750 ppmv
	Helium	11%	+ Traces: ammonia, water vapour etc.	
Saturn	Hydrogen	94%	Methane	4500 ppmv
	Helium	6%	+ Traces: ethylene, phosphine	

ppmv, parts per million volume.
Earth's data for carbon dioxide and methane have been updated to 2002 AD.
(Planetary data are from Taylor,[1] reproduced from Nunn[2] by permission of the Geologists' Association.)

Table 1.2 Average composition of gas evolved from Hawaiian volcanoes

Constituent	Percent
Water vapour	70.75
Carbon dioxide	14.07
Sulphur dioxide	6.40
Nitrogen	5.45
Sulphur trioxide	1.92
Carbon monoxide	0.40
Hydrogen	0.33
Argon	0.18
Sulphur	0.10
Chlorine	0.05

(Data are from reference 5, reproduced from Nunn[2] by permission of the Geologists' Association.)

The initial very high partial pressure of carbon dioxide, and probably some methane, would have provided a powerful greenhouse effect to offset the early minimal weak solar radiation, which was some 30% less than today (Figure 1.1). However, the sun commenced its main sequence of thermonuclear fusion of hydrogen to helium about 3000 Ma ago. Since then solar radiation has been increasing steadily as the sun proceeds remorselessly towards becoming a red giant, which will ultimately envelop the inner planets. It is fortunate that increasing solar radiation has been approximately offset by a diminishing greenhouse effect, due mainly to decreasing levels of carbon dioxide (see below). As a result, Earth's temperature has remained relatively stable, permitting the existence of surface water for the last 4000 Ma.

Significance of mass of Earth and distance from sun

Small bodies, such as Mercury and most of the planets' satellites, have a gravitational field that is too weak for the retention of any significant atmosphere (Figure 1.2). The gas giants (Jupiter, Saturn, Uranus and Neptune) have a gravitational field which is sufficiently strong to retain all gases, including helium and hydrogen, thereby ensuring the retention of a reducing atmosphere. The gravitational field of the earth is intermediate, resulting in a differential retention of the heavier gases (oxygen, carbon dioxide and nitrogen) while permitting the escape of hydrogen and helium. This is essential for the development of an oxidising atmosphere. Water vapour (molecular weight only 18) would be lost from the atmosphere were it not for the cold trap at the tropopause.

Surface temperature of a planetary body is crucial for the existence of liquid water, which is essential for life and therefore the composition of our atmosphere. To a first approximation, temperature is dependent on the distance of a planet from the sun and the intensity of solar radiation (see Figure 1.2). The major secondary factor is the greenhouse effect of any atmosphere that the planet may possess. Mercury and Venus have surface

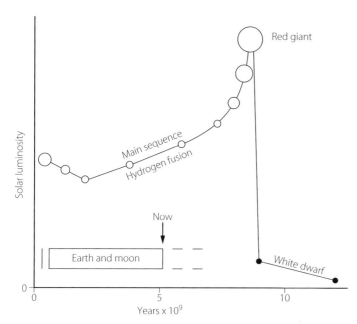

Figure 1.1 Solar luminosity plotted against the age of the sun, with the open circles giving a qualitative impression of the diameter of the sun. Superimposed is an indication of the life of Earth and its moon, which is now about halfway through the main sequence of the sun deriving its energy from hydrogen fusion to helium. The times can only be very approximate. (After reference 7.)

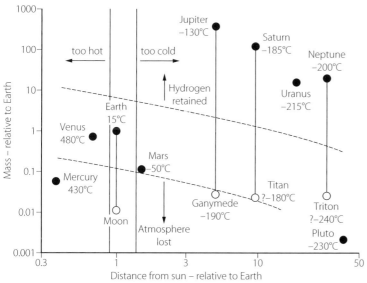

Figure 1.2 The planets and some of their larger satellites, plotted according to distance from the sun (abscissa) and mass (ordinate), both scales being logarithmic and relative to the Earth. Mean surface temperatures are shown. Potential for life as we know it exists only within the parallelogram surrounding the Earth.

temperatures far above the boiling point of water. All planets (and their satellites) which are further away from the sun than Earth have a surface temperature too cold for liquid water to exist today. However, there is now evidence that Mars had liquid surface water in the past,[8] though not at present.

Earth is the only planet in the solar system that has a mass permitting the retention of an oxidising atmosphere and a distance from the sun at which liquid water can today exist on its surface. It is difficult to see how there could be life as we know it anywhere in the solar system outside the small parallelogram in Figure 1.2.

However, an environment similar to that of the Earth may well exist on some planets of the vast number of other sun-like stars in the universe.

Origin of life and the development of photosynthesis

Amino acids and a wide range of organic compounds are found in a type of meteorite known as carbonaceous chondrites.[4] Therefore, whether or not such compounds were actually synthesised on the early Earth, as was formerly believed,[6] it is highly likely that a wide range of organic compounds were available on Earth when liquid oceans were formed.

It is less easy to explain the next stage in the evolution of life. An essential feature of all life is the synthesis of proteins using a ribonucleic acid (RNA) template, usually transcribed from the genetic code carried on deoxyribonucleic acid (DNA). There would appear to have been a classic 'chicken and egg' situation. Useful proteins could not be formed without the appropriate sequences in RNA or DNA: RNA and DNA could not be polymerised without appropriate enzymes, which are normally proteins. Nevertheless, life did appear, perhaps in the first instance with the genetic code carried on RNA or even the much simpler peptide nucleic acid (PNA).[9]

An essential requirement for life is the availability of bio-usable forms of energy. The forms of available energy and their location at the dawn of life remain a mystery. However, one cannot ignore the possibility of hydrothermal vents, such as the black smokers along the mid-ocean ridges at great depths, which still support very simple life forms on the basis of chemo-autotrophy. They are totally independent of sunlight and exploit the profound chemical disequilibrium between the emerging hot, reducing and acid water, containing hydrogen sulphide, methane, ammonia, phosphorus and a range of metals, and the surrounding sea water.[10] It is likely that there have been hydrothermal vents on Earth for as long as surface water has coexisted with volcanic activity. Chemo-autotrophs might therefore have appeared as early as 4000 Ma ago.

Hydrothermal vents provide an extremely constrained and hazardous environment for life, with energy supply depending on their continued existence. A much more attractive alternative was to utilise the limitless availability of energy in the form of solar visible light. The most familiar of such reactions is the oxygenic photosynthesis of glucose, summarised as follows:

$$6CO_2 + 6H_2O + energy = C_6H_{12}O_6 + 6O_2$$

The biochemical adaptation from thermal detection in hydrothermal vents to photosynthesis does not seem to have been insuperable[11] and there is strong evidence for the existence of photosynthesising cyanobacteria (blue-green algae) by 2700 Ma ago.[12] At a later date, cyanobacteria underwent symbiotic incorporation into the cells of certain eukaryotes to become chloroplasts, which then conferred the biochemical benefits of photosynthesis on their hosts, which include all plants.

The appearance of oxygen in the atmosphere

Oxygenic photosynthesis releases oxygen, apparently as a waste product. However, there was a delay of about 400 Ma between the development of photosynthesis and the appearance of oxygen in the atmosphere. Oxygen

Figure 1.3 Long-term changes in oxygen and carbon dioxide concentrations during the last 600 Ma. Broken horizontal lines show present atmospheric levels. The vertical broken line shows the Carboniferous/Permian boundary. The continuous horizontal lines with arrows show some oxygen limits suggested by the geological record of forest fires.[2] Geological periods shown by their capital letters are: Cambrian, Ordovician, Silurian, Devonian, Carboniferous and Permian (Palaeozoic Era), Triassic, Jurassic, Cretaceous (Mesozoic Era) and Tertiary. Recent research suggests levels of carbon dioxide may be slightly less than shown, but the nature of the changes is not in doubt. (From Nunn,[2] after Graham et al.[14] Reproduced by permission of the Geologists' Association.)

was consumed by oxidising methane and also soluble ferrous iron (Fe^{2+}), leached from basalt and deposited as ferric iron (Fe^{3+}) in the vast banded iron formations. This process prevented the appearance of detectable concentrations of oxygen in the atmosphere (10^{-5} bar) until about 2320 Ma ago.[12,13] After the atmosphere attained a higher but critical level of oxygen (about 1800 Ma ago), banded iron formations seldom appeared and iron was then deposited in red (ferric) beds.[2]

After 2320 Ma ago, oxygen accumulated in the oceans and atmosphere, probably reaching a peak 300 Ma ago[14] (Figure 1.3). It then decreased sharply, perhaps contributing to the mass extinction at the end of the Palaeozoic Era, about 250 Ma ago.[2] Thereafter it appears to have risen towards the present atmospheric level.

Biological consequences of an oxidising environment

It seems likely that the appearance of molecular oxygen in their environment would have been unwelcome to anaerobic organisms. Chapter 26 describes the toxicity of oxygen and its derived free radicals, against which primitive anaerobes would probably have had no defences. Three lines of response can be identified. Some anaerobes sought an anaerobic microenvironment in which to remain and survive. Others developed defences in depth against oxygen and its derived free radicals (page 355). The best response was the development of aerobic metabolism, which gave enormous energetic advantages over organisms relying on anaerobic metabolism (page 186). This required the symbiotic incorporation of purple bacteria that became mitochondria, but the increased availability of biological energy was essential for the evolution of all forms of life more complex than micro-organisms.

Photosynthesis and aerobic metabolism eventually established a cycle of energy exchange between plants and animals, with its ultimate energy input in the form of solar visible light, which was interrupted only under exceptional circumstances. Such circumstances included major meteorite strikes and exceptional volcanic activity, both of which can throw vast quantities of persistent dust into the atmosphere and cause extinctions by blocking photosynthesis.

Changes in carbon dioxide levels

After the major outgassing phase of the newly formed Earth, the concentration of carbon dioxide in the atmosphere probably exceeded 90% at high atmospheric pressure. It declined rapidly due to weathering and photosynthesis, reaching about 0.5% at the time of the beginning of the overt fossil record (Palaeozoic Era, from 570 Ma ago). A secondary major decline to near the present atmospheric level occurred during the Carboniferous period, when the coal-forming forests involved photosynthesis and carbon burial on a massive scale. A sharp increase occurred at the end of the Permian period (the last period of the Palaeozoic Era) about 250 Ma ago and carbon dioxide may have contributed to the end-Permian mass extinction. This coincided with the decrease in oxygen concentration mentioned above (see Figure 1.3).

Carbon dioxide and the ice ages

Carbon dioxide and global temperature reached levels well above those pertaining today from about 270 Ma until about 40 Ma ago. Thereafter, carbon dioxide and temperature declined, resulting in the formation of the Antarctic ice sheets (from about 35 Ma ago) and, at a later stage, the present phase of periodic ice ages interspersed with warmer interglacial periods. The fundamental causes of the periodicity appear to be astronomical (Milankovitch cycles), which cause variations in the heat received by Earth from the sun. The most influential seems to be the degree of ellipticity of the Earth's orbit, with a periodicity of about 100 thousand years (ka), and its effect is very clear in the mean global temperature record for the last 420 ka derived from Antarctic ice cores (Figure 1.4).[15]

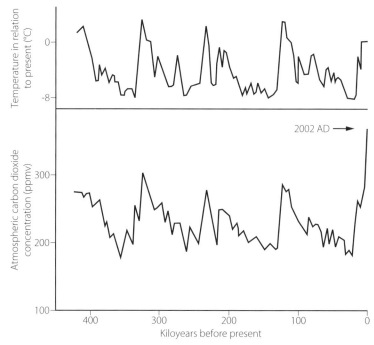

Figure 1.4 General trends for temperature and atmospheric carbon dioxide concentration, obtained from ice cores from Vostok, Antarctica, for the last 420 000 years. (Data from reference [15] and reproduced in part from reference 16, with the permission of the Editor of *The Optimum Population Trust Journal*.)

There is also a remarkably close correlation between temperature and atmospheric concentrations of both carbon dioxide and methane, which appear to have exerted positive feedback to the change in temperature initiated by the changes in ellipticity of our orbit. Carbon dioxide has ranged between about 180 parts per million, volume (ppmv) during glacials and 280 ppmv during interglacial periods until the start of the industrial revolution in AD 1750[15] (see Figure 1.4).

Casual inspection of Figure 1.4 suggests that the next glacial period is overdue. However, it appears that the rhythmic changes in global mean temperature shown for the last 420 ka will not continue, as we now enter a long phase when the Earth's orbit will remain almost circular. The 100 ka cycle will be in virtual abeyance for about 50 ka, during which there will be a prolonged interglacial.[17] However, it is highly unlikely that mean global temperature will remain constant, owing to the current unprecedented increase in the atmospheric carbon dioxide concentration.

Recent changes in carbon dioxide levels

Atmospheric carbon dioxide remained close to 280 ppmv from the start of the current interglacial until the start of the Industrial Revolution (AD 1750). In the next 200 years it increased to 310 ppmv (0.15 ppmv per year) (Table 1.3). Between AD 1992 and 2002 the increase was from 356.4 to 372.9 ppmv (1.65 ppmv per year). Over short periods, the increase approximates to a 'tearaway' exponential function, i.e. constant percentage increase per year as with compound interest (page 467, Appendix F). However, over a longer period it is clear that the annual percentage increase is not constant but is itself increasing as a second 'tear-away' exponential function.[16]

On this basis, extrapolation of trends from AD 1750 to the present suggests that the concentration should reach at least 1000 ppmv by the year AD 2100, rather than the 450 ppmv that was previously expected. The increased estimate is similar to the latest computed predictions based on analysis of the many primary factors governing atmospheric CO_2 concentrations. Thus we may expect to reach the highest concentration that has existed since the formation of the present polar ice sheets. Whether the rate of change continues to accelerate is critically dependent on the continued efficiency of the global carbon sinks and attempts to control emissions, with all the current political uncertainty. The only certain limitation on emissions would seem to be exhaustion of the world's fossil fuels. Global warming may have disturbing short-term effects on ocean currents, particularly a weakening of the north Atlantic conveyor (including the Gulf Stream).[18] This could result in a substantial cooling of north-western Europe.

THE GREENHOUSE EFFECT

The balance of heat gain from solar radiation is the difference between incoming radiation, mainly in the visible wavelengths, and outgoing radiation, which is largely infrared. The latter is partially trapped in the troposphere, mainly by water vapour (60%) and carbon dioxide (25%). Atmospheric water vapour concentration increases with rising global temperature and therefore provides positive feedback to global warming. It is estimated that the present greenhouse effect raises the mean surface temperature of the Earth by some 30°C. Carbon dioxide makes a major contribution to the very high surface temperature of Venus (480°C), hotter than Mercury but further from the sun.

Other greenhouse gases

There are no infrared absorption bands for water vapour and carbon dioxide between 7 and 13 μm wavelength and heat loss in this band is considerable. It follows that any gas or vapour with strong infrared absorption in this range will have a disproportionate greenhouse effect. Such a gas could be considered not so much as thickening the panes in the greenhouse as replacing a missing pane.

After water and carbon dioxide, the most important greenhouse gases are ozone (8% of total effect) and methane (3% of total effect), which is present in the atmosphere at a concentration of only 2 ppmv but rapidly increasing: it absorbs infrared some 25 times as effectively as carbon dioxide. The chlorofluorocarbons (2% of total effect) absorb infrared some 10 000 times as effectively as carbon dioxide but present atmospheric concentrations are only of the order of 0.003 ppmv. However, with their long half-life, they cannot be

Table 1.3 Recent changes in atmospheric carbon dioxide concentrations			
	Atmospheric CO_2		Rate of change
Date	Mass in Gt	ppmv	ppmv per year
18 ka ago	420	200	
10 ka ago	590	280	0.01
1750 AD	590	280	0
1950 AD	650	310	0.15
1995 AD	760	362	1.16

Gt, gigatonne; ka, thousand years; ppmv, parts per million, volume.
Data are from various sources. (Reproduced from Nunn[2] by permission of the Geologists' Association.)

ignored. Nitrous oxide, mainly of biological origin, also makes a small contribution.

With Earth in an approximately circular orbit for the next 50 ka and solar gain remaining reasonably constant, greenhouse gases are now the major factors governing global temperature. Carbon dioxide is rising rapidly towards the highest levels in the last 40 Ma and water vapour will increase with rising temperature. The mean global temperature is predicted to increase to within 90% confidence limits of 1.5–4.5°C by AD 2100. Temperature has already increased by 0.6°C in the last century, mostly since 1950.[19] Not the least serious consequence will be melting of polar ice, which has the ultimate potential to raise sea level by 67 m. Sea level has been rising at about 1.8 mm/year since AD 1850, without evidence of significant increase.[16] However, there is already retreat of Greenland and Alaskan glaciers and disruption of the western Antarctic ice sheets.

TURNOVER RATES OF ATMOSPHERIC GASES

Biological and geological turnover rates of carbon dioxide are quantitatively totally different.[2] Living organisms, the atmosphere and surface waters of the oceans contain about 2200 Gt (gigatonnes) of carbon. The annual exchange between photosynthesis and aerobic metabolism is approximately 100 Gt annually, with anthropogenic burning of fossil fuels and deforestation currently releasing about 8 Gt each year (Figure 1.5).

In stark contrast, geological stores (ocean depths, organic biomass and limestone) have a carbon content in excess of 30 000 000 Gt but with an annual turnover (volcanoes, weathering etc.) of less than 0.1 Gt per year. Thus, long-term changes are governed by the geological stores, while very rapid atmospheric changes can occur as a result of imbalance in the biomass or the anthropogenic activities outlined above.

Atmospheric stores of oxygen are almost 600 times greater than those for carbon dioxide. If oxygen decreased at the same rate as the current increase in carbon dioxide, it would take 40 000 years for sea level PO_2 to fall to the level which pertains in Denver today.

OXYGEN, OZONE AND ULTRAVIOLET SCREENING

In addition to its toxicity and potential for more efficient metabolism, oxygen had a profound effect on evolution by ultraviolet screening. Oxygen itself absorbs ultraviolet radiation to a certain extent but ozone (O_3) is far more effective. It is formed in the stratosphere from oxygen, which undergoes photodissociation, producing free oxygen atoms. The oxygen atoms then rapidly combine with oxygen molecules to form ozone thus:

$$O_2 \rightleftharpoons 2O$$
$$\downarrow$$
$$O + O_2 \rightleftharpoons O_3$$

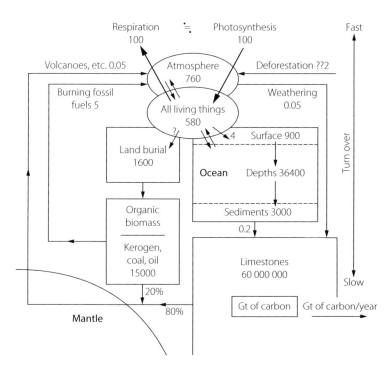

Figure 1.5 Stores and turnover of carbon dioxide (not to scale). Stores are in Gt (gigatonnes) and turnover in Gt per year. The burning of fossil fuels was 6.4 Gt per year and atmospheric carbon dioxide 783 Gt in 2002 AD: both are increasing rapidly. (After reference 2, where sources are cited. Reproduced by permission of the Geologists' Association.)

The absolute quantity is very small, being the equivalent of a layer of pure ozone only a few millimetres thick. A Dobson unit of ozone is defined as the equivalent of a layer of pure ozone 0.01 mm thick. About 10% of the total atmospheric ozone is in the troposphere, mainly as a pollutant. This also acts as an ultraviolet screen and may become relatively more important in the years to come.

Life evolved in water, which provided adequate screening from ultraviolet radiation. The first colonisation of dry land by plants and animals was in the late Silurian period about 400 Ma years ago and it has been suggested that this coincided with oxygen and ozone reaching concentrations at which the degree of ultraviolet shielding first permitted organisms to leave the shelter of an aqueous environment.

Ozone is in a state of dynamic equilibrium in the stratosphere and its concentration varies markedly from year to year, in addition to displaying a pronounced annual cycle. Ozone can be removed by the action of many free radicals, including chlorine and nitric oxide. Highly reactive chlorine radicals cannot normally pass through the troposphere to reach the stratosphere, but the situation was disturbed by the manufacture of chlorofluorocarbons (e.g. CF_2Cl_2) for use as propellants and refrigerants. These compounds are highly stable in the troposphere with a half-life of the order of 100 years. This permits their diffusion through the troposphere to reach the stratosphere, where they undergo photodissociation to release chlorine radicals, which then react with ozone as follows:

$$Cl + O_3 \rightarrow ClO + O_2$$
$$\uparrow \qquad \qquad \downarrow$$
$$Cl + O_2 \leftarrow ClO + O$$

Chlorine is recycled and it has been estimated that a single chlorine radical will destroy 10 000 molecules of ozone before it combines with hydrogen to form the relatively harmless hydrochloric acid. The Antarctic 'hole' in the ozone layer forms in October of each year, when spring sunlight initiates photochemical reactions. Minimal levels fell from 300 Dobson units in 1960 to 100 in 1994 and are still falling.[20]

EVOLUTION AND ADAPTATION

This chapter has outlined the environmental conditions and biological factors under which the atmosphere has evolved to its present composition. In the past, nothing has been permanent and we can expect a continuation of the interaction between organisms and their environment. What is new is that one species now has the power to cause major changes in the environment, and the atmosphere in particular. These will affect a wide range of organisms and result in the extinction of certain species.

REFERENCES

1. Taylor SR. *Solar system evolution*. Cambridge: Cambridge University Press, 1992.
*2. Nunn JF. Evolution of the atmosphere. *Proc Geol Assoc* 1998; **109**: 1–13.
3. Nisbet EG, Sleep NH. The habitat and nature of early life. *Nature* 2001; **409**: 1083–91.
4. Oró J. Early chemical stages in the origin of life. In: Bengston S, ed. *Early life on Earth*. Nobel symposium no. 84. New York: Columbia University Press, 1994; 48–59.
5. MacDonald GA, Hubbard DH. *Volcanoes of the national parks in Hawaii*, 6th edn. Honolulu: Hawaii Natural History Association, 1972.
6. Miller SL. A production of amino acids under possible primitive earth conditions. *Science* 1953; **117**: 528–9.
7. Chapman CR, Morrison D. *Cosmic catastrophes*. London: Plenum Press, 1989; 97.
8. Malin MC, Edgett KS. Evidence of persistent flow and aqueous sedimentation on early Mars. *Science* 2003; **302**: 1931–4.
9. Böhler C, Nielsen PE, Orgel LE. Template switching between PNA and RNA oligonucleotides. *Nature* 1995; **376**: 578–81.
10. Nisbet EG. Archaean ecology. In: Coward MP, Reis AC, eds. *Early Precambrian processes*. London: Geological Society, 1995; 27–51.
11. Nisbet EG. Origins of photosynthesis. *Nature* 1995; **373**: 479–80.
12. Kasting JF. The rise of atmospheric oxygen. *Science* 2001; **293**: 819–20.
13. Bekker A, Holland HD, Wang PL, *et al*. Dating the rise of atmospheric oxygen. *Nature* 2004; **427**: 117–20.
14. Graham JB, Dudley R, Aguilar NM, Gans C. Implications of the late Palaeozoic oxygen pulse for physiology amd evolution. *Nature* 1995; **375**: 117–20.
*15. Petit JR, Jouzel, R, Raynaud DS, *et al*. Climate and atmospheric history of the past 420,000 years from the Vostok ice core, Antarctica. *Nature* 1999; **399**: 429–36.
16. Nunn JF. Climate change and sea level in relation to overpopulation. *Optimum Population Trust Journal* 2004; **4**: 3–9.
*17. Loutre MF, Berger A. Future climatic changes: are we entering an exceptionally long interglacial? *Climatic Change* 2000; **46**: 61–90.
*18. Broecker WS. Thermohaline circulation, the Achilles heel of our climate system: will man-made CO_2

upset the current balance? *Science* 1997; **278**: 1582–8.

*19. Karl TR, Trenberth KE. Modern global climate change. *Science* 2003; **302**: 1719–23.

20. Jones AE, Shanklin JD. Continued decline of total ozone over Halley, Antarctica, since 1985. *Nature* 1995; **376**: 409–11.

KEY POINTS

- In addition to conducting air to and from the lungs, the nose, mouth and pharynx have other important functions, including speech, swallowing and airway protection.
- The respiratory epithelium lining the nose, pharynx, larynx and airways warms and humidifies inspired gases and prevents inhaled chemicals, particles and pathogens from reaching the alveoli.
- Starting at the trachea, the airway divides about 23 times, terminating in an estimated 30 000 pulmonary acini, each containing more than 10 000 alveoli.
- The alveolar wall is ideally designed to provide a minimal physical barrier to gas transfer, while also being structurally strong enough to resist the large mechanical forces applied to the lung.

This chapter is not a comprehensive account of respiratory anatomy but concentrates on those aspects that are most relevant to an understanding of function. The respiratory muscles are considered in Chapter 6.

MOUTH, NOSE AND PHARYNX

Breathing is normally possible through either the nose or the mouth, the two alternative air passages converging in the oropharynx. Nasal breathing is the norm and has two major advantages over mouth breathing: filtration of particulate matter by the vibrissae hairs and humidification of inspired gas. Humidification by the nose is highly efficient because the nasal septum and turbinates greatly increase the surface area of mucosa available for evaporation and produce turbulent flow, so increasing contact between the mucosa and air. However, the nose may offer more resistance to air flow than the mouth, particularly when obstructed by polyps, adenoids or congestion of the nasal mucosa. Nasal resistance may make

oral breathing obligatory, and many children and adults breathe only or partly through their mouths at rest.[1] With increasing levels of exercise in normal adults the respiratory minute volume increases, and at a level of about 35 l.min^{-1} the oral airway is brought into play.

Deflection of gas into either the nasal or the oral route is under voluntary control and accomplished with the soft palate, tongue and lips. These functions are best considered in relation to a midline sagittal section (Figure 2.1).

Part (a) shows the normal position for nose breathing, with the mouth closed by occlusion of the lips and the tongue lying against the hard palate. The soft palate is clear of the posterior pharyngeal wall.

Part (b) shows forced mouth breathing, as for instance when blowing through the mouth, without pinching the nose. The soft palate becomes rigid and is arched upwards and backwards by contraction of tensor and levator palati[2] to lie against a band of the superior constrictor of the pharynx known as Passavant's ridge which, together with the soft palate, forms the palatopharyngeal sphincter. Note also that the orifice of the pharyngotympanic (Eustachian) tube lies above the palatopharyngeal sphincter and the tubes can therefore be inflated by the subject only when the nose is pinched. As the mouth pressure is raised, this tends to force the soft palate against the posterior pharyngeal wall to act as a valve. The combined palatopharyngeal sphincter and valvular action of the soft palate is very strong and can easily withstand mouth pressures in excess of 10 kPa (100 cmH$_2$O).

Part (c) shows the occlusion of the respiratory tract during a Valsalva manoeuvre.

During swallowing the nasopharynx is occluded by contraction of both tensor and levator palati. The larynx is elevated 2–3 cm by contraction of the infrahyoid muscles, stylopharyngeus and palatopharyngeus, coming to lie under the epiglottis. In addition, the aryepiglottic folds are approximated, causing total occlusion of the entrance to the larynx. This extremely effective protection of the larynx is capable of withstanding pharyngeal pressures as high as 80 kPa (600 mmHg) that may be generated during swallowing.

a

b

c

Figure 2.1 Magnetic resonance imaging (MRI) scans showing median sagittal sections of the pharynx in a normal subject.
(a) Normal nasal breathing with the oral airway occluded by lips and tongue. (b) Deliberate oral breathing with the nasal airway occluded by elevation and backward movement of the soft palate. (c) A Valsalva manoeuvre in which the subject deliberately tries to exhale against a closed airway. The airway is occluded at many sites: the lips are closed, the tongue is in contact with the hard palate anteriorly, the palatopharyngeal sphincter is tightly closed, the epiglottis is in contact with the posterior pharyngeal wall and the vocal folds are closed, so becoming visible in this midline section. Data acquisition for scans (a) and (b) took 45 seconds so anatomical differences between inspiration and expiration will not be visible. Scanning a Valsalva manoeuvre required more rapid data acquisition so the texture of tissues in scan (c) is different from the previous two. I am grateful to the staff of the MRI unit at St James's Hospital for performing the scans and to Dr Mark Bellamy for being the subject. NC, nasal cavity; T, tongue; SP, soft palate; E, epiglottis; VF, vocal fold; L, larynx.

Figure 2.2 Normal acoustic reflectometry pattern of airway cross-sectional area during mouth breathing.[3,4]

Upper airway cross-sectional areas can be estimated from conventional radiographs, magnetic resonance imaging (MRI), as in Figure 2.1, or acoustic reflectometry. In the latter technique, a single sound pulse of 100 μs duration is generated within the apparatus and passes along the airway of the subject. Recording of the timing and frequency of sound waves reflected back from the airway allows calculation of cross-sectional area, which is then presented as a function of the distance travelled along the airway[3] (Figure 2.2). Acoustic reflectometry measurements correlate well with MRI scans of the airway[4] and the technique is now sufficiently developed for use in clinical situations with real-time results. For example, acoustic reflectometry has been used following the placement of a tracheal tube to differentiate between oesophageal and tracheal intubation.[5]

THE LARYNX

The larynx evolved in the lungfish for the protection of the airway during such activities as feeding and perfusion of the gills with water. While protection of the airway remains important, the larynx now has many other functions, all involving varying degrees of laryngeal occlusion.[6]

Speech.[7] Phonation, the laryngeal component of speech, requires a combination of changes in position, tension and mass of the vocal folds (cords). Rotation of the arytenoid cartilages by the posterior cricoarytenoid muscles opens the vocal folds, whilereas contraction of the lateral cricoarytenoid and oblique arytenoid muscles opposes this. With the vocal folds almost closed, the respiratory muscles generate a positive pressure of 5–35 cmH$_2$O which may then be released by slight opening of the vocal folds to produce sound waves. The cricothyroid muscle tilts the cricoid and arytenoid cartilages backwards and also moves them posteriorly in relation to the

thyroid cartilage. This produces up to 50% elongation and therefore tensioning of the vocal folds, an action opposed by the thyroarytenoid muscles, which draw the arytenoid cartilages forwards toward the thyroid and so shorten and relax the vocal folds. Tensioning of the cords results in both transverse and longitudinal resonance of the vocal fold, allowing the formation of complex sound waves. The deeper fibres of the thyroarytenoids comprise the vocales muscles, which exert fine control over pitch of the voice by slight variations in both the tension and mass of the vocal folds. A more dramatic example of the effect of vocal fold mass on voice production occurs with inflammation of the laryngeal mucosa and the resulting hoarse voice or complete inability to phonate.

Effort closure. Tighter occlusion of the larynx, known as effort closure, is required for making expulsive efforts. It is also needed to lock the thoracic cage and so to secure the origin of the muscles of the upper arm arising from the ribcage, thus increasing the power which can be transmitted to the arm. In addition to simple apposition of the vocal folds described above, the aryepiglottic muscles and their continuation, the oblique and transverse arytenoids, act as a powerful sphincter capable of closing the inlet of the larynx by bringing the aryepiglottic folds tightly together. The full process enables the larynx to withstand the highest pressures that can be generated in the thorax, usually at least 12 kPa (120 cmH$_2$O) and often more.[6] Sudden release of the obstruction is essential for effective coughing, when the linear velocity of air through the larynx is said to approach the speed of sound.

Swallowing. Effort closure is a part of the mechanism involved in the protection of the larynx during swallowing. In addition, the larynx is lifted towards the hyoid bone, elevating the epiglottis which becomes squeezed between the base of the tongue and the laryngeal inlet to deflect the food bolus backwards.

Laryngeal muscles are involved in controlling airways resistance, particularly during expiration, and this aspect of vocal fold function is described in Chapter 6.

THE TRACHEOBRONCHIAL TREE

An accurate and complete model of the branching pattern of the human bronchial tree remains elusive, though several different models have been described.[8] The most useful and widely accepted approach remains that of Weibel,[9,10] who numbered successive generations of air passages from the trachea (generation 0) down to the alveolar sacs (generation 23). This 'regular dichotomy' model assumes that each bronchus regularly divides into two approximately equal-sized daughter bronchi. As a rough approximation it may therefore be assumed that the number of passages in each generation is double that in the previous generation, and the number of air passages in each generation is approximately indicated by the number 2 raised to the power of the generation number. This formula indicates one trachea, two main bronchi, four lobar bronchi, 16 segmental bronchi etc. However, this mathematical relationship is unlikely to be true in practice, where bronchus length is variable, pairs of daughter bronchi are often unequal in size and trifurcations may be demonstrated.

Recent work using computed tomography to reconstruct, in three dimensions, the branching pattern of the airways has shown that a regular dichotomy system does occur for at least the first six generations.[11] Beyond this point, the same study demonstrated trifurcation of some bronchi and airways that terminated at generation 8.

Table 2.1 traces the characteristics of progressive generations of airways in the respiratory tract.

Trachea (generation 0)

The adult trachea has a mean diameter of 1.8 cm and length of 11 cm. It is supported by U-shaped cartilages which are joined posteriorly by smooth muscle bands. The part of the trachea in the neck is not subjected to intrathoracic pressure changes but it is very vulnerable to pressures arising in the neck due, for example, to tumours or haematoma formation after surgery. An external pressure of the order of 4 kPa (40 cmH$_2$O) is sufficient to occlude the trachea. Within the chest, the trachea can be compressed by raised intrathoracic pressure during, for example, a cough, when the decreased diameter increases the linear velocity of gas flow and therefore the efficiency of removal of secretions.

Main, lobar and segmental bronchi (generations 1–4)

The trachea bifurcates asymmetrically, with the right bronchus being wider and making a smaller angle with the long axis of the trachea. Foreign bodies therefore tend to enter the right bronchus in preference to the left. Main, lobar and segmental bronchi have firm cartilaginous support in their walls, U-shaped in the main bronchi but in the form of irregularly shaped and helical plates lower down with bronchial muscle between. Bronchi in this group (down to generation 4) are sufficiently regular to be individually named (Figure 2.3). Total cross-sectional area of the respiratory tract is minimal at the third generation (Figure 2.4).

These bronchi are subjected to the full effect of changes in intrathoracic pressure and will collapse when the intrathoracic pressure exceeds the intraluminar pressure by about 5 kPa (50 cmH$_2$O). This occurs in the larger bronchi during a forced expiration, so limiting peak expiratory flow rate (see Figure 4.7).

Small bronchi (generations 5–11)

The small bronchi extend through about seven generations with their diameter progressively falling from 3.5 to 1 mm. Down to the level of the smallest true bronchi, air passages lie in close proximity to branches of the pulmonary artery in a sheath containing pulmonary lymphatics, which can be distended with oedema fluid, giving rise to the characteristic 'cuffing' that is responsible for the earliest radiographic changes in pulmonary oedema. Because these air passages are not directly attached to the lung parenchyma they are not subject to direct traction and rely for their patency on cartilage within their walls and on the transmural pressure gradient, which is normally positive from lumen to intrathoracic space. In the normal subject this pressure gradient is seldom reversed, and even during a forced expiration the intraluminar pressure in the small bronchi rapidly rises to more than 80% of the alveolar pressure, which is more than the extramural (intrathoracic) pressure.

Bronchioles (generations 12–14)

An important change occurs at about the 11th generation where the internal diameter is about 1 mm. Cartilage disappears from the wall below this level and ceases to be a factor in maintaining patency. However, beyond this level the air passages are directly embedded in the lung parenchyma, the elastic recoil of which holds the air passages open like the guy ropes of a tent. Therefore the calibre of the airways below the 11th generation is influenced mainly by lung volume, since the forces holding their lumina open are stronger at higher lung volumes. The converse of this factor causes airway closure at reduced long volume (see Chapter 4). In succeeding generations, the number of bronchioles increases far more rapidly than the calibre diminishes (see Table 2.1). Therefore the total cross-sectional area increases until, in the terminal bronchioles, it is about 100 times the area at the level of the large bronchi (see Figure 2.4). Thus the flow resistance of these smaller air passages (less than 2 mm diameter) is negligible under normal conditions. However, the resistance of the bronchioles can increase to very high values when their strong helical muscular bands are contracted by the mechanisms described in Chapters 4 and 28. Down to the terminal bronchiole, the air passages derive their nutrition from the bronchial circulation and are thus influenced by systemic arterial blood gas levels. Beyond this point the smaller air passages rely upon the pulmonary circulation for their nutrition.

Table 2.1 Structural characteristics of the air passages[9,12]

	Generation (mean)	Number	Mean diameter (mm)	Area supplied	Cartilage	Muscle	Nutrition	Emplacement	Epithelium
Trachea	0	1	18	Both lungs	U-shaped	Links open end of cartilage	From the bronchial circulation	Within connective tissue sheath alongside arterial vessels	Columnar ciliated epithelium
Main bronchi	1	2	12	Individual lungs					
Lobar bronchi	2 → 3	4 → 8	8 → 5	Lobes					
Segmental bronchi	4	16	4	Segments	Irregular shaped	Helical bands			
Small bronchi	5 → 11	32 → 2 000	3 → 1	Secondary lobules					
Bronchioles Terminal bronchioles	12 → 14	4 000 → 16 000	1 → 0.7			Strong helical muscle bands		Embedded directly in the lung parenchyma	Cuboidal
Respiratory bronchioles	15 → 18	32 000 → 260 000	0.4	Pulmonary acinus	Absent	Muscle bands between alveoli	From the pulmonary circulation		Cuboidal to flat between alveoli
Alveolar ducts	19 → 22	520 000 → 4 000 000	0.3			Thin bands in alveolar septa		Form the lung parenchyma	Alveolar epithelium
Alveoli	23	8 000 000	0.2						

Right   Left

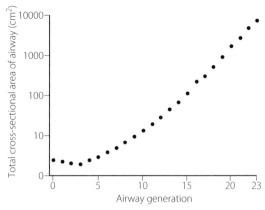

Figure 2.4 The total cross-sectional area of the air passages at different generations of the airways. Note that the minimum cross-sectional area is at generation 3 (lobar to segmental bronchi). The total cross-sectional area becomes very large in the smaller air passages, approaching a square metre in the alveolar ducts.

UPPER LOBE
1. Apical bronchus
2. Posterior bronchus
3. Anterior bronchus

Right   *Left*
MIDDLE LOBE   LINGULA
4. Lateral bronchus   4. Superior bronchus
5. Medial bronchus   5. Inferior bronchus

LOWER LOBE
6. Apical bronchus   6. Apical bronchus
7. Medial basal (cardiac)   8. Anterior basal bronchus
8. Anterior basal bronchus   9. Lateral basal bronchus
9. Lateral basal bronchus   10. Posterior basal bronchus
10. Posterior basal bronchus

Figure 2.3 Named branches of the tracheobronchial tree, viewed from the front. (Reproduced by permission of the Editors of *Thorax*.)

Alveolar ducts (generations 19–22)

Alveolar ducts arise from the terminal respiratory bronchioles, from which they differ by having no walls other than the mouths of mural alveoli (about 20 in number). The alveolar septa comprise a series of rings forming the walls of the alveolar ducts and containing smooth muscle. About half of the alveoli arise from ducts and some 35% of the alveolar gas resides in the alveolar ducts and the alveoli that arise directly from them.

Alveolar sacs (generation 23)

The last generation of the air passages differs from alveolar ducts solely in the fact that they are blind. It is estimated that about 17 alveoli arise from each alveolar sac and account for about half of the total number of alveoli.

Pulmonary acinus (*syn.* primary lobule, terminal respiratory unit)

The pulmonary acinus is usually defined as the zone supplied by a first-order respiratory bronchiole and includes the respiratory bronchioles, alveolar ducts and alveolar sacs distal to a single terminal bronchiole (Figure 2.5). This represents generations 15–23 above, but in practice the number of generations within a single acinus is quite variable, being between six and 12 divisions beyond the terminal bronchiole. A human lung contains about 30 000 acini,[12] each with a diameter of about 3.5 mm and containing in excess of 10 000 alveoli. A single pulmonary acinus is probably the equivalent of the alveolus when it is considered from a functional standpoint, as gas movement within the acinus is by diffusion rather than tidal ventilation. Acinar morphometry therefore

Respiratory bronchioles (generations 15–18)

Down to the smallest bronchioles, the functions of the air passages are solely conduction and humidification. Beyond this point there is a gradual transition from conduction to gas exchange. In the four generations of respiratory bronchioles there is a gradual increase in the number of alveoli in their walls. Like the bronchioles, the respiratory bronchioles are embedded in lung parenchyma; however, they have a well-defined muscle layer with bands that loop over the opening of the alveolar ducts and the mouths of the mural alveoli. There is no significant change in calibre of advancing generations of respiratory bronchioles (approximately 0.4 mm diameter).

a

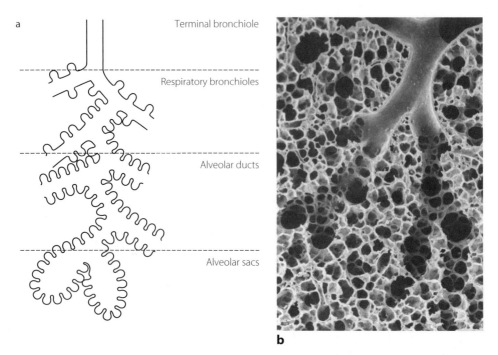

Terminal bronchiole

Respiratory bronchioles

Alveolar ducts

Alveolar sacs

b

Figure 2.5 (a) Schematic diagram of a single pulmonary acinus showing four generations between the terminal bronchiole and the alveolar sacs. The average number of generations in human lung is eight but may be as many as 12. (b) Thick section of rabbit lung showing respiratory bronchioles leading to alveolar ducts and sacs. Human alveoli would be considerably larger. (Photograph kindly supplied by Professor EM Weibel.)

becomes crucial,[13] in particular the path length between the start of the acinus and the most distal alveolus, which in humans is between 5 and 12 mm.[12]

RESPIRATORY EPITHELIUM[14]

From the nasal cavity to the bronchioles the respiratory tract is lined with a pseudo-stratified columnar ciliated epithelium containing many mucus-secreting (goblet) cells. In the bronchioles the cell height begins to reduce and tends toward cuboidal epithelial cells before gradually flattening further throughout the pulmonary acinus and merging with the alveolar epithelial cells. Goblet cells are present at a density of about 6000 per mm^2 (in the trachea) and are responsible, along with submucosal secretory cells, for producing the thick layer of mucus that lines all but the smallest conducting airways. Mucin, the principal glycoprotein in mucus, is released by rapid (<150 ms) exocytosis from the mucus-secreting cells in response to a range of stimuli including direct chemical irritation, inflammatory cytokines and neuronal stimulation, predominantly by cholinergic nerves.[15,16] Both goblet cell numbers and secretions increase in many airway diseases, such as asthma, bronchitis and cystic fibrosis (see Chapter 28).[15]

The mucous layer is propelled cephalad by the ciliated epithelial cells (Figure 2.6) at a rate of 4 mm.min^{-1} to be

Figure 2.6 Scanning electron micrograph of ciliated epithelial cells beating in the fluid layer beneath the mucus (Mu). (Kindly reproduced by permission of Dr PK Jeffery, Imperial College School of Science, Technology and Medicine, London, and the publishers of *Respiratory Medicine*.[14])

removed by expectoration on reaching the larynx. Each cell is topped by about 250 cilia which beat at a rate of 12–16 beats per second. Adjacent cells somehow coordinate their ciliar activity, probably by a physical linkage between cilia caused by the mucus above. Within the mucus there are two layers:[17] a periciliary or 'sol' layer, which is of low viscosity containing water and solutes and in which the cilia are embedded, and a mucus or 'gel' layer above, containing the viscous mucin in the underside of which the cilia tips intermittently 'grip' the mucous layer.

Other cell types found in the respiratory epithelium include the following.

Basal cells. These cells lie underneath the columnar cells, giving rise to the pseudo-stratified appearance, and are absent in the bronchioles and beyond. They are probably the stem cells responsible for producing new epithelial and goblet cells.

Mast cells. The lungs contain numerous mast cells which are located below the mucosa of the airways as well as in the alveolar septa. Some also lie free in the lumen of the airways and may be recovered by bronchial lavage. Their important role in bronchoconstriction is described in Chapter 28.

Non-ciliated bronchiolar epithelial (Clara) cells. These cells are found in the mucosa of the terminal bronchioles, where they may be the precursor of epithelial cells in the absence of basal cells. They are metabolically active,[18] secreting surfactant proteins A, B and D (page 26), antiprotease enzymes and a variety of other proteins whose functions are mostly unknown, though some are involved in the metabolism of chemical toxins.

APUD cells. These cells occur in bronchial epithelium and, from morphological considerations, are believed to be a part of the APUD series, so named because of their ability to undertake amine and **a**mine-**p**recursor **u**ptake and **d**ecarboxylation. APUD cells elsewhere are known to produce a range of hormones including ACTH, insulin, calcitonin and gastrin.

Functions of respiratory epithelium

Humidification.[19] The respiratory mucosa acts as a heat and moisture exchanger. During inspiration, relatively cool, dry air causes evaporation of surface water and cooling of the mucosa; then on expiration moisture condenses on the surface of the mucosa and warming occurs. Thus only about one-half of the heat and moisture needed to condition (fully warm and saturate) each breath is lost to the atmosphere. With quiet nasal breathing, air is conditioned before reaching the trachea, but as ventilation increases smaller airways are recruited until at minute volumes of over 50 l.min^{-1} airways of 1 mm diameter are involved in humidification.

Chemical barrier and particle clearance. The viscous mucus layer provides a physical barrier to chemical damage of the epithelium, with many inhaled irritants simply dissolving in the mucus until exhaled or removed by expectoration. Others are initially metabolised and then conjugated by the underlying cells (particularly Clara cells).[20] Inhaled particles are deposited in the airways either by inertial impaction or by sedimentation, depending on their size. Inertial impaction occurs when the airway has a sharp corner (e.g. the pharynx or nose) or when gas flow becomes turbulent (e.g. large bifurcations). Most particles above 8 μm impact on the pharyngeal walls, whereas those between 5 and 8 μm tend to be deposited near large airway divisions. In both cases the particles are either degraded by proteases in the mucosa or removed intact with the mucus. Sedimentation occurs in the respiratory bronchioles and alveoli where the velocity of gas flow becomes too low for the particle to remain suspended, so depositing particles smaller than 5 μm, which are then removed by macrophages.

Defence against infection. Respiratory epithelium is crucial in preventing infection from airborne pathogens. The first line of defence is physical removal of bacterial and viral particles by the mucus. Second, humoral defences within the mucus include immunoglobulins (particularly IgA), complement proteins, protease inhibitors (α_1-antitrypsin), lysozyme and transferrin (which binds iron, an essential cofactor for bacterial proliferation) and endogenous antibiotics (page 383). Third, cellular immunity is in evidence throughout the epithelium, with macrophages, neutrophils and lymphocytes all being commonly found during infection in the normal lung.

These functions require quite opposite mucus consistency. For humidification the mucus requires a high water content, whereas as a barrier it requires high viscosity and a high protein content. The epithelial cells are responsible for balancing these requirements by the secretion and reabsorption of water and solutes as appropriate, and this control must occur quickly to accommodate rapid changes in minute ventilation and air temperature and humidity. It seems likely that the epithelium in small airways secretes fluid into the mucus and that of large airways later absorbs any excess fluid before the mucus is removed from the lung.[17]

THE ALVEOLI

The mean total number of alveoli has recently been estimated as 480 million,[21] but ranges from about 270 million to 790 million, correlating with the height of the subject[22] and total lung volume.[21] The size of the alveoli is proportional to lung volume but owing to gravity they are normally larger in the upper part of the lung, except at maximal inflation, when the vertical gradient in size disappears. At functional residual capacity the mean diameter is 0.2 mm.

Figure 2.7 Scanning electron micrograph of the junction of three alveolar septa which are shown in both surface view and section showing the polyhedral structure. Two pores of Kohn are seen to the right of centre. Red blood cells are seen in the cut ends of the capillaries. The scale bar is 10 μm. (Reprinted by permission of the publisher from *The Pathway for Oxygen: Structure and Function in the Mammalian Respiratory System* by Ewald R. Weibel, pp. 245, 314, Cambridge, Mass.: Harvard University Press, Copyright © 1984 by the President and Fellows of Harvard College.)

Figure 2.8 Details of the interstitial space, the capillary endothelium and alveolar epithelium. Thickening of the interstitial space is confined to the left of the capillary (the 'service' side) while the total alveolar/capillary membrane remains thin on the right (the 'active' side) except where it is thickened by the endothelial nucleus. Alv, alveolus; BM, basement membrane; EN, endothelial nucleus; End, endothelium; Ep, epithelium; IS, interstitial space; RBC, red blood cell; FB, fibroblast process. (Electron micrograph kindly supplied by Professor ER Weibel.)

The alveolar septa

The septa are under tension generated partly by elastic fibres but more by surface tension at the air–fluid interface (page 26). They are therefore generally flat, making the alveoli polyhedral rather than spherical. The septa are perforated by small fenestrations known as the pores of Kohn (Figure 2.7), which provide collateral ventilation between alveoli. Direct communications have also been found between small bronchioles and neighbouring alveoli, adjacent pulmonary acini and occasionally intersegmental communications.[23]

On one side of the alveolar wall the capillary endothelium and the alveolar epithelium are closely apposed, with almost no interstitial space, such that the total thickness from gas to blood is about 0.3 μm (Figures 2.8 and 2.9). This may be considered the 'active' side of the capillary and gas exchange must be more efficient on this side. The other side of the capillary, which may be considered the 'service' side, is usually more than 1–2 μm thick and contains a recognisable interstitial space containing elastin and collagen fibres, nerve endings and occasional migrant polymorphs and macrophages. The distinction between the two sides of the capillary has considerable pathophysiological significance as the active side tends to be spared in the accumulation of both oedema fluid and fibrous tissue (see Chapter 29).

The fibre scaffold. The alveolar septum contains a network of fibres which forms a continuum between the peripheral fibres and the axial spiral fibres of the bronchioles. The septal fibre is in the form of a network, through which are threaded the pulmonary capillaries, which are themselves a network. Thus the capillaries pass repeatedly from one side of the fibre scaffold to the other (see Figure 2.7), the fibre always residing on the thick (or 'service') side of the capillary, allowing the other side to bulge into the lumen of the alveolus. The left side of the capillary in Figure 2.8 is the side with the fibres.

At the cellular level, the scaffolding for the alveolar septa is provided by the basement membrane, which provides the blood–gas barrier with enough strength to withstand the enormous forces applied to lung tissue.[26,27] At the centre of the basement membrane is a layer of type IV collagen, the lamina densa, approximately 50 nm thick and made up of many layers of a diamond-shaped matrix of collagen molecules. On each side of the lamina densa, the collagen layer is attached to the alveolar or endothelial cells by a series of proteins collectively known as laminins, of which seven subtypes are now known. The laminins are more than simple structural molecules, having complex interactions with membrane proteins and the intracellular cytoskeleton[28] to help regulate cell shape and permeability etc. These aspects of

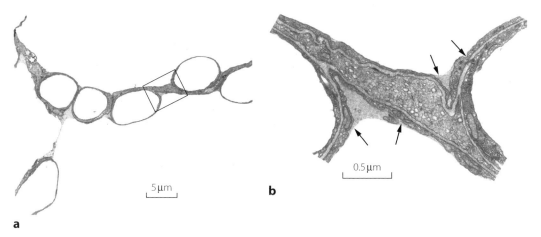

Figure 2.9 (a) Transmission electron micrograph of alveolar septum with lung inflated to 40% of total lung capacity. The section in the box is enlarged in (b) to show alveolar lining fluid, which has pooled in two concavities of the alveolar epithelium and has also spanned the pore of Kohn in (a). There is a thin film of osmophilic material (arrows), probably surfactant, at the interface between air and the alveolar lining fluid. (Reproduced from reference 25 by permission of the authors and the Editors of *Journal of Applied Physiology*.)

the function of the basement membrane are important. It has been shown that increases in the capillary transmural pressure gradient above about 3 kPa (30 cmH$_2$O) may cause disruption of endothelium and/or epithelium, whereas the basement membrane tends to remain intact, sometimes as the only remaining separation between blood and gas.[29]

ALVEOLAR CELL TYPES

Capillary endothelial cells. These cells are continuous with the endothelium of the general circulation and, in the pulmonary capillary bed, have a thickness of only 0.1 μm except where expanded to contain nuclei (see Figure 2.8). Electron microscopy shows the flat parts of the cytoplasm to be devoid of all organelles except for small vacuoles (caveolae or plasmalemmal vesicles) which may open onto the basement membrane or the lumen of the capillary or be entirely contained within the cytoplasm (see Figure 2.9). The endothelial cells abut against one another at fairly loose junctions which are of the order of 5 nm wide.[30] These junctions permit the passage of quite large molecules and the pulmonary lymph contains albumin at about half the concentration in plasma. Macrophages pass freely through these junctions under normal conditions and polymorphs can also pass in response to chemotaxis (page 413).

Recent work has begun to elucidate the complex systems responsible for controlling the passage of cells and molecules between adjacent endothelial cells (page 403).[28] A series of components outside the cell, in the cell membrane and in the cytoplasm interact in response to cytokines or mechanical forces such as shear stress.

Activation of these proteins causes further inflammatory activity and leads to contraction of the actin–myosin of the endothelial cell cytoskeleton, producing a physical change in cell shape and therefore permeability of the blood–gas barrier to large molecules and cells.

Alveolar epithelial cells – type I. These cells line the alveoli and also exist as a thin sheet approximately 0.1 μm thick, except where expanded to contain nuclei. Like the endothelium, the flat part of the cytoplasm is devoid of organelles except for small vacuoles. Epithelial cells each cover several capillaries and are joined into a continuous sheet by tight junctions with a gap of only about 1 nm.[30] These junctions may be seen as narrow lines snaking across the septa in Figure 2.7. The tightness of these junctions is crucial for prevention of the escape of large molecules, such as albumin, into the alveoli, thus preserving the oncotic pressure gradient essential for the avoidance of pulmonary oedema (see page 387). Nevertheless, these junctions permit the free passage of macrophages. Polymorphs may also pass in response to a chemotactic stimulus. Figure 2.9 shows the type I cell covered with a film of alveolar lining fluid, although it has been proposed that the surface is normally dry.[31] Type I cells are end cells and do not divide *in vivo*. However, they have been cultured *in vitro* with type II cells on a matrix secreted by the latter.[32] They are particularly sensitive to damage from high concentrations of oxygen (see Chapter 26).

Alveolar epithelial cells – type II. These are the stem cells from which type I cells arise.[33] They do not function as gas exchange membranes and are rounded in shape and situated at the junction of septa. They have large nuclei

Figure 2.10 Electron micrograph of a type II alveolar epithelial cell of dog. Note the large nucleus, the microvilli and the osmiophilic lamellar bodies thought to release surfactant. Alv, alveolus; C, capillary; LB, lamellar bodies; N, nucleus. (Reproduced from reference 35 by permission of Professor ER Weibel and the Editors of *Physiological Reviews*.)

Figure 2.11 Scanning electron micrograph of an alveolar macrophage advancing to the right over epithelial type I cells. The scale bar is 5 μm. (Reprinted by permission of the publisher from *The Pathway for Oxygen: Structure and Function in the Mammalian Respiratory System* by Ewald R. Weibel, Cambridge, Mass.: Harvard University Press, Copyright © 1984 by the President and Fellows of Harvard College.)

and microvilli (Figure 2.10). The cytoplasm contains characteristic striated osmiophilic organelles that contain stored surfactant (page 26).[34] Type II cells are also involved in pulmonary defence mechanisms in that they may secrete cytokines and contribute to pulmonary inflammation. Type II cells are easily grown in culture and tend to proliferate in lung explant tissue cultures. They are resistant to oxygen toxicity, tending to replace type I cells after prolonged exposure to high concentrations of oxygen (see Chapter 26).

Alveolar macrophages. The lung is richly endowed with these phagocytes which pass freely from the circulation, through the interstitial space and thence through the gaps between alveolar epithelial cells to lie on their surface within the alveolar lining fluid (Figure 2.11). They can re-enter the body but are remarkable for their ability to live and function outside the body. The macrophages are active in combating infection and scavenging foreign bodies such as small dust particles. They contain a variety of destructive enzymes but are also capable of generating oxygen-derived free radicals (see Chapter 26). These are highly effective bactericidal agents but their presence in lung tissue may rebound to damage the host. Dead macrophages release the enzyme trypsin, which may cause tissue damage in patients who are deficient in the protein α_1-antitrypsin.

THE PULMONARY VASCULATURE

Pulmonary arteries

Although the pulmonary circulation carries roughly the same flow as the systemic circulation, the arterial pressure and the vascular resistance are normally only one-sixth as great. The media of the pulmonary arteries is about half as thick as in systemic arteries of corresponding size. In the larger vessels it consists mainly of elastic tissue but in the smaller vessels it is mainly muscular, the transition being in vessels of about 1 mm diameter. Pulmonary arteries lie close to the corresponding air passages in connective tissue sheaths. Table 2.2 shows a scheme for consideration of the branching of the pulmonary arterial tree.[36] This may be compared with Weibel's scheme for the airways (see Table 2.1)

Pulmonary arterioles

The transition to arterioles occurs at an internal diameter of 100 μm. These vessels differ radically from their counterparts in the systemic circulation, being virtually devoid of muscular tissue. There is a thin media of elastic tissue separated from the blood by endothelium. Structurally there is no real difference between pulmonary arterioles and venules.

Pulmonary capillaries

Pulmonary capillaries tend to arise abruptly from much larger vessels, the pulmonary metarterioles. The capillaries form a dense network over the walls of one or more alveoli and the spaces between the capillaries are

Table 2.2 Dimensions of the branches of the human pulmonary artery

Orders	Numbers	Mean diameter (mm)	Cumulative volume (ml)
17	1	30	64
16	3	15	81
15	8	8.1	85
14	20	5.8	96
13	66	3.7	108
12	203	2.1	116
11	675	1.3	122
10	2 300	0.85	128
9	5 900	0.53	132
8	18 000	0.35	136
7	53 000	0.22	138
6	160 000	0.14	141
5	470 000	0.086	142
4	1 400 000	0.054	144
3	4 200 000	0.034	145
2	13 000 000	0.021	146
1	300 000 000	0.013	151

In contrast to the airways (Table 2.1), the branching is asymmetrical and not dichotomous. Singhal et al.[36] therefore grouped the vessels according to orders and not generation as in Table 2.1.

similar in size to the capillaries themselves (see Figure 2.7). In the resting state, about 75% of the capillary bed is filled but the percentage is higher in the dependent parts of the lungs. Inflation of the alveoli reduces the cross-sectional area of the capillary bed and increases resistance to blood flow (see Chapter 7). One capillary network is not confined to one alveolus but passes from one alveolus to another and blood traverses a number of alveolar septa before reaching a venule. This clearly has a bearing on the efficiency of gas exchange. From the functional standpoint it is often more convenient to consider the pulmonary microcirculation rather than just the capillaries. The microcirculation is defined as the vessels that are devoid of a muscular layer, and it commences with arterioles of diameter 75 μm and continues through the capillary bed as far as venules of diameter 200 μm. Special roles of the microcirculation are considered in Chapters 12 and 29.

Pulmonary venules and veins

Pulmonary capillary blood is collected into venules that are structurally almost identical to the arterioles. In fact, Duke obtained satisfactory gas exchange when an isolated cat lung was perfused in reverse.[37] The pulmonary veins do not run alongside the pulmonary arteries but lie some distance away, close to the septa that separate the segments of the lung.

Bronchial circulation[38]

Down to the terminal bronchioles, the air passages and the accompanying blood vessels receive their nutrition from the bronchial vessels that arise from the systemic circulation. The bronchial circulation therefore provides the heat required for warming and humidification of inspired air, and cooling of the respiratory epithelium causes vasodilation and an increase in the bronchial artery blood flow.[19] Part of the bronchial circulation returns to the systemic venous system but part mingles with the pulmonary venous drainage, thereby constituting a physiological shunt (page 122).

Pulmonary lymphatics

There are no lymphatics visible in the interalveolar septa, but small lymph vessels commence at the junction between alveolar and extraalveolar spaces. There is a well-developed lymphatic system around the bronchi and pulmonary vessels, capable of containing up to 500 ml of lymph and draining towards the hilum. Down to airway generation 11 the lymphatics lie in a potential space around the air passages and vessels, separating them from the lung parenchyma. This space becomes distended with lymph in pulmonary oedema and accounts for the characteristic butterfly shadow of the chest radiograph. In the hilum of the lung, the lymphatic drainage passes through several groups of tracheobronchial lymph glands, where they receive tributaries from the superficial subpleural plexus. Most of the lymph from the left lung usually enters the thoracic duct, whereas the right side drains into the right lymphatic duct. However, the pulmonary lymphatics often cross the midline and pass independently into the junction of the internal jugular and subclavian veins on the corresponding sides of the body.

REFERENCES

1. Rodenstein DO, Stanescu DC. The soft palate and breathing. *Am Rev Respir Dis* 1986; **134**: 311–25.
2. Hairston LE, Sauerland EK. Electromyography of the human palate: discharge patterns of the levator and tensor veli palatini. *Electromyogr Clin Neurophysiol* 1981; **21**: 287–97.
3. Hoffstein V, Fredberg JJ. The acoustic reflection technique for non-invasive assessment of upper airway area. *Eur Respir J* 1991; **4**: 602–11.
4. Marshall I, Maran NJ, Martin S, et al. Acoustic reflectometry for airway measurements in man:

implementation and validation. *Physiol Meas* 1993; **14**: 157–69.

5. Raphael DT. Acoustic reflectometry profiles of endotracheal and esophageal intubation. *Anesthesiology* 2000; **92**: 1293–9.

6. Bartlett D. Respiratory functions of the larynx. *Physiol Rev* 1989; **69**: 33–57.

7. Bannister LH. Anatomy of speech. In: Williams PL, ed. *Gray's anatomy*. London: Churchill Livingstone, 1995; 1651–2.

8. Phillips CG, Kaye SR, Schroter RC. A diameter-based reconstruction of the branching pattern of the human bronchial tree. Part I. Description and application. *Respir Physiol* 1994; **98**: 193–217.

9. Weibel ER. *Morphometry of the human lung*. Berlin: Springer, 1963.

10. Weibel ER. Why measure lung structure? *Am J Respir Crit Care Med* 2001; **163**: 314–15.

11. Sauret V, Halson PM, Brown IW, Fleming JS, Bailey AG. Study of the three-dimensional geometry of the central conducting airways in man using computed tomographic (CT) images. *J Anat* 2002; **200**: 123–34.

12. Haefeli-Bleuer B, Weibel ER. Morphometry of the human pulmonary acinus. *Anat Rec* 1988; **220**: 401–14.

13. Sapoval B, Filoche M, Weibel ER. Smaller is better – but not too small: a physical scale for the design of the mammalian pulmonary acinus. *Proc Natl Acad Sci USA* 2002; **99**: 10411–16.

14. Jeffery PK. Microscopic structure of normal lung. In: Brewis RAL, Corrin B, Geddes DM, Gibson GJ, eds. *Respiratory medicine*. London: WB Saunders, 1995; 54–72.

*15. Rogers DF. Airway goblet cells: responsive and adaptable frontline defenders. *Eur Respir J* 1994; **7**: 1690–706.

16. Rogers DF. Motor control of airway goblet cells and glands. *Respir Physiol* 2000; **125**: 129–44.

*17. Widdicombe JH, Widdicombe JG. Regulation of human airway surface liquid. *Respir Physiol* 1995; **99**: 3–12.

18. Singh G, Katyal SL. Clara cell proteins. *Ann N Y Acad Sci* 2000; **923**: 43–58.

19. McFadden ER Jr. Heat and water exchange in the human airways. *Am Rev Respir Dis* 1992; **146**: S8–10.

20. Dahl AR, Gerde P. Uptake and metabolism of toxicants in the respiratory tract. *Environ Health Perspect* 1994; **102**(Supp 11): 67–70.

21. Ochs M, Nyengaard JR, Jung L, *et al*. The number of alveoli in the human lung. *Am J Respir Crit Care Med* 2004; **169**: 120–4. .

22. Angus GE, Thurlbeck WM. Number of alveoli in the human lung. *J Appl Physiol* 1972; **32**: 483–5.

23. Topol M. Collateral respiratory pathways of pulmonary acini in man. *Folia Morphol* 1995; **54**: 61–6.

24. Weibel ER. *The pathway for oxygen.* Cambridge, Mass.: Harvard University Press, 1984.

25. Gil J, Bachofen H, Gehr P, Weibel ER. Alveolar volume–surface area relation in air and saline filled lungs fixed by vascular perfusion. *J Appl Physiol* 1979; **47**: 990–5.

*26. West JB. Structure, strength, failure and remodelling of the pulmonary blood–gas barrier. *Annu Rev Physiol* 1999; **61**: 543–72.

27. West JB. Pulmonary capillary stress failure. *J Appl Physiol* 2000; **89**: 2483–9.

*28. Dudek SM, Garcia JGN. Cytoskeletal regulation of pulmonary vascular permeability. *J Appl Physiol* 2001; **91**: 1487–500.

29. Tsukimoto K, Mathieu-Costello O, Prediletto R, Elliott AR, West JB. Ultrastructural appearances of pulmonary capillaries at high transmural pressures. *J Appl Physiol* 1991; **71**: 573–82.

30. DeFouw DO Ultrastructural features of alveolar epithelial transport. *Am Rev Respir Dis* 1983; **127**: S9–11.

31. Hills BA. An alternative view of the role(s) of surfactant and the alveolar model. *J Appl Physiol* 1999; **87**: 1567–83.

32. Schneeberger EE. Alveolar type I cells. In: Crystal RG, West JB, eds. *The lung, scientific foundations*. New York: Raven, 1991; 229.

33. Uhal BD. Cell cycle kinetics in the alveolar epithelium. *Am J Physiol* 1997; **272**: L1031–45.

34. Mason RJ, Williams MC. Alveolar type II cells. In: Crystal RG, West JB, eds. *The lung, scientific foundations*. New York: Raven, 1991; 235

35. Weibel ER. Morphological basis of alveolar-capillary gas exchange. *Physiol Rev* 1973; **53**: 419.

36. Singhal S, Henderson R, Horsfield K, Harding K, Cumming G. Morphometry of the human pulmonary arterial tree. *Circ Res* 1973; **33**: 190–7.

37. Duke HN. The site of action of anoxia on the pulmonary blood vessels of the cat. *J Physiol* 1954; **125**: 373.

38. Widdicombe J. Anatomy and physiology of the airway circulation. *Am Rev Respir Dis* 1992: **146**: S3–7.

3 Elastic forces and lung volumes

KEY POINTS

■ Inward elastic recoil of the lung opposes outward elastic recoil of the chest wall, and the balance of these forces determines static lung volumes.

■ Surface tension within the alveoli contributes significantly to lung recoil and is reduced by the presence of surfactant, though the mechanism by which this occurs is poorly understood.

■ Compliance is defined as the change in lung volume per unit change in pressure gradient and may be measured for lung, chest wall or both.

■ Various static lung volumes may be measured and the volumes obtained are affected by a variety of physiological and pathological factors.

An isolated lung will tend to contract until eventually all the contained air is expelled. In contrast, when the thoracic cage is opened it tends to expand to a volume about 1 litre greater than functional residual capacity (FRC). Thus in a relaxed subject with an open airway and no air flowing, for example at the end of expiration or inspiration, the inward elastic recoil of the lungs is exactly balanced by the outward recoil of the thoracic cage.

The movements of the lungs are entirely passive and result from forces external to the lungs. In the case of spontaneous breathing the external forces are the respiratory muscles, whereas artificial ventilation is usually in response to a pressure gradient that is developed between the airway and the environment. In each case, the pattern of response by the lung is governed by the physical impedance of the respiratory system. This impedance, or hindrance, has numerous origins, the most important of which are:

• elastic resistance of lung tissue and chest wall
• resistance from surface forces at the alveolar gas–liquid interface
• frictional resistance to gas flow through the airways

• frictional resistance from deformation of thoracic tissues (viscoelastic tissue resistance)
• inertia associated with movement of gas and tissue.

The last three may be grouped together as non-elastic resistance or respiratory system resistance; they are discussed in Chapter 4. They are measured while gas is flowing within the airways and work performed in overcoming this 'frictional' resistance is dissipated as heat and lost.

The first two forms of impedance may be grouped together as 'elastic' resistance. These are measured when gas is not flowing within the lung. Work performed in overcoming elastic resistance is stored as potential energy, and elastic deformation during inspiration is the usual source of energy for expiration during both spontaneous and artificial breathing.

This chapter is concerned with the elastic resistance afforded by lungs (including the alveoli) and chest wall, which will be considered separately and then together. When the respiratory muscles are totally relaxed, these factors govern the resting end-expiratory lung volume or FRC, and therefore lung volumes will also be considered in this chapter.

ELASTIC RECOIL OF THE LUNGS

Lung compliance is defined as the change in lung volume per unit change in transmural pressure gradient (i.e. between the alveolus and pleural space). Compliance is usually expressed in litres (or millilitres) per kilopascal (or centimetre of water) with a normal value of $1.5 \, l.kPa^{-1}$ ($150 \, ml.cmH_2O^{-1}$). Stiff lungs have a low compliance.

Compliance may be described as static or dynamic depending on the method of measurement (page 35). Static compliance is measured after a lung volume has been held at a fixed volume for as long as is practicable, whereas dynamic compliance is usually measured in the course of normal rhythmic breathing. Elastance is the reciprocal of compliance and is expressed in kilopascals per litre. Stiff lungs have a high elastance.

The nature of the forces causing recoil of the lung

For many years it was thought that the recoil of the lung was due entirely to stretching of the yellow elastin fibres present in the lung parenchyma. In 1929, von Neergaard (page 222) showed that a lung completely filled with and immersed in water had an elastance that was much less than the normal value obtained when the lung was filled with air. He correctly concluded that much of the 'elastic recoil' was due to surface tension acting throughout the vast air–water interface lining the alveoli.

Surface tension at an air–water interface produces forces that tend to reduce the area of the interface. Thus the gas pressure within a bubble is always higher than the surrounding gas pressure because the surface of the bubble is in a state of tension. Alveoli resemble bubbles in this respect, although the alveolar gas is connected to the exterior by the air passages. The pressure inside a bubble is higher than the surrounding pressure by an amount depending on the surface tension of the liquid and the radius of curvature of the bubble according to the Laplace equation:

$$P = \frac{2T}{R}$$

where P is the pressure within the bubble (dyn.cm^{-2}), T is the surface tension of the liquid (dyn.cm^{-1}) and R is the radius of the bubble (cm). In coherent SI units (see Appendix A), the appropriate units would be pressure in pascals (Pa), surface tension in newtons/metre (N.m^{-1}) and radius in metres (m).

On the left of Figure 3.1a is shown a typical alveolus of radius 0.1 mm. Assuming that the alveolar lining fluid has a normal surface tension of 20 mN.m^{-1} (= 20 dyn.cm^{-1}), the pressure within the alveolus will be 0.4 kPa (4 cmH$_2$O), which is rather less than the normal transmural pressure at FRC. If the alveolar lining fluid had the same surface tension as water (72 mN.m^{-1}), the lungs would be very stiff.

The alveolus on the right of Figure 3.1a has a radius of only 0.05 mm and the Laplace equation indicates that if the surface tension of the alveolus is the same, its pressure should be double the pressure in the left-hand alveolus. Thus gas would tend to flow from smaller alveoli into larger alveoli and that lung would be unstable which, of course, is not the case. Similarly, the retractive forces of the alveolar lining fluid would increase at low lung volumes and decrease at high lung volumes, which is exactly the reverse of what is observed. These paradoxes were clear to von Neergaard and he concluded that the surface tension of the alveolar lining fluid must be considerably less than would be expected from the properties of simple liquids and, furthermore, that its value must be variable. Observations 30 years later confirmed this when alveolar extracts were shown to have a surface

tension much lower than water and which varied in proportion to the area of the interface.[1] Figure 3.1b shows an experiment in which a floating bar is moved in a trough containing an alveolar extract. As the bar is moved to the right, the surface film is concentrated and the surface tension changes as shown in the graph on the right of the figure. During expansion, the surface tension increases to 40 mN.m^{-1}, a value which is close to that of plasma, but during contraction the surface tension falls to 19 mN.m^{-1}, a lower value than any other body fluid. The course of the relationship between pressure and area is different during expansion and contraction and a loop is described.

The consequences of these changes are very important. In contrast to a bubble of soap solution, the pressure within an alveolus tends to decrease as the radius of curvature is decreased. This is illustrated in Figure 3.1c, where the right-hand alveolus has a smaller diameter and a much lower surface tension than the left-hand alveolus. Gas tends to flow from the larger to the smaller alveolus and stability is maintained.

The alveolar surfactant[2]

The low surface tension of the alveolar lining fluid and its dependence on alveolar radius are due to the presence of a surface-active material known as the surfactant. Some 90% of surfactant consists of lipids, the remainder being proteins and small amounts of carbohydrate.[3] Most of the lipid is phospholipid, of which some 70–80% is dipalmitoyl phosphatidyl choline, the main constituent responsible for the effect on surface tension. The fatty acids are hydrophobic and generally straight, lying parallel to each other and projecting into the gas phase. The other end of the molecule is hydrophilic and lies within the alveolar lining fluid. The molecules are thus confined to the surface where, being detergents, they lower surface tension in proportion to the concentration at the interface.

Around 10% of surfactant obtained from bronchoalveolar lavage is protein, most of which are contaminating serum proteins such as albumin and globulin. Approximately 2% of surfactant by weight consists of surfactant proteins (SP), of which there are four types labelled A–D.[4–6] SP-B and SP-C are small proteins that are vital to the stabilisation of the surfactant monolayer (see below); a congenital lack of SP-B results in severe and progressive respiratory failure.[6,7] SP-A and, to a lesser extent, SP-D are involved in the control of surfactant release and possibly in preventing pulmonary infection (see below).[5,8]

Synthesis of surfactant. Surfactant is both formed in and liberated from the alveolar epithelial type II cell (page 21). The lamellar bodies (see Figure 2.10) contain stored

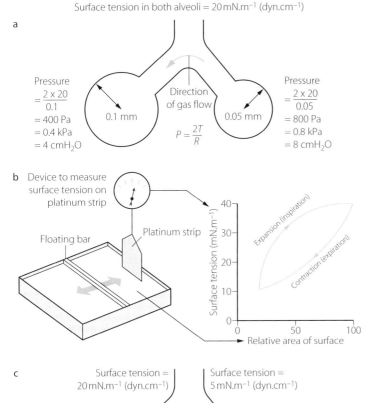

a

Surface tension in both alveoli = 20 mN.m^{-1} (dyn.cm^{-1})

Direction of gas flow

0.1 mm   0.05 mm

$P = \dfrac{2T}{R}$

Pressure
$= \dfrac{2 \times 20}{0.1}$
= 400 Pa
= 0.4 kPa
= 4 cmH$_2$O

Pressure
$= \dfrac{2 \times 20}{0.05}$
= 800 Pa
= 0.8 kPa
= 8 cmH$_2$O

b   Device to measure surface tension on platinum strip

Floating bar

Platinum strip

Surface tension (mN.m^{-1})

40
30
20
10
0

Expansion (inspiration)

Contraction (expiration)

0   50   100

Relative area of surface

c

Surface tension = 20 mN.m^{-1} (dyn.cm^{-1})

Surface tension = 5 mN.m^{-1} (dyn.cm^{-1})

Direction of gas flow

0.1 mm   0.05 mm

$P = \dfrac{2T}{R}$

Pressure
$= \dfrac{2 \times 20}{0.1}$
= 400 Pa
= 0.4 kPa
= 4 cmH$_2$O

Pressure
$= \dfrac{2 \times 5}{0.05}$
= 200 Pa
= 0.2 kPa
= 2 cmH$_2$O

Figure 3.1 Surface tension and alveolar transmural pressure. **(a)** Pressure relations in two alveoli of different size but with the same surface tension of their lining fluids. **(b)** The changes in surface tension in relation to the area of the alveolar lining film. **(c)** Pressure relations of two alveoli of different size when allowance is made for the probable changes in surface tension.

surfactant that is released into the alveolus by exocytosis in response to high-volume lung inflation, increased ventilation rate or endocrine stimulation. After release surfactant initially forms areas of a lattice structure termed tubular myelin, which is then reorganised into mono- or multilayered surface films. This conversion into the functionally active form of surfactant is believed to be critically dependent on surfactant proteins B and C (see below).[6,8] The alveolar half-life of surfactant is 15–30 hours, with most of its components being recycled by type II alveolar cells. Surfactant protein-A is intimately involved in controlling the surfactant present in the alveolus, with type II alveolar cells having SP-A surface receptors, stimulation of which exerts a negative feedback on surfactant secretion and increases reuptake of surfactant components into the cell.

Action of surfactant. To maintain the stability of alveoli as shown in Figure 3.1, surfactant must alter the surface

tension in the alveoli as their size varies with inspiration and expiration. A simple explanation of how this occurs is that during expiration, as the surface area of the alveolus diminishes, the surfactant molecules are packed more densely and so exert a greater effect on the surface tension, which then decreases, as shown in Figure 3.1b. In reality, the situation is considerably more complex and at present poorly elucidated.[6] Surfactant phospholipid is known to exist *in vivo* in both monolayer and multilayer forms[4] and it is possible that in some areas of the alveoli the phospholipid alternates between these two forms as alveolar size changes during the respiratory cycle. This aspect of surfactant function is entirely dependent on the presence of SP-B, a small hydrophobic protein which can be incorporated into a phospholipid monolayer, and SP-C, a larger protein with a hydrophobic central portion allowing it to span a lipid bilayer.[6] When alveolar size reduces and the surface film is compressed, SP-B molecules may be squeezed out of the lipid layer, so changing its surface properties, while SP-C may serve to stabilise bilayers of lipid to act as a reservoir from which the surface film may re-form when alveolar size increases.

Other effects of surfactant. Pulmonary transudation is also affected by surface forces. Surface tension causes the pressure within the alveolar lining fluid to be less than the alveolar pressure. Since the pulmonary capillary pressure in most of the lung is greater than the alveolar pressure (page 388), both factors encourage transudation, a tendency that is checked by the oncotic pressure of the plasma proteins. Thus the surfactant, by reducing surface tension, diminishes one component of the pressure gradient and helps to prevent transudation.

Surfactant may also play an important part in the immunology of the lung.[2,5,9] The lipid component of surfactant has antioxidant activity and thus may attenuate lung damage from a variety of causes and also suppress some groups of lymphocytes, so theoretically protecting the lungs from autoimmune damage. *In vitro* studies have shown that SP-A or SP-D can bind to a wide range of pulmonary pathogens, including viruses, bacteria, fungi, *Pneumocystis carinii* and *Mycobacterium tuberculosis*. Both SP-A and SP-D activate alveolar macrophages or neutrophils, acting via specific surface receptors. However, the contribution of surfactant to *in vivo* pulmonary defences remains unclear.[5]

Alternative models to explain lung recoil

Treating surfactant-lined alveoli as bubbles that obey Laplace's law has aided the understanding of lung recoil in health and disease for many decades (page 222). However, some workers are now beginning to challenge this explanation[10,11] and evidence is mounting that the real situation is much more complex. Arguments against the bubble model include:

- in theory, differing surface tensions in adjacent alveoli cannot occur if the liquid lining the alveoli is connected by a continuous liquid layer
- when surfactant layers are compressed at 37°C multilayered 'rafts' of dry surfactant form, though the inclusion of surfactant proteins reduces this physicochemical change
- alveoli are not shaped like perfect spheres with a single entrance point: they are variable polyhedrons with convex bulges in their walls where pulmonary capillaries bulge into them (see Figure 2.7).

These are just some of the arguments used to challenge the conventional description of the alveolar component of lung recoil. Two very different alternative models have been proposed.

Morphological model. Hills has for many years claimed that the surfactant lining alveoli results in a 'discontinuous' liquid lining.[12,13] Based on knowledge of the physical chemistry of surfactants, Hills' model shows that surfactant phospholipids are adsorbed directly onto the epithelial cell surface, so causing patches of the surface to become less 'wettable', these patches being interspersed with fluid pools. Surface forces generated by the interaction between the 'dry' areas of surfactant and the areas of liquid are theoretically large enough to maintain alveolar stability.

Foam model. Scarpelli has developed new techniques for preparing lung tissue for microscopy.[14] By maintaining tissue in a more natural state than previous studies, including keeping lung volume close to normal, he has described a 'new anatomy' for alveoli. Scarpelli's findings seem to show that *in vivo* alveoli have bubble films across their entrances, with similar lipid bilayer films also existing across alveolar ducts and respiratory bronchioles (Figure 3.2). In this model, each acinus may be considered as a series of interconnected but closed bubbles, so forming a stable 'foam'. The bubble films are estimated to be less than 7 nm thick and so will offer little resistance to gas diffusion, the normal mechanism by which gas movement occurs in a single pulmonary acinus (page 17).

More research is clearly needed to either confirm or refute each of these models. It would therefore be premature to consign the well-established bubble model of alveolar recoil to the history books, but physiologists should be aware that cracks have begun to appear in a long-standing physiological concept.

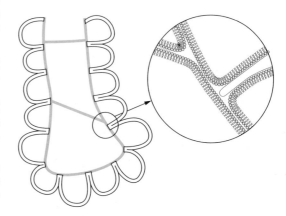

Figure 3.2 Scarpelli's 'foam' model of alveolar structure.[14] Surfactant lines the alveoli and forms films (blue) that span both the alveolar openings and the alveolar ducts. Inset: detail of the surfactant layer showing connection between phospholipid monolayer and bilayer (not to scale).

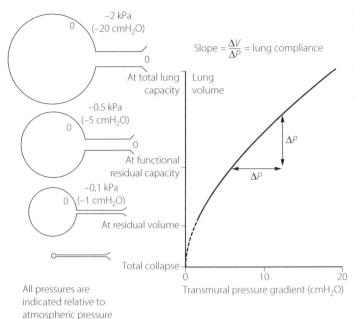

Slope $= \dfrac{\Delta V}{\Delta P} =$ lung compliance

Figure 3.3 Relationship between lung volume and the difference in pressure between the alveoli and the intrathoracic space (transmural pressure gradient). The relationship is almost linear over the normal tidal volume range. The calibre of small air passages decreases in parallel with alveolar volume. Airways begin to close at the closing capacity and there is widespread airway closure at residual volume. Values in the diagram relate to the upright position and to *decreasing* pressure. The opening pressure of a closed alveolus is not shown.

All pressures are indicated relative to atmospheric pressure

The transmural pressure gradient and intrathoracic pressure

The transmural pressure gradient is the difference between intrathoracic (or 'intrapleural') and alveolar pressure. The pressure within an alveolus is always greater than the pressure to the surrounding interstitial tissue except when the volume has been reduced to zero. With increasing lung volume, the transmural pressure gradient steadily increases, as shown for the whole lung in Figure 3.3. If an appreciable pneumothorax is present, the pressure gradient from alveolus to pleural cavity provides a measure of the overall transmural pressure gradient. Otherwise the oesophageal pressure may be used to indicate the pleural pressure, but there are conceptual and technical difficulties. The technical difficulties are considered at the end of this chapter, and some of the conceptual difficulties are indicated in Figure 3.4.

The alveoli in the upper part of the lung have a larger volume than those in the dependent part except at total lung capacity. The greater degree of expansion of the alveoli in the upper part results in a greater transmural pressure gradient, which decreases steadily down the lung at about 0.1 kPa (or 1 cmH₂O) per 3 cm of vertical height; such a difference is indicated in Figure 3.4a. Since the pleural cavity is normally empty, it is not strictly correct to speak of an intrapleural pressure and, furthermore, it would not be constant throughout the pleural 'cavity'. One should think rather of the relationship shown in Figure 3.3 as applying to various horizontal strata of the lung, each with its own volume and therefore its own transmural pressure gradient on which

its own 'intrapleural' pressure would depend. The transmural pressure gradient has an important influence on many aspects of pulmonary function and so its horizontal stratification confers a regional difference on many features of pulmonary function, including airway closure, ventilation/perfusion ratios and therefore gas exchange. These matters are considered in detail in the appropriate chapters of this book.

At first sight it might be thought that the subatmospheric intrapleural pressure would result in the accumulation of gas evolved from solution in blood and tissues. In fact, the total of the partial pressures of gases dissolved in blood, and therefore tissues, is always less than one atmosphere (see Table 26.2), and this factor keeps the pleural cavity free of gas.

Time dependence of pulmonary elastic behaviour

If an excised lung is rapidly inflated and then held at the new volume, the inflation pressure falls exponentially from its initial value to reach a lower level that is attained after a few seconds. This also occurs in the intact subject and is readily observed during an inspiratory pause in a patient receiving artificial ventilation (page 37). It is broadly true to say that the volume change divided by the initial change in transmural pressure gradient corresponds to the dynamic compliance, whereas the volume change divided by the ultimate change in transmural pressure gradient (i.e. measured after it has become steady) corresponds to the static compliance. Static compliance will thus be greater than the dynamic

a

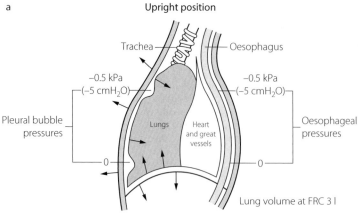

Upright position

Trachea — Oesophagus

−0.5 kPa (−5 cmH₂O)

−0.5 kPa (−5 cmH₂O)

Pleural bubble pressures

Lungs

Heart and great vessels

Oesophageal pressures

0

0

Lung volume at FRC 3 l

b

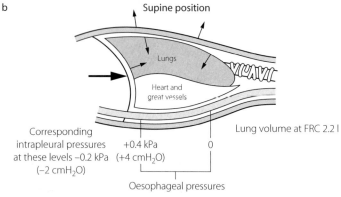

Supine position

Lungs

Heart and great vessels

Lung volume at FRC 2.2 l

Corresponding intrapleural pressures at these levels −0.2 kPa (−2 cmH₂O)

+0.4 kPa (+4 cmH₂O)

0

Oesophageal pressures

c

Mechanical analogy of static relationships

Spring representing lungs

Tension recorded on spring balance representing intrathoracic pressure

Spring representing thoracic cage

10   5   0 cm H₂O
1   0.5   0 kPa

Figure 3.4 Intrathoracic pressures: static relationships in the resting end-expiratory position. The lung volume corresponds to the functional residual capacity (FRC). The figures in (a) and (b) indicate the pressure relative to ambient (atmospheric). The arrows show the direction of elastic forces. The heavy arrow in (b) indicates displacement by the abdominal viscera. In (c) the tension in the two springs is the same and will be indicated on the spring balance. In the supine position: (1) the FRC is reduced; (2) the intrathoracic pressure is raised; (3) the weight of the heart raises the oesophageal pressure above the intrapleural pressure.

compliance by an amount determined by the degree of time dependence in the elastic behaviour of a particular lung. The respiratory frequency has been shown to influence dynamic pulmonary compliance in the normal subject but frequency dependence is much more pronounced in the presence of pulmonary disease.

Hysteresis. If the lungs are slowly inflated and then slowly deflated, the pressure/volume curve for static points during inflation differs from that obtained during deflation. The two curves form a loop, which becomes progressively broader as the tidal volume is increased (Figure 3.5). Expressed in words, the loop in Figure 3.5 means that rather more than the expected pressure is required during inflation and rather less than the expected recoil pressure is available during deflation.

This resembles the behaviour of perished rubber or polyvinyl chloride, both of which are reluctant to accept deformation under stress but, once deformed, are again reluctant to assume their original shape. This phenomenon is present to a greater or lesser extent in all elastic bodies and is known as elastic hysteresis.

Causes of time dependence of pulmonary elastic behaviour

There are many possible explanations of the time dependence of pulmonary elastic behaviour, the relative importance of which may vary in different circumstances.

Changes in surfactant activity. It has been explained above that the surface tension of the alveolar lining fluid

Figure 3.5 Static plot of lung volume against transmural pressure gradient (intra-oesophageal pressure relative to atmospheric at zero air flow). Note that inspiratory and expiratory curves form a loop that gets wider the greater the tidal volume. These loops are typical of elastic hysteresis. For a particular lung volume, the elastic recoil of the lung during expiration is always less than the distending transmural pressure gradient required during inspiration at the same lung volume.

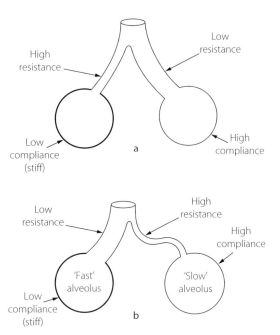

Figure 3.6 Schematic diagrams of alveoli to illustrate conditions under which static and dynamic compliance may differ. **(a)** represents a theoretically ideal state in which there is a reciprocal relationship between resistance and compliance, resulting in gas flow being delivered preferentially to the most compliant regions, regardless of the state of inflation. Static and dynamic compliance are equal. This situation is probably never realised even in the normal subject. **(b)** illustrates a state that is typical of many patients with respiratory disease. The alveoli can conveniently be divided into 'fast' and 'slow' groups. The direct relationship between compliance and resistance results in inspired gas being delivered preferentially to the stiff alveoli if the rate of inflation is rapid. An end-inspiratory pause then permits redistribution from the fast alveoli to the slow alveoli.

is greater at larger lung volumes and also during inspiration than at the same lung volume during expiration (see Figure 3.1b). This is probably the most important cause of the observed hysteresis in the intact lung (see Figure 3.5).

Stress relaxation. If a spring is pulled out to a fixed increase in its length, the resultant tension is maximal at first and then declines exponentially to a constant value. This is an inherent property of elastic bodies, known as stress relaxation. Thoracic tissues display stress relaxation, and these 'viscoelastic' properties contribute significantly to the difference between static and dynamic compliance[15] as well as forming a component of pulmonary resistance (page 42). The crinkled structure of collagen in the lung is likely to favour stress relaxation, and excised strips of human lung show stress relaxation when stretched.[16]

Redistribution of gas. In a lung consisting of functional units with identical time constants[†]of inflation, the distribution of gas should be independent of the rate of

inflation and there should be no redistribution when the lungs are held inflated. However, if different parts of the lungs have different time constants, the distribution of inspired gas will be dependent on the rate of inflation and redistribution ('pendelluft') will occur when inflation is held. This problem is discussed in greater detail on page 111, but for the time being we can distinguish 'fast' and 'slow' alveoli (the term 'alveoli' here referring to functional units rather than the anatomical entity).

The 'fast' alveolus has a low airway resistance and/or low compliance (or both), whereas the 'slow' alveolus has a high airway resistance and/or a high compliance (Figure 3.6b). These properties give the fast alveolus a shorter time constant so it is preferentially filled during a short inflation. This preferential filling of alveoli with low compliance gives an overall higher pulmonary transmural pressure gradient. A slow or sustained inflation permits increased distribution of gas to slow alveoli and

---

[†]Time constants are used to describe the exponential filling and emptying of a lung unit. One time constant is the time taken to achieve 63% of maximal inflation or deflation of the lung unit. See Appendix F for details.

so tends to distribute gas in accord with the compliance of the different functional units. There should then be a lower overall transmural pressure and no redistribution of gas when inflation is held. The extreme difference between fast and slow alveoli shown in Figure 3.6b applies to diseased lungs, and no such differences exist in normal lungs. Gas redistribution is therefore unlikely to be a major factor in healthy subjects, but it can be important in patients with increased airway obstruction, particularly in emphysema, asthma and chronic obstructive pulmonary disease.

Recruitment of alveoli. Below a certain lung volume, some alveoli tend to close and only reopen at a considerably greater lung volume, in response to a much higher transmural pressure gradient than that at which they closed. Recruitment of closed alveoli appears at first sight to be a plausible explanation of all the time-dependent phenomena described above, but there are two reasons why this is unlikely. First, the pressure required for reopening a closed unit is very high and is unlikely to be achieved during normal breathing. Secondly, there is no histological evidence for collapsed alveoli in normal lungs at functional residual capacity. In the presence of pathological lung collapse, a sustained deep inflation may well cause re-expansion and an increased compliance, e.g during anaesthesia (page 306). Cyclical opening and closing of alveoli during a normal respiratory cycle is unlikely in normal lungs but does occur in injured lungs (page 438).

Displacement of pulmonary blood. A sustained inflation might be expected to displace blood from the lungs and so to increase compliance by reducing the splinting effect of the pulmonary vasculature. The importance of this factor is not known, but experiments with excised lung indicate that all the major time-dependent phenomena are present when the pulmonary vasculature is empty.

Factors affecting lung compliance

Lung volume. It is important to remember that compliance is related to lung volume. This factor may be excluded by relating compliance to FRC to yield the specific compliance (i.e. compliance/FRC), which in humans is almost constant for both sexes and all ages down to neonatal. The relationship between compliance and lung volume is true not only within an individual lung but also between species. Larger animal species have thicker alveolar septae containing increased amounts of collagen and elastin, resulting in larger alveolar diameters,[17] so reducing the pressure needed to expand them. An elephant therefore has larger alveoli and hence a higher compliance than a mouse.

Posture. Lung volume, and therefore compliance, changes with posture (page 34). There are, however, problems in the measurement of intrapleural pressure in the supine position, and when this is taken into account it seems unlikely that changes of posture have any significant effect on the specific compliance.

Pulmonary blood volume. The pulmonary blood vessels probably make an appreciable contribution to the stiffness of the lung. Pulmonary venous congestion from whatever cause is associated with reduced compliance.

Age. One would have expected age to influence the elasticity of the lung, as of other tissues in the body. However, no correlation has ever been found between age and compliance, even after allowing for predicted changes in lung volume. This accords with the concept of lung 'elasticity' being largely determined by surface forces.

Restriction of chest expansion. Elastic strapping of the chest reduces both lung volume and compliance. However, when lung volume is returned to normal, either by removal of the restriction or by a more forceful inspiration, the compliance remains reduced. Normal compliance can be restored by taking a single deep breath.[18]

Recent ventilatory history. A period of hypoventilation without periodic deep breaths may lead to a reduction of compliance, particularly in pathological states. Compliance may usually be restored by one or more large breaths corresponding to sighs. This was first observed during artificial ventilation of patients with respiratory paralysis[19] and these observations led to the introduction of artificial ventilators that periodically administer 'sighs'. There can be no doubt of the importance of periodic expansion of the lungs during prolonged artificial ventilation of diseased lungs, but the case for 'sighs' while ventilating normal lungs (e.g. during anaesthesia) is less convincing.

Bronchial smooth muscle tone. Animal studies[20] have shown that an infusion of methacholine sufficient to result in a doubling of airway resistance decreases *dynamic* compliance by 50%. The airways might contribute to overall compliance or, alternatively, bronchoconstriction could enhance time dependence and so reduce dynamic but perhaps not static compliance (see Figure 3.6).

Disease. Important changes in lung pressure/volume relationships are found in some lung diseases and these are described in the relevant chapters in Part 3.

ELASTIC RECOIL OF THE THORACIC CAGE

The thoracic cage comprises the ribcage and the diaphragm. Each is a muscular structure and can be considered as an elastic structure only when the muscles are relaxed, and that is not easy to achieve except under conditions of paralysis. Relaxation curves have been prepared relating pressure and volumes in the supposedly relaxed subject, but it is now doubted whether total relaxation was ever achieved. For example, it seems that the diaphragm is not fully relaxed at the end of expiration *in the supine position* but maintains a resting tone to prevent the abdominal contents pushing the diaphragm cephalad.[21]

Compliance of the thoracic cage is defined as change in lung volume per unit change in the pressure gradient between atmosphere and the intrapleural space. The units are the same as for pulmonary compliance. The measurement is seldom made but the value is of the order of $2\ l.kPa^{-1}$ ($200\ ml.cmH_2O^{-1}$).

Factors influencing compliance of the thoracic cage

Anatomical factors include the ribs and the state of ossification of the costal cartilages. Obesity and even pathological skin conditions may have an appreciable effect. In particular, scarring of the skin overlying the front of the chest may result from scalding in children and this may embarrass the breathing.

In terms of compliance, a relaxed diaphragm simply transmits pressure from the abdomen, which may be increased by obesity and abdominal distension. Posture clearly has a major effect and this is considered below in relation to FRC. Compared with the supine position, thoracic cage compliance is 30% greater in the seated subject and the total static compliance of the respiratory system is reduced by 60% in the prone position owing to the diminished elasticity of the ribcage and diaphragm in the prone position.

PRESSURE/VOLUME RELATIONSHIPS OF THE LUNG PLUS THORACIC CAGE

Compliance is analogous to electrical capacitance and in the respiratory system the compliances of lungs and thoracic cage are in series. Therefore the total compliance of the system obeys the same relationship as for capacitances in series, in which reciprocals are added to obtain the reciprocal of the total value, thus:

$$\frac{1}{\text{total compliance}} =$$
$$\frac{1}{\text{lung compliance}} + \frac{1}{\text{thoracic cage compliance}}$$

typical static values ($l.kPa^{-1}$) for the supine paralysed patient being:

$$\frac{1}{0.85} = \frac{1}{1.5} + \frac{1}{2}$$

Instead of compliance, we may consider its reciprocal, elastance. The relationship is then much simpler:

Total elastance =
           lung elastance + thoracic cage elastance

Corresponding values ($kPa.l^{-1}$) are then:

$$1.17 = 0.67 + 0.5$$

Relationship between alveolar, intrathoracic and ambient pressures

At all times the alveolar–ambient pressure gradient is the sum of the alveolar–intrathoracic (or transmural) and intrathoracic–ambient pressure gradients. This relationship is independent of whether the patient is breathing spontaneously or being ventilated by intermittent positive pressure. Actual values depend on compliances, lung volume and posture and typical values are shown for the upright conscious relaxed subject in Figure 3.7. The values in the illustration are static and relate to conditions when no gas is flowing.

LUNG VOLUMES

Certain lung volumes, particularly the FRC, are determined by elastic forces. This is therefore a convenient point at which to consider the various lung volumes and their subdivision (Figure 3.8).

Total lung capacity (TLC). This is the volume of gas in the lungs at the end of a maximal inspiration. TLC is achieved when the maximal force generated by the inspiratory muscles is balanced by the forces opposing expansion. It is rather surprising that *expiratory* muscles are also contracting strongly at the end of a maximal inspiration.

Residual volume (RV). This is the volume remaining after a maximal expiration. In the young, RV is governed by the balance between the maximal force generated by expiratory muscles and the elastic forces opposing reduction of lung volume. However, in older subjects closure of small airways may prevent further expiration.

Functional residual capacity. This is the lung volume at the end of a normal expiration.

Within the framework of TLC, RV and FRC, other capacities and volumes shown in Figure 3.8 are self-explanatory.

Spontaneous respiration

FRC   FRC + 0.5 litre   FRC + 1 litre

Intermittent positive-pressure ventilation

FRC   FRC + 0.5 litre   FRC + 1 litre
Figures denote pressure relative to atmosphere (kPa)

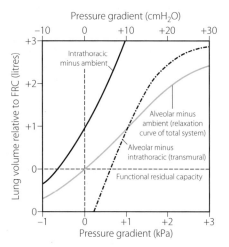

Figure 3.7 Static pressure/volume relations for the intact thorax for the conscious subject in the upright position. The transmural pressure gradient bears the same relationship to lung volume during both intermittent positive-pressure ventilation and spontaneous breathing. The intrathoracic-to-ambient pressure difference, however, differs in the two types of ventilation due to muscle action during spontaneous respiration. At all times:

alveolar/ambient pressure difference = alveolar/intrathoracic pressure difference + intrathoracic/ambient pressure difference (due attention being paid to the sign of the pressure difference).

Factors affecting the FRC

So many factors affect the FRC that they require a special section of this chapter. The actual volume of the FRC has particular importance because of its relationship to the closing capacity (see below).

Body size. FRC is linearly related to height. Estimates range[22,23] from an increase in FRC of 32 to 51 ml.cm^{-1}. Obesity causes a marked reduction in FRC compared with lean subjects of the same height.

Sex. For the same body height, females have an FRC about 10% less than males.[23]

Age. FRC increases slightly with age,[22] increasing by around 16 ml per year.

Diaphragmatic muscle tone. FRC has in the past been considered to be simply the volume at which there is a balance between the elastic forces represented by the inward retraction of the lungs and the outward expansion of the thoracic cage. However, as explained above, it now appears that residual end-expiratory muscle tone is a major factor in the supine position, maintaining the FRC about 400 ml above the volume in the totally relaxed subject, which in practice means paralysed during anaesthesia.

Posture. Figures 3.4 and 3.9 show the reduction in FRC in the supine position, which may be attributed to the increased pressure of the abdominal contents on the diaphragm. Values of FRC in these figures and Table 3.1 are typical for a subject of 168–170 cm height and reported mean differences between supine and upright positions range from 500 to 1000 ml. Teleologically, end-expiratory diaphragmatic tone can be seen as a protection against the weight of the abdominal contents causing an unacceptable reduction of lung volume in the supine position. Values for FRC in other positions are shown in Table 3.1.

Lung disease. The FRC will be reduced by increased elastic recoil of the lungs, chest wall or both. Possible causes include fibrosing alveolitis, organised fibrinous pleurisy, kyphoscoliosis, obesity and scarring of the thorax following burns. Conversely, elastic recoil of the lungs is diminished in emphysema and asthma and the FRC is usually increased (see Chapter 28). This is beneficial, since airway resistance decreases as the lung volume increases.

FRC in relation to closing capacity

In Chapter 4 it is explained how reduction in lung volume below a certain level results in airway closure with relative or total underventilation in the dependent parts of the lung. The lung volume below which this effect becomes apparent is known as the closing capacity (CC). With increasing age, CC rises until it equals FRC at about 66 years in the upright position but only 44 in the supine position (Figure 3.10). This is a

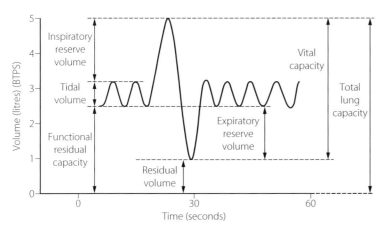

Figure 3.8 Static lung volumes of Dr Nunn in 1990. The 'spirometer curve' indicates the lung volumes that can be measured by simple spirometry. These are tidal volume, inspiratory reserve volume, expiratory reserve volume and vital capacity. The residual volume, total lung capacity and functional residual capacity cannot be measured by observation of a spirometer without further elaboration of methods. BTPS, body temperature and pressure, saturated.

Figure 3.9 Studies by Dr Nunn and his coworkers of the functional residual capacity in various body positions.

major factor in the decrease of arterial PO_2 with age (page 180).

PRINCIPLES OF MEASUREMENT OF COMPLIANCE

Compliance is measured as the change in lung volume divided by the corresponding change in the appropriate pressure gradient, there being no gas flow when the two measurements are made. For lung compliance the appropriate pressure gradient is alveolar–intrapleural (or intrathoracic) and for the total compliance alveolar–ambient. Measurement of compliance of the thoracic cage is seldom undertaken but the appropriate pressure gradient would then be intrapleural–ambient. This would be meaningless for measurement of compliance if there were any tone in the respiratory muscles.

Volume may be measured with a spirometer, a body plethysmograph, or by integration of a flow rate obtained from a pneumotachogram. Points of zero air flow are best

indicated by a pneumotachogram. Static pressures can be measured with a simple water manometer but electrical transducers are now more usual. Intrathoracic pressure is normally measured as oesophageal pressure which, in the upright subject, is different at different levels. The pressure rises as the balloon descends, the change being roughly in accord with the specific gravity of the lung (0.3 g.ml^{-1}). It is convention to measure the pressure 32–35 cm beyond the nares, the highest point at which the measurement is free from artefacts due to mouth pressure and tracheal and neck movements. In the supine position the weight of the heart may introduce an artefact (see Figure 3.4) but there is usually a zone some 32–40 cm beyond the nares where the oesophageal pressure is close to atmospheric and probably only about 0.2 kPa (2 cmH$_2$O) above the neighbouring intrathoracic pressure. Alveolar pressure equals mouth pressure when no gas is flowing: it cannot be measured directly.

Static compliance. In the conscious subject, a known volume of air is inhaled from FRC and the subject then relaxes against a closed airway. The various pressure gradients are then measured and compared with the resting values at FRC. It is, in fact, very difficult to ensure that the respiratory muscles are relaxed, but the measurement of lung compliance is valid since the static alveolar–intrathoracic pressure difference is unaffected by any muscle activity.

In the paralysed subject there are no difficulties about muscular relaxation and it is very easy to measure static compliance of the whole respiratory system simply using recordings of airway pressure and respiratory volumes. However, due to the uncertainties about interpretation of the oesophageal pressure in the supine position (see Figure 3.4), there is usually some uncertainty about the pulmonary compliance. For static compliance it is therefore easier to measure *lung* compliance in the upright

Table 3.1 Effect of posture on some aspects of respiratory function[24]

Position	FRC (litres) (BTPS)	Ribcage breathing* (%)	Forced expiratory volume in 1 second (litres) (BTPS)
Sitting	2.91	69.7	3.79
Supine	2.10	32.3	3.70
Supine (arms up)	2.36	33.0	3.27
Prone	2.45	32.6	3.49
Lateral	2.44	36.5	3.67

Data for 13 healthy males aged 24–64.
* Proportion of breathing accounted for by movement of the ribcage.

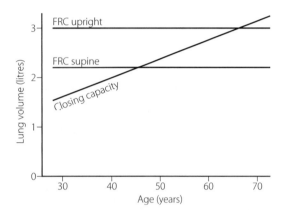

Figure 3.10 Functional residual capacity and closing capacity as a function of age. (Data from reference 25.)

position and *total* compliance in the anaesthetised paralysed patient, who will usually be in the supine position.

Dynamic compliance. These measurements are made during rhythmic breathing, but compliance is calculated from pressure and volume measurements made when no gas is flowing, usually at end-inspiratory and end-expiratory 'no-flow' points. The usual method involves creation of a pressure/volume loop by displaying simultaneously as X and Y coordinates the required pressure gradient and the respired volume. In the resultant loop, as in Figure 3.11, the 'no-flow' points are where the trace is horizontal and the dynamic compliance is the slope of the line joining these points.

Automated measurement of compliance

In a spontaneously breathing awake patient lung compliance measurement is difficult because of the requirement to place an oesophageal balloon. However, in anaesthetised patients or those receiving intermittent positive-pressure ventilation (IPPV) in intensive care,

the measurement of compliance is considerably easier. Many ventilators and anaesthetic monitoring systems now routinely measure airway pressure and tidal volume. This enables a pressure/volume loop to be displayed (Figure 3.11a), from which the dynamic compliance of the respiratory system may be calculated on a continuous breath-by-breath basis. When no gas is flowing during IPPV (at the end of inspiration and expiration) the airway pressure equals alveolar pressure. At this point, the airway pressure recorded by the ventilator therefore equals the difference between alveolar and atmospheric pressure, allowing derivation of the total compliance.

Some ventilators will also measure static compliance. The microprocessor will inflate the lung with the patient's usual tidal volume and then pause at end-inspiration for between 0.5 and 2 seconds, until the airway pressure falls to a plateau lasting 300 ms (Figure 3.11b). Static compliance is then calculated from the volume delivered and pressure recorded during the plateau and may be easily compared with dynamic compliance.

PRINCIPLES OF MEASUREMENT OF LUNG VOLUMES

Vital capacity, tidal volume, inspiratory reserve and expiratory reserve can all be measured with a simple spirometer (see Figure 3.8). Total lung capacity, functional residual capacity and residual volume all contain a fraction (the residual volume) that cannot be measured by simple spirometry. However, if one of these volumes is measured (most commonly the FRC), the others may easily be derived.

Measurement of FRC

Three techniques are available. The first employs nitrogen wash-out by breathing 100% oxygen. Total quantity of nitrogen eliminated is measured as the product of the expired volume collected and the concentration of nitro-

a

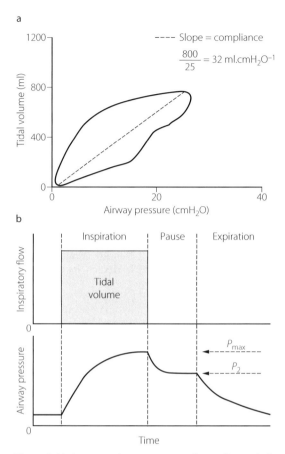

---- Slope = compliance

$$\frac{800}{25} = 32 \text{ ml.cmH}_2\text{O}^{-1}$$

b

Inspiratory flow

Inspiration | Pause | Expiration

Tidal volume

0

Airway pressure

P_{max}

P_2

0

Time

Figure 3.11 Automated measurement of compliance during intermittent positive-pressure ventilation. **(a)** Dynamic compliance. Simultaneous measurement of tidal volume and airway pressure creates a pressure/volume loop. End-expiratory and end-inspiratory 'no-flow' points occur when the trace is horizontal. At this point, airway pressure and alveolar pressure are equal, so the pressure gradient is the difference between alveolar and atmospheric pressure. Total respiratory system compliance is therefore the slope of the line between these points. Note that in this patient compliance is markedly reduced. **(b)** Static compliance. Following an end-inspiratory pause the plateau pressure is recorded (P_2) and along with tidal volume the static compliance easily derived. This manoeuvre also provides an assessment of respiratory system resistance by recording the pressure drop ($P_{max} - P_2$) and the inspiratory flow immediately before the inspiratory pause (see page 51).

gen. If, for example, 4 l of nitrogen are collected and the initial alveolar nitrogen concentration was 80%, then the initial lung volume was 5 l.

The second method uses the wash-in of a tracer gas such as helium, the concentration of which may be relatively easily measured by catharometry.[26] If, for example, 50 ml of helium are introduced into the lungs and the helium concentration is then found to be 1%,

the lung volume is 5 l. Helium is used for this method because of its low solubility in blood. For the technique to be accurate, the measurement must be made rapidly or helium dissolving in the tissues and blood will introduce errors.

The third method uses the body plethysmograph. The subject is totally contained within a gas-tight box and attempts to breathe against an occluded airway. Changes in alveolar pressure are recorded at the mouth and compared with the small changes in lung volume, derived from pressure changes within the plethysmograph. Application of Boyle's law then permits calculation of lung volume.

The last method is the only technique for FRC measurement that includes gas trapped within the lung distal to closed airways.

REFERENCES

1. Brown ES, Johnson RP, Clements JA. Pulmonary surface tension. *J Appl Physiol* 1959; **14**: 717–20.
2. Hamm H, Kroegel C, Hohlfeld J. Surfactant: a review of its functions and relevance in adult respiratory disorders. *Respir Med* 1996; **90**: 251–70.
3. van Gold LMG, Batenburg JJ, Robertson B. The pulmonary surfactant system: biochemical aspects and functional significance. *Physiol Rev* 1988; **68**: 374–455.
*4. Whitsett JA, Weaver TE. Hydrophobic surfactant proteins in lung function and disease. *N Engl J Med* 2002; **347**: 2141–8.
5. Mason RJ, Greene K, Voelker DR. Surfactant protein A and surfactant protein D in health and disease. *Am J Physiol* 1998; **275**: L1–13.
*6. Weaver TE, Conkright JJ. Functions of surfactant proteins B and C. *Annu Rev Physiol* 2001; **63**: 555–78.
7. Nogee LM, DeMello DE, Dehner LP, Colten HR. Brief report: deficiency of pulmonary surfactant protein B in congenital alveolar proteinosis. *N Engl J Med* 1993; **328**: 406–10.
8. Hawgood S, Poulain FR. The pulmonary collectins and surfactant metabolism. *Annu Rev Physiol* 2001; **63**: 495–519.
9. Crouch E, Wright JR. Surfactant proteins A and D and pulmonary host defense. *Annu Rev Physiol* 2001; **63**: 521–54.
10. Dorrington KL, Young JD. Development of the concept of a liquid pulmonary alveolar lining layer. *Br J Anaesth* 2001; **86**: 614–17.
*11. Scarpelli EM, Hills BA. Opposing views on the alveolar surface, alveolar models and the role of surfactant. *J Appl Physiol* 2000; **89**: 408–12.
12. Hills BA. What forces keep the airspaces of the lung dry? *Thorax* 1982; **37**: 713–17.

13. Hills BA. An alternative view of the role(s) of surfactant and the alveolar model. *J Appl Physiol* 1999; **87**: 1567–83.

14. Scarpelli EM. The alveolar surface network: A new anatomy and its physiological significance. *Anat Rec* 1998; **251**: 491–527.

15. Milic-Emili J, Robatto FM, Bates JHT. Respiratory mechanics in anaesthesia. *Br J Anaesth* 1990; **65**: 4–12.

16. Sugihara T, Hildebrandt J, Martin CJ. Viscoelastic properties of alveolar wall. *J Appl Physiol* 1972; **33**: 93–8.

17. Mercer RE, Russell ML, Crapo JD. Alveolar septal structure in different species. *J Appl Physiol* 1994; **77**: 1060–6.

18. Caro CG, Butler J, DuBois AB. Some effects of restriction of chest cage expansion on pulmonary function in man. *J Clin Invest* 1960; **39**: 573–83.

19. Butler J, Smith BH. Pressure–volume relationships of the chest in the completely relaxed anaesthetised patient. *Clin Sci* 1957; **16**: 125–46.

20. Mitzner W, Blosser S, Yager D, Wagner E. Effect of bronchial smooth muscle contraction on lung compliance. *J Appl Physiol* 1992; **72**: 158–67.

21. Muller N, Volgyesi G, Becker L, Bryan MH, Bryan AC. Diaphragmatic muscle tone. *J Appl Physiol* 1979; **47**: 279–84.

22. Cotes JE. *Lung function. Assessment and application in medicine.* Oxford: Blackwell Scientific, 1993.

23. Bates DV, Macklem PT, Christie RV. *Respiratory function in disease.* London: WB Saunders, 1971.

24. Lumb AB, Nunn JF. Respiratory function and ribcage contribution to ventilation in body positions commonly used during anesthesia. *Anesth Analg* 1991; **73**: 422–6.

25. Leblanc P, Ruff F, Milic-Emili J. Effects of age and body position on 'airway closure' in man. *J Appl Physiol* 1970; **28**: 448–53.

26. Hewlett AM, Hulands GH, Nunn JF, Minty KB. Functional residual capacity, I: Methodology. *Br J Anaesth* 1974; **46**: 479–85.

Respiratory system resistance

KEY POINTS

■ Gas flow in the airways is a mixture of laminar and turbulent flow, becoming more laminar in smaller airways.

■ Respiratory system resistance is a combination of resistance to gas flow in the airways and resistance to deformation of tissues of both the lung and chest wall.

■ In smaller airways smooth muscle controls airway diameter under the influence of neural, humoral and cellular mechanisms.

■ The respiratory system can rapidly compensate for increases in either inspiratory or expiratory resistance.

Elastic resistance, which occurs when no gas is flowing, results from only two of the numerous causes of impedance to inflation of the lung (considered in the previous chapter). This chapter considers the remaining components, which together are referred to as non-elastic resistance or respiratory system resistance. Most non-elastic resistance is provided by frictional resistance to air flow and thoracic tissue deformation (both lung and chest wall), with small contributions from the inertia of gas and tissue and compression of intrathoracic gas.[1] Unlike elastic resistance, work performed against non-elastic resistance is not stored as potential energy (and therefore recoverable) but is lost and dissipated as heat.

PHYSICAL PRINCIPLES OF GAS FLOW AND RESISTANCE

Gas flows from a region of high pressure to one of lower pressure. The rate at which it does so is a function of the pressure difference and the resistance to gas flow, thus and is analogous to the flow of an electrical current (Figure 4.1). The precise relationship between pressure difference and flow rate depends on the nature of the

flow, which may be laminar, turbulent or a mixture of the two. It is useful to consider laminar and turbulent flow as two separate entities but mixed patterns of flow usually occur in the respiratory tract. With a number of important caveats, similar basic considerations apply to the flow of liquids through tubes, which is considered in Chapter 7.

Laminar flow

With laminar flow, gas flows along a straight unbranched tube as a series of concentric cylinders that slide over one another, with the peripheral cylinder stationary and the central cylinder moving fastest, the advancing cone forming a parabola (Figure 4.2a).

The advancing cone front means that some fresh gas will reach the end of a tube while the volume entering the tube is still less than the volume of the tube. In the context of the respiratory tract, this is to say that there may be significant alveolar ventilation when the tidal volume is less than the volume of the airways (the anatomical dead space), a fact that is very relevant to high-frequency ventilation (page 429). For the same reason, laminar flow is relatively inefficient for purging the contents of a tube.

In theory, gas adjacent to the tube wall is stationary, so friction between fluid and the tube wall is negligible. The physical characteristics of the airway or vessel wall should therefore not affect resistance to laminar flow. Similarly, the composition of gas sampled from the periphery of a tube during laminar flow may not be representative of the gas advancing down the centre of the tube. To complicate matters further, laminar flow requires a critical length of tubing before the characteristic advancing cone pattern can be established. This is known as the entrance length and is related to the diameter of the tube and the Reynolds' number of the fluid (see below).

Quantitative relationships. With laminar flow the gas flow rate is directly proportional to the pressure gradient along the tube (Figure 4.2b), the constant thus being defined as resistance to gas flow:

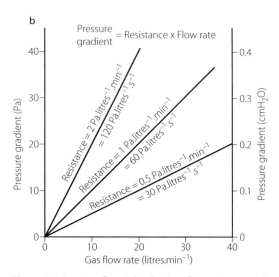

$$Resistance = \frac{Pressure\ difference}{flow\ rate}$$

Figure 4.1 Electrical analogy of gas flow. Resistance is pressure difference per unit flow rate. Resistance to gas flow is analogous to electrical resistance (provided that flow is laminar). Gas flow corresponds to electrical current (amps); gas pressure corresponds to potential (volts); gas flow resistance corresponds to electrical resistance (ohms); Poiseuille's law corresponds to Ohm's law.

$$\Delta P = flow\ rate \times resistance$$

where ΔP = pressure gradient.

In a straight unbranched tube, the Hagen–Poiseuille equation allows gas flow to be quantified:

$$Flow\ rate = \frac{\Delta P \times \pi \times (radius)^4}{8 \times length \times viscosity}$$

By combining these two equations:

$$Resistance = \frac{8 \times length \times viscosity}{\pi \times (radius)^4}$$

In this equation the fourth power of the radius of the tube explains the critical importance of narrowing of air passages. With constant tube dimensions, viscosity is the only property of a gas that is relevant under conditions of laminar flow. Helium has a low density but a viscosity close to that of air and will not therefore improve gas flow if the flow is laminar (page 42).

In the Hagen–Poiseuille equation, the units must be coherent. In CGS units, $dyn.cm^{-2}$ (pressure), $ml.s^{-1}$ (flow) and cm (length and radius) are compatible with the unit of poise for viscosity ($dyn.sec.cm^{-2}$). In SI units, with pressure in kilopascals, the unit of viscosity is $newton.second.metre^{-2}$ (see Appendix A). However, in practice it is still customary to express gas pressure in cmH_2O and flow in $l.s^{-1}$. Resistance therefore continues

Figure 4.2 Laminar flow. **(a)** In laminar flow gas moves along a straight tube as a series of concentric cylinders of gas, with the central cylinder moving fastest and the outside cylinder theoretically stationary. This gives rise to a 'cone front' of gas velocity across the tube. **(b)** The linear relationship between gas flow rate and pressure gradient. The slope of the lines indicates the resistance (1 Pa= 0.01 cmH$_2$O).

to be expressed usually as cmH_2O per litre per second ($cmH_2O.l^{-1}.s$).

Turbulent flow

High flow rates, particularly through branched or irregular tubes, result in a breakdown of the orderly flow of gas described above. An irregular movement is superimposed on the general progression along the tube (Figure 4.3a), with a square front replacing the cone front of laminar flow. Turbulent flow is almost invariably present when high resistance to gas flow is a problem.

The square front means that no fresh gas can reach the end of a tube until the amount of gas entering the tube is almost equal to the volume of the tube. Turbulent flow is more effective than laminar flow in purging the contents of a tube and also provides the best conditions for drawing a representative sample of gas from the periphery of a tube. Frictional forces between the tube wall and fluid become more important in turbulent flow.

Quantitative relationships. The relationship between driving pressure and flow rate differs from the relation-

a

(i) High flow rates

(ii) Sharp angles

(iii) Changes in diameter

(iv) Branches

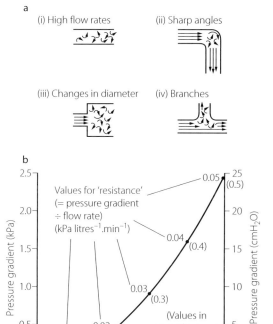

b

Figure 4.3 Turbulent flow. (a) Four circumstances under which gas flow tends to be turbulent. (b) The square law relationship between gas flow rate and pressure gradient when flow is turbulent. Note that the value for 'resistance', calculated as for laminar flow, is quite meaningless during turbulent flow.

ship described above for laminar flow in three important respects.

1. The driving pressure is proportional to the square of the gas flow rate.
2. The driving pressure is proportional to the density of the gas and is independent of its viscosity.
3. The required driving pressure is, in theory, inversely proportional to the fifth power of the radius of the tube (Fanning equation).

The square law relating driving pressure and flow rate is shown in Figure 4.3b. Resistance, defined as pressure gradient divided by flow rate, is not constant as in laminar flow but increases in proportion to the flow rate. Units such as $cmH_2O.l^{-1}.s$ should therefore be used only when flow is entirely laminar. The following methods of quantification of 'resistance' should be used when flow is totally or partially turbulent.

(a) Two constants. This method considers resistance as comprising two components, one for laminar flow and one for turbulent flow. The simple relationship for laminar flow given above would then be extended as follows:

$$\text{Pressure gradient} = k_1(\text{flow}) + k_2(\text{flow})^2$$

k_1 contains the factors of the Hagen–Poiseuille equation and represents the laminar flow component, whereas k_2 includes factors in the corresponding equation for turbulent flow. Mead and Agostoni[2] summarised studies of normal human subjects in the following equation:

$$\text{Pressure gradient (kPa)} = 0.24\,(\text{flow}) + 0.03\,(\text{flow})^2$$

(b) The exponent n. Over a surprisingly wide range of flow rates, the equation above may be condensed into the following single-term expression with little loss of precision:

$$\text{Pressure gradient} = K\,(\text{flow})^n$$

In this equation n has a value ranging from 1, with purely laminar flow, to 2, with purely turbulent flow, the value of n being a useful indication of the nature of the flow. The constants for the normal human respiratory tract are:

$$\text{Pressure gradient (kPa)} = 0.24\,(\text{flow})^{1.3}$$

(c) The graphical method. It is often convenient to represent 'resistance' as a graph of pressure difference against gas flow rate, on either linear or logarithmic coordinates. Logarithmic coordinates have the advantage that the plot is usually a straight line whether flow is laminar, turbulent or mixed, and the slope of the line indicates the value of n in the equation above.

Reynolds' number

In the case of long straight unbranched tubes, the nature of the gas flow may be predicted from the value of Reynolds' number, which is a non-dimensional quantity derived from the following expression:

$$\frac{\text{Linear velocity of gas} \times \text{tube diameter} \times \text{gas density}}{\text{Gas viscosity}}$$

The property of the gas that affects Reynolds' number is the ratio of density to viscosity. When Reynolds' number is less than 2000, flow is predominantly laminar, whereas above a value of 4000, flow is mainly turbulent.[3] Between these values, both types of flow coexist. Reynolds' number also affects the entrance length, that is, the distance required for laminar flow to become established, which is derived from:

Entrance length =
0.03 × tube diameter × Reynolds' number

Thus for gases with a low Reynolds' number not only will resistance be less during turbulent flow, but laminar flow

Table 4.1 Physical properties of clinically used gas mixtures relating to gas flow

	Viscosity relative to air	Vapour density relative to air	Vapour density Viscosity
Oxygen	1.11	1.11	1.00
70% N$_2$O/30% O$_2$	0.89	1.41	1.59
80% He/20% O$_2$	1.08	0.33	0.31

will become established more quickly after bifurcations, corners and obstructions.

Values for some gas mixtures that a patient may inhale are shown relative to air in Table 4.1. Viscosities of respirable gases do not differ greatly but there may be very large differences in density.

RESPIRATORY SYSTEM RESISTANCE

Airway resistance

This results from frictional resistance in the airways. In the healthy subject, the small airways make only a small contribution to total airway resistance because their aggregate cross-sectional area increases to very large values after about the eighth generation (see Figure 2.4). Overall airway resistance is therefore dominated by the resistance of the larger airways.

Gas flow along pulmonary airways is very complex compared to the theoretical tubes described above, and consists of a varying mixture of both laminar and turbulent flow. Both the velocity of gas flow and airway diameter (and therefore Reynolds' number) decrease in successive airway generations, from a maximum in the trachea to almost zero at the start of the pulmonary acinus (generation 15). In addition, there are frequent divisions with variable lengths of approximately straight airway between. Finally, in large-diameter airways entrance length is normally greater than the length of the individual airway. As a result of these purely physical factors, laminar flow cannot become established until approximately the 11th airway generation.[4] Predominantly turbulent flow in the conducting airways has two practical implications. First, the physical characteristics of the airway lining will influence frictional resistance more with turbulent than with laminar flow, so changes in mucus consistency that occur in many airway diseases will have a significant effect (see Chapter 28). Second, gas mixtures containing helium (low Reynolds' number) are more beneficial in overcoming increased resistance in large airways and of less benefit in small airways disease such as asthma.

Figure 4.4 The spring and dashpot model of D'Angelo *et al.*[5] Inflation of the lungs is represented by the bar moving upwards. The springs represent elastance (reciprocal of compliance) and the dashpots resistance. The spring and dashpot in series on the right confers time dependence, which is due to viscoelastic tissue resistance.

Tissue resistance

In 1955 Mount identified a component of the work of breathing which he attributed to the resistance caused by tissue deformation.[4] D'Angelo *et al.*[5] subsequently described how, in anaesthetised and paralysed subjects, the viscoelastic 'tissue' component of respiratory resistance may be measured.

Figure 4.4 shows the 'spring and dashpot' model, which D'Angelo *et al.*[5] used to illustrate this component of respiratory resistance. Dashpots here represent resistance and springs elastance (reciprocal of compliance). Upward movement of the upper bar represents an increase in lung volume, caused by contraction of the inspiratory muscles or the application of inflation pressure as shown in the diagram. There is good evidence that, in humans, the left-hand dashpot represents predominantly airway resistance. The spring in the middle represents the static elastance of the respiratory system. On the right there is a spring and dashpot arranged in series. With a rapid change in lung volume, the spring is extended while the piston rises more slowly in the dashpot. In due course (approx. 2–3 seconds) the spring returns to its original length and so ceases to exert any influence on pressure/volume relationships. This spring therefore represents the time-dependent element of elastance. While it is still under tension at end-inspiration, the combined effect of the two springs results in a high elastance of which the reciprocal is the dynamic compliance. If inflation is held for a few seconds and movement of the piston through the right-hand dashpot is completed, the right-hand spring ceases to exert any tension and the total elastance is reduced to that caused by the spring in the middle. The reciprocal of this elastance is the static compliance, which is therefore greater than the dynamic compliance. D'Angelo et al.[5] stress that the system shown in Figure 4.4 is only a simplified scheme to which many further components could be added; nevertheless, the model accords well with experimental findings.

The time-dependent change in compliance represented by the spring and dashpot in series could be due to many factors. Redistribution of gas makes only a negligible contribution in normal man, the major component being due to viscoelastic flow resistance in tissue.[1,5] In anaesthetised healthy subjects tissue resistance is of the order of half of the respiratory system resistance[5] and seems to be largely unaffected by end-expiratory pressure or tidal volume.[6] Tissue resistance originates from both lung and chest wall tissues, with a significant proportion originating in the chest wall.[6–8] The magnitude and importance of this component, particularly in lung disease, have often been underestimated and it is clearly important to distinguish airway resistance from that afforded by the total respiratory system. Separate measurement of tissue resistance is described below.

Inertance as a component of respiratory system resistance

Respired gases, the lungs and the thoracic cage all have appreciable mass and therefore inertia, which must offer an impedance to change in direction of gas flow, analogous to electrical inductance. This component, termed inertance, is extremely difficult to measure, but inductance and inertance offer an impedance that increases with frequency.[9] Therefore, although inertance is generally believed to be negligible at normal respiratory frequencies, it may become appreciable during high-frequency ventilation (see Chapter 32).

FACTORS AFFECTING RESPIRATORY RESISTANCE

In normal lungs respiratory resistance is controlled by changes in airway diameter, mainly in small airways and bronchioles. This would be expected to alter only the airways component of respiratory resistance, but animal studies suggest that contraction of bronchial smooth muscle also causes changes in tissue resistance. It is

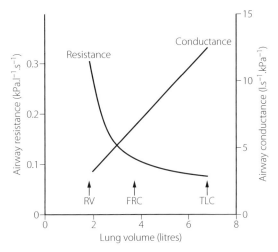

Figure 4.5 Airway resistance and conductance as a function of lung volume (upright posture). The resistance curve is a hyperbola. Specific conductance (sG_{aw}) is the gradient of the conductance line. RV, residual volume; FRC, functional residual capacity; TLC, total lung capacity.

thought that airway constriction distorts the surrounding tissue sufficiently to alter its viscoelastic properties.[10] Airway calibre may be reduced either by physical compression (due to a reversal of the normal transluminal pressure leading to airway collapse) or by contraction of the smooth muscle in the airway wall.

Volume-related airway collapse

Effect of lung volume on resistance to breathing. When the lung volume is reduced, there is a proportional reduction in the volume of all air-containing components, including the air passages. Thus, if other factors (such as bronchomotor tone) remain constant, airway resistance is an inverse function of lung volume (Figure 4.5) and there is a direct relationship between lung volume and the maximum expiratory flow rate that can be attained (see below). Quantifying airway diameter is difficult from these curves. It is therefore more convenient to refer to conductance, which is the reciprocal of resistance and usually expressed as litres per second per cmH_2O. Specific airway conductance (sG_{aw}) is the airway conductance relative to lung volume[11] or the gradient of the line showing conductance as a function of lung volume (see Figure 4.5). Because it takes into account the important effect of lung volume on airway resistance, it is a useful index of bronchomotor tone.

Gas trapping. At low lung volumes, flow-related airway collapse (see below) occurs more readily because airway calibre and the transmural pressure are less. Expiratory airway collapse gives rise to a 'valve' effect and gas becomes trapped distal to the collapsed airway, leading to an increase in residual volume and FRC. Thus, in general, increasing lung volume reduces airway resistance and helps to prevent gas trapping. This is most conveniently achieved by the application of continuous positive airway pressure (CPAP) to the spontaneously breathing subject or positive end-expiratory pressure (PEEP) to the paralysed ventilated patient (see Chapter 32). Many patients with obstructive airways disease acquire the habit of increasing their expiratory resistance by exhaling through pursed lips. Alternatively, premature termination of expiration keeps the lung volume above FRC (intrinsic PEEP, page 431). Both manoeuvres have the effect of enhancing airway transmural pressure gradient and so reducing airway resistance and preventing trapping.

The closing capacity. In addition to the overall effect on airway resistance shown in Figure 4.5, there are important regional differences. This is because the airways and alveoli in the dependent parts of the lungs are always smaller than those at the top of the lung, except at total lung capacity or at zero gravity when all are the same size. As the lung volume is reduced towards residual volume, there is a point at which dependent airways begin to close and the lung volume at which this occurs is known as the closing capacity (CC). The alternative term, closing volume (CV), equals the closing capacity minus the residual volume (RV) (Figure 4.6). Closing capacity increases with age and is less than FRC in young adults, but increases to become equal to FRC at a mean age of 44 years in the supine position and 66 years in the upright position (see Figure 3.10). The closing capacity seems to be independent of body position but the FRC changes markedly with position (see Figure 3.9).

When the FRC is less than the closing capacity, some of the pulmonary blood flow will be distributed to alveoli with closed airways, usually in the dependent parts of the lungs. This will constitute a shunt (page 122) and must increase the alveolar–arterial PO_2 gradient. If the alveolar PO_2 remains the same, the arterial PO_2 must be decreased. This can be seen when volunteers breathe below their FRC and is particularly marked in older subjects who have a greater closing capacity. Shunting of blood through areas of the lung with closed airways is an important cause of decreasing arterial PO_2 with increasing age (page 180) and changes of position (page 305). Reduction in FRC is closely related to the increased alveolar–arterial PO_2 gradient seen during anaesthesia (page 311).

Flow-related airway collapse

All the airways can be compressed by reversal of the normal transmural pressure gradient to a sufficiently high level. The cartilaginous airways have considerable structural resistance to collapse but even the trachea may be compressed with an external pressure in the range 5–7 kPa (50–70 cmH$_2$O). Airways beyond generation 11 have no structural rigidity (see Table 2.1) and rely instead on the traction on their walls from elastic recoil of the lung tissue in which they are embedded. They can be collapsed by a reversed transmural pressure gradient that is considerably less than that which closes the cartilaginous airways.

Reversal of the transmural pressure gradient may be caused by high levels of air flow during expiration. During all phases of normal breathing, the pressure in the lumina of the air passages should always remain well

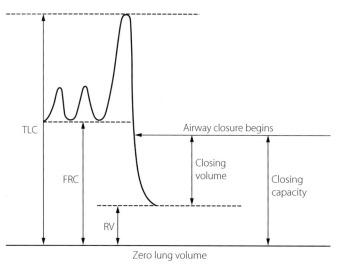

Figure 4.6 Spirogram to illustrate the relationship between closing volume and closing capacity. This example would be in a young adult with closing capacity less than functional residual capacity (FRC). RV, residual volume; TLC, total lung capacity.

above the subatmospheric pressure in the thorax, so the airways remain patent. During a maximal forced expiration, the intrathoracic pressure rises to well above atmospheric, resulting in high gas flow rates. Pressure drops as gas flows along the airways and there will therefore be a point at which airway pressure equals the intrathoracic pressure. At that point (the equal pressure point) the smaller air passages are held open only by the elastic recoil of the lung parenchyma in which they are embedded or, if it occurs in the larger airways, by their structural rigidity. Downstream of the equal pressure point, the transmural pressure gradient is reversed and at some point may overcome the forces holding the airways open, resulting in airway collapse. This effect is also influenced by lung volume (see above) and the equal pressure point moves progressively down towards the smaller airways as lung volume is decreased.

Flow-related collapse is best demonstrated on a flow–volume plot. Figure 4.7 shows the normal rela-tionship between lung volume on the abscissa and instantaneous respiratory flow rate on the ordinate. Time is not directly indicated. In part (a) of the figure the small loop shows a normal tidal excursion above FRC and with air flow rate either side of zero. Arrows show the direction of the trace. At the end of a maximal expiration the black square indicates residual volume. The lower part of the large curve then shows the course of a maximal inspiration to TLC (black circle). There follow four expiratory curves, each with different expiratory effort and each attaining a different peak expiratory flow rate. Within limits, the greater the effort, the greater is the resultant peak flow rate. However, all the expiratory curves terminate in a final common pathway, which is independent of effort. In this part of the curves, the flow rate is limited by airway collapse and the maximal air flow rate is governed by the lung volume (abscissa). The greater the effort, the greater the degree of airway collapse and the resultant gas flow rate remains the

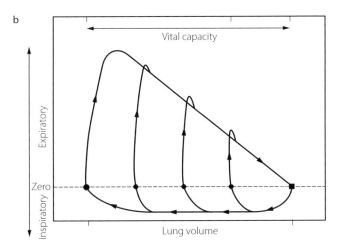

Figure 4.7 Normal flow/volume curves. Instantaneous air flow rate (ordinate) is plotted against lung volume (abscissa). **(a)** The normal tidal excursion is shown as the small loop. In addition, expiration from total lung capacity at four levels of expiratory effort are shown. Within limits, peak expiratory flow rate is dependent on effort, but during the latter part of expiration all curves converge on an effort-independent section where flow rate is limited by airway collapse. **(b)** The effect of forced expirations from different lung volumes. The pips above the effort-independent section probably represent air expelled from collapsed airways.

same. Figure 4.7b shows the importance of a maximal inspiration before measurement of peak expiratory flow rate.

MUSCULAR CONTROL OF AIRWAY DIAMETER

Small airways are the site of most of the important causes of obstruction in a range of pathological conditions, described in Chapter 28. Four pathways are involved in controlling muscle tone in small bronchi and bronchioles.

1. Neural pathways
2. Humoral (via blood) control
3. Direct physical and chemical effects
4. Local cellular mechanisms.

These may conveniently be considered as discrete mechanisms but in practice there is considerable interaction between them, particularly in disease. Neural control is the most important in normal lung, with direct stimulation and humoral control contributing under some circumstances. Cellular mechanisms, particularly mast cells, have little influence under normal conditions but are important in airway disease (see Chapter 28).

Neural pathways[12,13]

Parasympathetic system.[3] This system is of major importance in the control of bronchomotor tone, and when activated can completely obliterate the lumina of small airways.[13] Both afferent and efferent fibres travel to the lung in the vagus nerve with efferent ganglia in the walls of small bronchi. Afferents arise from receptors under the tight junctions of the bronchial epithelium and respond either to noxious stimuli acting directly on the receptors (see below) or cytokines released by cellular mechanisms such as mast cell degranulation. Efferent nerves release acetylcholine (ACh), which acts at M_3 muscarinic receptors to cause contraction of bronchial smooth muscle, while also stimulating M_2 prejunctional muscarinic receptors to exert negative feedback on ACh release.[3] A complex series of second messengers is involved in bringing about smooth muscle contraction in response to ACh (see below). Stimulation of any part of the reflex arc results in bronchoconstriction. Some degree of resting tone is normally present and may therefore permit some degree of bronchodilation when vagal tone is reduced, in a similar fashion to vagal control of heart rate.

Sympathetic system. In contrast to the parasympathetic system, the sympathetic system is poorly represented in the lung and not yet proven to be of major importance in humans. Indeed, it appears unlikely that there is any direct sympathetic innervation of the airway smooth muscle, although there may be an inhibitory effect on cholinergic neurotransmission in some species.

Non-adrenergic non-cholinergic (NANC) system.[14] The airways are provided with a third autonomic control which is neither adrenergic nor cholinergic. This is the only potential bronchodilator nervous pathway in man, though the exact role of the NANC system in humans remains uncertain. The efferent fibres run in the vagus nerve and pass to the smooth muscle of the airway where they cause prolonged relaxation of bronchi. The neurotransmitter is vasoactive intestinal peptide (VIP), which produces airway smooth muscle relaxation by promoting the production of nitric oxide (NO). How NO brings about smooth muscle relaxation in the airway is not as fully understood as its effect on vascular smooth muscle. It seems likely that NO has its effect without having to cross the cell membrane by some form of cell surface interaction that produces activation of guanylate cyclase to produce cyclic GMP and muscle relaxation.[15] Resting airway tone does involve bronchodilation by NO, but whether this is from local cellular production of NO or NANC and VIP-mediated release of NO is not clear.[13]

There is also a bronchoconstrictor part of the NANC system. Non-myelinated C-fibres are found in the airway close to, but separate from, the parasympathetic nerves. They are sensory fibres, reacting to direct stimulation by irritants such as cigarette smoke. In addition to their sensory actions, when stimulated the neurones also manufacture and secrete both substance P and neurokinin A, which are potent bronchoconstrictors in normal lung.[15] Although of significance in airways disease, the contribution of this system to normal airway tone is unknown.

Humoral control[3,16]

In spite of the minimal significance of sympathetic innervation, bronchial smooth muscle has plentiful β_2-adrenergic receptors, which are highly sensitive to circulating adrenaline and once again act via complex second messenger systems described below.[17] Basal levels of adrenaline probably do not contribute to bronchial muscle tone, but this mechanism is brought into play during exercise or during the sympathetic 'stress response'. There are a few α-adrenergic receptors which are bronchoconstrictors but these are unlikely to be of clinical significance.

Physical and chemical effects

Direct stimulation of the respiratory epithelium activates the parasympathetic reflex described above, causing bronchoconstriction. Activation of the bronchoconstrictor path of the NANC system may also play a part. Physical factors known to produce bronchocon-

Table 4.2 Mediators involved in alteration of bronchial smooth muscle tone during airway inflammation[19,20]

Source	Bronchoconstriction		Bronchodilation	
	Mediator	*Receptor*	*Mediator*	*Receptor*
Mast cells & other pro-inflammatory cells	Histamine	H_1	Prostaglandin E_2	EP
	Prostaglandin D_2	TP		EP
	Prostaglandin $F_{2\alpha}$	TP	Prostacyclin (PGI_2)	
	Leukotrienes $C_4 D_4 E_4$	$CysLT_1$		
C-fibres (e-NANC)	PAF	PAF		
	Bradykinin	B_2		
Endothelial & epithelial cells	Substance P	NK_2		
	Neurokinin A	NK_2		
	CGRP	CGRP		
	Endothelin	ET_B		

PAF, platelet-activating factor; CGRP, calcitonin gene-related peptide; e-NANC, excitatory non-adrenergic non-cholinergic.

striction include mechanical stimulation of the upper air passages by laryngoscopy and the presence of foreign bodies in the trachea or bronchi. Inhalation of particulate matter, an aerosol of water or just cold air may cause bronchoconstriction, the latter being used as a simple provocation test.[18] Many chemical stimuli result in bronchoconstriction, including liquids with low pH such as gastric acid and gases such as sulphur dioxide, ammonia, ozone and nitrogen dioxide.

Local cellular mechanisms

Inflammatory cells in the lung include mast cells, eosinophils, neutrophils, macrophages and lymphocytes and the role of these cells in lung infection and inflammation is described in Chapters 28, 30 and 31. These inflammatory cells are all stimulated by a variety of pathogens, but some may also be activated by the direct physical factors described in the previous paragraph. Once activated, cytokine production causes amplification of the response and a variety of mediators are released that can cause bronchoconstriction (Table 4.2). These mediators are produced in normal individuals, but patients with airway disease are usually 'hyperresponsive' and so develop symptoms of bronchospasm more easily.

DRUG EFFECTS ON AIRWAY SMOOTH MUSCLE

β₂-agonists

Non-specific β-adrenoreceptor agonists (e.g. isoprenaline) were the first bronchodilator drugs to be widely used for treating asthma. However, cardiac effects from β₁-receptor stimulation in the heart were believed to be responsible for an increase in mortality during acute asthma and the development of β₂-specific drugs (e.g. salbutamol, terbutaline) soon followed. Recent developments have involved the introduction of long-acting β₂-agonists (e.g. salmeterol).[21] The therapeutic effect of β₂-agonists is more complex than simple relaxation of airway smooth muscle, as they are also known to inhibit the secretion of inflammatory cytokines and most of the bronchoconstrictor mediators shown in Table 4.2.[22] Controversy associated with β₂-agonists still continues today – their effect on inflammatory cells and their ability to downregulate β₂-receptors are both claimed to be potentially harmful in asthmatic patients,[23] and this has contributed to the gradual move away from these drugs in asthma therapy (page 378).

The β₂-receptor. The molecular basis of the functional characteristics of the β-adrenoceptor is now clearly elucidated.[24–26] It contains 413 amino acids and has seven transmembrane helices (Figure 4.8). The agonist binding site is within this hydrophobic core of the protein, which sits within the lipid bilayer of the cell membrane. This affects the interaction of drugs at the binding site in that more lipophilic drugs form a depot in the lipid bilayer from which they can repeatedly interact with the binding site of the receptor, producing a much longer duration of action than hydrophilic drugs.[21] Receptors exist in either activated or inactivated form, the former state occurring when the third intracellular loop (see Figure 4.8) is bound to guanosine triphosphate and the α-subunit of the Gs-protein. β₂-receptor agonists probably do not induce a significant conformational change in the protein structure but simply stabilise the activated form, allowing this to predominate.

Activation of the G-protein by the β₂-receptor in turn activates adenylate cyclase to convert adenosine

Figure 4.8 Molecular mechanisms of β_2-adrenoceptor stimulation. The receptor exists in activated and inactivated states according to whether or not the α-subunit of the G-protein is bound to adenyl cyclase (AC). The agonist binds to three amino acid residues on the third and fifth transmembrane domains and by doing so stabilises the receptor G-protein complex in the activated state. The intracellular C-terminal region of the protein (blue) is the area susceptible to phosphorylation by intracellular kinases causing inactivation of the receptor and downregulation.

triphosphate to cyclic adenosine monophosphate (cAMP).[24] Cyclic AMP causes relaxation of the muscle cell by inhibition of calcium release from intracellular stores and probably also activates protein kinase A to phosphorylate some of the regulatory proteins involved in the actin–myosin interaction.

Two β_2-receptor genes are present in humans, with a total of 13 polymorphisms described,[27] giving rise to a large number of possible phenotypes. Studies of these phenotypes are at an early stage, but some genetic differences have been shown to be associated with worse nocturnal falls in peak flow and varying degrees of receptor desensitisation by β_2-agonists.[24]

Phosphodiesterase inhibitors

After its production following β_2-receptor stimulation, cAMP is rapidly hydrolysed by the intracellular enzyme phosphodiesterase (PDE), inhibition of which will therefore prolong the smooth muscle relaxant effect of β_2-receptor stimulation. Seven subgroups of PDE have now been identified, with subgroups PDE3 and PDE4 occurring in airway smooth muscle, but the PDE inhibitors currently used in asthma, such as theophylline, are nonspecific for the different subgroups.[19] This lack of specificity of currently used PDE inhibitors also accounts for their wide-ranging side effects, which continue to limit their therapeutic potential. In addition, recent work has also shown that their major therapeutic effect in airways diseases does not arise solely from PDE inhibition, with theophylline potentially causing bronchodilation by a variety of routes not involving cAMP and by having anti-inflammatory effects.[28]

Anticholinergic drugs

The ACh receptor. Stimulation of M_3 ACh receptors also activates a G-protein, characterised as Gq. This in turn activates phospholipase C to stimulate the production of inositol triphosphate (IP_3), which then binds to sarcoplasmic reticulum receptors causing the release of calcium from intracellular stores. The elevation of intracellular calcium activates myosin light chain kinase, which phosphorylates part of the myosin chain to activate myosin ATPase and initiate crossbridging between actin and myosin.[19] IP_3 is converted into the inactive inositol diphosphate by IP_3 kinase. Tachykinin, histamine and leukotriene receptors responsible for bronchoconstriction from other mediators (see Table 4.2) act by a very similar mechanism, being linked to G-protein–phospholipase C complexes, which lead to IP_3 formation.[29]

There are now believed to be many molecular interactions between the IP_3 and cAMP signalling pathways. Activation of phospholipase C by protein Gq also liberates intracellular diacylglycerol, which activates another membrane-bound enzyme, protein kinase C. This enzyme is able to phosphorylate a variety of proteins, including G-proteins and the β_2-receptor itself (see Figure 4.8), causing uncoupling of the receptor from the G-protein and downregulation of the transduction pathway.[19,24]

Anticholinergic drugs used in the airway are classified into short-acting (e.g. ipratropium) or long-acting (e.g. tiotropium) types. They are more useful in treating chronic obstructive pulmonary disease than asthma (see Chapter 28), because only in the former disease is increased parasympathetic activity thought to contribute to symptoms. These drugs have similar binding affinities for both M_2 and M_3 receptors, giving rise to opposing effects on the degree of stimulation of airway smooth muscle. Differences in relative numbers of M_2 and M_3 receptors between individuals and in different disease states[13] will therefore explain the variability in response seen with inhaled anticholinergic drugs. Tiotropium, a recently introduced anticholinergic, has a long duration of therapeutic effect because of faster dissociation of the

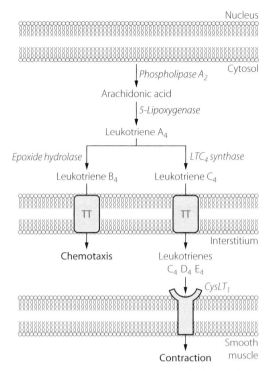

Figure 4.9 The leukotriene pathway in the lung. Inflammatory mediators stimulate phospholipase A_2 to produce arachidonic acid from the phospholipid of the nuclear membrane. Leukotrienes B_4 and C_4 leave the cell via a specific transmembrane transporter (TT) protein. Non-specific peptidases in the interstitium convert leukotriene C_4 into D_4 and E_4, all of which stimulate the CysLT receptor to cause intense bronchoconstriction. (After reference 31.)

drug from M_2 than from M_3 receptors, leaving only the M_3 receptors antagonised.[30]

Leukotriene antagonists[31]

Even in non-asthmatic individuals leukotrienes are potent bronchoconstrictors, so the therapeutic potential of leukotriene antagonists has been extensively investigated. Activation of phospholipase A_2 by inflammatory cells initiates the pathway, which ultimately produces three leukotrienes (see Table 4.2; Figure 4.9). In the lung, these all act via a single receptor ($CysLT_1$) on airway smooth muscle cells to cause contraction via the G-protein–IP_3 system described above. Leukotrienes have a wide range of activities apart from bronchoconstriction, in particular amplification of the inflammatory response by chemotaxis of eosinophils.

As may be predicted from their actions, antagonists of the $CysLT_1$ receptor (e.g. montelukast, zafirlukast) are not effective in treating acute bronchoconstriction, but are useful in situations when the leukotriene pathway has been activated by stimulation of inflammatory cells. They are therefore most likely to be of benefit in the prevention of bronchospasm in chronic asthma, but their place in asthma therapy remains uncertain.

COMPENSATION FOR INCREASED RESISTANCE TO BREATHING

Inspiratory resistance. The normal response to increased inspiratory resistance is increased inspiratory muscle effort with little change in the FRC. Accessory muscles may be brought into play according to the degree of resistance.

There are two principal mechanisms of compensation for increased inspiratory resistance. The first operates immediately and even during the first breath in which resistance is applied. It seems probable that the muscle spindles indicate that the inspiratory muscles have failed to shorten by the intended amount, and their afferent discharge then augments the activity in the motor neurone pool of the anterior horn. This is the typical servo operation of the spindle system, with which the intercostal muscles are richly endowed (page 82). With a severe increase in resistance (added resistance of 8.3 $kPa.l^{-1}.s$), a second compensatory mechanism develops over about 90 seconds[32] and overacts for a similar period when the resistance is removed.[33] This mechanism is driven by a slight elevation of arterial PCO_2.

Expiratory resistance. Expiration against a pressure of up to 1 kPa (10 cmH_2O) does not usually result in activation of the expiratory muscles in conscious or anaesthetised subjects. The additional work to overcome this resistance is, in fact, performed by the inspiratory muscles. The subject augments his inspiratory force until he achieves a lung volume (FRC) at which the additional elastic recoil is sufficient to overcome the expiratory

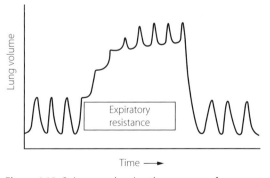

Figure 4.10 Spirogram showing the response of an anaesthetised patient to the sudden imposition of an expiratory resistance. Note that there is an immediate augmentation of the force of contraction of the inspiratory muscles. This continues with successive breaths until the elastic recoil is sufficient to overcome the expiratory resistance.[33]

resistance (Figure 4.10). The mechanism for resetting the FRC at a higher level probably requires accommodation of the intrafusal fibres of the spindles to allow for an altered length of diaphragmatic muscle fibres caused by the obstructed expiration. This would reset the developed inspiratory tension in accordance with the increased FRC.[33] The conscious subject normally uses his expiratory muscles to overcome expiratory pressures in excess of about 1 kPa (10 cmH$_2$O).

Patients show a remarkable capacity to compensate for acutely increased resistance, such that arterial PCO$_2$ is usually normal. However, the efficiency of these mechanisms in maintaining alveolar ventilation carries severe physiological consequences. In common with other muscles the respiratory muscles can become fatigued,[34] and this is a major factor in the onset of respiratory failure. A raised PCO$_2$ in a patient with increased respiratory resistance is therefore always serious. Intrathoracic pressure will rise during acutely increased expiratory resistance and so impede venous return and reduce cardiac output (page 435) to the point that syncope may occur.

PRINCIPLES OF MEASUREMENT OF RESPIRATORY RESISTANCE AND CLOSING CAPACITY

Respiratory system resistance

Resistance is determined by the simultaneous measurement of gas flow rate and the driving pressure gradient. In the case of the respiratory tract, the difficulty centres the measurement of the pressure gradient between mouth and alveolus. Problems also arise because of varying nomenclature and different methods for measuring different components of respiratory system resistance (Table 4.3).[35,36] In all cases, apparatus resistance

must be measured separately and subtracted from the value obtained in the subject.

Normal values for total respiratory system resistance are variable because of the large changes with lung volume and methodological differences. Typical values obtained in a normal population at FRC are between 0.14 and 0.4, but values below 0.84 kPa.l^{-1}.s are considered normal.[37]

Pressure–flow technique. In Chapter 3 it was shown how simultaneous measurement of tidal volume and intrathoracic (oesophageal) pressure yielded the dynamic compliance of the lung (see Figure 3.11). For this purpose, pressures were selected at the times of zero air flow when pressures were uninfluenced by air flow resistance. The same apparatus may be employed for the determination of flow resistance by subtracting the pressure component used in overcoming elastic forces (Figure 4.11). The shaded areas in the pressure trace indicate the components of the pressure required to overcome flow resistance, and these may be related to the concurrent gas flow rates.

Alternatively, the intrathoracic-to-mouth pressure gradient and respired volume may be displayed as X and Y coordinates of a loop. Figure 3.11 showed how dynamic compliance could be derived from the no-flow points of such a loop. The area of the loop is a function of the work performed against flow resistance.

The use of an oesophageal balloon makes the method a little invasive, but it does allow continuous measurement of resistance. By measuring intrathoracic pressure, the chest wall component of resistance is excluded, so providing a measure of pulmonary resistance, which is airways resistance plus the lung component of tissue resistance.

Table 4.3 Components of respiratory system resistance[35]

	Mouth and pharynx	Larynx and large airways	Small airways <3 mm diameter	Alveoli and lung tissue	Chest wall	Total
Contribution (kPa.l^{-1}.s)	0.05	0.05	0.02	0.02	0.12	0.26
Airway resistance		Body plethysmograph Interrupter technique				0.12
Pulmonary resistance		Pressure flow technique				0.14
Respiratory system resistance		Oscillating air flow technique End-inspiratory interruption				0.26

Shaded areas indicate which components contribute to each form of resistance, and the text in the shaded boxes states the methodology used to measure each form of resistance.

Figure 4.11 The measurement of pulmonary resistance and dynamic compliance by simultaneous measurement of air flow and intrathoracic-to-mouth differential pressure. The spirogram is conveniently obtained by integration of the pneumotachogram. In the pressure trace, the dotted line shows the pressure changes that would be expected in a hypothetical patient with no pulmonary resistance. Compliance is derived as shown in Figure 3.11. Pulmonary resistance is derived as the difference between the measured pressure differential and that which is required for elastic forces (shaded area) compared with the flow rate shown in the pneumotachogram. Note that the pneumotachogram is a much more sensitive indicator of the no-flow points than the spirogram.

Oscillating air flow. In this technique, a high-frequency oscillating air flow is applied to the airways, with measurement of the resultant pressure and air flow changes. By application of alternating current theory it is possible to derive a continuous measurement of airway resistance.[38,39] The technique measures total respiratory resistance and may be used throughout a vital capacity manoeuvre and so display resistance as a function of lung volume and derive specific airway conductance.

The body plethysmograph. During inspiration, alveolar pressure falls below ambient as a function of airway resistance and the alveolar gas expands in accord with Boyle's law. The increased displacement of the body is then recorded as an increase in pressure in the body plethysmograph. Airway resistance may be derived directly from measurements of air flow and pressure changes. The method requires the subject to perform either a 'panting' respiratory manoeuvre or to deliberately breathe with a small tidal volume, but is generally non-invasive and FRC may be measured at the same time.[35,40]

The interrupter technique. A single manometer may be used to measure both mouth and alveolar pressure if the air passages distal to the manometer are momentarily interrupted with a shutter. The method is based on the assumption that, while the airway is interrupted, the mouth pressure comes to equal the alveolar pressure. Resistance is then determined from the relationship between flow rate (measured before interruption) and the pressure difference between mouth (measured before interruption) and alveoli (measured at the end of the interruption). Duration of interruption must be short enough to avoid disturbing the subject's breathing pattern but long enough to allow equilibration of pressure along the airway. In practice, interruption is for 50–100 ms, occurring repeatedly throughout the respiratory cycle. The technique is adequate for measuring resistance in normal lungs but it is doubtful whether equilibration occurs fully in subjects with diseased airways.[40] The interrupter method measures airway resistance and excludes tissue resistance.

End-inspiratory interruption. This method is now widely used for measuring the tissue component of respiratory system resistance.[5–8,41] The method may only be used in anaesthetised paralysed subjects receiving artificial ventilation with accurate control of the respiratory cycle. Following a constant flow inflation of the lung, the airway is occluded for 0.5–3 s before a passive exhalation occurs. To prevent artefacts during the inspiratory pause, numerous successive breaths may be averaged.[7] Figure 4.12 shows the changes in gas flow, transpulmonary pressure (P_L), oesophageal pressure and lung volume averaged over 33 breaths. Immediately before occlusion, P_L reaches a value of P_{max}, which is governed by both elastic and non-elastic resistance. The fall in pressure following occlusion is biphasic. Immediately after airway occlusion, the P_L falls rapidly to P_1 and $P_{max} - P_1$ is referred

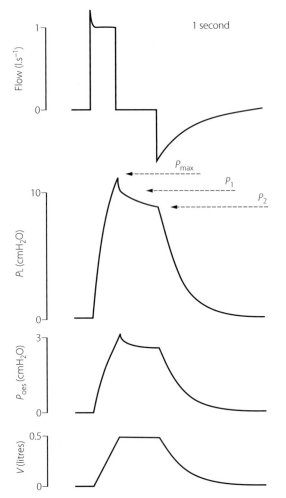

Figure 4.12 End-inspiratory interruption method of measuring resistance. Following a constant-flow positive-pressure breath, there is an end-inspiratory pause of almost 1s before passive exhalation. The peak airway pressure (P_{max}) falls initially very quickly to P_1 and thereafter more slowly to a plateau P_2. Tissue resistance, airway resistance and total resistance can then all be calculated (see text for details). In this example, showing the average of 33 consecutive breaths, both transpulmonary (tracheal minus oesophageal) pressure and oesophageal pressure relative to atmosphere have been measured, allowing lung and chest wall components of tissue resistance to be calculated separately. Flow, airway flow rate; P_L, transpulmonary pressure; P_{oes}, oesophageal pressure; V, change in lung volume. (After reference 7.)

to as interrupter resistance and believed to reflect airway resistance as in the interrupter method already described.

$$\text{Airway resistance} = \frac{P_{max} - P_1}{\text{Flow rate of inflation}}$$

In the second phase, a slower decay in pressure occurs from P_1 to P_2, which represents the loss of the time-dependent element of tissue compliance (due to visco-elastic behaviour) and therefore represents tissue resistance.

$$\text{Tissue resistance} = \frac{P_1 - P_2}{\text{Flow rate of inflation}}$$

In practice, the pressure signal may be converted into digital form and computer analysis calculates the three pressures.[7]

Where these pressures are recorded determines which component of tissue resistance is measured. In Figure 4.12, transpulmonary pressure (tracheal minus oesophageal pressure) is recorded, so allowing calculation of the tissue resistance of the lung alone. Oesophageal pressure is also recorded, so allowing calculation of the thoracic cage component of tissue resistance. In theory, for oesophageal pressure recordings there should be no contribution from airway resistance and so the pressure decay following interruption should not be biphasic, with P_{max} being equal to P_1. For many years this was thought to be the case,[5,8] until averaging of multiple breaths to remove cardiac artefacts showed a smoother and biphasic oesophageal pressure trace (see Figure 4.12). The initial pressure drop is believed to represent 'stress adaptation' of the chest wall.[7]

Finally, measurement of tracheal to atmospheric pressure gradient allows calculation of total respiratory resistance:

$$\text{Respiratory system resistance} = \frac{P_{max} - P_2}{\text{Flow rate of inflation}}$$

This technique is utilised by the current generation of ventilators to calculate respiratory system resistance. The same static respiratory manoeuvre described in the previous chapter for calculation of static compliance (see Figure 3.11b) also allows measurement of P_{max} and P_2, from which respiratory system resistance is calculated (see Figure 4.12).

Measurement of closing capacity[35]

This is perhaps the most convenient place to outline the measurement of closing capacity. It is the maximal lung volume at which airway closure can be detected in the dependent parts of the lungs (page 44). The measurement is made during expiration and is based on having different concentrations of a tracer gas in the upper and lower parts of the lung. This may be achieved by inspiration of a bolus of tracer gas at the commencement of an inspiration from residual volume, at which time airways are closed in the dependent part of the lungs (Figure 4.13). The tracer gas will then be preferentially

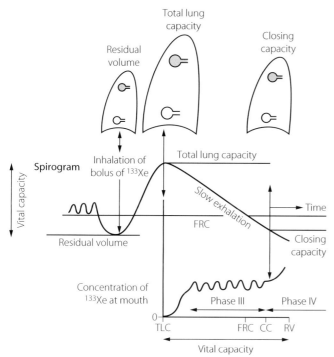

Total lung
capacity

Residual
volume

Closing
capacity

Spirogram

Inhalation of
bolus of [133]Xe

Total lung capacity

Slow exhalation

Time

FRC

Residual volume

Closing
capacity

Concentration of
[133]Xe at mouth

Phase III

Phase IV

0

TLC

FRC CC RV

Vital capacity

Figure 4.13 Measurement of closing capacity by the use of a tracer gas such as [133]Xe. The bolus of tracer gas is inhaled near residual volume and, due to airway closure, is distributed only to those alveoli whose air passages are still open (shown shaded in the diagram). During expiration, the concentration of the tracer gas becomes constant after the dead space is washed out. This plateau (phase III) gives way to a rising concentration of tracer gas (phase IV) when there is closure of airways leading to alveoli that did not receive the tracer gas.

distributed to the upper parts of the lungs. After a maximal inspiration to total lung capacity, the patient slowly exhales while the concentration of the tracer gas is measured at the mouth. When lung volume reaches the closing capacity and airways begin to close in the dependent parts, the concentration of the tracer gas will rise (phase IV) above the alveolar plateau (phase III). Suitable tracers are ^{133}Xe or 100% oxygen (measured as a fall in nitrogen concentration). The technique can be undertaken in the conscious subject who performs the ventilatory manoeuvres spontaneously, or in the paralysed subject in whom ventilation is artificially controlled.

REFERENCES

*1. Milic-Emili J, Robatto FM, Bates JHT. Respiratory mechanics in anaesthesia. *Br J Anaesth* 1990; **65**: 4–12.
2. Mead J, Agostini E. Dynamics of breathing. In: Fenn WO, Rahn H, eds. *Handbook of physiology; section 3, volume 1– Respiration.* Washington DC: American Physiological Society,1964.
3. Burwell DR, Jones JG. The airways and anaesthesia – 1: anatomy, physiology and fluid mechanics. *Anaesthesia* 1996; **51**; 849–57.
4. Mount LE. The ventilation flow-resistance and compliance of rat lungs. *J Physiol* 1955; **127**: 157–67.
5. D'Angelo E, Calderini E, Torri G, Robatto FM, Bonon D, Milic-Emili J. Respiratory mechanics in anaesthetized paralyzed humans: effects of flow, volume and time. *J Appl Physiol* 1989; **67**: 2556–64.
6. D'Angelo E, Tavola M, Milic-Emili J. Volume and time dependence of respiratory system mechanics in normal anaesthetized paralysed humans. *Eur Respir J* 2000; **16**: 665–72.
7. D'Angelo E, Prandi E, Tavola M, Calderini E, Milic-Emili J. Chest wall interrupter resistance in anaesthetized paralyzed humans. *J Appl Physiol* 1994; **77**: 883–7.
*8. D'Angelo E, Robatto FM, Calderini E, *et al.* Pulmonary and chest wall mechanics in anaesthetized paralyzed humans. *J Appl Physiol* 1991; **70**: 2602–10.
9. Dorbin HL, Luchen KR, Jackson AC. Human respiratory input impedance from 4 to 200 Hz: physiologic and modelling considerations. *J Appl Physiol* 1988; **64**; 823–31.
10. Kimmel E, Seri M, Fredberg JJ. Lung tissue resistance and hysteretic modelling of lung parenchyma. *J Appl Physiol* 1995; **79**: 461–6.
11. Lehane JR, Jordan C, Jones JG. Influence of halothane and enflurane on respiratory air flow resistance and specific conductance in man. *Br J Anaesth* 1980; **52**: 773–80.
12. Jordan D. Central nervous pathways and control of the airways. *Respir Physiol* 2001; **125**: 67–81.
13. Canning BJ, Fischer A. Neural regulation of airway smooth muscle tone. *Respir Physiol* 2001; **125**: 113–27.

14. Widdicombe JG. Autonomic regulation: i-NANC/ e-NANC. *Am J Respir Crit Care Med* 1998; **158**: S171–5.
15. Drazen JM, Gaston B, Shore SA. Chemical regulation of pulmonary airway tone. *Annu Rev Physiol* 1995; **57**: 151–70.
16. Thomson NC, Dagg KD, Ramsay SG. Humoral control of airway tone. *Thorax* 1996; **51**: 461–64.
17. Hakonarson H, Grunstein MM. Regulation of second messengers associated with airway smooth muscle contraction and relaxation. *Am J Respir Crit Care Med* 1998; **158**: S115–22.
18. Heaton RW, Henderson AF, Costello JF. Cold air as a bronchial provocation technique. *Chest* 1984; **86**: 810–14.
*19. Barnes PJ. Pharmacology of airway smooth muscle. *Am J Respir Crit Care Med* 1998; **158**: S123–32.
20. Thirstrup S. Control of airway smooth muscle tone. I – Electrophysiology and contractile mediators. *Respir Med* 2000; **94**: 328–36.
21. Kips JC, Pauwels RA. Long-acting inhaled β$_2$-agonist therapy in asthma. *Am J Respir Crit Care Med* 2001; **164**: 923–32.
22. Barnes PJ. Effect of β-agonists on inflammatory cells. *J Allergy Clin Immunol* 1999; **104**: S10–17.
23. Bernstein IL. β$_2$-agonists: déjà vu all over again. The second generation controversy. *Chest* 2002; **122**: 763–5.
*24. Johnson M. The β-adrenoceptor. *Am J Respir Crit Care Med* 1998; **158**: S146–53.
25. Thirstrup S. Control of airway smooth muscle tone: II - Pharmacology of relaxation. *Respir Med* 2000; **94**: 519–28.
26. Liggett SB. Molecular and genetic basis of β$_2$-adrenergic receptor function. *J Allergy Clin Immunol* 1999; **104**: S42–6.
27. Palmer LJ, Silverman ES, Weiss ST, Drazen JM. Pharmacogenetics of asthma. *Am J Respir Crit Care Med* 2002; **165**: 861–6.
28. Barnes PJ. Theophylline. New perspectives for an old drug. *Am J Respir Crit Care Med* 2003; **167**: 813–18.
29. Reynolds PN, Holmes MD, Scicchitano R. Role of tachykinins in bronchial hyper-responsiveness. *Clin Exp Pharmacol Physiol* 1997; **24**: 273–80.
30. Barnes PJ. The pharmacological properties of tiotropium. *Chest* 2000; **117**: 63S–66S.
31. Drazen JM, Isreal E, O'Byrne PM. Treatment of asthma with drugs modifying the leukotriene pathway. *N Engl J Med* 1999; **340**: 197–206.
32. Nishino T, Kochi T. Breathing route and ventilatory responses to inspiratory resistive loading in humans. *Am J Respir Crit Care Med* 1994; **150**: 742–6.
33. Nunn JF, Ezi-Ashi TI. The respiratory effects of resistance to breathing in anaesthetized man. *Anesthesiology* 1961; **22**: 174–85.
34. Moxham J. Respiratory muscle fatigue; mechanisms, evaluation and therapy. *Br J Anaesth* 1990; **65**: 43–53.
35. Cotes JE. *Lung function: assessment and application in medicine.* Oxford: Blackwell Scientific Publications, 1993.
36. Phagoo SB, Watson RA, Silverman M, Pride NB. Comparison of four methods of assessing air flow resistance before and after induced airway narrowing. *J Appl Physiol* 1995; **79**: 518–25.
37. van Altena R, Gimeno F. Respiratory resistance measured by flow-interruption in a normal population. *Respiration* 1994; **61**: 249–54.
38. Hyatt RE, Zimmerman IR, Peters GM, Sullivan WJ. Direct write out of total respiratory resistance. *J Appl Physiol* 1970; **28**: 675–8.
39. Goldman M, Knudson RJ, Mead J, Paterson N, Schwaber JR, Wohl ME. A simplified measurement of respiratory resistance by forced oscillation. *J Appl Physiol* 1970; **28**: 113–16.
40. Freedman S. Mechanics of ventilation. In: Brewis RAL, Corrin B, Gedded DM, Gibson GJ, eds. *Respiratory medicine.* London: WB Saunders, 1995; 116–19.
41. Jonson B, Beydon L, Brauer K, Mansson C, Valind S, Grytzell H. Mechanics of the respiratory system in healthy anesthetized humans with an emphasis on viscoelastic properties. *J Appl Physiol* 1993; **75**: 132–40.

KEY POINTS

- The respiratory centre in the medulla generates the respiratory rhythm using an oscillating network of six groups of interconnecting neurones.
- Many other diverse areas of the central nervous system influence respiratory control, these connections being coordinated by the pons.
- Irritant and stretch receptors in the lungs and diaphragm are involved in a series of reflex actions on the respiratory centre to influence respiratory activity.
- Central chemoreceptors respond to changes in pH caused by alterations in carbon dioxide partial pressure, rapidly increasing ventilation in response to elevated arterial $P\text{CO}_2$.
- Peripheral chemoreceptors, principally in the carotid body, increase ventilation in response to reduced arterial $P\text{O}_2$.

Early in pregnancy the foetal brainstem develops a 'respiratory centre', which produces uninterrupted rhythmic breathing activity for many years.[1] Throughout life the subject is mostly unaware of this action, which is closely controlled by a combination of chemical and physical reflexes. In addition, when required, breathing may (within limits) be completely overridden by voluntary control or interrupted by swallowing and involuntary non-rhythmic acts such as sneezing, vomiting, hiccuping or coughing. The control system is highly complex, with its automatic ability to adapt the action of the respiratory muscles to the changing demands of posture, speech, voluntary movement, exercise and innumerable other circumstances that alter the respiratory requirement or influence the performance of the respiratory muscles.

THE ORIGIN OF THE RESPIRATORY RHYTHM[2]

Early attempts to find the site of respiratory control used an anatomical approach involving the removal or stimu-

lation of specific areas of the brainstem (page 223). More recent approaches have included the application of modern imaging techniques such as magnetic resonance imaging (MRI)[3] and positron emission tomography (PET)[4] to localise respiratory regions in normal human subjects, and these studies confirm that much of the historical animal work does apply to humans. The anatomical approach to understanding respiratory patterns has also been succeeded by the biochemical approach. New research methods and the possibility of therapeutic intervention have led to an explosion of interest in the chemical interactions between and within respiratory neurones.

Anatomical location of the 'respiratory centre'

The medulla is accepted as the area of brain where the respiratory pattern is generated and where the various voluntary and involuntary demands on respiratory activity are coordinated. There are many neuronal connections both into and out of the medulla, as summarised in Figure 5.1, the functions of which are described below.

Respiratory neurones in the medulla are mainly concentrated in two anatomical areas, the ventral and dorsal respiratory groups, which have numerous interconnections (Figure 5.2).

The *dorsal* respiratory group lies in close relation to the nucleus tractus solitarius, where visceral afferents from cranial nerves IX and X terminate (see Figure 5.2). It is predominantly composed of inspiratory neurones with upper motor neurones passing to the inspiratory anterior horn cells of the opposite side. The dorsal group is primarily concerned with timing of the respiratory cycle.

The *ventral* respiratory group comprises four nuclei. The most caudal is the nucleus retroambigualis, which is predominantly expiratory with upper motor neurones passing to the expiratory muscles of the other side. The nucleus ambiguus controls the dilator functions of larynx, pharynx and tongue. The nucleus paraambigualis (lying parallel to it) is mainly inspiratory and controls the force of contraction of the inspiratory muscles of

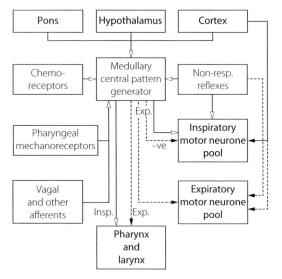

Figure 5.1 Afferent and efferent connections to and from the medullary central pattern generator. The broken lines are expiratory pathways, which normally remain silent during quiet breathing.

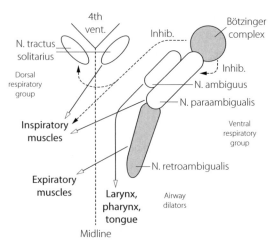

Figure 5.2 Dorsal view of the organisation of the respiratory neurones in the medulla. The dorsal respiratory group (nucleus tractus solitarius) is shown on both sides. For clarity, the ventral respiratory group (Bötzinger complex, nucleus ambiguus, nucleus paraambigualis and nucleus retroambigualis) is shown only on the right side. Areas with predominantly expiratory activity are shaded. Fibres that decussate are shown crossing the midline. The broken lines are expiratory pathways that inhibit inspiratory neurones. See text for details.

the opposite side. The Bötzinger complex (within the nucleus retrofacialis) has widespread expiratory functions.

Central pattern generation (CPG)[2,5]

It is no longer sufficient to consider the generation of the respiratory rhythm to be simply oscillating networks of uniform populations of inspiratory and expiratory neurones. The respiratory pattern depends on a complex interaction of at least six groups of neurones with identifiable firing patterns spread throughout the medulla. These include early inspiratory neurones, inspiratory augmenting neurones (Iaug), late inspiratory interneurones (putative 'off-switch' neurones), early expiratory decrementing neurones, expiratory augmenting neurones and late expiratory (preinspiratory) neurones. Typical firing patterns and the resulting muscle group activity are shown schematically in Figure 5.3. The resultant respiratory cycle may be divided into three phases.

Inspiratory phase. A sudden onset is followed by a ramp increase in Iaug neurones resulting in motor discharge to the inspiratory muscles, including the pharyngeal dilator muscles. Pharyngeal dilator muscles start to contract shortly before the start of inspiration, possibly by activation of late expiratory (preinspiratory) neurones.

Postinspiratory or expiratory phase I. This is characterised by declining discharge of the Iaug neurones and

therefore motor discharge to the inspiratory muscles. Early expiratory decrementing neurones also produce declining activity in the laryngeal adductor muscles. This phase therefore represents passive expiration with a gradual let-down of inspiratory muscle tone and an initial braking of the expiratory gas flow rate (page 77) by the larynx.

Expiratory phase II. The inspiratory muscles are now silent, and if required, expiratory augmenting neurones will be activated to produce a gradual increase in expiratory muscle activity.

Alterations in the rate at which spontaneous neuronal activity increases or decreases and the point at which the next group of neurones are activated allow an infinite variety of respiratory patterns. For example, during quiet breathing in the supine position, early expiratory neurones will reduce activity slowly and expiratory augmenting neurones will be active only briefly, resulting in almost totally passive exhalation. The converse situation will arise following exercise or at a minute volume in excess of about $40\,\mathrm{l.min^{-1}}$, when expiration will be immediately and almost totally active.

In practice, many such rhythm-generating networks are represented in parallel, so that it is difficult to destroy the respiratory rhythm by isolated electrical or cold lesions.[6] The system is thus very robust.

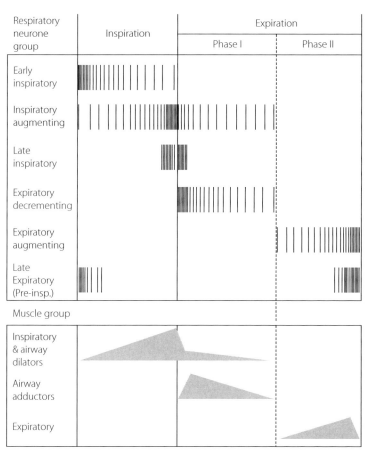

Figure 5.3 Firing patterns of the respiratory neurone groups involved in central pattern generation and the corresponding respiratory muscle group activity. Note that expiration is divided into two phases representing passive (phase I) and active (phase II) expiration. See text for details.

Cellular mechanisms of central pattern generation.[2] Respiratory neurones that exhibit spontaneous activity achieve this by a combination of intrinsic membrane properties and excitatory and inhibitory feedback mechanisms requiring neurotransmitters. In practice, neurotransmitters (both inhibitory and excitatory) have a dual effect – they recruit other cells by direct activation and modulate the spontaneous activity of a single cell by effects on its own membrane ion channels.

In a similar fashion to rhythm generation in cardiac tissue, a combination of potassium and calcium ion channels is involved. For instance, in a single Iaug neurone slow membrane depolarisation occurs, so producing a spontaneous discharge. These cells then 'recruit' other Iaug cells by excitatory postsynaptic potentials (EPSPs) and a crescendo of Iaug activity develops. Calcium-dependent potassium channels then begin to be activated and repolarise the cells, so 'switching off' the Iaug respiratory group. Activation of other cell groups, for instance expiratory augmenting neurones, will result in activation of inhibitory postsynaptic potentials (IPSPs) on the Iaug neurones to hyperpolarise the neurone and inhibit the next wave of inspiratory activity. Similar membrane effects occur in all the respiratory neurone groups shown in Figure 5.3.

Neurotransmitters involved in CPG and respiratory control[2,7,8]

These are summarised in Figure 5.4.

Central pattern generation requires a combination of excitatory and inhibitory neurotransmitters. Excitatory amino acids (usually glutamate) activate several different receptors. These are divided into two groups, N-methyl-D-aspartate (NMDA) receptors, which are fast-acting ion channels, and non-NMDA receptors, which are slower reacting receptors involving G-protein mediated effects. Inhibitory neurotransmitters include glycine and γ-aminobutyric acid (GABA) acting via specific glycine receptors and GABA$_A$ receptors respectively to hyperpolarise the neurone and thereby inhibit its activity. These two inhibitory transmitters act quite independently during different phases of CPG.

Neuromodulators are substances that can influence the CPG output, but are not themselves involved in rhythm generation. There are numerous neuromodulators of

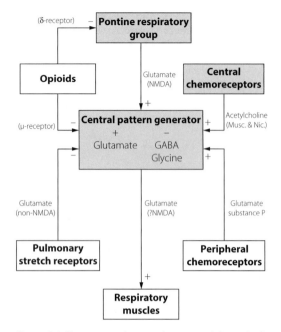

Figure 5.4 Neurotransmitters and neuromodulators in the respiratory centre. Boxes indicate functional neuronal groups and bold type represents other influences on the respiratory centre. Substances involved in neurotransmission are shown with the most likely receptor subtype, in parentheses, if known. + indicates excitatory effect increasing respiratory activity; – indicates inhibitory activity decreasing respiration. Many of the connections shown may not be active during normal resting conditions. (After references 2 and 6.)

respiration, many of which have several subtypes of receptor. Their exact role in normal human respiration remains unclear, but they are of undoubted relevance in both normal and abnormal breathing. For example, exogenous opioids are known to have an enormous effect in depressing respiratory activity in humans (page 70), indicating the presence of opioid receptors in the respiratory centre,[7] but administration of the opioid antagonist naloxone has no effect on respiration in resting normal subjects. Other neuromodulators include acetylcholine, which acts via both muscarinic and nicotinic receptors to mediate the effect of central chemoreceptors on respiration. Serotonin (5-hydroxytryptamine, 5HT) has many conflicting effects on respiration as a result of the numerous receptor subtypes present. Glutamate acts as a neuromodulator via both NMDA and non-NMDA receptors to mediate the pontine influence on CPG, and is also involved in the influence of pulmonary stretch receptors and peripheral chemoreceptors on the respiratory pattern. Substance P also has an excitatory influence resulting in an increase in tidal volume in response to peripheral chemoreceptor activ-

ity. This diverse collection of neuromodulators probably all ultimately act via a common intracellular signalling pathway within CPG neurones, involving protein kinases A and C which in turn influence the activity of GABA, glycine and glutamate-linked potassium and chloride channels.[9]

Efferent pathways from the respiratory centre

Respiratory motor neurones in the brainstem are pooled into two separate areas, corresponding to inspiratory and expiratory muscle activity (see Figure 5.1). The complex integration of respiratory control seen in the CPG neurones continues to take place at the junction of the upper motor neurone with the anterior horn cell of the lower motor neurone. Three groups of upper motor neurones converge on the anterior horn cells supplying the respiratory muscles. The first group of upper motor neurones is from the dorsal and ventral respiratory groups of the medulla and is concerned with both inspiratory and expiratory output from the CPG. The second group is concerned with voluntary control of breathing (speech, respiratory gymnastics etc.) and the third group with involuntary non-rhythmic respiratory control (swallowing, cough, hiccup etc.). Each group of upper motor neurones occupies a specific anatomical location within the spinal cord. Neuronal control of the respiratory muscles is described in Chapter 6.

CENTRAL NERVOUS SYSTEM CONNECTIONS TO THE RESPIRATORY CENTRE

The pons[2]

There is no doubt of the existence of pontine neurones firing in synchrony with different phases of respiration, now referred to as the pontine respiratory group (PRG). Previously known as the pneumotaxic centre, three groups of neurones were identified (inspiratory, expiratory and phase spanning) that were believed to be involved in controlling the timing of the respiratory cycle. The PRG is no longer considered to be essential for the generation of the respiratory rhythm, but does nevertheless influence the medullary respiratory neurones via a multisynaptic pathway contributing to fine control of the respiratory rhythm as, for example, in setting the lung volume at which inspiration is terminated. There are many central afferent pathways into the PRG, including connections to the hypothalamus, the cortex and the nucleus tractus solitarius. These connections suggest that the pons coordinates the respiratory effects of numerous CNS activities, including cortical control, peripheral sensory information (odour, temperature) and visceral/cardiovascular inputs.

Cerebral cortex[10]

Breathing can be interrupted voluntarily and the pattern of respiratory movements altered within limits determined mainly by changes in arterial blood gas tensions. This is essential for such acts as speech, singing, sniffing, coughing, expulsive efforts and the performance of tests of ventilatory function. There is now some evidence that the neurones involved in this cortical 'override' of respiration may completely bypass the respiratory centre and act directly on the respiratory muscle lower motor neurones.[11]

Volitional changes in respiration are common and under some circumstances overcome the usual chemical control of respiration. For example, conscious respiratory drive may well maintain breathing in subjects following voluntary hyperventilation, when the P_{CO_2} is below the apnoeic threshold (page 63), since apnoea may be consistently produced by only moderate hypocapnia in anaesthetised patients.[12]

There are usually minor changes in the respiratory pattern when subjects focus their attention on their breathing, as when physiological mouth pieces or breathing masks are used.[13]

In addition to volitional changes in the pattern of breathing, there are numerous other suprapontine reflex interferences with respiration, such as sneezing, swallowing and coughing. Reflex control of respiration during speech is a complex process.[14] During prolonged conversation, respiratory rate and tidal volume must be maintained approximately normal to prevent biochemical disturbance. In addition, for speech to be easily understood, pauses to allow inspiration must occur at appropriate boundaries in the text, for example between sentences. To achieve this, the brain performs complex assessments of the forthcoming speech to select appropriate-sized breaths to prevent cumbersome interruptions. This is easier to achieve during reading aloud, when 88% of breaths are taken at appropriate boundaries in the text,[15] compared with a figure of only 63% during spontaneous speech.[14]

Ondine's curse (primary alveolar hypoventilation syndrome)

In 1962 Severinghaus and Mitchell[16] described three patients who exhibited long periods of apnoea, even when awake, but who breathed on command. They termed the condition 'Ondine's curse' from its first description in German legend. The water nymph Ondine, having been jilted by her mortal husband, took from him all automatic functions, requiring him to remember to breathe. When he finally fell asleep, he died. The condition is seen in adults with primary alveolar hypoventilation occurring as a feature of many different diseases, including chronic poliomyelitis and cerebrovascular accidents.[17] Characteristics include a raised P_{CO_2} in the absence of pulmonary pathology, a flat CO_2/ventilation response curve and periods of apnoea which may be central or obstructive. A similar condition is also produced by overdosage with opiates.

Ondine's curse is also used to describe the rare condition of congenital central hypoventilation syndrome, in which babies are born with a permanent defect in automatic respiratory control, leading to apnoea and hypoventilation during sleep.[18,19] In addition, these children have abnormal respiratory responses to exercise[20] and, in keeping with the German legend, also have abnormalities of cardiac control.[21] In spite of such severe abnormalities, non-invasive methods of nocturnal ventilation and diaphragmatic pacing have led to almost normal lives in many of these children.[19]

PERIPHERAL INPUT TO THE RESPIRATORY CENTRE AND NON-CHEMICAL REFLEXES

Reflexes arising from the upper respiratory tract[22,23]

Nose. Water and stimulants such as ammonia or cigarette smoke may cause apnoea as part of the diving reflex (page 285). Irritants can initiate sneezing which, unlike coughing, cannot be undertaken voluntarily. There are also cold receptors that initiate bronchoconstriction in sensitive subjects.

Pharynx. Mechanoreceptors that respond to pressure play a major role in activation of the pharyngeal dilator muscles (page 76). There is ample evidence that local anaesthesia of the pharynx impairs their action. Irritants may cause bronchodilation, hypertension, tachycardia and secretion of mucus in the lower airway.

Larynx. The larynx has a dense sensory innervation with fibres from the subglottic region in the recurrent laryngeal nerve and those from the supraglottic region in the internal branch of the superior laryngeal nerve. Most reflexes arise from the supraglottic area, as section of the latter nerve abolishes almost all reflex activity. There are three groups of receptors. Mechanoreceptors respond to changes in transmural pressure or laryngeal motion and result in increased pharyngeal dilator muscle activity, particularly during airway obstruction. Cold receptors are found superficially on the vocal folds and activation generally results in depression of ventilation. The importance of this reflex in adult humans is uncertain, but these receptors may produce bronchoconstriction in susceptible individuals (see Chapter 27). Irritant receptors respond to many substances, such as distilled water, cigarette smoke and inhaled anaesthetics and, in a similar fashion to direct mechanical stimulation of the larynx, cause cough, laryngeal closure and bronchoconstriction.

The cough reflex may be elicited by chemical or mechanical stimuli arising in the larynx, trachea, carina or main bronchi. Which of these sites is responsible for the initiation of a cough is difficult to determine. For chemical stimuli the larynx may be of less importance, as superior laryngeal nerve block has little effect on cough stimulated by citric acid inhalation,[24] and in patients following heart–lung transplant inhalation of the normally potent stimulant distilled water results in little or no cough.[25] Coughing can be undertaken voluntarily, but the reflex is complex and comprises three main stages.

1. An inspiration, which takes into the lungs a volume of air sufficient for the expiratory activity.
2. Build-up of pressure in the lungs by contraction of expiratory muscles against a closed glottis.
3. Forceful expiration through narrowed airways, resulting in high linear velocity of gas flow, which sweeps irritant material up towards the pharynx.

Transient changes of pressure up to 40 kPa (300 mmHg) may occur in the thorax, arterial blood and the cerebrospinal fluid (CSF) during the act of coughing.

Reflexes arising in the lung

Pulmonary stretch receptors and their associated reflexes.[26] There are a large number of different types of receptor in the lungs sensitive to inflation, deflation, and mechanical and chemical stimulation, afferents from which are mostly conducted by the vagus, although some fibres may be carried in the sympathetic nerves. Slowly adapting stretch receptors (SARs) are found predominantly in the airways rather than in the alveoli and are closely associated with the tracheobronchial smooth muscle. Lung inflation stimulates the SARs, which are named 'slowly adapting' owing to their ability to maintain their firing rate when lung inflation is maintained, thus acting as a form of lung volume sensor. Conversely, rapidly adapting stretch receptors (RARs) are located in the superficial mucosal layer[22] and are stimulated by changes in tidal volume, respiratory frequency or lung compliance.[26] The RARs also differ from SARs in being nociceptive and chemosensitive, responding to a wide range of chemical irritants, mechanical stimuli and inflammatory mediators.

The reflexes associated with pulmonary stretch receptors have attracted much attention since the associated inflation and deflation reflexes were described by Hering and Breuer in 1868.[27] Breuer was a clinical assistant to Professor Hering, but apparently the work was at his own instigation. However, Hering, who was a corre-

sponding member of the Vienna Academy of Science, published Breuer's work under his own name, in accordance with the custom of the time. Breuer's role was clearly stated in Hering's paper but he was not a co-author. Later the same year, Breuer published a much fuller account of his work under his own name.

The inflation reflex consists of inhibition of inspiration in response to an increased pulmonary transmural pressure gradient (as in sustained inflation of the lung). An exactly similar effect may be obtained by obstructing expiration so that an inspiration is retained in the lungs.

The significance of the Hering–Breuer reflex in humans is controversial.[28] There appears to be an important species difference between laboratory animals, in which the reflex is easy to demonstrate, and humans, in whom the reflex is very weak.[29] This is borne out in studies showing no effect of bilateral vagal block on breathing patterns in volunteers,[30] and it is also clear that patients have essentially normal ventilatory patterns after bilateral lung transplant, when both lungs must be totally denervated (see Chapter 33). Although the Hering–Breuer inflation reflex therefore appears to have minimal functional significance in man, its existence has been demonstrated in adults[29,31] and it is widely accepted as being present in neonates and infants.[32]

The deflation reflex consists of an augmentation of inspiration in response to deflation of the lung and can be demonstrated in man.[33] These results are consistent with the hypothesis that lung deflation has a reflex excitatory effect on breathing, but that the threshold is higher in man than for other mammalian species.

Head's paradoxical reflex. Head, working in Professor Hering's laboratory, described a reversal of the inflation reflex.[34] Many authors have reported that, with normal vagal conduction, sudden inflation of the lungs of many species may cause a transient inspiratory effort before the onset of apnoea due to the inflation reflex.[29] A similar response may also be elicited in newborn infants,[35] but it has not been established whether this 'gasp reflex' is analogous to Head's paradoxical reflex. All anaesthetists are aware that, after the administration of respiratory depressants, transient increases in airway pressure often cause an immediate deep gasping type of inspiration. There is a possible relationship between the reflex and the mechanism of sighing, which may be considered a normal feature of breathing.[36]

Other pulmonary afferents

C-fibre endings lie in close relationship to the capillaries; one group is in relation to the bronchial circulation and the other to the pulmonary microcirculation. The latter correspond to Paintal's juxtapulmonary capillary receptors (J receptors, for short).[22,37]

These receptors are relatively silent during normal breathing but are stimulated under various pathological conditions. They are similar to RARs described above, being nociceptive and activated by tissue damage, accumulation of interstitial fluid and release of various mediators. In the laboratory they can be activated by intravascular injection of capsaicin to produce the so-called pulmonary chemoreflex, which comprises bradycardia, hypotension, apnoea or shallow breathing, bronchoconstriction and increased mucus secretion.[22] They may well be concerned in the dyspnoea of pulmonary vascular congestion and the ventilatory response to exercise and pulmonary embolisation. C-fibre endings have been characterised in physiological studies but have never been identified histologically, although non-myelinated nerve fibres are seen in the alveolar walls.

Reflexes arising from outside the airway and lungs

Phrenic nerve afferents.[38] Approximately one-third of neurones in the phrenic nerve are afferent, with the majority arising from muscle spindles and tendon organs forming the spinal reflex arc described on page 82. However, some afferent neurones continue through the ipsilateral spinal cord to the brainstem and somatosensory cortex. Experimental stimulation of phrenic afferent fibres generally results in a reduction of respiratory efferent activity known as phrenic-to-phrenic inhibition, but stimulation of some smaller afferent fibres has the opposite effect. Thus the physiological role of phrenic afferents remains obscure, but it is unlikely that they have any influence on normal breathing. The sensory information provided by phrenic afferents is believed to be important in the perception of, and compensation for, increased inspiratory loads, and these afferents are important in the 'breaking point' following a breath hold (page 69).

Baroreceptor reflexes. The most important groups of arterial baroreceptors are in the carotid sinus and around the aortic arch. These receptors are primarily concerned with regulation of the circulation, but a large decrease in arterial pressure produces hyperventilation, whereas in animals a substantial rise in arterial pressure causes respiratory depression and, ultimately, apnoea.

Afferents from the musculoskeletal system. A variety of mechanical stimuli applied to the gastrocnemius muscle of the dog can produce a reflex increase in ventilation.[39] Afferents from the musculoskeletal system probably do not contribute to normal resting ventilation but have an important role in the hyperventilation of exercise (see Chapter 15).

THE INFLUENCE OF CARBON DIOXIDE ON RESPIRATORY CONTROL[40,41]

For many years it was believed that the respiratory centre itself was sensitive to carbon dioxide. However, it is now known that the central chemoreceptors are actually separate from the respiratory neurones of the medulla although located only a short distance away. About 85% of the total respiratory response to inhaled carbon dioxide originates in these medullary chemoreceptors.[42]

Localisation of the central chemoreceptors

Anatomical studies in animals indicate that central chemosensitive areas are located on the anterolateral surfaces of the medulla, close to the origins of the glossopharyngeal and vagus nerves.[43] More recently, c-fos immunochemistry has been used in animals to identify the medullary neurones that responded to stimulation by carbon dioxide.[44] Evidence of stimulation was found in the rostral and caudal areas of the anterior medulla and the most stimulated cells lay within 0.2 mm of the surface. In addition, MRI and PET scanning techniques during CO_2-stimulated breathing in humans have confirmed that the surface of the anterior medulla is the primary site of chemosensitive neurone activity.[3,4] Other areas of the CNS that display increased neural activity with CO_2 stimulation include other areas of the medulla, the midline pons, small areas in the cerebellum and the limbic system,[3,4] though the contribution of these areas to respiratory control is unclear.

Mechanism of action

An elevation of arterial P_{CO_2} causes an approximately equal rise of CSF, cerebral tissue and jugular venous P_{CO_2}, which are all about 1.3 kPa (10 mmHg) more than the arterial P_{CO_2}. Over the short term and without change in CSF bicarbonate, a rise in CSF P_{CO_2} causes a fall in CSF pH. The blood–brain barrier (operative between blood and CSF) is permeable to carbon dioxide but not hydrogen ions, and in this respect resembles the membrane of a P_{CO_2}-sensitive electrode (page 161). In both cases, carbon dioxide crosses the barrier and hydrates to carbonic acid, which then ionises to give a pH inversely proportional to the log of the P_{CO_2}. A hydrogen ion sensor is thus made to respond to P_{CO_2}. This accords with the old observation that the ventilatory response to respiratory acidosis is greater than to a metabolic acidosis with the same change in *blood* pH. Ventilation is, in fact, a single function of CSF pH in both conditions.[45]

The precise mechanism by which a change in pH causes stimulation of chemoreceptor neurones is not firmly established, but it could clearly influence the action of an enzyme. Decreased pH inhibits the metabolism of acetylcholine by cholinesterase and it has been observed that atropine blocks the CO_2 sensitivity of the central chemoreceptors, an effect mediated by M_2 muscarinic receptors.[46]

Compensatory bicarbonate shift in the CSF. If the PCO_2 of CSF is maintained at an abnormal level, the CSF pH gradually returns towards normal over the course of many hours as a result of changes in the CSF bicarbonate concentration. This is analogous to, and proceeds in parallel with, the partial restoration of blood pH in patients with chronic hyper- or hypocapnia. Compensatory changes in bicarbonate concentrations are similar in both CSF and blood, suggesting a common mechanism.[47,48] Bicarbonate shift in CSF could therefore result simply from passive ion distribution, although the possibility of active ion transfer cannot be completely excluded.

A shift in CSF bicarbonate occurs during prolonged periods of hypocapnic artificial ventilation and contributes to the early partial reversal of the hypocapnia that occurs in response to hypoxia at altitude (page 257). As would be expected from a passive ion transfer system, the speed at which bicarbonate shift compensates the CSF pH depends on the magnitude of the change in PCO_2. After commencing passive hyperventilation the CSF bicarbonate would in theory be significantly reduced after only 1 hour[49] and CSF pH has been reported to have returned to normal after 30 hours of hyperventilation in humans following cerebrovascular accidents.[50] In animal studies a substantial resetting of the CSF pH occurs within 4.5 hours of a step increase in ventilation.[51] This offers one reason why patients receiving artificial hyper-

ventilation often continue to hyperventilate after resumption of spontaneous breathing.

Compensatory changes in CSF bicarbonate and the restoration of its pH are not confined to respiratory alkalosis, but are also found in chronic respiratory acidosis and metabolic acidosis and alkalosis. In a study of patients with a variety of pathological acid–base disturbances, values of CSF pH did not differ by more than 0.011 units from the normal value (7.326) in spite of mean arterial pH values ranging from 7.334 to 7.523.[52]

If the bicarbonate concentration in CSF is itself altered by pathological factors, the pH is changed and ventilatory disturbances follow. For example, after intracranial haemorrhage patients may spontaneously hyperventilate,[53] and in these patients the CSF pH and bicarbonate have been shown to be below the normal values. It was postulated that this was due to the metabolic breakdown products of blood that contaminated the CSF, and the correction of hyperventilation by intrathecal administration of 3–5 mmol of bicarbonate has been reported.[54]

The PCO_2/ventilation response curve

Following a rise in arterial PCO_2, respiratory depth and rate increase until a steady state of hyperventilation is achieved after a few minutes. The response is linear over the range that is usually studied and may therefore be defined in terms of two parameters: slope and intercept (see Appendix F):

$$\text{Ventilation} = S(PCO_2 - B)$$

where S is the slope (l.min^{-1}.kPa^{-1} or l.min^{-1}.mmHg^{-1}) and B is the intercept at zero ventilation (kPa or mmHg). The blue line in Figure 5.5 is a typical normal curve with

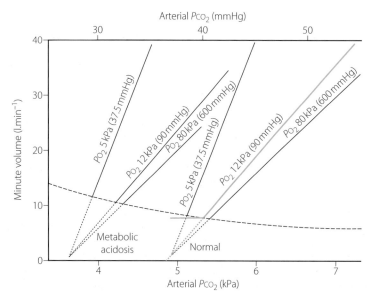

Figure 5.5 Two fans of PCO_2/ventilation response curves at different values of PO_2. The right-hand fan is at normal metabolic acid–base state (zero base excess). The left-hand fan represents metabolic acidosis. The broken line represents the PCO_2 produced by the indicated ventilation for zero inspired PCO_2, at basal metabolic rate. The intersection of the broken curve and any response curve indicates the resting PCO_2 and ventilation for the relevant metabolic acid–base state and PO_2. The blue curve is the normal response. See text for details.

an intercept (*B*) of about 4.8 kPa (36 mmHg) and a slope (*S*) of about 15 l.min^{-1}.kPa^{-1} (2 l.min^{-1}.mmHg^{-1}). There is in fact a very wide individual variation in P_{CO_2}/ventilation response curves, including a circadian variation within individuals,[55] and the response may be decreased by normal hormonal changes, disease or drugs. The dashed curve in Figure 5.5 shows the effect of changing ventilation on arterial P_{CO_2} when the inspired carbon dioxide concentration is negligible and is a section of a rectangular hyperbola. The normal resting P_{CO_2} and ventilation are indicated by the intersection of this curve with the normal P_{CO_2}/ventilation response curve, which is usually obtained by varying the carbon dioxide concentration in the inspired gas.

When subjects hyperventilate voluntarily and reduce their P_{CO_2} below the threshold for CO_2 stimulation of respiration a variety of responses are seen, varying from apnoea to normal respiration or even hyperventilation.[56] Figure 5.5 shows two possible extensions to the normal response curve (in blue) below the threshold for CO_2 stimulation (dashed line). The first is an extrapolation of the curve to intersect the *x* axis (zero ventilation) at a P_{CO_2} known as the apnoeic threshold (dotted lines in Figure 5.5). If P_{CO_2} is depressed below this point apnoea may result, and this is seen in some subjects. The second type of extension (shown on the blue line) is horizontal and to the left, like a hockey stick, representing the response of a subject who continues to breathe regardless of the fact that his P_{CO_2} has been reduced. The resting arterial point at resting ventilation is normally approximately 0.3 kPa to the left of the extrapolated response curve,[57] supporting the idea of a hockey stick-shaped response curve. When breathing below this threshold for the onset of CO_2-stimulated ventilation (the angle of the hockey stick) hypoxia seems to have no influence.[56] This variable ventilatory response to low P_{CO_2} almost certainly arises from the cortical control of respiration maintaining breathing despite a lack of chemical drive.

As P_{CO_2} is raised, a point of maximal ventilatory stimulation is reached, probably within the range 13.3–26.7 kPa (100–200 mmHg), beyond which respiratory fatigue and CO_2 narcosis intervene (see Chapter 23). The ventilatory stimulation is reduced until, at very high P_{CO_2}, the ventilation is actually depressed below the control value and finally apnoea results, at least in animals and almost certainly in humans as well.

The P_{CO_2}/ventilation response curve is the response of the entire respiratory system to the challenge of a raised P_{CO_2}. Apart from reduced sensitivity of the central chemoreceptors, the overall response may be blunted by partial neuromuscular blockade or by obstructive or restrictive lung disease. These factors must be taken into account in drawing conclusions from a reduced response, and diffuse airway obstruction is a most important consideration. Nevertheless, the slope of the P_{CO_2}/ventilation response curve remains one of the most valuable parameters in the assessment of the responsiveness of the respiratory system to carbon dioxide and its depression by drugs.

Time course of P_{CO_2}/ventilation response.[58] As described above, the initial ventilatory response to elevated P_{CO_2} is extremely rapid, occurring within just a few minutes, at which time about 75% of the final ventilatory response has occurred. With sustained hypercapnia, the minute ventilation continues to increase for a further hour before reaching a plateau, which is sustained for at least 8 hours in healthy subjects.

THE INFLUENCE OF OXYGEN ON RESPIRATORY CONTROL

As for carbon dioxide, it was initially thought that hypoxia stimulated respiration by a direct effect on the respiratory centre. However, around 1930 the histological studies of de Castro[59] led him to suggest a chemoreceptor function for the carotid bodies, and the respiratory role of the peripheral chemoreceptors was established by Heymans,[60] who received a Nobel prize for his work.

Peripheral chemoreceptors

The peripheral chemoreceptors are fast-responding monitors of the arterial blood, responding to a fall in Pa_{O_2}, a rise in Pa_{CO_2} or H$^+$ concentration, or a fall in their perfusion rate. An increase in ventilation is the result of stimulation. The bilaterally paired carotid bodies, rather than the aortic bodies, are almost exclusively responsible for the respiratory response. Each is only about 6 mm^3 in volume and they are located close to the bifurcation of the common carotid artery. The carotid bodies undergo hypertrophy and hyperplasia under conditions of chronic hypoxia and are usually lost in the operation of carotid endarterectomy (see below).

Histology. The carotid bodies contain large sinusoids with a very high rate of perfusion – about ten times the level that would be proportional to their metabolic rate, which is itself very high. Therefore the arterial/venous P_{O_2} difference is small. This accords with their role as a sensor of arterial blood gas tensions and their rapid response, which is within the range 1–3 seconds.[61]

At the cellular level, the main feature is the glomus or type 1 cell, which is in synaptic contact with nerve endings derived from an axon with its cell body in the petrosal ganglion of the glossopharyngeal nerve (Figure 5.6). These endings are mainly postsynaptic to the glomus cell. Type I cells are partly encircled by type II or sheath cells, whose function is still obscure.[55] Effer-

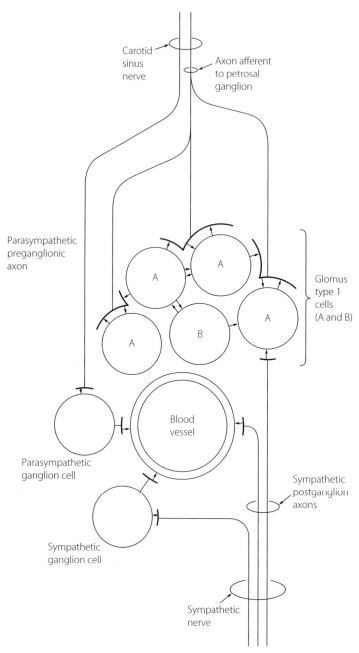

Figure 5.6 Schematic representation of the histology of the carotid bodies. Glomus type I cells are grouped around a blood vessel in the carotid body. Numerous nerve cells are also shown. This grouping would be surrounded by a sheath cell (not shown) which is sometimes termed a glomoid.

ent nerves, which are known to modulate receptor afferent discharge, include preganglionic sympathetic fibres from the superior cervical ganglion, amounting to 5% of the nerve endings on the glomus cell.

Discharge rate in the afferent nerves from the carotid body increases in response to the following forms of stimulation.

Decrease of arterial Po₂. Stimulation is by decreased P_{O_2} and not by reduced oxygen content (at least down

to about half the normal value). Thus there is little stimulation in anaemia, carboxyhaemoglobinaemia or methaemoglobinaemia. Quantitative aspects of the hypoxic ventilatory response are described in detail below.

Decrease of arterial pH. Acidaemia of perfusing blood causes stimulation, the magnitude of which is the same whether it is due to respiratory or metabolic acidosis. Quantitatively, the change produced by elevated P_{CO_2}

on the peripheral chemoreceptors is only about one-sixth of that caused by the action on the central chemosensitive areas (see below). This response does, however, occur very rapidly[58] and only develops when a 'threshold' value of arterial PCO_2 is exceeded.[56]

Hypoperfusion of peripheral chemoreceptors causes stimulation, possibly by causing a 'stagnant hypoxia' of the chemoreceptor cells. Hypoperfusion may result from severe systemic hypotension.

Blood temperature elevation causes stimulation of breathing via the peripheral chemoreceptors. In addition, the ventilatory responses to both hypoxia and CO_2 are enhanced by a modest (1.4°C) rise in body temperature.[62]

Chemical stimulation by a wide range of substances is known to cause increased ventilation through the medium of the peripheral chemoreceptors. These substances fall into two groups. The first comprises agents such as nicotine and acetylcholine that stimulate sympathetic ganglia. The second group of chemical stimulants comprises substances such as cyanide and carbon monoxide which block the cytochrome system and so prevent oxidative metabolism. Drugs that stimulate respiration via the peripheral chemoreceptors are described below.

Mechanism of action of peripheral chemoreceptors[63]

In type I cells arterial hypoxaemia causes a reduction in the intracellular level of adenosine triphosphate (ATP) at levels of PO_2 that have little effect elsewhere in the body. In addition, in response to hypoxia there is a graded increase in intracellular calcium concentration following its release from mitochondria.[64] Oxygen-sensitive potassium channels have been described, as have haem-based mitochondrial cytochromes that respond to changes in local PO_2.[63,65] Stimulation of the chemoreceptors by an increased arterial PCO_2 is dependent on carbonic anhydrase (present in the type I cell) and there is therefore the possibility of both raised PCO_2 and decreased arterial pH acting through an increase in intracellular hydrogen ion concentration. However, for hypoxia, raised PCO_2 and decreased pH the full transductive cascade of events between the stimulus and activation of the carotid sinus nerve afferents is not yet clear.

Various neurotransmitters have been identified within the carotid body, including dopamine, noradrenaline, acetylcholine, substance P and enkephalins, but the role of each is uncertain. For example, dopamine is abundant in type I cells and released in a calcium-dependent

fashion, and both carotid sinus nerve endings and type I cells have dopamine D_2 receptors. Exogenous low-dose dopamine inhibits carotid sinus nerve activity and reduces the acute hypoxic ventilatory response,[66] and selective D_2 dopamine antagonists augment the response to hypoxia,[67] indicating that dopamine has an inhibitory or 'regulatory' role in the carotid bodies. Similarly, the α_2-adrenoceptor agonist clonidine reduces the ventilatory response to acute hypoxia, indicating that noradrenaline also has an inhibitory effect.[68] It is therefore impossible at this stage to define any one critical neurotransmitter between the type I cell and the carotid sinus nerve endings.[63] No single receptor blocker prevents the hypoxic ventilatory response.

The gain of the carotid bodies is under nervous control. There is an efferent pathway in the sinus nerve which, on excitation, decreases chemoreceptor activity. Excitation of the sympathetic nerve supply to the carotid body causes an increase in activity.

Other effects of stimulation. Apart from the well-known increase in depth and rate of breathing, peripheral chemoreceptor stimulation causes a number of other effects, including bradycardia, hypertension, increase in bronchiolar tone and adrenal secretion. Stimulation of the carotid bodies has predominantly respiratory effects, whereas the aortic bodies have a greater influence on the circulation.

Time course of the ventilatory response to sustained hypoxia[69]

By controlling the concentration of inhaled oxygen, arterial oxygen saturation can be reduced and then maintained at a constant level of hypoxia, usually with an Sa_{O_2} of about 80%. In order to separate the effects on ventilation of hypoxia and PCO_2 most studies use isocapnic conditions, where the subject's alveolar PCO_2 is maintained at their control (resting ventilation) level by addition of CO_2 to the inspired gas. The interaction of PCO_2 and hypoxia in ventilatory control is discussed below. With a moderate degree of sustained hypoxia the ventilatory response is triphasic, as shown in Figure 5.7. The three phases are described separately.

Acute hypoxic response. This is the first immediate and rapid increase in ventilation. Sudden imposition of hypoxia results in stimulation of ventilation within the lung-to-carotid body circulation time (about 6 s), but in most studies the response appears slower owing to the delay between reducing inspired oxygen and the reduction in alveolar and arterial PO_2. Ventilation continues to increase for between 5 and 10 minutes, rapidly reaching high levels.

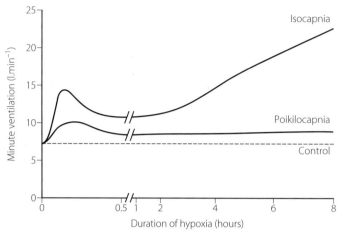

Figure 5.7 Time course of the ventilatory response to hypoxia ($Sa_{O_2} \approx 80\%$). Practical problems prevent the continuous and rapid measurement of minute volume and respiratory gases for 8 hours, so the curves are produced by combining the data from three studies. When arterial P_{CO_2} is maintained at normal levels (isocapnia) the response is triphasic. When arterial P_{CO_2} is not controlled (poikilocapnia) the magnitude of the response is damped because the hypoxia-induced hyperventilation reduces P_{CO_2} and therefore respiratory drive. See Figure 17.3 for respiratory effects of prolonged hypoxia. (After references 70, 71 and 72.)

Many factors affect the acute ventilatory response. There are wide variations between individuals, within an individual on different days,[73] between male and female subjects and with the hormonal changes of the menstrual cycle.[74] A small number of otherwise normal subjects lack a measurable ventilatory response to hypoxia when studied at normal P_{CO_2}. This is of little importance under normal circumstances, because the P_{CO_2} drive from the central chemoreceptors will normally ensure a safe level of P_{O_2}. However, in certain therapeutic and abnormal environmental circumstances, it could be dangerous. Such people would certainly do badly at high altitude.

Hypoxic ventilatory decline (HVD). Shortly after the acute hypoxic response reaches a peak, minute ventilation begins to decline, reaching a plateau level, still above the resting ventilation, after 20–30 minutes (see Figure 5.7). The degree of HVD in a single subject correlates with the acute hypoxic response – the greater the initial increase in ventilation, the greater the subsequent decline.[71] Though not yet completely elucidated, the mechanism of HVD appears to have a significant centrally mediated component[75] and represents a change in ventilatory drive rather than a decline in the sensitivity of the receptors to hypoxia.[76] In neonates, HVD is reversed by naloxone, but this effect is not seen in adults.[77] In animals, central glutamate release is involved in the acute hypoxic response, whereas GABA is implicated in producing HVD.[78] Whether the trigger for release of these transmitters is from the peripheral chemoreceptors or a direct central effect of hypoxia remains unclear.

Ventilatory response to sustained hypoxia. Once HVD is complete, continued isocapnic hypoxia results in a second, slower rise in ventilation over several hours (see Figure 5.7).[72] Ventilation continues to increase for

at least 8 hours[72] and reaches a plateau by 24 hours.[79] Species differences in this response again make elucidation of the mechanism in humans difficult, but the most likely explanation is a direct effect of hypoxia on the carotid bodies.[72]

Hypoxia for more than 2–3 days only occurs following ascent to altitude and the effects of this are described in Chapter 17. Finally, over many years there is a loss of hypoxic drive, which is grossly attenuated in residents at very high altitudes.[80]

Ventilatory response to progressive hypoxia

Instead of maintaining a constant degree of hypoxia, ventilation may be measured during a progressive reduction in P_{O_2}. Once again, by controlling inspired gas concentrations, alveolar P_{O_2} may be reduced from 16 to 5 kPa (120 to 40 mmHg) over 15 minutes[81] and ventilation increases progressively throughout this period. The response under these circumstances probably equates to the acute hypoxic response. If alveolar P_{O_2} is plotted against minute ventilation a P_{O_2}/ventilation response curve is produced (Figure 5.8). A P_{O_2}/ventilation response curve approximates to a rectangular hyperbola (see Appendix F), asymptotic to the ventilation at high Pa_{O_2} (zero hypoxic drive) and to the Pa_{O_2} at which ventilation theoretically becomes infinite (known as 'C' and about 4.3 kPa). Figure 5.8 shows a typical example but there are very wide individual variations. Note that there is a small but measurable difference in ventilation between normal and very high P_{O_2}.

The initial ventilatory response to P_{O_2} may be expressed as:

$$\frac{W}{Pa_{O_2} - C}$$

where W is a multiplier (i.e. the gain of the system) and partly dependent upon the P_{CO_2}. The ventilatory

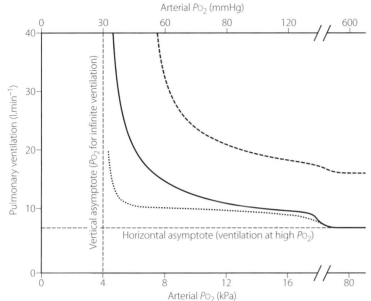

Figure 5.8 Ventilatory response to progressive hypoxia. The heavy curve represents the normal P_{O_2}/ventilation response under isocapnic conditions, that is, with P_{CO_2} maintained at the resting value. It has the form of a rectangular hyperbola asymptotic to the ventilation at high P_{O_2} and the P_{O_2} at which ventilation becomes infinite. The curve is displaced upwards by both hypercapnia and exercise at normal P_{CO_2} (dashed line). Hypocapnia displaces the curve downwards (dotted line) regardless of whether the hypocapnia results from not controlling P_{CO_2} (poikilocapnia) or from deliberately reducing P_{CO_2}. (Data from references 81, 82 and 83.)

response here is the difference between the actual ventilation and the ventilation at high P_{O_2}, P_{CO_2} being unchanged.

The inconvenience of the non-linear relationship between ventilation and P_{O_2} may be overcome by plotting ventilation against oxygen saturation. The relationship is then linear with a negative slope, at least down to a saturation of 70%.[84] This approach is the basis of a simple non-invasive method of measurement of the hypoxic ventilatory response (see below).

Iatrogenic loss of peripheral chemoreceptor sensitivity[85]

Nerves from the carotid bodies are usually divided during bilateral carotid endarterectomy,[86] which provides evidence that the carotid bodies are not essential for the maintenance of reasonably normal breathing under conditions of rest and mild exercise. Indeed, there is some evidence that the common finding of atheromatous disease at the carotid bifurcation may itself reduce chemoreceptor function and that a careful, 'nerve-sparing' carotid endarterectomy can increase the ventilatory response to hypoxia.[87] Deliberate abolition of the hypoxic ventilatory response by carotid endarterectomy has been advocated as a treatment for incapacitating dyspnoea in severe respiratory disease.[88]

Central hypoxic depression of breathing

In addition to its effects on peripheral chemoreceptors, hypoxia also has a direct effect on the respiratory centre. Central respiratory neurone activity is depressed by hypoxia and apnoea follows severe medullary hypoxia whether due to ischaemia or to hypoxaemia. With denervated peripheral chemoreceptors, phrenic motor activity becomes silent when the medullary P_{O_2} falls to about 1.7 kPa (13 mmHg).[89] More intense hypoxia causes a resumption of breathing with an abnormal pattern, possibly driven by a 'gasping' centre. This pattern of central hypoxic depression appears to be particularly marked in neonates and may be the relic of a mechanism to prevent the fetus from attempting to breathe *in utero*.

Mechanisms of hypoxic depression of ventilation. Medullary P_{CO_2}, and therefore ventilation, may be reduced by increased cerebral blood flow induced by hypoxia, and severe hypoxia causes depletion of high-energy phosphates. However, it has also been shown that neonatal hypoxia results in decreased levels of excitatory neurotransmitters (glutamate and aspartate) and increased levels of inhibitory substances, particularly GABA and endogenous opioids, both powerful respiratory depressants.

INTEGRATION OF THE CHEMICAL CONTROL OF BREATHING

The two main systems contributing to chemical control of breathing have been described quite separately, but in the intact subject this is not possible. For example, the peripheral chemoreceptors respond (slightly) to changes in P_{CO_2}, and hypoxia affects the respiratory centre directly as well as via the carotid body receptors. An overall view of the chemical control of breathing is shown schematically in Figure 5.9.

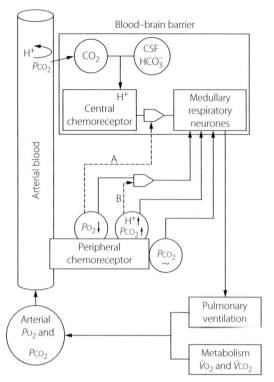

Figure 5.9 Scheme of connections between individual aspects of chemical control of breathing. See text for details.

It was originally thought that the various factors interacted according to the algebraic sum of the individual effects caused by changes of P_{CO_2}, P_{O_2}, pH etc. Hypoxia and hypercapnia were, for example, thought to be simply additive in their effects, but it is now realised that this was a very simplistic view of a complex system.

Effects of P_{CO_2} and pH on the hypoxic ventilatory response[81]

The acute hypoxic response is enhanced at elevated P_{CO_2} as shown by the upper dashed curve in Figure 5.8, the mechanism being indicated by broken line B in Figure 5.9. This interaction contributes to the ventilatory response in asphyxia being greater than the sum of the response to be expected from the rise in P_{CO_2} and the fall in P_{O_2} if considered separately.

Responses to both acute and prolonged hypoxia are depressed by hypocapnia, as shown in the lower dotted curve in Figure 5.8. This results from opposing effects on the CPG of increased chemoreceptor input and decreased central chemoreceptor drive. On prolonged exposure to hypoxia at altitude, this effect continues until acclimatisation takes place (page 257).

Poikilocapnic conditions occur when no attempt is made to control P_{CO_2} during hypoxic ventilation and the hypoxia-induced hyperventilation immediately gives rise to hypocapnia. Though rarely studied, this situation is important as poikilocapnia will occur in clinical situations. Early studies of the effects of P_{CO_2} on hypoxic ventilation showed that without control of P_{CO_2}, the hypoxia-driven increase in ventilation is almost exactly counteracted by the P_{CO_2}-driven depression of ventilation, resulting in no change in minute volume until breathing less than 10% oxygen.[82,83] Many earlier studies were, however, performed before technology allowed elucidation of the time course of hypoxic ventilation, and may have been measuring the plateau of ventilation after hypoxic ventilatory decline rather than the acute hypoxic response. More recent studies have shown that poikilocapnic conditions attenuate, but do not abolish, the first two phases of the ventilatory response to constant hypoxia (see Figures 5.8 and 5.9).[70,71] Increased ventilation with sustained (over 1 hour) hypoxia is abolished during poikilocapnia but the minute volume does remain above resting levels (see Figure 5.7).[72]

Exercise enhances the response to hypoxia even if the P_{CO_2} is not raised,[90] possibly due to lactic acidosis, oscillations of arterial P_{CO_2}, afferent input from muscle or perhaps to catecholamine secretion. The upper broken curve in Figure 5.8 would also correspond to the response during exercise at an oxygen consumption of about 800 ml.min^{-1}. It is important to note that the slope of the curve at normal P_{O_2} is considerably increased in both these circumstances, so there will then be an appreciable 'hypoxic' drive to ventilation at normal P_{O_2}. Enhanced response to P_{O_2} during exercise seems to be an important component in the overall ventilatory response to exercise (see Chapter 15).

Effects of Pa_{O_2} and pH on central chemoreceptor response[56]

The broken line (A) in Figure 5.9 shows the influence of the peripheral chemoreceptor drive on the gain of the central ventilatory response to P_{CO_2}. Typical quantitative relationships are shown in Figure 5.5, with hypoxia at the left of each fan and hyperoxia on the right. The curve marked P_{O_2} 80 kPa represents total abolition of chemoreceptor drive obtained by the inhalation of 100% oxygen.

Metabolic acidosis displaces the whole fan of curves to the left, as shown in Figure 5.5. The intercept (B) is reduced but the slope of the curves at each value of P_{O_2} is virtually unaltered. Display of the fan of P_{CO_2}/ventilation response curves at different P_{O_2} is a particularly complete method of representing the state of respiratory control in a patient, but it is unfortunately laborious to determine.

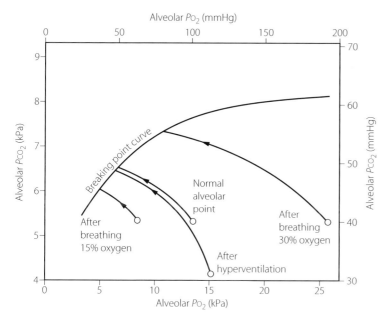

Figure 5.10 The 'breaking point' curve defines the coexisting values of alveolar P_{O_2} and P_{CO_2}, at the breaking point of breath holding, starting from various states. The normal alveolar point is shown and the curved arrow shows the changes in alveolar gas tensions that occur during breath holding. Starting points are displaced to the right by preliminary breathing of oxygen-enriched gases and to the left by breathing mixtures containing less than 21% oxygen. Hyperventilation displaces the point representing alveolar gas to the right and downwards. The length of arrows from starting point to the breaking point curve gives an approximate indication of the duration of breath hold. This can clearly be prolonged by oxygen breathing or by hyperventilation, maximal duration occurring after hyperventilation with 100% oxygen.

BREATH HOLDING

Influence of P_{CO_2} and P_{O_2}

When the breath is held after air breathing, the arterial and alveolar P_{CO_2} are remarkably constant at the breaking point and values are normally close to 6.7 kPa (50 mmHg). This does not mean that P_{CO_2} is the sole or dominant factor and concomitant hypoxia is probably more important. Preliminary oxygen breathing delays the onset of hypoxia and breath-holding times may be greatly prolonged, with consequent elevation of P_{CO_2} at the breaking point. The relationship between P_{CO_2} and P_{O_2} at breaking point, after starting from different levels of oxygenation, is shown in Figure 5.10. The breaking point curve is displaced upwards and to the left by carotid body resection.[91]

On the basis of changing blood gas tensions and the great variability of individuals' responses, it might be predicted that subjects with 'flat' ventilatory responses to oxygen and carbon dioxide would be able to hold their breath longer. Elite breath-hold divers (page 271) have been shown to have a blunted response to carbon dioxide but not to hypoxia.[92]

Effect of lung volume

Breath-holding time is directly proportional to the lung volume at the onset of breath holding, partly because this has a major influence on oxygen stores. There are, however, other effects of lung volume and its change, which are mediated by afferents arising from the chest wall, the diaphragm and the lung itself. Prolongation of

breath-holding times is seen after bilateral vagal and glossopharyngeal nerve block[93] and following complete muscular paralysis of conscious subjects.[94,95] These studies suggest that much of the distress leading to the termination of breath holding is caused by frustration of the involuntary contractions of the respiratory muscles, which increase progressively during breath holding. Fowler's experiment in 1954 easily demonstrates the importance of frustration of involuntary respiratory movements.[96] After normal air breathing, the breath is held until breaking point. If the expirate is then exhaled into a bag and immediately reinhaled, there is a marked sense of relief although it may be shown that the rise of P_{CO_2} and fall of P_{O_2} are uninfluenced.

Extreme durations of breath holding may be attained after hyperventilation and preoxygenation. Times of 14 minutes have been reached and the limiting factor is then reduction of lung volume to residual volume, as oxygen is removed from the alveolar gas.

DRUG EFFECTS ON THE CONTROL OF BREATHING

Considering the therapeutic potential of drugs that could specifically influence respiratory drive, it is surprising that so few drugs affecting respiratory control have been developed.[97] Elucidation of the mechanisms for the control of breathing described in this chapter is a relatively recent event, particularly when considering the neurotransmitters and neuromodulators involved. The large number of different receptors involved in normal respiratory control (see Figure 5.4) means that drugs affecting a single receptor may have little effect, or unpredictable effects, on respiration and so be of little use clinically. In addition, the neurotransmitters and neuromodulators involved are widely distributed throughout the central nervous system (CNS), so agonists or antagonists of their receptors are likely to have diverse effects resulting in unacceptable adverse effects.

Many other factors apart from the drug itself affect respiratory activity, so the effect that a drug exerts on the respiration of an individual patient is complex and unpredictable. For example, in a healthy patient recovering from surgery under general anaesthesia, pain, anxiety, stress and changes in blood chemistry will be stimulating breathing, whereas sedation, sleep and residual anaesthetic or analgesic agents will all be tending to depress respiration.

Respiratory depressants

Any drug that depresses CNS activity may depress respiration, either individually or in combination with other CNS depressants such as alcohol. Almost all general anaesthetic agents reduce ventilation in a dose-dependent fashion and are described in detail on page 297. Two specific groups of drugs that have well-documented depressant effects on ventilation are opioid analgesics and benzodiazepines.

Opioids.[98,99] Figure 5.4 shows that both μ- and δ-opioid receptors are present in the respiratory centre. As indicated above, the role of these receptors in normal respiratory control is unknown. Some recent animal work suggests that μ-receptors may be involved in normal respiratory control. A study involving mice lacking the gene for the μ-opioid receptors found an increased resting ventilation and a complete resistance to the respiratory effects of morphine in those mice with no μ-receptors.[100] In humans, the evidence is less clear. In healthy subjects, administration of the non-specific opioid receptor antagonist naloxone has no effect on respiration,[98] although in some patients with respiratory disease naloxone does stimulate ventilation.[97]

Agonists of μ-opioid receptors, such as morphine, cause dose-dependent depression of respiration, normally characterised by a slow respiratory rate, but tidal volume is also commonly reduced. Female subjects show a greater susceptibility to the respiratory depression seen with opioids.[101] Ventilatory responses to hypoxia and hypercapnia are also severely impaired, removing the physiological safety mechanism for patients. Partial agonists at the μ-receptor, such as nalbuphine and buprenorphine, have a ceiling effect for their analgesic efficacy that is associated with a lesser effect on ventilation than with full agonists. Most of the analgesic effects of clinically used opioids are also mediated by the μ-receptor,

so the respiratory depressant effect of opioid drugs is inseparable from their therapeutic effect. Equi-analgesic doses of different opioids show similar degrees of respiratory depression but the speed of onset of the drug does affect the clinical pattern of respiratory depression that occurs. With rapidly acting opioids such as fentanyl, apnoea normally follows its intravenous administration, but when an equi-analgesic dose of the slower acting morphine is administered, apnoea is unusual because hypercapnia develops to counteract the respiratory depression.[102]

δ-Opioid receptors are normally present in the pontine respiratory group (see Figure 5.4) and stimulation of these receptors reduces ventilation by a decreasing respiratory rate. Thus opioid drugs with δ-receptor activity again depress respiration in parallel with their analgesic effects. σ-Opioid receptors may be respiratory stimulants, but these receptors are poorly understood. κ Receptors are believed to have no influence on respiratory control despite still having analgesic effects, so this receptor subgroup offers some hope, in the future, for opioid analgesia without respiratory depression.

Benzodiazepines. Benzodiazepines exert their effect by binding directly to $GABA_A$ receptors and increasing the inhibitory effect of endogenous GABA.[103] Figure 5.4 shows that GABA is involved in respiratory central pattern generation, so it is unsurprising that benzodiazepines affect respiration. Parenterally administered benzodiazepine drugs, such as midazolam or diazepam, cause a dose-dependent reduction in resting ventilation and reduce the ventilatory response to hypoxia[104] and hypercapnia.[98] The degree of respiratory impairment seen correlates well with their effect on consciousness. Reduced resting ventilation with midazolam can be reversed with the benzodiazepine antagonist flumazenil, though the responses to hypoxia and hypercapnia may still be abnormal despite the subjects no longer being sedated.[105,106] Unlike for opioids, the respiratory depressant effects of benzodiazepines seem to have a ceiling effect, with massive overdoses of these drugs rarely causing life-threatening respiratory depression unless other CNS depressants, commonly alcohol, are ingested simultaneously.[103]

Respiratory stimulants

Non-specific CNS stimulant drugs have existed for many years and, as part of their general stimulant effects, also increase respiratory drive. Early drugs of this type, such as nikethamide and almitrine, were used as respiratory stimulants[97] but at effective doses they had an unacceptably high incidence of CNS toxicity, such as headache, agitation, muscle spasms or convulsions.

Doxapram is the only currently used respiratory stimulant and seems to be more specific for respiratory stimulation than its predecessors, although it still has a high incidence of CNS side effects. Animal studies[107] and indirect evidence from humans[108] both indicate that doxapram stimulates the peripheral chemoreceptors to increase respiratory drive, this effect occurring at lower doses than those causing more generalised CNS stimulation. In healthy subjects, infusion of a standard dose of doxapram approximately doubles resting minute volume and also substantially increases the ventilatory responses to hypoxia and hypercapnia.[109,110] Despite this impressive action on respiratory control, when used to treat patients with type 2 ventilatory failure (page 365) generalised CNS stimulation undoubtedly contributes to the therapeutic effect by reversing the sedative effects of hypercapnia (page 328) and increasing the patient's perception of their breathlessness.[111]

METHODS FOR ASSESSMENT OF FACTORS IN CONTROL OF BREATHING

In assessing the control of breathing under ideal conditions, arterial blood gas tensions would be measured continuously. In practice, this is invasive and rapid measurements are impossible, so in almost all cases end-tidal gas concentrations are measured and converted to partial pressure. In normal healthy subjects with reasonable slow respiratory rates, these measurements will equate well to alveolar and therefore arterial tension, but this may not be the case in patients.

Sensitivity to carbon dioxide

A lack of ventilatory response to carbon dioxide may result from impaired function of the respiratory system anywhere between the medullary neurones and the mechanical properties of the lung (see Figure 27.2). Thus it cannot be assumed that a decreased ventilation/PCO_2 response is necessarily due to failure of central chemoreceptor mechanism.

Steady-state method. This technique requires the simultaneous measurement of minute volume and PCO_2 after PCO_2 has been raised by increasing the concentration of carbon dioxide in the inspired gas. The ventilation is usually reasonably stable after 5 minutes of inhaling a fixed concentration of carbon dioxide. Severinghaus's pseudo steady-state method[112] measures ventilation after 4 minutes and is a useful compromise, giving highly repeatable results.[57] Several points are needed to define the PCO_2/ventilation response curve and it is a time-consuming process, which may be distressing to some patients.

Rebreathing method. Introduced by Read in 1967, this technique greatly simplified determination of the slope of the PCO_2/ventilation response curve.[113] The subject rebreathes for up to 4 minutes from a 6-l bag originally containing 7% carbon dioxide and about 50% oxygen, the remainder being nitrogen. The carbon dioxide concentration rises steadily during rebreathing, but the oxygen concentration should remain above 30%. Thus there should be no appreciable hypoxic drive and ventilation is driven solely by the rising arterial PCO_2, which should be very close to the PCO_2 of the gas in the bag. Ventilation is measured by any convenient means and plotted against the PCO_2 of the gas in the bag. An automated technique may be used by which the PCO_2/ventilation response curve is automatically determined and presented on an X-Y plotter.[114]

The PCO_2/ventilation response curve measured by the rebreathing technique is displaced to the right by about 0.7 kPa (5 mmHg) compared with the steady-state method, but the slope agrees closely with the steady-state method.[57,113]

Sensitivity to hypoxia

There is often some reluctance to test sensitivity to hypoxia because of the reduction in PO_2 to which the patient is exposed. Various approaches to the problem have been described, of which three are used (albeit rarely) in practice.

Steady-state method. This is the classic technique and is best undertaken by preparing PCO_2/ventilation response curves at different levels of PO_2, which are presented as a fan (see Figure 5.5). The spread of the fan is an indication of peripheral chemoreceptor sensitivity but it is also possible to present the data in the form of a rectangular hyperbola (see Figure 5.8) by plotting the ventilatory response for different values of PO_2 at the same PCO_2 (intercepts of components of the fan with a vertical line drawn through a particular value of PCO_2). The parameters of the hyperbola may then be derived as outlined above. A minimum of 5 minutes is required to reach a steady state for PCO_2 although it is possible to speed up the process by varying PO_2 while keeping PCO_2 constant. Nevertheless, it is a laborious undertaking to determine the oxygen response by these methods and patients may be distressed, particularly by the run at low PO_2 and high PCO_2.

Rebreathing method. Read's rebreathing method is described above and has been adapted to measure the response to hypoxia.[84] The oxygen concentration of the rebreathed gas is reduced by the oxygen consumption of the subject, but active steps have to be taken to maintain the PCO_2 at a constant level. Calculation of the response is greatly simplified by measuring the oxygen saturation (usually non-invasively by means of a pulse oximeter) and plotting the response as ventilation against saturation. This normally approximates to a straight line and the slope is a function of the chemoreceptor sensitivity. However, even if $P\text{CO}_2$ is held constant, the response is directly influenced by the patient's sensitivity to $P\text{CO}_2$.

Intermittent inhalation of high oxygen concentration. This method avoids exposing subjects to hypoxia. Temporary withdrawal of peripheral chemoreceptor drive by inhalation of oxygen should reduce ventilation by about 15%. This may be used as an indication of the existence of carotid body activity but clearly it is much less sensitive than the steady-state method.

REFERENCES

1. Blanco CE. Maturation of fetal breathing activity. *Biol Neonate* 1994; **65**: 182–8.
2. Bianchi AL, Denavit-Saubie M, Champagnat J. Central control of breathing in mammals: neuronal circuitry, membrane properties and neurotransmitters. *Physiol Rev* 1995; **75**: 1–31.
3. Gozal D, Hathout GM, Konrad AT, *et al.* Localization of putative neural respiratory regions in the human by functional magnetic resonance imaging. *J Appl Physiol* 1994; **76**: 2076–83.
4. Corfield DR, Fink GR, Ramsay SC, *et al.* Evidence for limbic system activation during CO_2-stimulated breathing in man. *J Physiol* 1995; **488**: 77–84.
*5. Richter DW, Ballanyi K, Schwarzacher S. Mechanisms of respiratory rhythm generation. *Curr Opin Neurobiol* 1992: **2**; 788–93.
6. Speck DF, Beck ER. Respiratory rhythmicity after extensive lesions of the dorsal and ventral respiratory groups in the decerebrate cat. *Brain Res* 1989; **482**: 387–92.
7. Bonham AC. Neurotransmitters in the CNS control of breathing. *Respir Physiol* 1995: **101**; 219–30.
*8. Ramirez JM, Telgkamp P, Elsen FP, Quellmalz UJA, Richter DW. Respiratory rhythm generation in mammals: synaptic and membrane properties. *Respir Physiol* 1997; **110**: 71–85.
9. Richter DW, Lalley PM, Pierrefiche O, *et al.* Intracellular signal pathways controlling respiratory neurons. *Respir Physiol* 1997; **110**: 113–23.
10. Horn EM, Waldrop TG. Suprapontine control of respiration. *Respir Physiol* 1998; **114**: 201–11.
11. Corfield DR, Murphy K, Guz A. Does the motor cortical control of the diaphram 'bypass' the brain stem respiratory centres in man? *Respir Physiol* 1998; **114**: 109–17.
12. Hanks EC, Ngai SH, Fink BR. The respiratory threshold for carbon dioxide in anesthetized man. *Anesthesiol* 1961; **22**: 393–7.
13. Western PJ, Patrick JM. Effects of focussing attention on breathing with and without apparatus on the face. *Respir Physiol* 1988: **72**; 123–30.
14. Winkworth AL, Davis PJ, Adams RD, Ellis E. Breathing patterns during spontaneous speech. *J Speech Hear Res* 1995: **38**; 124–44.
15. Winkworth AL, Davis PJ, Ellis E, Adams RD. Variability and consistency in speech breathing during reading: lung volumes, speech intensity and linguistic factors. *J Speech Hear Res* 1994; **37**: 535–6.
16. Severinghaus JW, Mitchell RA. Ondine's curse: failure of respiratory centre automaticity while asleep. *Clin Res* 1962; **10**: 122.
17. Vingerhoets F, Bogousslavsky J. Respiratory dysfunction in stroke. *Clin Chest Med* 1994; **15**: 729–37.
18. Commare MC, Francois B, Estournet B, Barois A. Ondine's curse: a discussion of five cases. *Neuropediatrics* 1993; **24**: 313–18.
19. Weese-Mayer DE, Silvestri JM, Menzies LJ, Morrow-Kenny AS, Hunt CE, Hauptman SA. Congenital central hypoventilation syndrome: diagnosis, management and long-term outcome in thirty-two children. *J Pediatr* 1992; **120**: 381–7.
20. Silvestri JM, Weese-Mayer DE, Flanagan EA. Congenital central hypoventilation syndrome: cardiorespiratory responses to moderate exercise, simulating daily activity. *Pediatr Pulmonol* 1995; **20**: 89–93.
21. Woo MS, Woo MA, Gozal D, Jansen MT, Keens TG, Harper RM. Heart rate variability in congenital central hypoventilation syndrome. *Pediatr Res* 1992; **31**: 291–6.
*22. Widdicombe JG. Afferent receptors in the airways and cough. *Respir Physiol* 1998; **114**: 5–15.
23. Sant'Ambrogio G, Tsubone H, Sant'Ambrogio FB. Sensory information from the upper airway: role in the control of breathing. *Respir Physiol* 1995; **102**: 1–16.
24. Stockwell M, Lang S, Yip R, Zintel T, White C, Gallagher CG. Lack of importance of the superior laryngeal nerves in citric acid cough in humans. *J Appl Physiol* 1993; **75**: 613–17.
25. Higginbottam T, Jackson M, Woolman P, Lowry R, Wallwork J. The cough response to ultrasonically nebulised distilled water in heart-lung transplantion patients. *Am Rev Respir Dis* 1989; **140**: 58–61.
*26. Widdicombe J. Airway receptors. *Respir Physiol* 2001; **125**: 3–15.
27. Ullman E. About Hering and Breuer. In: Porter R, ed. *Breathing: Hering-Breuer Centenary Symposium.* Edinburgh: Churchill Livingstone, 1970: 3.
28. Gaudy JH. The Hering-Breuer reflex in man? *Br J Anaesth* 1991; **66**: 627–8.

29. Widdicombe JG. Respiratory reflexes in man and other mammalian species. *Clin Sci* 1961; **21**: 163–70.

30. Guz A, Noble MIM, Trenchard D, Cochrane HL, Makey AR. Studies on the vagus nerves in man: their role in respiratory and circulatory control. *Clin Sci* 1964; **27**: 293–304.

31. Gautier H, Bonora M, Gaudy JH. Breuer–Hering inflation reflex and breathing pattern in anaesthetized humans and cats. *J Appl Physiol* 1981; **51**: 1162–8.

32. Rabbette PS, Fletcher ME, Dezateux CA, Soriano-Brucher H, Stocks J. Hering–Breuer reflex and respiratory system compliance in the first year of life: a longitudinal study. *J Appl Physiol* 1994; **76**: 650–6.

33. Guz A, Noble MIM, Eisle JH, Trenchard D. The effect of lung deflation on breathing in man. *Clin Sci* 1971; **40**: 451–61.

34. Head H. On the regulation of respiration. *J Physiol (Lond)* 1889; **10**: 1–70.

35. Cross KW, Klaus M, Tooley WH, Weisser K. The response of the new-born baby to inflation of the lungs. *J Physiol (Lond)* 1960; 151: 551–65.

36. Bendixen HH, Smith GM, Mead J. Pattern of ventilation in young adults. *J Appl Physiol* 1964; **19**: 195–8.

*37. Paintal AS. Some recent advances in studies on J receptors. *Adv Exp Med Biol* 1995; **381**: 15–25.

38. Frazier DT, Revelette WR. Role of phrenic nerve afferents in the control of breathing. *J Appl Physiol* 1991; **70**: 491–6.

39. Kalia M, Senapati JM, Parida B, Panda A. Reflex increase in ventilation by muscle receptors with nonmedullated fibers (C-fibers). *J Appl Physiol* 1972; **32**: 189–93.

40. Bledsoe SW, Hornbein TF. Central chemosensors and the regulation of their chemical environment. In: Hornbein TF, ed. *Regulation of breathing, part I.* New York: Marcel Dekker, 1981.

41. Loeschcke HH. Central chemoreceptors. In: Pallot DJ, ed. *Control of respiration.* London: Croom Helm, 1983.

42. Cunningham DJC. The control system regulating breathing in man. *Q Rev Biophys* 1974; **6**: 433–83.

43. Schlafke ME, Pokorski M, See WR, Prill RK, Loeschcke HH. Chemosensitive neurons on the ventral medullary surface. *Bull Physio-Pathol Respir* 1975; **11**: 277.

44. Sato M, Severinghaus JW, Basbaum AI. Medullary CO_2 chemoreceptor neuron identification by c-fos immunochemistry. *FASEB J* 1991; **5**: A1120.

45. Fencl V, Miller TB, Pappenheimer JR. Studies on the respiratory response to disturbances of acid–base balance, with deductions concerning the ionic composition of cerebral interstitial fluid. *Am J Physiol* 1966; **210**: 459–72.

46. Dev NB, Loeschcke HH. Topography of the respiratory and circulatory responses to acetylcholine and nicotine of the ventral surface of the medulla oblongata. *Pflüger's Archiv* 1979; **379**: 19–27.

47. Dempsey JA, Forster HV, DOPico GA. Ventilatory acclimatization to moderate hypoxaemia in man. *J Clin Invest* 1974; **53**: 1091–100.

48. Forster HV, Dempsey JA, Chosy LW. Incomplete compensation of CSF [H^+] in man during acclimatization to high altitude. *J Appl Physiol* 1975; **38**: 1067–72.

49. Semple SLG. Respiration and the cerebrospinal fluid. *Br J Anaesth* 1965; **37**: 262–7.

50. Christensen MS. Acid-base changes in cerebrospinal fluid and blood and blood volume changes, following prolonged hyperventilation in man. *Br J Anaesth* 1974; **46**: 348–57.

51. Hornbein TF, Pavlin EG. Distribution of H^+ and HCO_3^- between CSF and blood during respiratory alkalosis in dogs. *Am J Physiol* 1975; **228**: 1149–54.

52. Mitchell RA, Carman CT, Severinghaus JW, Richardson BW, Singer MM, Snider S. Stability of cerebrospinal fluid pH in chronic acid–base disturbances in blood. *J Appl Physiol* 1965; **20**: 443–52.

53. Froman C, Crampton-Smith A. Hyperventilation associated with low pH of cerebrospinal fluid after intracranial haemorrhage. *Lancet* 1966; **1**: 780–2.

54. Froman C. Correction of cerebrospinal fluid metabolic acidosis by intrathecal injection of bicarbonate. *Br J Anaesth* 1966; **39**: 90.

55. Spengler CM, Czeisler CA, Shea SA. An endogenous circadian rhythm of respiratory control in humans. *J Physiol* 2000; **526**: 683–94.

*56. Mohan R, Duffin J. The effect of hypoxia on the ventilatory resonse to carbon dioxide in man. *Respir Physiol* 1997; **108**: 101–15.

57. Lumb AB, Nunn JF. Ribcage contributions to CO_2 response during rebreathing and steady state methods. *Respir Physiol* 1991; **85**: 97–110.

58. Tansley JG, Pedersen MEF, Clar C, Robbins PA. Human ventilatory response to 8 h of euoxic hypercapnia. *J Appl Physiol* 1998; **84**: 431–4.

59. de Castro F. Sur la structure et l'innervation de la glande intercarotidienne. *Trab Lab Invest Biol Univ Madrid* 1926; **26**: 365.

60. Heymans C, Bouckaert JJ, Dautrebande L. Sinus carotidien et réflexes respiratoire. *Arch Int Pharmacodyn Ther* 1930; **39**: 400.

61. Ponte J, Purves MJ. Frequency response of carotid body chemoreceptors in the cat to changes of PaO_2, $PaCO_2$ and pH_a. *J Appl Physiol* 1974; **37**: 635–47.

62. Petersen ES, Vejby-Christenson H. Effects of body temperature on ventilatory response to hypoxia and breathing pattern in man. *J Appl Physiol* 1977; **42**: 492–500.

*63. Prabhakar NR. Oxygen sensing by the carotid body chemoreceptors. *J Appl Physiol* 2000; **88**: 2287–95.

64. Biscoe TJ, Duchen MR. Cellular basis of transduction in carotid chemoreceptors. *Am J Physiol* 1990; **258**: L271–L278.

65. Acker H. Cellular oxygen sensors. *Ann N Y Acad Sci* 1994; **718**: 3–10.

66. Ward DS, Bellville JW. Reduction of hypoxic ventilatory drive by dopamine. *Anesth Analg* 1982; **61**: 333–7.

67. Delpierre S, Fornaris M, Guillot C, Grimaud C. Increased ventilatory chemosensitivity induced by domperidone, a dopamine antagonist, in healthy humans. *Bull Eur Physiopath Respir* 1987; **23**: 31–5.

68. Foo IT, Warren PM, Drummond GB. Influence of oral clonidine on the ventilatory response to acute and sustained isocapnic hypoxia in human males. *Br J Anaesth* 1996; **76**: 214–20.

69. Powell FL, Milsom WK, Mitchell GS. Time domains of the hypoxic ventilatory response. *Respir Physiol* 1998; **112**: 123–34.

70. Huang SY, Alexander JK, Grover RF, *et al.* Hypocapnia and sustained hypoxia blunt ventilation on arrival at high altitude. *J Appl Physiol* 1984; **56**: 602–6.

71. Easton PA, Slykerman LJ, Anthonisen NR. Ventilatory response to sustained hypoxia in normal adults. *J Appl Physiol* 1986; **61**: 906–11.

72. Howard LSGE, Robbins PA. Ventilatory response to 8 h of isocapnic and poikilocapnic hypoxia in humans. *J Appl Physiol* 1995; **78**: 1092–7.

73. Sahn SA, Zwillich CW, Dick N, McCullough RE, Lakshminarayan S, Weil JV. Variability of ventilatory responses to hypoxia and hypercapnia. *J Appl Physiol* 1977; **43**: 1019–25.

74. White DP, Douglas NJ, Picket CK, Weil JV, Zwillich CW. Sexual influence on the control of breathing. *J Appl Physiol* 1983; **54**: 874–9.

75. Robbins PA. Hypoxic ventilatory decline: site of action. *J Appl Physiol* 1995; **78**: 373–4.

76. Garcia N, Hopkins SR, Elliott AR, Aaron EA, Weinger MB, Powell FL. Ventilatory response to 2-h sustained hypoxia in humans. *Respir Physiol* 2000; **124**: 11–22.

77. Kagawa S, Stafford MJ, Waggener TB, Severinghaus JW. No effect of naloxone on hypoxia-induced ventilatory depression in adults. *J Appl Physiol* 1982; **52**: 1030–4.

78. Soto-Arape I, Burton MD, Kazemi H. Central amino acid neurotransmitters and the hypoxic ventilatory response. *Am J Respir Crit Care Med* 1995; **151**: 1113–20.

79. Cruz JC, Reeves JT, Grover RF, *et al.* Ventilatory acclimatization to high altitude is prevented by CO_2 breathing. *Respiration* 1980; **39**: 121–30.

80. Weil JVW, Byrne-Quinn E, Sodal IE, Filley GF, Grover RF Acquired attenuation of chemoreceptor function in chronically hypoxic man at high altitude. *J Clin Invest* 1971; **50**: 186–95.

81. Weil JV, Byrne-Quinn E, Sodal IE, *et al.* Hypoxic ventilatory drive in normal man. *J Clin Invest* 1970; **49**: 1061–72.

82. Dripps RD, Comroe JH. The effect of the inhalation of high and low oxygen concentrations on respiration, pulse rate, ballistocardiogram and arterial oxygen saturation (oximeter) of normal individuals. *Am J Physiol* 1947; **149**: 277–91.

83. Cormack RS, Cunningham DJC, Gee JBL. The effect of carbon dioxide on the respiratory response to want of oxygen in man. *Q J Exp Physiol* 1957; **42**: 303–16.

84. Rebuck AS, Campbell EJM. A clinical method for assessing the ventilatory response to hypoxia. *Am Rev Respir Dis* 1974; **109**: 345–50.

*85. Timmers HJLM, Wieling W, Karemaker JM, Lenders JWM. Denervation of carotid and baro-chemoreceptors in humans. *J Physiol* 2003; **553**: 3–11.

86. Wade JG, Larson CP, Hickey RF, Ehrenfeld WK, Severinghaus JW. Effect of carotid endarterectomy on carotid chemoreceptor and baroreceptor function in man. *N Engl J Med* 1970; **282**: 823–9.

87. Vanmaele RG, De Backer WA, Willeman MJ, *et al.* Hypoxic ventilatory response to carotid endarterectomy. *Eur J Vasc Surg* 1992; **6**: 241–4.

88. Vanmaele RG, De Leersnijder, Bal J, Van Kerkhoven W, Bongaerts P, Vaerenberg C. One year follow-up after bilateral carotid body resection for COPD. *Eur J Respir Dis* 1983; **64** (Supp 126): 470.

89. Edelman NH, Neubauer JA. Hypoxic depression of breathing. In: Crystal RG, West JB, eds. *The lung, scientific foundations*. New York: Raven, 1991; 1341.

90. Weil JVW, Byrne-Quinn E, Sodal IE, Kline JS, McCullough RE, Filley GF. Augmentation of chemosensitivity during mild exercise in normal man. *J Appl Physiol* 1972; **33**: 813–19.

91. Davidson JT, Whipp BJ, Wasserman K, Koyal SN, Lugliani R. Role of carotid bodies in breath holding. *N Engl J Med* 1974; **290**: 819–22.

92. Grassi B, Ferretti G, Costa M, *et al.* Ventilatory responses to hypercapnia and hypoxia in elite breath-hold divers. *Respir Physiol* 1994; **97**: 323–32.

93. Guz A, Noble MIM, Widdicombe JG, Trenchard D, Mushin WW, Makey AR. The role of the vagal and glossopharyngeal afferent nerves in respiratory sensation, control of breathing and arterial pressure regulation in conscious man. *Clin Sci* 1966; **30**: 161–70.

94. Campbell EJM, Freedman S, Clark TJH, Robson JG, Norman J. The effect of muscular paralysis induced by tubocurarine on the duration and sensation of breath holding. *Clin Sci* 1967; **32**: 425–32.

95. Campbell EJM, Godfrey S, Clark TJH, Freedman S, Norman J. The effect of muscular paralysis induced by tubocurarine on the duration and sensation of

breath holding during hypercapnia. *Clin Sci* 1969; **36**: 323–8.

96. Fowler WS. Breaking point of breath-holding. *J Appl Physiol* 1954; **6**: 539–45.

97. Casaburi R. Pharmacological modulators of respiratory control. *Monaldi Arch Chest Dis* 1998; **53**: 287–93.

98. Shook J, Watkins WD, Camporesi EM. Differential roles of opioid receptors in respiration, respiratory disease and opiate-induced respiratory depression. *Am Rev Respir Dis* 1990; **142**: 895–909.

*99. Dahan A, Teppema LJ. Influence of anaesthesia and analgesia on the control of breathing. *Br J Anaesth* 2003; **91**: 40–9.

100. Forster A, Gardaz J-P, Suter P, Gemperie M. Respiratory depression by midazolam and diazepam. *Anesthesiology* 1980; **53**: 494–7.

101. Sarton E, Teppema L, Dahan A. Sex differences in morphine-induced ventilatory depression reside within the peripheral chemoreflex loop. *Anesthesiology* 1999; **90**: 1329–38.

102. Gross JB. When you breathe in you inspire, when you don't breathe, you . . . expire. *Anesthesiol* 2003; **99**: 767–70.

103. Charney DS, Mihic SJ, Harris RA. Hypnotics and sedatives. In: Hardman JG, Limbird LE, Goodman Gilman A, eds. *Goodman and Gilman's the pharmacological basis of therapeutics*. New York: McGraw-Hill, 2001.

104. Alexander CM, Gross JB. Sedative doses of midazolam depress hypoxic ventilatory response in humans. *Anesth Analg* 1988; **67**: 377–82.

105. Gross JB, Weller RS, Conard P. Flumazenil antagonism of midazolam-induced ventilatory depression. *Anesthesiology* 1991; **75**: 179–85.

106. Gross JB, Blouin RT, Zandsberg S, Conard PF, Häussler J. Effect of flumazenil on ventilatory drive during sedation with midazolam and alfentanil. *Anesthesiology* 1996; **85**: 713–20.

107. Mitchell RA, Herbert DA. Potencies of doxapram and hypoxia in stimulating carotid-body chemoreceptors and ventilation in anaesthetised cats. *Anesthesiology* 1975; **42**: 559–66.

108. Scott RM, Whitwam JG, Chakrabarti MK. Evidence of a role for the peripheral chemoreceptors in the ventilatory response to doxapram in man. *Br J Anaesth* 1977; **49**: 227–31.

109. Calverley PMA, Robson RH, Wraith PK, Prescott LF, Flenley DC. The ventilatory effects of doxapram in normal man. *Clin Sci* 1983; **65**: 65–9.

110. Burki NK. Ventilatory effects of doxapram in conscious human subjects. *Chest* 1984; **85**: 600–4.

111. Ebihara S, Ogawa H, Sasaki H, Hida W, Kikuchi Y. Doxapram and perception of dyspnea. *Chest* 2002; **121**: 1380–1.

112. Severinghaus JW. Proposed standard determination of ventilatory responses to hypoxia and hypercapnia in man. *Chest* 1976; **70**: 129s.

113. Read DJC. A clinical method for assessing the ventilatory response to carbon dioxide. *Australas Ann Med* 1967; **16**: 20–32.

114. Milledge JS, Minty KB, Duncalf D. On-line assessment of ventilatory response to carbon dioxide. *J Appl Physiol* 1974; **37**: 596–9.

KEY POINTS

- Pharyngeal and laryngeal muscles display both tonic and phasic contraction to maintain airway patency and to regulate air flow.
- The diaphragm, intercostals and some neck muscles bring about inspiration by a complex combination of actions, these varying with different postures.
- Expiration is normally passive, except during exercise or at minute volumes several times higher than normal, when intercostal and abdominal wall muscle contraction causes active expiration.
- The 'work of breathing' describes the power needed to overcome both the elastic recoil of the respiratory system and the non-elastic resistance to gas flow and is normally generated by the respiratory muscles used for inspiration.

Breathing consists of rhythmic changes in lung volume brought about by the medullary respiratory neurones described in Chapter 5. Several muscle groups are involved in effecting the change in lung volume. First, muscles of the pharynx and larynx control upper airway resistance; second, the diaphragm, ribcage, spine and neck muscles bring about inspiration; and finally, muscles of the abdominal wall, ribcage and spine are used when active expiration is required. Many of these muscle groups have common origins and attachments such that their activity is complex and dependent both on each other and on many non-respiratory factors, such as posture, locomotion and voluntary activity.

UPPER AIRWAY MUSCLES

During inspiration through the nose, the pressure in the pharynx must fall below atmospheric by an amount equal to the product of inspiratory gas flow rate and the flow resistance afforded by the nose (see Figure 4.1).

This development of only a few kilopascals of subatmospheric pressure in the pharynx tends to cause the pharynx to collapse.

Pharyngeal obstruction in response to these pressure changes during inspiration is opposed by reflex contraction of the pharyngeal dilator muscles during inspiration. The afferent side of the reflex arises from mechanoreceptors in the pharynx and larynx. These pressure receptors respond in a graded manner to subatmospheric pressure and have myelinated afferent fibres to facilitate a rapid response.[1,2] Based on the observation that the pharyngeal dilator reflex is less active during sleep (page 247), the reflex pathway is believed to involve higher centres of the brain.[3] Nevertheless, the reflex is extremely rapid, with both genioglossus[1] and tensor palati[4] electromyographic (EMG) activity increasing less than 50 ms after a negative pressure is applied to the pharynx. This compares with a reaction time for voluntary tongue movements of 190 ms.[1] The efferent side of the reflex involves most of the pharyngeal dilator muscles, which display tonic contraction and/or phasic inspiratory activity. Airway diameters are well maintained down to pressures of 1.5 kPa (15 cmH$_2$O) below atmospheric during active but not passive breathing manoeuvres.[5] Pulmonary stretch receptors may also contribute to the reflex as pharyngeal cross-sectional area correlates directly with lung volume.[6]

There is no significant narrowing of the airway when changing from the erect to the supine posture in the normal subject.[7] Genioglossus EMG activity is increased by 34% in the supine position, presumably to counteract the effect of gravity on the tongue.[8,9] Anatomical considerations suggest that patency of the nasopharynx in the supine position is maintained by tensor palati, palatoglossus and palatopharyngeus, and tonic but not phasic respiratory activity has been detected in levator palati.[10] Without contraction of these muscles the soft palate tends to fall back against the posterior pharyngeal wall in the supine position.

Failure of the various mechanisms that preserve pharyngeal airway patency may occur during sleep, hypoxia or anaesthesia; their occurrence and prevention are discussed in Chapters 16 and 22.

Laryngeal control of airway resistance. During quiet breathing, movement of the vocal folds is used as a choke for fine control of airway resistance.[11] On inspiration, phasic activity of the posterior cricoarytenoid muscles, acting by rotating the arytenoid cartilages, abducts the vocal cords to minimise resistance.[12] A greater effect occurs during expiration, when phasic electrical activity in the thyroarytenoid muscles indicates adduction of the vocal cords[13] and hence an increase in resistance. This may help to prevent collapse of the lower airways (page 44).

RESPIRATORY MUSCLES OF THE TRUNK

Nomenclature in this area can be confusing, with different authors using different terms. The trunk (referred to as the chest wall by some studies) may be divided into ribcage and abdomen. These two compartments are separated by the diaphragm and both are therefore greatly influenced by its activity.

The diaphragm

The diaphragm is a membranous muscle separating the abdominal cavity and chest and in adults has a total surface area[14] of approximately 900 cm^2. It is the most important inspiratory muscle, with motor innervation solely from the phrenic nerves (C3, 4, 5). In comparison with other skeletal muscles, the diaphragm is extremely active. Muscle fibres within the diaphragm can reduce their length by up to 40% between residual volume and total lung capacity,[14] and spend 45% of each day contracting, compared with only 14% for the soleus muscle.[15] The diaphragm has considerable reserve of function and unilateral phrenic block causes little decrement of overall ventilatory capacity. Despite the importance of the diaphragm to respiration, bilateral phrenic interruption is still compatible with good ventilatory function.[16]

Mechanics of diaphragmatic function. The origins of the crural part of the diaphragm are the lumbar vertebrae and the arcuate ligaments, whereas the costal parts arise from the lower ribs and xiphisternum. Both parts are inserted into the central tendon. Recent studies of human subjects using CT scans, illustrated in Figure 6.1, have enabled the *in vivo* actions of the diaphragm to be better defined.[14,17–19] Under normal circumstances, a zone of apposition exists around the outside of the diaphragm where it is in direct contact with the internal

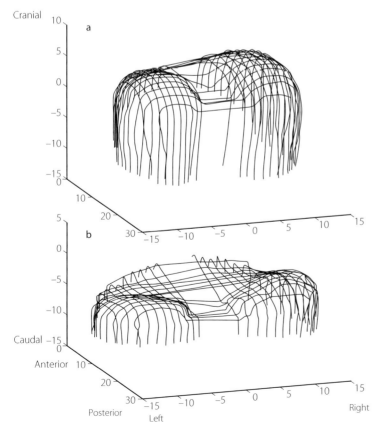

Figure 6.1 Three-dimensional reconstructions of the human diaphragm at functional residual capacity using fast computed tomography scanning (dimensions in cm). **(a)** Normal subject showing extensive zone of apposition and normal curvature of the diaphragm domes. **(b)** Patient with hyperinflated chest as a result of chronic obstructive pulmonary disease (page 380). Note the reduced zone of apposition and the flattened diaphragm domes. (Reproduced with permission from Cassart M, Pettiaux N, Gevenois PA et al. Effect of chronic hyperinflation on diaphragm length and surface area. *Am J Respir Crit Care Med* 1997; 156(2 pt 1): 504–8.)

a b c d

Figure 6.2 'Piston in a cylinder' analogy of the mechanisms of diaphragm actions on the lung volume. **(a)** Resting end-expiratory position. **(b)** Inspiration with pure piston-like behaviour. **(c)** Inspiration with pure non-piston-like behaviour. **(d)** Combination of piston-like and non-piston-like behaviour in an expanding cylinder, which equates most closely with inspiration *in vivo*. ZA, zone of apposition.

aspect of the ribcage, with no lung in between, but the parietal pleura still allowing free movement of the diaphragm. At upright FRC in humans, approximately 55% of the diaphragm surface area is in the zone of apposition.[14,17]

There are many ways by which diaphragm contraction may bring about an increase in lung volume[20] and these are illustrated schematically in Figure 6.2. They may be considered using a 'piston in a cylinder' analogy, the trunk representing the cylinder and the diaphragm the piston (Figure 6.2a). Figure 6.2b illustrates the first possible mechanism, involving downward movement of the diaphragm simply by shortening the zone of apposition around the whole cylinder and leaving the dome shape unchanged. This is a pure 'piston-like' action and has the advantage of very efficient conversion of diaphragm muscle fibre shortening into changes in lung volume. Figure 6.2c illustrates 'non-piston like' behaviour, in which the zone of apposition remains unchanged but an increase in the tension of the diaphragm dome reduces the curvature, so expanding the lung. In this situation, the diaphragm behaves like a bubble and Laplace's law dictates the change in transdiaphragmatic pressure (or lung volume) with changes in diaphragmatic tension. This is likely to be less efficient than piston-like behaviour because much of the muscle tension developed simply opposes the opposite side of the diaphragm rather than moving the diaphragm downwards, such that in theory, when the diaphragm becomes flat, further contraction will have no effect on lung volume. Finally, Figure 6.2d incorporates both types of behaviour already described but also now includes expansion of the lower ribcage that occurs with diaphragmatic contraction (known as 'piston in an expanding cylinder') and so represents a simple description of the *in vivo* situation.

In the supine position, diaphragm action is a combination of all the above mechanisms as well as a change in shape involving a tilting and flattening of the diaphragm in the anteroposterior direction.[14]

Ribcage muscles[21]

As already described, the ribcage may be regarded as a cylinder with length governed primarily by the diaphragm and secondarily by flexion and extension of the spine. The cross-sectional area of the cylinder is governed by movement of the ribs. This movement involves mainly rotation of the neck of the rib about the axis of the costovertebral joints and their shape is such that elevation of the ribs in this way increases both the lateral and anteroposterior diameter of the ribcage.[22] Elevation of the ribs by the intercostal muscles tends to result in a 'bucket-handle' action, whereas elevation of the anterior ribcage by, for example, the sternomastoid muscle elevating the sternum results in a 'pump-handle' type of movement. These two actions tend to occur together and depend also on other requirements, such as posture and upper limb movements. Upper ribs are inserted into the sternum and do not necessarily behave in quite the same way as the lower 'floating' ribs, which are inserted into the more flexible costal cartilage.

The intercostal muscles are divided into the external group (deficient anteriorly), the less powerful internal group (deficient posteriorly) and the feeble strands of intercostalis intima. The internal intercostal muscles of the upper ribcage become thicker anteriorly, where they are known as the parasternal intercostal muscles. In 1749, mechanical considerations led Hamberger to suggest that the external intercostals were primarily inspiratory and the internal intercostals primarily expiratory.[23] Though an oversimplification,[22] this has generally been confirmed by electromyography. The parasternal portion of the internal intercostals is inspiratory in both humans and animals[24] and the inspiratory activity of external intercostals, though minimal during quiet breathing,[21] becomes increasingly important during stimulated breathing. Posture plays an important role in intercostal activity in humans. For example, during the rather extreme postural challenge of rotating the trunk, which changes the mechanical properties of the ribs, the respiratory activity of internal and external intercostals is reversed, with internal intercostals becoming expiratory and vice versa.[25]

Scalene muscles are active in inspiration during quiet breathing in humans,[24] particularly when upright. Their role is to elevate the ribcage and this counteracts the tendency of the diaphragm to cause inward displacement of the upper ribs. Innervation is from C1 to C5.

Accessory muscles. These are silent in normal breathing in humans but as ventilation increases, the inspiratory muscles contract more vigorously and accessory muscles are recruited. Considerable hyperventilation (about 50 $l.min^{-1}$) or severe increases in respiratory loading are usually present before the accessory muscles become active. Accessory muscles include the sternocleidomastoids, extensors of the vertebral column, pectoralis minor, trapezius and the serrati muscles. Many of these muscles, for example the pectorals, reverse their usual origin/insertion and help to expand the chest, provided the arms and shoulder girdle are fixed by grasping a suitable support.

Abdominal muscles

With the exception of gas within the bowel lumen, the abdomen is an incompressible volume held between the diaphragm and the abdominal muscles. Contraction of either will cause a corresponding passive displacement of the other. Thus abdominal muscles are generally expiratory.

Rectus abdominis, external oblique, internal oblique and tranversalis muscles are the most important expiratory muscles, whereas the muscles of the pelvic floor have a supportive role. Contraction of this muscle group results in an increase in abdominal pressure, displacing the diaphragm in a cephalad direction. In addition, their insertion into the costal margin results in a caudad movement of the ribcage, so assisting expiration by opposing the ribcage muscles. External obliques are usually monitored as an indication of expiratory muscle activity, but gastric pressure is a valuable index of their activity because they cannot contract without causing an increase in intraabdominal pressure.

In the supine position, the abdominal muscles are normally inactive during quiet breathing and become active only when the minute volume exceeds about 40 $l.min^{-1}$, in the face of substantial expiratory resistance, during phonation or when making expulsive efforts. When upright, their use in breathing is complicated by their role in the maintenance of posture.

INTEGRATION OF RESPIRATORY MUSCLE ACTIVITY[22]

Breathing

Figure 6.3 shows the radiographic appearance of the ribcage at residual volume, the normal expiratory level and at maximal inspiration, and illustrates the enormous range of movement within the semi-rigid ribcage. Expiration normally proceeds passively to the functional residual capacity (FRC), which may be considered as the equilibrium position governed by the balance of elastic forces, unless modified by residual end-expiratory tone in certain muscle groups. Inspiration is the active phase, entering the inspiratory capacity but normally leaving a substantial volume unused (the inspiratory reserve volume). Similarly, there is a substantial volume (the expiratory reserve volume) between FRC and the residual volume (see Figure 3.8). By voluntary effort it is possible to effect a satisfactory tidal exchange anywhere within the vital capacity, but the work of breathing is minimal at FRC.

Although we tend to think of the respiratory muscles individually, it is important to remember that they act together in an extraordinarily complex interaction that is influenced by factors including posture, minute volume, respiratory load, disease and anaesthesia. Figure 6.4 illustrates some features of this interaction.[25,26]

Inspiration. In Figure 6.4 it can be seen that the ribcage inspiratory muscles (external intercostals and scalenes)

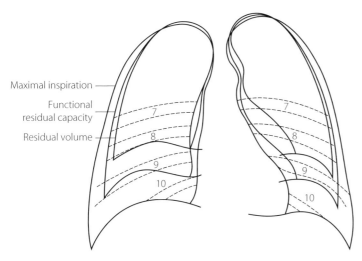

Figure 6.3 Outlines of chest radiographs of a normal subject at various levels of lung inflation. The numbers refer to ribs as seen in the position of maximal inspiration. (With thanks to Dr RL Marks, who was the subject.)

Maximal inspiration

Functional residual capacity

Residual volume

7

7

8

8

9

9

10

10

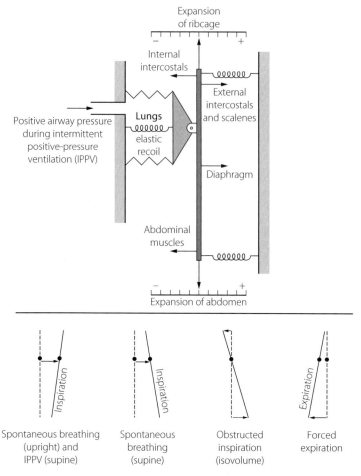

Figure 6.4 A model of the balance of static and dynamic forces acting on the respiratory system. The central bar, attached to the lungs, is floating freely, held in equilibrium by the elastic forces at the end-expiratory position as shown. It may be displaced by the actions of the various muscles shown, with movement to the right generally indicating inspiration and vice versa. Action of the various inspiratory or expiratory muscles causes changes, not only in the lung volume but also in the inclination of the bar, which represents relative changes in the cross-sectional area of the ribcage and abdomen. See text for details. (Derived from references 26 and 27.)

Spontaneous breathing (upright) and IPPV (supine)

Spontaneous breathing (supine)

Obstructed inspiration (isovolume)

Forced expiration

The broken line represents FRC

and diaphragm act in parallel to inflate the lungs, with posture affecting which muscle group is dominant (see below). In either position, diaphragm activity alone results in a widening of the lower ribcage and an indrawing of the upper ribcage (often seen with spontaneous respiration during general anaesthesia), which must be countered by the intercostal and neck muscles contracting simultaneously.

Expiration requires no muscular activity during quiet breathing in the supine position, because the elastic recoil of the lungs provides the energy required, aided by the weight of the abdominal contents pushing the diaphragm in a cephalad direction. In the upright posture and during stimulated ventilation the internal intercostal muscles and the abdominal wall muscles are active in returning the ribcage and diaphragm to the resting position. In extreme hyperventilation, for example following exercise, the expiratory muscles become progressively

more important until ventilation assumes a quasi sine-wave push–pull pattern.

Separation of volume contributions of ribcage and abdomen

Konno and Mead originally proposed that the separate contributions to tidal volume of changes in ribcage (RC) and abdominal (AB) compartments could be measured.[28] Essentially similar results may be obtained by measuring either anteroposterior distance (magnetometers), circumference (strain gauge) or cross-sectional area (respiratory inductance plethysmography, RIP[29]). Once initially calibrated to convert measurements of trunk dimensions into volumes, the sum of RC and AB movements correlates well with tidal volume and provides an excellent non-invasive measure of ventilation. RC/(RC + AB) indicates the proportion of tidal volume that can be attributed to expansion of the ribcage (usually expressed

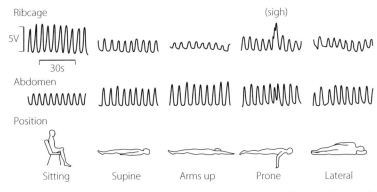

Ribcage

(sigh)

Abdomen

Position

Sitting   Supine   Arms up   Prone   Lateral

Figure 6.5 Normal respiratory inductance plethysmography (RIP) traces. The amplitude (in volts) of the RIP signal reflects the cross-sectional area of the ribcage (RC) and abdomen (AB). The sum of the RC and AB signals correlates closely with tidal volume. The figure shows normal breathing in five different positions, demonstrating the predominantly RC contribution when upright and AB contribution in all horizontal positions. Note the spontaneous sigh occurring in the prone position, resulting entirely from ribcage expansion. (Reproduced with permission from Lumb AB, Nunn JF. Respiratory function and ribcage contribution to ventilation in body positions commonly used during anaesthesia. *Anesth Analg* 1991; **73**: 422–6.)

as %RC). However, such is the complexity of the muscular system described above that changes in %RC cannot be attributed to changes in the force of contraction of any particular muscle. Figure 6.5 shows RIP traces during normal breathing in different positions.

Effect of posture on respiratory muscles

Upright posture, whether standing or sitting, is associated with greater expansion of the ribcage[30] such that %RC is around 67% (see Figure 6.5). To account for this, increased EMG activity has been demonstrated in the scalene muscles[31] and the parasternal intercostals,[32] and probably therefore also occurs in the external intercostals.

Supine position. When supine, the weight of the abdominal contents pushes the diaphragm upwards, so that in the supine position the diaphragm tends to lie some 4 cm higher, which accords with the reduction in FRC when supine (see Figure 3.9). With the diaphragm higher in the chest, its fibre length is greater and it can therefore contract more effectively, counteracting the tendency to airway closure at the reduced FRC. The dimensions of the ribcage are probably little altered and the increased diaphragm activity therefore results in a reduced %RC of about 33% in the supine position.[30] In the prone and lateral positions, RC contribution does not differ significantly from that in the supine position (see Figure 6.5).[30]

Lateral position. In this position (Figure 6.6) only the lower dome of the diaphragm is pushed higher into the chest by the weight of the abdominal contents,

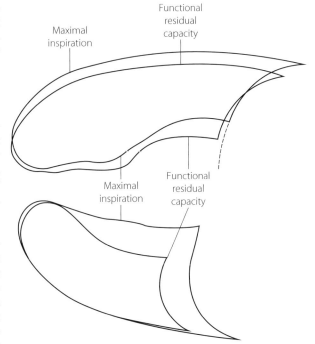

Figure 6.6 Radiographic outlines of the lungs at two levels of lung volume in a conscious subject during spontaneous breathing in the lateral position (right side down). This is the same subject as in Figure 6.3: comparison will show that, in the lateral position at FRC, the lower lung is close to residual volume whereas the upper lung is close to inspiratory capacity. The diaphragm therefore lies much more cephalad in the lower half of the chest. Both these factors contribute to the greater volume changes that occur in the lower lung during inspiration.

whereas the upper dome is flattened. It follows that the lower dome can contract more effectively than the upper, and the ventilation of the lower lung is about twice that of the upper. This is fortunate since gravity causes a preferential perfusion of the lower lung (page 114). As in other horizontal positions, abdominal expansion is predominant in the lateral position (see Figure 6.5).

Chemoreceptor activation

In animals, clear differences have been demonstrated in the respiratory muscle response to hyperventilation induced by either hypoxia or hypercapnia.[33] For an equivalent minute volume, hypoxia stimulates mostly inspiratory muscles, whereas hypercapnia stimulates both inspiratory and expiratory groups. Similar responses occur in humans, with diaphragm EMG activity increasing in response to both hypercapnia and hypoxia, but more rapidly in the latter, and expiratory muscle activity increasing almost exclusively during hypercapnic hyperventilation.[31,34] Hyperventilation in response to hypercapnia in the supine position results in a small increase in RC contribution (0.13% per kPa P_{CO_2} or 1% per mmHg P_{CO_2}).[35]

NEURONAL CONTROL OF RESPIRATORY MUSCLES

The respiratory muscles, in common with other skeletal muscles, have their tension controlled by a servo mechanism mediated by muscle spindles. They appear to play a more important role in the intercostal muscles than in the diaphragm, and there was some doubt about the existence of spindles in the human diaphragm until a small number were demonstrated.[36] Their function is largely inferred from knowledge of their well-established role in other skeletal muscles not concerned with respiration.

Two types of cell can be distinguished in the motor neurone pool of the anterior horn cell. The alpha motor neurone has a thick efferent fibre (12–20 μm diameter) and passes in the ventral root directly to the neuromuscular junction of the muscle fibre (Figure 6.7a). The gamma motor neurone has a thin efferent fibre (2–8 μm), which also passes in the ventral root but terminates in the intrafusal fibres of the muscle spindle. Contraction of the intrafusal fibres alone (without overall shortening of the muscle) increases the tension in the central part of the spindle (the nuclear bag), causing stimulation of the annulospiral endings. Impulses so generated are then transmitted via fibres that lie in the dorsal root to reach the anterior horn where they have an excitatory effect on the alpha motor neurones. Using this system, an efferent impulse transmitted by the gamma system causes reflex contraction of the main muscle mass by means of an arc through the annulospiral afferent and the alpha motor neurone. Thus contrac-

tion of the whole muscle may be controlled entirely by efferents travelling in the gamma fibres, and this is believed to occur in relation to breathing.[37]

Alternatively, muscle contraction may in the first instance result from discharge of both the alpha and gamma motor neurones. If shortening of the muscle is unopposed, main (extrafusal) and intrafusal fibres will contract together and the tension in the nuclear bag of the spindle will be unchanged. If, however, the shortening of the muscle is opposed, the intrafusal fibres will shorten more than the extrafusal fibres, causing the nuclear bag to be stretched (Figure 6.7b). The consequent stimulation of the annulospiral endings results in afferent activity that raises the excitatory state of the motor neurones, causing the main muscle fibres to increase their tension until the resistance is overcome, allowing the muscle to shorten and the tension in the nuclear bag of the spindle to be reduced (Figure 6.7c).

By this mechanism, fine control of muscle contraction is possible. The message from the upper motor neurone is in the form: 'muscles should contract with whatever force may be found necessary to effect such and such a shortening' and not simply: 'muscles should contract with such and such a force'. The former message is typical of input into a servo system and far more satisfactory when the load is not known in advance.

For respiratory muscles, a servo system is very advantageous. The message conveyed by the efferent tract from the inspiratory neurones of the medulla would be in the form: 'inspiratory muscles should contract with whatever force may be necessary to effect such and such a change in length (corresponding to a certain tidal volume)' and not simply: 'inspiratory muscles should contract with such and such a force'. A servo system also provides an excellent mechanism for rapid response to sudden changes in airway resistance. The nature and magnitude of the response of the inspiratory muscles to added resistance to breathing are described in Chapter 4 and the immediate effectiveness of the response is easily explicable in terms of muscle spindles.

Neuronal firing patterns[38]

Respiratory muscles are also similar to other skeletal muscle with respect to the action potential (AP) patterns in their motor neurones. The tension generated in a muscle is directly related to the frequency of APs in the motor nerve. Even in supine resting subjects, nerves supplying the parasternal intercostals display a continuous 'train' of APs at a frequency of 8 Hz during expiration, increasing to 12 Hz during inspiration. Occasionally superimposed on this pattern are 'doublets' of APs, which are pairs of APs only 8 ms apart. In non-respiratory muscle, doublets are believed to cause a sudden step increase in muscle tension, but their role in

a
Relaxed position

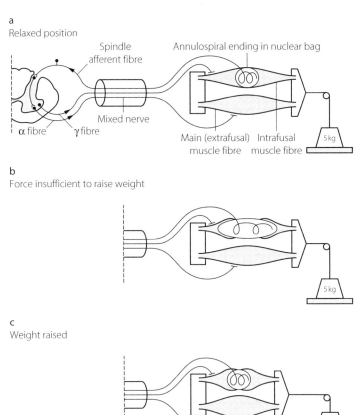

b
Force insufficient to raise weight

c
Weight raised

Figure 6.7 Diagrammatic representation of the servo mechanism mediated by the muscle spindles. **(a)** The resting state with muscle and intrafusal fibres of spindle relaxed. **(b)** The muscle is attempting to lift the weight following discharge of both alpha and gamma systems. The force developed by the muscle is insufficient: the weight is not lifted and the muscle cannot shorten. However, the intrafusal fibres are able to shorten and stretch the annulospiral endings in the nuclear bag of the spindle. Afferent discharge causes increased excitation of the motor neurone pool in the anterior horn. **(c)** Alpha discharge is augmented and the weight is finally lifted by the more powerful contraction of the muscle. When the weight is lifted, the tension on the nuclear bag is relieved and the afferent discharge from the spindle ceases. This series of diagrams relates to the lifting of a weight, but it is thought that a similar action of spindles is brought into play when inspiratory muscles contract against increased airways resistance.

respiration is unclear and they may be related only to voluntary chest movements.

Muscle fibre subtypes[39]

Respiratory muscles, like all skeletal muscle, contain different types of fibre classified according to which isoform of myosin heavy chain (MHC) is expressed. Table 6.1 shows the three fibre types known to exist in human respiratory muscles and their contractile and biochemical features. Which isoform of MHC is expressed in a muscle fibre determines the velocity of contraction (see Table 6.1). Different isoforms of enzymes involved in muscle relaxation also exist in the different fibre types and so influence the rate at which relaxation occurs and therefore the ability of the cell to maintain a tetanic contraction. Type I fibres contract and relax slowly, but can maintain tension for long periods using aerobic metabolic pathways and are fatigue resistant. In contrast, type IIb fibres rely mainly on glycolytic metabolic pathways for energy supply, contraction is quicker and stronger in bursts of activity, and they fatigue easily. Type IIa fibres have properties intermediate between these two extreme. The proportions of different fibre types in a muscle therefore reveal the sort of work normally undertaken by the muscle; for example, in muscles mainly involved in maintaining posture, type I fibres predominate, whereas in those requiring intermittent activity, such as hand muscle, type IIa or IIb fibres predominate.

Relative proportions of the different fibre types in human respiratory muscle are shown in Table 6.1, but it is unclear which type are responsible for different respiratory muscle activities. In animal respiratory muscles, which tend to have fewer type II fibres than humans, both eupnoeic and stimulated breathing can be achieved solely by using type I fibres and type II fibres are only required for expulsive efforts such as sneezing and coughing.[15] A high proportion of type I fibres (45% in human diaphragm) indicates that they are probably responsible for both posture and respiration in humans, and that type II fibres are again only required for expulsive efforts and active movements such as running, jumping etc. Respiratory disease, drugs and artificial ventilation all cause changes in the relative proportions of different fibre types in respiratory muscles (see Table 6.1).

Table 6.1 Properties of muscle fibre types found in human respiratory muscle and their relative proportions in normal and pathological situations[39–41]

	Type I	Type IIa	Type IIb
Contractile properties:			
Velocity of shortening	+	+ +	+ + + +
Tetanic force	+	+	+ +
Fatigue resistance	+ + + +	+ + +	+
Biochemical properties:			
Mitochondrial density	+ + +	+ + +	+
ATP consumption rate	+	+ +	+ + + +
Oxidative enzymes	+ + +	+ + +	+
Glycolytic enzymes	+	+ +	+ + + +
Glycogen content	+	+ +	+ + +
Relative proportions in:			
Normal subjects	45%	39%	16%
COPD	↑↑	↓	↓↓
Steroid myopathy	↔	↔	↓↓↓
Artificial ventilation[†]	↓	↑	↔

[†] Animal studies only. COPD, chronic obstructive pulmonary disease (Chapter 28); ATP, adenosine triphosphate.

RESPIRATORY MUSCLE FATIGUE AND DISUSE[39,42]

The diaphragm, like other striated muscles, is subject to fatigue, defined as an inability to sustain tension with repeated activity.[42] For non-respiratory skeletal muscle, fatigue may be 'central', that is, the subject is not trying hard enough (either consciously or subconsciously), but this is unlikely to be significant in respiration because subjects with respiratory failure usually have a high central respiratory drive. Peripheral fatigue occurs when the frequency of motor nerve APs becomes chronically increased in an attempt to increase muscle tension. Eventually, when working against an unsustainable load, striated muscle shows a progressive loss of the high-frequency component of the EMG relative to lower frequencies. A reduction in the high/low frequency ratio of the EMG is an indication of impending fatigue. Finally, relaxation of the muscle fibre, the energy-requiring part of contraction, becomes excessively prolonged and the muscle is unable to respond to the next AP in order to generate the required tension. In the diaphragm, resistive loads less than 40% of maximum may be sustained indefinitely, but loads greater than 40% of maximum can only be sustained for a short time.[43]

Blood supply to respiratory muscles may be important in fatigue.[44,45] Animal studies have shown that increased cardiac output and diaphragmatic blood flow (stimulated with noradrenaline) augment the contractility of fatigued diaphragm. In addition, patients with severe congestive cardiac failure, and therefore low cardiac output, have weakened respiratory muscles compared to matched controls, despite having similar muscle strength in the arms.[46] The high rate of activity of respiratory muscles seems to leave them more susceptible to weakness in the face of reduced oxygen supply compared with other muscles, a situation that often causes problems in intensive care when trying to wean patients from artificial ventilation before their cardiovascular function is adequate (page 430).

Effect of disuse[15]

The diaphragm may be rested by artificial ventilation with or without neuromuscular blockade and the effect on diaphragmatic performance is clearly important. Animal studies have found that after only 18 hours of controlled ventilation, protein degradation has begun in all muscle fibre types and diaphragm mass is reduced by 10%.[47] Similarly, changes in the expression of major histocompatibility complex (MHC) occur within 24 hours of artificial ventilation,[40] and within days diaphragm strength is substantially reduced (see Table 6.1).[39,48] Extrapolation of the results of these animal studies to humans is difficult, as there are numerous factors affecting respiratory muscle strength in critically ill patients receiving artificial ventilation. Even so, it seems safe to assume that complete inactivity of the normally very active respiratory muscles will be detrimental to their function and recent developments in artificial ventilation have mostly focused on supporting, rather than replacing, the activity of the patient's respiratory muscles (see Chapter 32).

THE WORK OF BREATHING[49]

When expiration is passive during quiet breathing, the work of breathing is performed entirely by the inspiratory muscles. Approximately half of this work is dissipated during inspiration as heat in overcoming the frictional forces opposing inspiration. The other half is stored as potential energy in the deformed elastic tissues of lung and chest wall. This potential energy is thus available as the source of energy for expiration and is then dissipated as heat in overcoming the frictional forces resisting expiration. Energy stored in deformed elastic tissue thus permits the work of *expiration* to be transferred to the *inspiratory* muscles. This remains true with moderate increases of either inspiratory or expiratory resistance, lung volume and therefore elastic recoil being increased in the latter condition (page 49).

The actual work performed by the respiratory muscles is very small in the healthy resting subject. Under these circumstances the oxygen consumption of the respiratory muscles is only about 3 ml.min^{-1} or less than 2% of the metabolic rate. Furthermore, the efficiency of the respiratory muscles is only about 10%. The efficiency is further reduced in many forms of respiratory disease, certain deformities, pregnancy, and when the minute volume is increased (Figure 6.8) When maximal ventilation is approached, the efficiency falls to such a low level that additional oxygen made available by further increases in ventilation will be entirely consumed by the respiratory muscles.

Units of measurement of work

Work is performed when a force moves its point of application and the work is equal to the product of force and distance moved. Similarly, work is performed when force is applied to the plunger of a syringe, raising the pressure of gas contained therein. In this case the work is equal to the product of the mean pressure and the change in volume or, alternatively, the product of the mean volume and the change in pressure. The units of work are identical whether the product is *force × distance* or *pressure × volume*. A multiplicity of units have been used for measuring work and are listed in Appendix A.

Power is a measure of the rate at which work is being (or can be) performed. The term 'work of breathing', as it is normally used and when expressed in watts, is thus a misnomer because we are referring to the rate at which

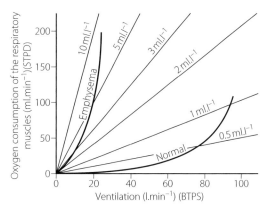

Figure 6.8 Oxygen consumption of the respiratory muscles plotted against minute volume of respiration. The isopleths indicate the oxygen cost of breathing in millilitres of oxygen consumed per litre of minute volume. The curve obtained from the normal subject shows the low oxygen cost of breathing up to a minute volume of 70 l.min^{-1}. Thereafter the oxygen cost rises steeply. In a patient with chronic obstructive pulmonary disease the oxygen cost of breathing is not only much higher at the resting minute volume but also rises more steeply as ventilation increases. At a minute volume of 20 l.min^{-1}, the respiratory muscles are consuming 200 ml of oxygen per minute and a further increase of ventilation would consume more oxygen than it would make available to the rest of the body. (After reference 50 by permission of the *Journal of Applied Physiology*.)

work is being performed, so *power* is the correct term. 'Work of breathing' would be appropriate for a single event such as one breath, and joules would then be the appropriate units.

Dissipation of the work of breathing

The work of breathing overcomes two main sources of impedance. The first is the elastic recoil of the lungs and chest wall (see Chapter 3) and the second is the non-elastic resistance to gas flow (see Chapter 4).

Work against elastic recoil. When an elastic body is deformed, no work is dissipated as heat and all work is stored as potential energy. Figure 6.9a shows a section of the alveolar pressure/volume plot for the total respiratory system, showing only the straight part of the curve from near FRC (see Figure 3.7). As the lungs are inflated, the plot forms the hypotenuse of a triangle, whose area represents the work done against elastic resistance. The area of the triangle (half the base times the height) will thus equal either half the tidal volume times the pressure change or the mean pressure times the volume change. Either product has the units of work or energy (joules) and represents the potential energy available for expiration. In Figure 6.9b, the pressure/volume curve is

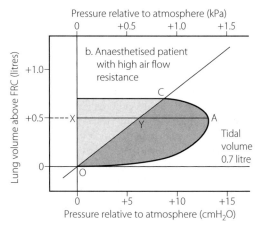

Figure 6.9 Work of breathing against elastic resistance during passive inflation. The lines show pressure/volume plots of the lungs of anaesthetised patients (conscious subjects are shown in Figure 3.7). The length of the pressure/volume curve covered during inspiration forms the hypotenuse of a right-angled triangle whose area equals the work performed against elastic resistance. Note that the area is greater when the pressure/volume curve is flatter (indicating stiffer or less compliant lungs).

Figure 6.10 Work of breathing against air flow resistance during passive inflation. The sloping line OYC is the alveolar pressure/volume curve. The curve OAC is the mouth pressure/volume curve during inflation of the lungs. The darker shaded area indicates the work of inspiration performed against air flow resistance. This work is increased in the patient with high resistance **(b)**. At the point when 500 ml gas has entered the patient, XY represents the pressure distending the lungs, while YA represents the pressure overcoming air flow resistance. XA is the inflation pressure at that moment. The lighter shaded areas represent the work done against elastic resistance (see Figure 6.9).

flatter, indicating stiffer or less compliant lungs. For the same tidal volume, the area of the triangle is increased. This indicates the greater amount of work performed against elastic resistance and the greater potential energy available for expiration.

Work against resistance to gas flow. Frictional resistance was ignored in Figure 6.9. Additional pressure is required to overcome frictional resistance to gas flow that is reflected in the mouth pressure, which, during inspiration, is above the alveolar pressure by the driving pressure required to overcome frictional resistance. When mouth pressure is plotted as in Figure 6.10, the inspiratory curve is bowed to the right and the darker shaded

area to the right of the pressure/volume curve indicates the additional work performed in overcoming inspiratory frictional resistance. Figure 6.10b represents a patient with increased airway resistance. The expiratory curve, not shown in Figure 6.10, would be bowed to the left as the mouth-to-alveolar pressure gradient is reversed during expiration.

The minimal work of breathing

For a constant minute volume, the work performed against elastic resistance is increased when breathing is

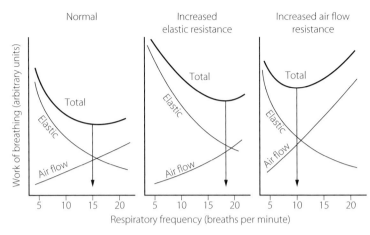

Figure 6.11 Minimal work of breathing. The diagrams show the work done against elastic and air flow resistance separately and summated to indicate the total work of breathing at different respiratory frequencies. The total work of breathing has a minimum value at about 15 breaths per minute under normal circumstances. For the same minute volume, minimum work is performed at higher frequencies with stiff (less compliant) lungs and at lower frequencies when the air flow resistance is increased.

slow and deep. Conversely, the work performed against air flow resistance is increased when breathing is rapid and shallow. If the two components are summated and the total work is plotted against respiratory frequency, it will be found that there is an optimal frequency at which the total work of breathing is minimal (Figure 6.11). If there is increased elastic resistance (as in patients with pulmonary fibrosis), the optimal frequency is increased, whereas in the presence of increased air flow resistance, the optimal frequency is decreased. Humans and animals tend to select a respiratory frequency close to that which minimises respiratory work. This applies to different species, different age groups and also to pathological conditions.

MEASUREMENT OF VENTILATION

Volume may be measured either directly or by the continuous integration of instantaneous gas flow rate (Figure 6.12).

Direct measurement of respired volumes

Inspiratory and expiratory tidal volumes (and therefore minute volume) may be markedly different and the difference is important in calculations of gas exchange. The normal respiratory exchange ratio of about 0.8 means that inspiratory minute volume is about 50 ml larger than the expiratory minute volume in the resting subject. Much larger differences can arise during exercise and during uptake or wash-out of an inert gas such as nitrogen or, to a greater extent, nitrous oxide.

Water-sealed spirometers provide the reference method for the measurement of ventilation (see Figure 6.12) and may be precisely calibrated by water displacement. They provide negligible resistance to breathing and, by suit-able design, may have a satisfactory frequency response up to very high respiratory frequencies.

Dry spirometers are hinged bellows, usually with electronic displays of both volume and instantaneous flow rate. Their accuracy approaches that of a water-filled spirometer and they are far more convenient in use.

Dry gas meters are based on two bellows that alternately drive a spindle by means of cranks. The principle is similar to the long-established design of meters used for measuring domestic gas consumption. They are not accurate for small volumes such as a single tidal volume but are very reliable for the measurement of larger volumes such as the volume exhaled over a few minutes.

Impellers and turbines. The best known of these instruments is the respirometer developed by Wright in 1955.[51] Alternating gas flow is mechanically rectified and the dead space (22 ml) is sufficiently small for the patient to breathe to and fro through it. The essential mechanism is entirely mechanical with indication of volume on a dial, but the output may be converted to an electrical signal to indicate either tidal volume or minute volume. In general the respirometer is accurate and tends to read low at low minute volumes and high at high minute volumes.[52] Departure from normality is thus exaggerated and the instrument is essentially safe.

Respiratory inductance plethysmography. Reference has been made above (page 80) to this method of measuring the cross-sectional area of the ribcage (RC) and abdomen (AB).[29] The sum of RC and AB signals correlates well with lung volume and, following calibration against a spirometer, changes in the summated signals provide a very useful non-invasive method of measuring ventilation, uninfluenced by the presence of a mouth piece or mask and feasible during sleep (see Figure 6.5).

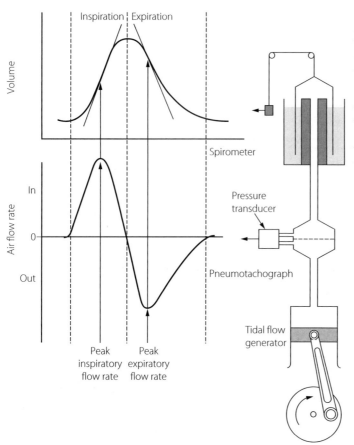

Figure 6.12 Relationship between volume and flow rate. The upper graph shows volume plotted against time; this type of tracing is obtained from a spirometer. The lower graph shows instantaneous air flow rate plotted against time; this type of tracing is obtained from a pneumotachograph. At any instant, the flow rate trace indicates the slope of the volume trace, whereas the volume trace indicates the cumulative area under the flow rate trace. *Flow* is the differential of volume; *volume* is the integral of flow rate. Differentiation of the spirometer trace gives a 'pneumotachogram'; integration of the pneumotachogram gives a 'spirometer' trace.

Measurement of ventilatory volumes by integration of instantaneous gas flow rate

Electronics have made measurement of ventilatory volumes by integration of instantaneous flow rate a widespread technique in clinical environments. There are many methods for measuring rapidly changing gas flow rates, of which the original was pneumotachography. This employs measurement of the pressure gradient across a laminar resistance, which ensures that the pressure drop is directly proportional to flow rate. This is illustrated in Figure 6.12, where the resistance is a wire mesh screen. It is necessary to take precautions to prevent errors due to different gas compositions and temperatures, and to prevent condensation of moisture on the screen. The pressure drop need not exceed a few millimetres of water and the volume can be very small. The pneumotachograph should not therefore interfere with respiration.

Most ventilators and anaesthetic machines currently in use can measure respiratory volumes. A pneumotachograph or electronic turbine system is used, normally on the expired limb of the breathing system and designed to be of very low resistance to allow measurements during spontaneous respiration. In this way each expired tidal volume may be measured, from which respiratory rate and minute volume can be derived and a useful method of detecting apnoea or disconnection is therefore provided.

MEASUREMENT OF VENTILATORY CAPACITY

Measurement of ventilatory capacity is the most commonly performed test of respiratory function. The ratio of ventilatory capacity to actual ventilation is a measure of ventilatory reserve and of the comfort of breathing.

Maximal breathing capacity (MBC)

Also referred to as maximal voluntary ventilation, MBC is defined as the maximum minute volume of ventilation that the subject can maintain for 15 seconds. In the normal subject MBC is about 15–20 times the resting minute volume. The subject simply breathes in and out of a spirometer without the need for removal of carbon dioxide; although simple, the test is exhausting to perform and is now seldom used. The average fit young male adult should have an MBC of about 170 l.min^{-1} but normal values depend upon body size, age and sex, the range being 47–253 l.min^{-1} for men and 55–139 l.min^{-1} for women.[53]

Forced expiration

A more practical test of ventilatory capacity is the forced expiratory volume in 1 second (FEV$_1$), which is the maximal volume exhaled in the first second starting from a maximal inspiration. A simple spirometer is all that is required. It is far more convenient to perform than the MBC and less exhausting for the patient. It correlates well with the MBC, which is normally about 35 times the FEV$_1$.

Peak expiratory flow rate

Most convenient of all the indirect tests of ventilatory capacity is the peak expiratory flow rate. This can be measured with simple and inexpensive hand-held devices, usually based on the Wright peak flow meter.[54] Interpretation of measurements of maximal expirations may be misleading. It should be remembered that these tests measure active expiration, which plays no part in normal breathing. They are most commonly performed as a measure of airway obstruction and are extensively used in patients with asthma and chronic obstructive airway disease. However, the results also depend on many other factors, including chest restriction, motivation and muscular power. The measurements may also be inhibited by pain. A more specific indication of airway resistance is the ratio of FEV$_1$ to vital capacity. This should exceed 75% in the normal subject.

ASSESSMENT OF THE RESPIRATORY MUSCLES[55,56]

Severe abnormalities of muscle function may be assessed by simple observation of spontaneous breathing. During inspiration, paradoxical movements of the trunk may occur, such as inward displacement of the abdominal wall (diaphragm failure) or inward movement of the upper chest (intercostal failure). Fluoroscopy or ultrasound imaging of the diaphragm provides a more subtle form of observation and is helpful in detecting phrenic nerve damage, particularly if unilateral, when the body surface changes will be less obvious.

Vital capacity (VC; see Figure 3.8) is now accepted as the best 'bedside' monitor of respiratory muscle function, particularly when performed supine.[55] Performance of a VC manoeuvre requires patient cooperation and coordination and a single low reading is non-specific. However, repeated measurement allows the observation of a trend in VC to be followed and a 25% reduction is unequivocally abnormal. In spite of the many causes of a reduced VC, this method of assessing respiratory muscle function is very useful for monitoring the development of progressive muscle weakness in conditions such as myasthenia gravis and Guillain–Barré syndrome (page 367).

Pressure measurements, when breathing against an imposed resistance, are used to assess both inspiratory and expiratory muscle strength. All require some patient compliance and involve a degree of respiratory discomfort so these tests, though more specific than VC for respiratory muscle function, are not widely used. Mouth pressure may be measured while a slow inspiration or expiration is performed against a moderate respiratory resistance, or during a rapid 'sniff' procedure in which the nasal airway acts as the resistance. Finally, using either of the above imposed resistances, the more invasive oesophageal and intragastric pressures may be measured to obtain transdiaphragmatic pressure, which is the best assessment of diaphragm force generation.

REFERENCES

1. Horner RL, Innes JA, Guz A. Reflex pharyngeal dilator muscle activation by stimuli of negative airway pressure in awake man. *Sleep* 1993; **16**(Suppl 8): S85–6.
*2. Widdicombe J. Airway receptors. *Respir Physiol* 2001; **125**: 3–15.
3. Remmers JE. Wagging the tongue and guarding the airway. Reflex control of the genioglossus. *Am J Respir Crit Care Med* 2001; **164**: 2013–15.
4. Wheatley JR, Tangel DJ, Mezzanotte WS, White DP. Influence of sleep on response to negative airway pressure of tensor palatini muscle and retropalatal airway. *J Appl Physiol* 1993; **75**: 2117–24.
5. Wheatley JR, Kelley WT, Tully A, Engel LA. Pressure–diameter relationships in the upper airway in awake supine subjects. *J Appl Physiol* 1991; **70**: 2242–51.
6. Burger CD, Stanson AW, Daniels BK, Sheedy PF, Shepard JW. Fast CT evaluation of the effect of lung volume on upper airway size and function in normal men. *Am Rev Respir Dis* 1992; **146**: 335–9.
7. Yildirim N, Fitzpatrick MF, Whyte KF, Jalleh R, Wightman AJA, Douglas NJ. The effect of posture on upper airway dimensions in normal subjects and in patients with the sleep apnea/hypopnea syndrome. *Am Rev Respir Dis* 1991; **144**: 845–7.
8. Douglas NJ, Jan MA, Yildirim N, Warren PM, Drummond GB. Effect of posture and breathing route on genioglossal EMG activity in normal subjects and in patients with the sleep apnea/hypopnea syndrome. *Am Rev Respir Dis* 1993; **148**: 1341–5.

9. Pae EK, Lowe AA, Sasaki K, Price C, Tsuchiya M, Fleetham JA. A cephalometric and electromyographic study of upper airway structures in the upright and supine positions. *Am J Orthod Dent Facial Orthop*1991; **106**: 52–9.

10. Tangel DJ, Mezzanotte WS, White DP. Influence of sleep on tensor palatini EMG and upper airway resistance in normal men. *J Appl Physiol* 1991; **70**: 2574–81.

11. Gal TJ. Is glottic function the key to improved gas exchange? *Chest* 1990; **98**: 9–10.

12. Brancatisano TP, Dodd DS, Engel LA. Respiratory activity of posterior cricoarytenoid muscle and vocal cords in humans. *J Appl Physiol* 1984; **57**: 1143–9.

13. Kuna ST, Insalaco G, Woodson GE. Thyroarytenoid muscle activity during wakefulness and sleep in normal adults. *J Appl Physiol* 1988; **65**: 1332–9

*14. Gauthier AP, Verbanck S, Estenne M, Segebarth C, Macklem PT, Paiva M. Three-dimensional reconstruction of the in vivo human diaphragm shape at different lung volumes. *J Appl Physiol* 1994; **76**: 495–506.

15. Sieck GC. Physiological effects of diaphragm muscle denervation and disuse. *Clin Chest Med* 1994; **15**: 641–59.

16. Eisele JH, Noble MIM, Katz J, Fung DL, Hickey RF. Bilateral phrenic nerve block in man. *Anesthesiology* 1972; **37**: 64–9.

17. Paiva M, Verbanck S, Estenne M, Poncelet B, Segebarth C, Macklem PT. Mechanical implications of in vivo human diaphragm shape. *J Appl Physiol* 1992; **72**: 1407–12.

18. Loring SH. Invited editorial on "Three-dimensional reconstruction of the in vivo human diaphragm shape at different lung volumes". *J Appl Physiol* 1994; **79**: 493–4.

19. Cassart M, Pettiaux N, Gevenois PA, Paiva M, Estenne M. Effect of chronic hyperinflation on diaphragm length and surface area. *Am J Respir Crit Care Med* 1997; **156**: 504–8.

20. Petroll WM, Knight H, Rochester DF. A model approach to assess diaphragmatic volume displacement. *J Appl Physiol* 1990; **69**: 2175–82.

21. Han JN, Gayan-Ramirez G, Dekhuijzen R, Decramer M. Respiratory function of the ribcage muscles. *Eur Respir J* 1993; **6**: 722–8.

22. De Troyer A. Respiratory muscle function. In: Brewis RAL, Corrin B, Gedded DM, Gibson GJ, eds. *Respiratory medicine*. London: WB Saunders, 1995; 125–33.

23. Hamberger GE. *De Respirirationis Mechanismo et usu genuino*. Jena, 1749.

24. De Troyer, Estenne M. Coordination between ribcage muscles and diaphragm during quiet breathing in humans. *J Appl Physiol* 1984; **57**: 899–906.

25. Rimmer KP, Ford GT, Whitelaw WA. Interaction between postural and respiratory control of human intercostal muscles. *J Appl Physiol* 1995; **79**: 1556–61.

26. Hillman DR, Finucane KE. A model of the respiratory pump. *J Appl Physiol* 1987; **63**: 951–61.

27. Drummond GB. Chest wall movements in anaesthesia. *Eur J Anaesthiol* 1989; **6**: 161–96.

28. Konno K, Mead J. Measurement of the separate volume changes of ribcage and abdomen during breathing. *J Appl Physiol* 1967: **22**: 407–22.

29. Milledge JS, Stott FD. Inductive plethysmography – a new respiratory transducer. *J Physiol (Lond)* 1977; **267**: 4–5P.

30. Lumb AB, Nunn JF. Respiratory function and ribcage contribution to ventilation in body positions commonly used during anaesthesia. *Anesth Analg* 1991; **73**: 422–6.

31. Xie S, Takasaki Y, Popkin J, Orr D, Bradley TD. Chemical and postural influence on scalene and diaphragmatic activation in humans. *J Appl Physiol* 1991; **70**: 658–64.

32. Druz WS, Sharp JT. Activity of respiratory muscles in upright and recumbent humans. *J Appl Physiol* 1981; **51**: 1552–61.

33. Cooke IRC, Soust M, Berger PJ. Differential recruitment of inspiratory muscles in response to chemoreceptor drive. *Respir Physiol* 1993; **92**: 167–81.

34. Takasaki Y, Orr D, Popkin J, Xie A, Bradley TD. Effect of hypercapnia and hypoxia on respiratory muscle activation in humans. *J Appl Physiol* 1989; **67**: 1776–84.

35. Lumb AB, Nunn JF. Ribcage contribution to CO_2 response during rebreathing and steady state methods. *Respir Physiol* 1991; **85**: 97–110.

36. Muller N, Volgyesi G, Becker L, Bryan MH, Bryan AC. Diaphragmatic muscle tone. *J Appl Physiol* 1979; **47**: 279–84.

37. Robson JG. The respiratory centres and their responses. In: Evans FT, Gray TC, eds. *Modern trends in anaesthesia – 3*. London: Butterworths, 1967.

38. Whitelaw WA, Watson TWJ. Spike trains from single motor units in human parasternal intercostal muscles. *Respir Physiol* 1992; **88**: 289–98.

*39. Laghi F, Tobin MJ. Disorders of the respiratory muscles. *Am J Respir Crit Care Med* 2003; **168**: 10–48.

40. Gayan-Ramirez G, Decramer M. Effects of mechanical ventilation on diaphragm function and biology. *Eur Respir J* 2002; **20**: 1579–86.

41. Levine S, Kaiser L, Leferovich J, Tikunov B. Cellular adaptations in the diaphragm in chronic obstructive pulmonary disease. *N Engl J Med* 1997; **337**: 1799–806.

42. Moxham J. Respiratory muscle fatigue: mechanisms, evaluation and therapy. *Br J Anaesth* 1990; **65**: 43–53.

43. Roussos C, Macklem PT. Diaphragmatic fatigue in man. *J Appl Physiol* 1977; **43**: 189–97.

44. Fujii Y, Toyooka H, Amaha K. Diaphragmatic fatigue and its recovery are influenced by cardiac output. *J Anaesth* 1991; **5**: 17–23.

45. Supinski GS, Di Marco AF, Gonzalez J, Altose MD. Effect of norepinephrine on diaphragm contractility and blood flow. *J Appl Physiol* 1990; **69**: 2019–28.

46. Hammond MD, Bauer KA, Sharp JT, Rocha RD. Respiratory muscle strength in congestive cardiac failure. *Chest* 1990; **98**: 1091–4.

47. Shanely RA, Zergeroglu MA, Lennon SL, *et al.* Mechanical ventilation-induced diaphragmatic atrophy is associated with oxidative injury and increased proteolytic activity. *Am J Respir Crit Care Med* 2002; **166**: 1369–74.

48. Zhan W, Sieck GC. Adaptations of diaphragm and medial gastrocnemius muscles to inactivity. *J Appl Physiol* 1992; **72**: 1445–53.

49. Milic-Emili J. Work of breathing. In: Crystal RG, West JB, eds. *The lung, scientific foundations*. New York: Raven, 1991; 1065–75.

50. Campbell EJM, Westlake EK, Cherniak RM. Simple methods of estimating oxygen consumption and the efficiency of the muscles of breathing. *J Appl Physiol* 1957; **11**: 303–8.

51. Wright BM. A respiratory anemometer. *J Physiol* 1955; **127**: 25P.

52. Nunn JF, Ezi-Ashi TI. The accuracy of the respirometer and ventigrator. *Br J Anaesth* 1962; **34**: 422–32.

53. Cotes JE. *Lung function: assessment and application in medicine*. Oxford: Blackwell Scientific Publications, 1993; 122.

54. Wright BM, McKerrow CB. Maximum forced expiratory flow rate as a measure of ventilatory capacity. *Br Med J* 1959; **2**: 1041–7.

*55. Polkey MI, Green M, Moxham J. Measurement of respiratory muscle strength. *Thorax* 1995; **50**: 1131–5.

56. Clanton TL, Diaz PT. Clinical assessment of the respiratory muscles. *Phys Ther* 1995; **75**: 983–95.

The pulmonary circulation

KEY POINTS

■ Pulmonary blood flow approximates to cardiac output and can increase severalfold with little change in pulmonary arterial pressure.

■ Passive distension and recruitment of closed pulmonary capillaries, particularly in the upper zones of the lung, allow pulmonary vascular resistance to fall as blood flow increases.

■ Active control of pulmonary vascular resistance has only a minor role in controlling pulmonary vascular resistance and involves intrinsic responses in vascular smooth muscle, modulated by numerous neural and humoral factors.

■ Hypoxic pulmonary vasoconstriction of pulmonary arterioles is a fundamental difference from the systemic circulation, though the mechanism of this response to hypoxia remains uncertain.

Evolution first led to the development of a separate pulmonary circulation in amphibians, though in this case both systemic and pulmonary circulations are supplied by a single ventricle and there is therefore a great deal of mixing of blood between the two. The occurrence of warm-blooded animals led to a tenfold increase in oxygen requirements, which may only be achieved through having a pulmonary circulation almost completely separate from the systemic circulation.[1]

The entire blood volume passes through the lungs during each circulation. This is an ideal arrangement for gas exchange but is equally suitable for the filtering and metabolic functions of the lungs, which are considered in Chapter 12.

PULMONARY BLOOD FLOW

The flow of blood through the pulmonary circulation is approximately equal to the flow through the whole of the systemic circulation. It therefore varies from about 6 l.min^{-1} under resting conditions to as much as 25 l.min^{-1} in severe exercise. It is remarkable that such an increase can normally be achieved with a minimal increase in pressure. Pulmonary vascular pressures and vascular resistance are much less than those of the systemic circulation. Consequently the pulmonary circulation has only limited ability to control the regional distribution of blood flow within the lungs and is markedly affected by gravity, which results in overperfusion of the dependent parts of the lung fields. Maldistribution of the pulmonary blood flow has important consequences for gaseous exchange, and these are considered in Chapter 8.

In fact, the relationship between the inflow and outflow of the pulmonary circulation is much more complicated (Figure 7.1). The lungs receive a significant quantity of blood from the bronchial arteries, which usually arise from the arch of the aorta. Blood from the bronchial circulation returns to the heart in two ways. From a plexus around the hilum, blood from the pleurohilar part of the bronchial circulation returns to the superior vena cava via the azygos veins and this fraction may thus be regarded as normal systemic flow, neither arising from nor returning to the pulmonary circulation. However, another fraction of the bronchial circulation, distributed more peripherally in the lung, passes through postcapillary anastomoses to join the pulmonary veins, constituting an admixture of venous blood with the arterialised blood from the alveolar capillary networks.[2]

The situation may be further complicated by blood flow through precapillary anastomoses from the bronchial arteries to the pulmonary arteries. These communications (so-called 'sperr arteries') have muscular walls and are thought to act as sluice gates, opening when increased pulmonary blood flow is required.[3] Their functional significance in normal subjects is unknown, but in diseased lungs flow through these anastomoses may be crucial. For example, in situations involving pulmonary oligaemia (e.g. pulmonary artery stenosis, pulmonary embolism) blood from the bronchial arteries will flow through the anastomoses to supplement pulmonary arte-

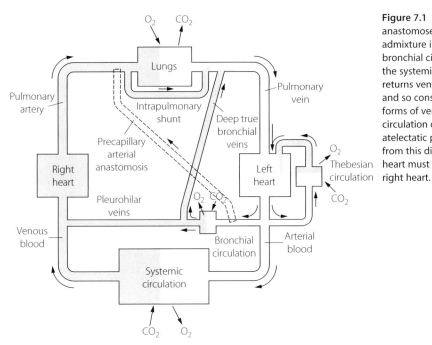

Figure 7.1 Schema of bronchopulmonary anastomoses and other forms of venous admixture in the normal subject. Part of the bronchial circulation returns venous blood to the systemic venous system while another part returns venous blood to the pulmonary veins and so constitutes venous admixture. Other forms of venous admixture are the Thebesian circulation of the left heart and flow through atelectatic parts of the lungs. It will be clear from this diagram why the output of the left heart must be slightly greater than that of the right heart.

rial flow.[4] It should be noted that a Blalock–Taussig shunt operation achieves the same purpose for palliation of patients with cynanotic congenital heart disease.

PULMONARY BLOOD VOLUME

As a first approximation the right heart pumps blood into the pulmonary circulation while the left heart pumps away the blood that returns from the lungs. Therefore, provided that the output of the two sides is the same, the pulmonary blood volume will remain constant. However, very small differences in the outputs of the two sides must result in large changes in pulmonary blood volume if they are maintained for more than a few beats.

Factors influencing pulmonary blood volume

Posture. Change from the supine to the erect position decreases the pulmonary blood volume by almost one-third, which is about the same as the corresponding change in cardiac output. Both changes result from pooling of blood in dependent parts of the systemic circulation.

Systemic vascular tone. Because the systemic circulation has much greater vasomotor activity than the pulmonary circulation, an overall increase in vascular tone will tend to squeeze blood from the systemic into the pulmonary circulation. This may result from the administration of vasoconstrictor drugs, from release of endogenous catecholamines or from passive compression of the body in

a G-suit. The magnitude of the resulting volume shift will depend on many factors, such as position, overall blood volume and activity of the numerous humoral and nervous mechanisms controlling pulmonary vascular tone at the time (see below). Conversely, it seems likely that pulmonary blood volume would be diminished when systemic tone is diminished, as for example following regional anaesthesia when systemic vascular resistance is decreased with no effect on the autonomic supply to the pulmonary vasculature.

Left heart failure. Pulmonary venous hypertension (due, for example, to mitral stenosis) would be expected to result in an increased pulmonary blood volume. There has, however, been difficulty in the experimental demonstration of any significant change.

PULMONARY VASCULAR PRESSURES

Pulmonary arterial pressure is only about one-sixth of systemic arterial pressure, although the capillary and venous pressures are not greatly different for the two circulations (Figure 7.2). There is thus only a small pressure drop along the pulmonary arterioles and therefore a reduced potential for active regulation of the distribution of the pulmonary blood flow. This also explains why there is little damping of the arterial pressure wave and the pulmonary capillary blood flow is markedly pulsatile.

Consideration of pulmonary vascular pressures carries a special difficulty in the selection of the reference pressure. Systemic pressures are customarily measured with reference to ambient atmospheric pressure but this is not always appropriate when considering the pulmonary arterial pressure, which is relatively small in comparison with the intrathoracic and pulmonary venous pressures. This may be important in two circumstances. First, the extravascular (intrathoracic) pressure may have a major influence on the intravascular pressure and should be taken into account. Second, the driving pressure through the pulmonary circulation may be markedly influenced by the pulmonary venous pressure, which must be taken into account when measuring pulmonary vascular resistance. We must therefore distinguish between pressures within the pulmonary circulation expressed in the three different forms listed below. Measurement techniques may be adapted to indicate these pressures directly (Figure 7.3).

Intravascular pressure is the pressure at any point in the circulation relative to atmosphere. This is the customary way of expressing pressures in the systemic circulation and is also the commonest method of indicating pulmonary vascular pressures.

Transmural pressure is the difference in pressure between the inside of a vessel and the tissue surrounding the vessel. In the case of the larger pulmonary vessels, the outside pressure is the intrathoracic pressure (commonly measured as the oesophageal pressure, as shown in Figure 7.3). This method should be used to exclude the physical effect of major changes in intrathoracic pressure.

Driving pressure is the difference in pressure between one point in the circulation and another point downstream. The driving pressure of the pulmonary circulation as a whole is the pressure difference between pulmonary artery and left atrium. This is the pressure that overcomes the flow resistance and should be used for determination of vascular resistance.

Systemic circulation				Pulmonary circulation	
mmHg	cmH$_2$O			mmHg	cmH$_2$O
90	120	Arteries		17	22
		Arterioles			
30	40			13	17
		Capillaries			
10	13			9	12
		Veins			
2	3	Atria		6	8

Figure 7.2 Comparison of typical mean pressure gradients along the systemic and pulmonary circulations. (Mean pressures relative to atmosphere.)

Figure 7.3 Normal values for pressures in the pulmonary circulation relative to atmospheric (cmH$_2$O). Systolic and diastolic pressures are shown for the right ventricle and pulmonary trunk, and mean pressures elsewhere. Note the effect of gravity on pressures at different levels in the lung fields. Three different manometers are shown connected to indicate driving pressure, intravascular pressure and transmural pressure.

These differences are far from being solely academic. For example, an increase in intrathoracic pressure due to positive-pressure ventilation will increase the pulmonary arterial intravascular pressure but will also similarly increase pulmonary venous intravascular pressure, and therefore driving pressure (and therefore flow) remains unchanged. Similarly, if the primary problem is a raised left atrial pressure, blood will 'back up' through the pulmonary circulation and pulmonary arterial intravascular pressure will also be raised but the driving pressure will again not be increased. Therefore, for assessing pulmonary blood flow (and so resistance), driving pressure is the correct measurement, but this requires pulmonary venous (left atrial) pressure to be recorded, which is difficult to achieve continuously (page 105). Pulmonary arterial intravascular pressure is usually measured and the value must therefore be interpreted with caution.

Typical normal values for pressures within the pulmonary circulation are shown in Figure 7.3. The effect of gravity on the pulmonary vascular pressure may be seen and it will be clear why pulmonary oedema is most likely to occur in the lower zones of the lungs where the intravascular pressures and the transmural pressure gradients are highest.

Effect of intraalveolar pressure

Alteration of intraalveolar pressure causes changes in intrathoracic pressure according to the following relationship:

Intrathoracic pressure =

alveolar pressure – alveolar transmural pressure

Alveolar transmural pressure is a function of lung volume (see Figure 3.7), and when the lungs are passively inflated the intrathoracic pressure will normally increase by rather less than half the inflation pressure. The increase will be even less if the lungs are stiff, and thus a low compliance protects the circulation from inflation pressure (page 436). Intravascular pressures are normally increased directly and instantaneously by the effects of changes in intrathoracic pressure, and this explains the initial rise in systemic arterial pressure during a Valsalva manoeuvre (page 434). It also explains the cyclical changes in pulmonary arterial pressure during spontaneous respiration, with pressures greater during expiration than during inspiration. Such changes would not be seen if transmural pressure were measured (see Figure 7.3).

In addition to the immediate physical effect of an increase in intrathoracic pressure on intravascular pressures, there is a secondary physiological effect due to interference with venous filling. This accounts for the secondary decline in systemic pressure seen in the Valsalva manoeuvre.

PULMONARY VASCULAR RESISTANCE

Vascular resistance is an expression of the relationship between driving pressure and flow, as in the case of resistance to gas flow. It may be expressed in similar terms as follows:

Pulmonary vascular resistance

$$= \frac{\text{Pulmonary driving pressure}}{\text{Cardiac output}}$$

There are, however, important caveats and the concept of pulmonary vascular resistance is not a simple parallel to Ohm's law, appropriate to laminar flow (page 40). When gases flow through rigid tubes the flow is laminar or turbulent, or a mixture of the two. In the first case, pressure increases in direct proportion to flow rate and the resistance remains constant (Poiseuille's law). In the second case pressure increases according to the square of the flow rate and the resistance increases with flow. When the type of flow is mixed, the pressure rises in proportion to the flow rate raised to a power between one and two.

The circumstances are two stages more complicated in the case of blood. First, the tubes through which the blood flows are not rigid but tend to expand as flow is increased, particularly in the pulmonary circulation with its low vasomotor tone. Consequently, the resistance tends to fall as flow increases, and the plot of pressure against flow rate is neither linear (see Figure 4.2) nor curved with the concavity upwards (see Figure 4.3) but curved with the concavity downwards. The second complication is that blood is a non-newtonian fluid (owing to the presence of the corpuscles) and its viscosity varies with the shear rate, which is a function of its linear velocity.

Vascular resistance in the lung. Although the relationship between flow and pressure in blood vessels is far removed from simple linearity, there is a widespread convention that pulmonary vascular resistance should be expressed in a form of the equation above. This is directly analogous to electrical resistance, as though there were laminar flow of a newtonian fluid though rigid pipes. It would, of course, be quite impractical in the clinical situation to measure pulmonary driving pressure at different values of cardiac output to determine the true nature of their relationship.

Vascular resistance is expressed in units derived from those used for expression of pressure and flow rate. Using conventional units, vascular resistance is usually expressed in units of mmHg per litre per minute. In absolute CGS units, vascular resistance is usually expressed in units of dynes/square centimetre per cubic centimetre/second (i.e. $dyn.s.cm^{-5}$). The appropriate SI units will probably be kPa.l^{-1}.minute. Normal values for the pulmonary circulation in the various units are as follows.

	Driving pressure	Pulmonary blood flow	Pulmonary vascular resistance
SI units	1.2 kPa	5 l.min^{-1}	0.24 kPa.l^{-1}.min
Conventional units	9 mmHg	5 l.min^{-1}	1.8 mmHg.l^{-1}.min
Absolute CGS units	12 000 dyn.cm^{-2}	83 cm^3.s^{-1}	144 dyn.s.cm^{-5}

Localisation of the pulmonary vascular resistance. In the systemic circulation the greatest part of resistance is in the arterioles, along which the pressure falls from a mean value of about 12 kPa (90 mmHg) down to about 4 kPa (30 mmHg) (see Figure 7.2). This pressure drop largely obliterates the pulse pressure wave and the systemic capillary flow is not pulsatile to any great extent. In the pulmonary circulation, the pressure drop along the arterioles is very much smaller than in the systemic circulation and, as an approximation, the pulmonary vascular resistance is equally divided between arteries, capillaries and veins. Pulmonary arteries and arterioles, with muscular vessel walls, are mostly extraalveolar and involved in active control of pulmonary vascular resistance by mechanisms such as nervous, humoral or gaseous control. In contrast, pulmonary capillaries are intimately associated with the alveolus (see Figure 2.7), so resistance of these vessels is therefore greatly influenced by alveolar pressure and volume. Thus in the pulmonary circulation, vessels without the power of active vasoconstriction play a major role in governing total vascular resistance and the distribution of the pulmonary blood flow.

PASSIVE CHANGES IN PULMONARY VASCULAR RESISTANCE

Effect of pulmonary blood flow (cardiac output)

The pulmonary circulation can adapt to large changes in cardiac output with only small increases in pulmonary arterial pressure. Thus pulmonary vascular resistance must decrease as flow increases. Reduced resistance implies an increase in the total cross-sectional area of the pulmonary vascular bed, and particularly the capillaries. These adaptations to increased flow occur partly by passive distension of vessels and partly by recruitment of collapsed vessels, the former being the most important factor.[5]

Recruitment of previously unperfused pulmonary vessels occurs in response to increased pulmonary flow. This is particularly true of the capillary bed, which is devoid of any vasomotor control, so allowing the opening of new passages in the network of capillaries lying in the alveolar septa, and is most likely to occur in the upper part of the lung where capillary pressure is lowest (zone 1, see below). Capillary recruitment was first described in histological studies involving sections cut in lungs rapidly frozen while perfused with blood, which showed that the number of open capillaries increased with rising pulmonary arterial pressure, particularly in the mid-zone of the lung.[6] Recruitment of capillaries in the intact lung remains poorly understood. Animal studies have found that pulsatile blood flow results in greater capillary recruitment than constant flow at the same pressures.[7] Studies using colloidal gold particles in the circulation demonstrate that there is perfusion in all pulmonary capillaries, including in zone 1, during normal ventilation.[8] A similar study using fluorescent-labelled albumin but with airway pressure increased above pulmonary capillary pressure showed no flow in almost two-thirds of capillaries in zone 1.[9] It therefore seems that with increased alveolar pressure (e.g. during positive-pressure ventilation) unperfused capillaries are available for recruitment but that under normal circumstances, with low airway pressures, there is flow in all capillaries. However, the studies using colloidal particles cannot discriminate between plasma or blood flow and have led to speculation that some, *almost* collapsed capillaries may contain only plasma ('plasma skimming') or even blood flow from the bronchial circulation.[10]

Distension in the entire pulmonary vasculature occurs in response to increased transmural pressure gradient and is again most likely to occur in capillaries devoid of muscular control. In one study, capillary diameter increased from 5 to 10 μm as the transmural pressure increased from 0.5 to 2.5 kPa (5 to 25 cmH$_2$O).[11] As described in the previous section, it now seems likely that capillaries never collapse completely and therefore passive distension is clearly the more important adaptation to increased flow.[5]

A striking example of the ability of the pulmonary vasculature to adapt to changing flow occurs after pneumonectomy, when the remaining lung will normally take the entire resting pulmonary blood flow without a rise in pulmonary arterial pressure. There is, inevitably, a limit to the flow that can be accommodated without an increase in pressure, and this will be less if the pulmonary vascular bed is diminished by disease or surgery. The most important pathological cause of increased flow is left-to-right shunting through a patent ductus arteriosus or through atrial or ventricular septal defects. Under these circumstances the pulmonary blood flow may be several times greater than the systemic flow before pulmonary hypertension develops. Despite this, secondary changes in pulmonary vessels commonly result in an

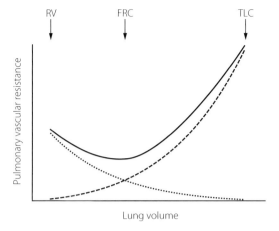

Figure 7.4 Relationship between pulmonary vascular resistance (PVR) and lung volume. The solid line represents total PVR and is minimal at the functional residual capacity (FRC). Compression of alveolar capillaries (dashed line) is responsible for the increased PVR as lung volume approaches total lung capacity (TLC). Increasing PVR as lung volume approaches residual volume (RV) may result from compression of corner capillaries (dotted line) or extraalveolar vessels, or hypoxia-induced vasoconstriction in collapsed lung units. It should be noted that this graph is derived from studies mainly involving isolated animal lungs and may not be applicable to the intact subject.

increase in vascular resistance, causing an earlier and more severe rise in pulmonary arterial pressure.

Effect of lung inflation

Reference has been made above to the effect of alveolar pressure on pulmonary vascular pressures. The effect on pulmonary vascular resistance is complex. Confusion has arisen in the past because of failure to appreciate that pulmonary vascular resistance must be derived from driving pressure and not from pulmonary arterial or transmural pressure (see Figure 7.3). This is important because inflation of the lungs normally influences the pressure in the oesophagus, pulmonary artery and left atrium and so can easily conceal the true effect on vascular resistance.

When pulmonary vascular resistance is correctly calculated from the driving pressure, there is reasonable agreement that the pulmonary vascular resistance is minimal at FRC and that changes in lung volume in either direction cause a small increase in resistance, particularly at high lung volumes (Figure 7.4). These observations may be explained by considering pulmonary capillaries as belonging to three distinct groups.[12]

Alveolar capillaries are sandwiched between two adjacent alveolar walls, usually bulging into one alveolus (see

Figure 2.7) and supported from collapse only by the pressure in the capillary and flimsy septal fibrous tissue. Expansion of the alveolus will therefore compress these capillaries and increase their contribution to pulmonary vascular resistance. If the lung consisted entirely of alveolar capillaries then pulmonary vascular resistance would be directly related to lung volume.

Corner capillaries lie within the junction between three or more alveoli and are not therefore sandwiched between alveolar walls. In this area, the alveolar wall is believed to form 'pleats' during lung deflation, which are then stretched out longitudinally (rather than expanded outwards) during inspiration and so have little effect on the blood vessels nearby. Indeed, blood vessels in this area are generally uninfluenced by alveolar pressure but may expand at high lung volume and constrict at very small lung volumes, possibly secondary to local hypoxia surrounding the collapsed alveoli.

Extraalveolar vessels provide an additional explanation for the increased pulmonary vascular resistance at small lung volumes. Compression of larger pulmonary vessels at low lung volumes may result in reduced flow in dependent parts of the lung (page 114) and this is likely to contribute to the overall change in pulmonary vascular resistance.

The anatomical difference between these capillaries is undoubted, whereas the effect of the anatomical features on physiology is unproven. Much of the work has involved mathematical modelling based on animal studies in the open-chested or isolated preparation, and the relevance of these to the intact human is as yet uncertain.

Effect of gravity on alveolar and vascular pressures

The vascular weir. The interplay of alveolar pressure, flow rate and vascular resistance is best considered by dividing the lung field into three zones.[13,14] Figure 7.5 shows behaviour as a Starling resistor and also as the analogy of a weir. A Starling, or threshold, resistor can be visualised as a length of compressible tubing within a rigid chamber, such that flow occurs only when the upstream pressure (left gauges in Figure 7.5) exceeds the pressure within the chamber (middle gauges), and a reduction in the downstream pressure (right gauges) cannot initiate flow. In zone 1 of Figure 7.5, the pressure within the arterial end of the collapsible vessels is less than the alveolar pressure and therefore insufficient to open the vessels that remain collapsed, as in a Starling resistor. The upstream water is below the top of the weir and so there can be no flow. The downstream (venous) pressure is irrelevant. Zone 1 corresponds to conditions that may apply in the uppermost parts of the lungs.

Comparable behaviour
of a Starling resistor

Analogy of
the weir

Zone 1
$P_A > P_a > P_v$

No flow

Zone 2
$P_a > P_A > P_v$

Flow α P_a–P_A

Zone 3
$P_a > P_v > P_A$

Flow α P_a–P_v

Figure 7.5 The effect of gravity on pulmonary vascular resistance is shown by comparison with a Starling resistor (left) and with a weir (right). P_a, pulmonary artery pressure; P_A, alveolar pressure; P_v, pulmonary venous pressure (all pressures relative to atmosphere). See text for full discussion.

In the mid-zone of the lungs (zone 2 of Figure 7.5), the pressure at the arterial end of the collapsible vessels exceeds the alveolar pressure and, under these conditions, a collapsible vessel, behaving like a Starling resistor, permits flow in such a way that the flow rate depends on the arterial–alveolar pressure difference. Resistance in the Starling resistor is concentrated at the point marked with the arrow in Figure 7.5. The greater the difference between arterial and alveolar pressure, the more widely the collapsible vessels will open and the greater will be the flow. Note that the venous pressure is still not a factor that affects flow or vascular resistance. This condition is still analogous to a weir, the upstream depth (head of pressure) corresponding to the arterial pressure and the height of the weir corresponding to alveolar pressure. Flow depends solely on the difference in height between the upstream water level and the top of the weir. The depth of water below the weir (analogous to venous pressure) cannot influence the flow of water over the weir unless it rises above the height of the weir.

In the lower zone of the lungs (zone 3 of Figure 7.5) the pressure in the venous end of the capillaries is above the alveolar pressure, and under these conditions a collapsible vessel behaving like a Starling resistor will be held wide open and the flow rate will, as a first approximation, be governed by the arterial–venous pressure difference (the driving pressure) in the normal manner for the systemic circulation. However, as the intravascular pressure increases in relation to the alveolar pressure, the collapsible vessels will be further distended and their resistance will be correspondingly reduced. Returning to the analogy of the weir, the situation is now one in which the downstream water level has risen until the weir is completely submerged and offers little resistance to the flow of water, which is largely governed by the difference in the water level above and below the weir. However, as the levels rise further, the weir is progressively more and more submerged and what little resistance it offers to water flow is diminished still further.

ACTIVE CONTROL OF PULMONARY VASCULAR RESISTANCE

In addition to the passive mechanisms described, pulmonary blood vessels are also able to control vascular resistance by active vasoconstriction and vasodilation, and there is now evidence that the pulmonary vasculature is normally kept in a state of active vasodilation.[15]

Cellular mechanisms controlling pulmonary vascular tone[16-18]

There are many mechanisms by which pulmonary vascular tone may be controlled (Table 7.1), but the role of many of these in the human lung is uncertain. Some of the receptor–agonist systems in Table 7.1 have only been demonstrated *in vitro* using animal tissue, but may eventually emerge as important in humans either for normal maintenance of pulmonary vascular tone or during lung injury (see Chapter 31). Activity of some, though not all, of the mechanisms listed in Table 7.1 is dependent on the endothelial lining of the pulmonary blood vessels. It seems likely that many basic control mechanisms occur within the smooth muscle cell, whereas the endothelium acts as a modulator of the response. Some control mechanisms, such as the autonomic nervous system and hypoxic pulmonary vasoconstriction, have

Table 7.1 Receptors and agonists involved in active control of pulmonary vascular tone

Receptor group	Subtypes	Principal agonists	Responses	Endothelium dependent?
Adrenergic	α_1	Noradrenaline	Constriction	no
	α_2	Noradrenaline	Dilation	yes
	β_2	Adrenaline	Dilation	yes
Cholinergic	M_3	Acetylcholine	Dilation	yes
Amines	H_1	Histamine	Variable	yes
	H_2	Histamine	Dilation	no
	$5HT_1$	5HT	Variable	variable
Purines	P_{2x}	ATP	Constriction	no
	P_{2y}	ATP	Dilation	yes
	A_1	Adenosine	Constriction	no
	A_2	Adenosine	Dilation	no
Eicosanoids	TP	Thromboxane A_2	Constriction	no
	?	Prostacyclin (PGI_2)	Dilation	?
Peptides	NK_1	Substance P	Dilation	yes
	NK_2	Neurokinin A	Constriction	no
	?	VIP	Relaxation	variable
	AT	Angiotensin	Constriction	no
	ANP	ANP	Dilation	no
	B_2	Bradykinin	Dilation	yes
	ET_A	Endothelin	Constriction	no
	ET_B	Endothelin	Dilation	yes
	?	Adrenomedullin	Dilation	?
	V_1	Vasopressin	Dilation	yes

The existence of many of the substances listed is at present only established in animals and their physiological or pathological relevance in humans therefore remains uncertain. From references 16 and 17. 5HT, 5-hydroxytryptamine; ATP, adenosine triphosphate; VIP, vasoactive intestinal peptide; ANP, atrial natriuretic peptide.

been extensively investigated in humans and are described separately below.

Receptors. Endothelial and smooth muscle cells of the pulmonary vasculature each have numerous receptor types and the agonists for these receptors may originate from nerve endings (e.g. acetylcholine, noradrenaline), be produced locally (e.g. eicosanoids) or arrive via the blood (e.g. peptides). In addition, many similar or identical compounds produce opposing effects by their actions on differing subgroups of receptors, for example α_1 (vasoconstrictor) and β_2 (vasodilator) adrenergic receptors. There remains therefore a large number of poorly understood systems acting together to bring about control of pulmonary vascular smooth muscle.

Second messengers. Pulmonary vasodilators that act directly on the smooth muscle, such as prostaglandins, vasoactive intestinal peptide, and under some circum-

stances β_2-agonists, mostly activate adenyl cyclase to produce cyclic adenosine 3′,5′ monophosphate (cAMP) as a second messenger. In turn, cAMP causes a host of intracellular activities via activation of protein kinase enzymes that reduce both the phosphorylation of myosin and intracellular calcium levels to bring about relaxation of the muscle cell.[19]

Receptors that cause contraction of pulmonary vascular smooth muscle are usually G-protein coupled. Activation produces a second messenger, inositol 1,4,5-triphosphate (IP_3), which releases calcium from intracellular stores and activates myosin phophorylation to produce contraction.

Role of the endothelium and nitric oxide.[16,20,21] Furchgott and Zawadzki in 1980 were the first to demonstrate that endothelial cells were required for acetylcholine (ACh)-induced relaxation in isolated aortic tissue.[22] The messenger passing between the endothelium and smooth muscle cells was termed endothelium-derived relaxing factor (EDRF),[23] the major part of which was subsequently shown to be nitric oxide (NO).[21] Many pulmonary vasodilator mechanisms have been shown to be endothelium dependent (see Table 7.1), and it seems likely that NO is a common pathway for producing relaxation of vascular smooth muscle from a variety of stimuli. Nitric oxide is not the only form of EDRF, with some species showing a quite separate messenger termed endothelium-derived hyperpolarising factor (EDHF).[24-26] The chemical nature of EDHF remains uncertain; current candidates include a metabolite of arachidonic acid, a cannabinoid or a simple change in extracellular potassium concentration. So far, EDHF has only been investigated in the systemic vasculature and there is currently no evidence for its existence in the pulmonary circulation.

Nitric oxide synthase (NOS) produces NO by the conversion of L-arginine to L-citrulline, via a highly reactive hydroxyarginine intermediate (Figure 7.6). NOS is involved in both stages and requires many cofactors, including calmodulin and NADPH and probably other flavine-derived factors, such as flavine adenine dinucleotide. Control of NOS activity depends on the availability of the substrate, arginine, and the concentrations of the various cofactors. Citrulline produced by NOS enters the urea cycle and is converted back into arginine (see Figure 7.6). This pathway utilises ammonia derived from the conversion of amino acids into energy-producing substrates such as pyruvate and provides a mechanism by which ammonium ions may be converted into relatively harmless nitrates (via NO). The biological disposal of nitric oxide is described on page 180.

Nitric oxide synthase exists in two forms, known as constitutive and inducible. Inducible NO synthase (iNOS) is produced in many cells but only in response to activation by inflammatory mediators and other cytokines and, once activated, can produce large amounts of NO for long periods. Constitutive NO synthase (cNOS) is permanently present in some cells, including pulmonary endothelium, and produces short bursts of low levels of NO in response to changes in calcium and calmodulin levels. In systemic vessels, sheer stress of the blood vessel wall may directly activate calcium-dependent potassium channels to activate cNOS, but in the pulmonary circulation receptor stimulation is the usual source of altered calcium levels and cNOS activation.

The mechanism by which receptor activation leads to muscle relaxation is illustrated in Figure 7.7. Nitric oxide diffuses from the site of production to the smooth muscle cell, where it activates guanylate cyclase to produce cyclic guanosine 3',5' monophosphate (cGMP), which in turn activates a protein kinase enzyme. This system is similar to the cAMP pathway described above and causes relaxation by a combination of effects on cytosolic calcium levels and the activity of enzymes controlling myosin activity.

Figure 7.6 Biochemical production of nitric oxide (NO). Nitric oxide synthase (NOS) acts as a catalyst for a two-stage reaction to convert arginine to citrulline. Oxygen is required at both stages and NADPH, calmodulin and flavine adenine dinucleotide (FAD) are required as cofactors for the first stage, and are believed to control the rate of NO production. Citrulline produced in this reaction may then enter the urea cycle and, using ammonia derived from amino acid metabolism, is converted back into arginine.

Figure 7.7 Schematic pathway for the activation of constitutive nitric oxide synthase and the action of nitric oxide in the pulmonary vasculature. There are many different receptors thought to act via this mechanism to bring about vasodilation. See text for details.

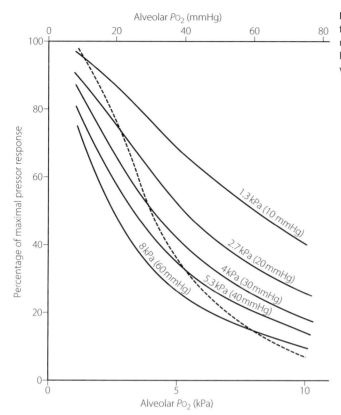

Figure 7.8 Pulmonary vasoconstriction (ordinate) as a function of alveolar P_{O_2} (abscissa) for different values of mixed venous P_{O_2} (indicated for each curve). The broken line shows the response when the alveolar and mixed venous P_{O_2} are identical. (Data from reference 30.)

There is now good evidence that basal production of NO occurs in normal human lungs and contributes to the maintenance of low pulmonary vascular resistance.[15,27] Both of these studies have used N^G-monomethyl-L-arginine (L-NMMA), a NOS inhibitor, to demonstrate reduced global or regional pulmonary blood flow.

Hypoxic pulmonary vasoconstriction

When vasoconstriction occurs in response to hypoxia, pulmonary blood vessels are displaying their fundamental difference from all systemic vessels. Hypoxic pulmonary vasoconstriction (HPV) is mediated both by mixed venous (pulmonary arterial) P_{O_2} and alveolar P_{O_2} (Figure 7.8), the greater influence being from the alveolus. The overall response to P_{O_2} is non-linear. This may be deduced from Figure 7.8 by noting the pressure response for different values of the isobaric P_{O_2} (the broken line), and it will be seen that the general shape of the response curve resembles an oxyhaemoglobin dissociation curve with a P_{50} of about 4 kPa (30 mmHg). The combined effect of hypoxia in alveolar gas and mixed venous blood may be considered as acting at a single point,[28] which exerts a 'stimulus' P_{O_2} as follows:

$$P\text{(stimulus)}_{O_2} = P\bar{v}_{O_2}^{0.375} \times P_{A_{O_2}}^{0.626}$$

In addition to the effect of mixed venous and alveolar P_{O_2}, the bronchial arterial P_{O_2} influences tone in the larger pulmonary arteries via the vasa vasorum.[29]

Regional hypoxic pulmonary vasoconstriction is beneficial as a means of diverting the pulmonary blood flow away from regions in which the oxygen tension is low and is an important factor in the optimisation of ventilation/perfusion relationships (see Chapter 8). It is also important in the foetus to minimise perfusion of the unventilated lung. However, overall chronic or intermittent hypoxic pulmonary vasoconstriction results in pulmonary hypertension and this response is disadvantageous in a range of clinical conditions (see Chapter 29).

The pressor response to hypoxia results from constriction of small arterioles of 30–200 μm in diameter.[31] Animal studies have shown that HPV begins within a few seconds of the P_{O_2} decreasing.[32] In humans, hypoxia in a single lobe of the lung results in a rapid decline in perfusion of the lobe, such that after 5 minutes regional blood flow is half that during normoxia.[33] In vitro and animal studies have shown that with prolonged hypoxia HPV is biphasic.[34] The first phase is similar to that seen in the human study already described, being rapid in onset with a maximum vasoconstriction after 5–10 minutes of hypoxia before rapidly returning to almost baseline levels of vascular activity. A second phase then develops involving a slow and sustained vasoconstriction that reaches a plateau after 40 minutes.

Mechanism of HPV.[35-37] Neural connections to the lung are not required, as HPV occurs in isolated lung preparations and in humans following lung transplantation.[38] There is no evidence for release of a vasoconstrictor substance in response to acute hypoxia, although almost all the vasoconstrictor substances listed in Table 7.1 have at some time been implicated, but with no subsequent confirmation.[31] With systemic arterial hypoxaemia some pulmonary vasoconstriction may result from hypoxic stimulation of the peripheral chemoreceptors (page 63) by way of sympathetic efferent pathways, but this is manifestly less important than the local effect.

Attempts to elucidate the mechanism of HPV have been hampered by species differences, the multitude of systems affecting pulmonary vascular tone and a lack of appreciation of the biphasic nature of the response. There remain many hypotheses on the cellular mechanism of HPV, based on either the inhibition of a vasodilator mechanism or stimulation of vasoconstriction. Proposed mechanisms include the following.

- Hypoxia may inhibit endothelial NO production and so induce vasoconstriction. This assumes a high level of normal NO production and although basal NO production does occur, its inhibition cannot alone explain HPV. Results of studies of NO and HPV are contradictory[34] and it is likely that NO is involved in modulation of HPV rather than being the underlying mechanism. Furthermore, it has been suggested that NO may be responsible for opposing HPV to maintain some perfusion of hypoxic regions.[36,39]
- Cyclooxygenase activity is inhibited by hypoxia, which may diminish the effects of vasodilator products such as prostacyclin (PGI$_2$), but again there are contradictory studies implying that this pathway is also involved only in modulation of HPV.[36]
- Hypoxia promotes the production of endothelin, a vasoconstrictor peptide, which has a prolonged effect on pulmonary vascular tone such that this mechanism is probably involved in the second slow phase of HPV and is likely to be important in the development of pulmonary hypertension with chronic hypoxia.[34,40]
- There is continuing interest in the possibility of a direct effect of hypoxia on pulmonary vascular smooth muscle cells. Pulmonary blood vessels, unlike systemic ones, have voltage-gated potassium channels (Kv) which under hypoxic conditions alter the membrane potential of the smooth muscle cell and so allow voltage-gated calcium channels to open and produce contraction.[35,37,41] It remains unclear whether hypoxia has a direct effect on Kv channels or whether an as yet unidentified oxygen sensor is required. Potential oxygen sensors that may fulfil this role include the β-subunit of the Kv channel itself,[41] reactive oxygen species from the mitochondria (page 353)[42] or intracellular ATP concentration.[43] Whether or not these direct ion channel mechanisms alone are sufficient to produce HPV *in vivo* is unclear, but it does show the origin of the fundamental difference between pulmonary and systemic blood vessels.

Hypoxic pulmonary vasoconstriction is therefore almost certainly multifactorial in origin and likely to result from a combination of direct effects of hypoxia on smooth muscle modulated by endothelium-dependent factors.

Other factors influencing pulmonary vascular resistance

Hypercapnia and acidosis. Elevated $P\text{CO}_2$ has a slight pressor effect. For example, hypoventilation of one lobe of a dog's lung reduces perfusion of that lobe, although its ventilation/perfusion ratio is still reduced.[44] Both respiratory and metabolic acidosis augment HPV.[12,45]

Hypocapnia and alkalosis. Alkalosis, whether respiratory or metabolic in origin, causes pulmonary vasodilation[12] and reduces[46] or even abolishes[47] HPV.

Neural control

There are three systems involved in autonomic control of the pulmonary circulation,[16,17] which are similar to those controlling airway tone (page 46).

Adrenergic sympathetic nerves originate from the first five thoracic nerves and travel to the pulmonary vessels via the cervical ganglia and a plexus of nerves around the trachea and smaller airways. They act mainly on the smooth muscle of arteries and arterioles down to a diameter of less than 60 μm.[12,16] There are both α$_1$-receptors which mediate vasoconstriction, usually in response to noradrenaline release, and β$_2$-receptors which produce vasodilation mainly in response to circulating adrenaline. Finally, pulmonary blood vessels contain α$_2$-receptors which cause vasodilation, either presynaptically where they inhibit noradrenaline release, or postsynaptically on endothelial cells, where they increase NO production (see Figure 7.7).[48] Overall, α$_1$ effects predominate and sympathetic stimulation increases pulmonary vascular resistance.[16] The influence of the sympathetic system is not as strong as in the systemic circulation and seems to have little influence under resting conditions. There is no obvious disadvantage in this respect in patients with lung transplant (see Chapter 33).

Cholinergic nerves of the parasympathetic system travel in the vagus nerve and cause pulmonary vasodilation by release of ACh and stimulation of M_3 muscarinic receptors.[16] Acetylcholine-mediated vasodilation is now accepted as being endothelium and NO dependent,[15,22] and in the absence of endothelium ACh is a vasoconstrictor. The significance of cholinergic nerves in humans is less clear than that of adrenergic systems. Infusion of ACh into the pulmonary artery in normal subjects results in vasodilation,[15] so ACh receptors clearly exist, but cholinergic nerve fibres have not been demonstrated histologically around human pulmonary vessels.[16]

Non-adrenergic, non-cholinergic (NANC)[16] nerves are closely related anatomically to the other autonomic mechanisms but with different neurotransmitters, and are similar to the NANC nerves controlling airway smooth muscle (page 46). In the lung, most NANC nerves are inhibitory, causing vasodilation via release of NO, possibly in conjunction with peptides (see Table 7.1). The functional significance of this system is unknown.

Humoral control

Pulmonary vascular endothelium is involved in the metabolism of many circulating substances (see Chapter 12), some of which cause changes in vascular tone (see Table 7.1). Which of these are involved in the control of normal pulmonary vascular resistance is unclear and it is quite possible that very few are, but some are undoubtedly involved in pulmonary vascular disease (see Chapter 29).

Catecholamines. Circulating adrenaline following sympathetic stimulation acts on both α- and β-receptors and results in a predominantly vasoconstrictor response. Exogenous adrenaline and related inotropes such as dopamine have a similar effect.

Eicosanoids. Arachidonic acid metabolism via the cyclooxygenase pathway (to prostaglandins and thromboxane) and lipoxygenase pathway (to leukotrienes) has been demonstrated in pulmonary vessels in animals. The products of arachidonic acid metabolism have diverse biological effects in many physiological systems and the pulmonary vasculature is no exception. Arachidonic acid itself, thromboxane A_2, $PGF_{2\alpha}$, PGD_2, PGE_2 and LTB_4 are all vasoconstrictors, whereas PGI_2 (prostacyclin) is usually a vasodilator. These pathways are believed to be involved in pathological pulmonary hypertension resulting from sepsis, reperfusion injury or congenital heart disease.[16]

Amines. Histamine relaxes pulmonary vascular smooth muscle during adrenaline-induced constriction but constricts resting smooth muscle. Constriction is in response to H_1 stimulation on smooth muscle cells, whereas relaxation occurs either via H_1 receptors on endothelium (NO dependent) or H_2 receptors on smooth muscle cells. 5-hydroxytryptamine (serotonin) is liberated from activated platelets and is a potent vasoconstrictor. It may be involved in pulmonary hypertension secondary to emboli (page 393).

Peptides. Numerous peptides that are vasoactive in the pulmonary circulation are shown in Table 7.1. Responses are again diverse, many systems producing vasodilation via endothelium receptors and vasoconstriction via direct effects on smooth muscle (e.g. substance P and neurokinin A).[16]

Purine nucleosides such as adenosine and ATP are highly vasoactive, again with variable responses according to the amount of tone in the pulmonary blood vessel.[16] Adenosine is a pulmonary vasodilator in normal subjects.[49]

DRUG EFFECTS ON THE PULMONARY CIRCULATION

A higher than normal pulmonary arterial pressure occurs rarely as a primary disease but commonly develops as a secondary consequence of chronic hypoxia from a variety of lung diseases (see Chapter 29). Pulmonary hypertension often leads to right-sided heart failure (cor pulmonale) and is a major cause of morbidity and mortality in patients with respiratory disease. Considering the wide range of receptor–agonist systems present in the pulmonary vasculature (see Table 7.1) it is surprising that there are few effective drugs available. One reason for this is the non-specific nature of many of the receptors found in the pulmonary vasculature, such that drugs acting on these receptors have widespread effects elsewhere in the body that make them therapeutically unacceptable. Another problem with pulmonary vasodilators in respiratory disease is that abolishing HPV removes the body's main mechanisms for compensating for poor respiratory function. For example, nifedipine administered sublingually in patients with severe airways disease causes a significant reduction in pulmonary hypertension, but this is associated with a worsening of arterial hypoxaemia.[50] As a way of avoiding both these problems, delivering drugs by inhalation has had some success,[51] particularly if the drug is inactivated before reaching the systemic circulation.

Inhaled drugs

Nitric oxide. Inhaled NO (iNO) in patients with severe lung disease is a selective pulmonary vasodilator, with the systemic circulation being unaffected owing to its rapid inactivation by haemoglobin (page 180). Nitric oxide therefore increases blood flow to well-ventilated areas of the lung and so diverts blood flow away from poorly ventilated areas,[52] thereby decreasing ventilation/perfusion mismatch and improving arterial oxygenation. In addition to its role in modulating vascular tone and oxygenation, NO may play a significant role as an immunomodulator; for example, by reducing leucocyte adhesion and activation[53] it may attenuate lung inflammation (see Chapter 31).

Inhaled NO in the presence of oxygen is rapidly oxidised to NO_2, the rate of oxidation being directly related to oxygen concentration and the square of NO concentration. NO_2 can react with water to form highly injurious nitric and nitrous acids that can cause severe pneumonitis and pulmonary edema. Hence to minimise the production of NO_2 both the concentration of oxygen and NO, and the contact time between the two, should be minimised. Practical guidelines for the safe use of iNO have been published.[54] Some of the beneficial effects of iNO may be short-lived, out rapid discontinuation of iNO leads to a rebound phenomenon, probably due to inhibition of endogenous NO, with decreased oxygenation and increased pulmonary artery pressures. Hence iNO should be withdrawn in a slow stepwise fashion. Despite these numerous drawbacks, in some groups of patients with acute lung injury therapeutic iNO does seem to produce improved clinical outcomes.[55]

Prostacyclin.[51] Intravenous prostacyclin (PGI_2) has been used for many years in critically ill patients to reduce PA pressure, but its lack of selectivity for the pulmonary vasculature causes significant adverse effects. When delivered by inhalation, metabolism of PGI_2 by the lung is negligible, so systemic absorption occurs. However, the dose required by inhalation is very small, so despite its systemic absorption clinically significant adverse effects are minimal. Compared with iNO, inhaled PGI_2 has the advantage of not producing toxic metabolites and early clinical studies are encouraging.[51]

Systemic drugs[56]

Angiotensin-converting enzyme inhibitors reduce pulmonary vascular resistance in patients with pulmonary hypertension secondary to lung disease, but only with long-term treatment. These drugs are believed to reduce pulmonary vascular remodelling, a pathological process that occurs with long-term hypoxia and involving smooth muscle cell proliferation and a loss of elasticity in the pulmonary blood vessels. Losartan, an angiotensin II receptor antagonist, reduces pulmonary artery pressure within hours of administration, without detriment to the patient's oxygen saturation.[57]

Phosphodiesterase inhibitors such as amrinone and milrinone can inhibit the breakdown of both cAMP and cGMP and so enhance the activity of these cellular messengers that bring about vascular smooth muscle cell relaxation from a variety of pathways (see above). These drugs have been used to reduce pulmonary hypertension by both the intravenous and the inhaled routes.

Calcium antagonists such as nifedipine reduce secondary pulmonary hypertension in a dose-dependent fashion. However, as described above, in some patient groups hypoxaemia may worsen and at the large doses often needed to reduce pulmonary hypertension, the negative inotropic effects of calcium antagonists become significant and right heart failure caused by the pulmonary hypertension can deteriorate.

Endothelin receptor antagonists are a new class of drugs that competitively antagonise both ET_A and ET_B receptors, though in the clinical situation ET_B effects seem to predominate and reduce PA pressure. Endothelin has been implicated in vascular remodelling of pulmonary vessels with chronic hypoxia, so these drugs may slow this process. Bosentan, a non-selective oral endothelin antagonist, has not yet been studied in patients with pulmonary hypertension secondary to respiratory disease, but has shown some benefit in patients with primary pulmonary hypertension (page 396).[58] Sitaxsentan is a recently introduced endothelin antagonist which is highly specific for ET_A receptors and so may prove particularly useful for treating pulmonary hypertension.[59]

PRINCIPLES OF MEASUREMENT OF THE PULMONARY CIRCULATION

Detailed consideration of haemodynamic measurement techniques lies outside the scope of this book. The following section presents only the broad principles of measurement such as may be required in relation to respiratory physiology.

Pulmonary blood volume

Available methods are based on the technique used for measurement of cardiac output by dye dilution (see below). The flow rate so obtained is multiplied by the interval between the time of injection of the dye and its mean arrival time at the sampling point. This product indicates the amount of blood lying between injection and sampling sites and the volume result obtained therefore depends very much on exactly where sampling occurs. Total pulmonary blood volume may be measured by sampling from the proximal pulmonary artery and the pulmonary vein (or left atrium). Typical values are of the order of 0.5–1.0 l or 10–20% of total blood volume in an adult.

Table 2.2 shows the anatomical distribution of the pulmonary blood volume within the pulmonary arterial tree, which has a volume of the order of 150 ml. Pulmonary capillary volume may be calculated from measurements of diffusing capacity (see Chapter 9) and this technique yields values of the order of 80 ml. The pulmonary veins therefore contain over half of the pulmonary blood volume, as they possess much less vasomotor tone than the pulmonary arteries.

Pulmonary vascular pressures

Pressure measurements within the pulmonary circulation are almost always made with electronic pressure transducers, which measure pressure in a column of liquid in continuity with a blood vessel compared with atmospheric pressure. If the system is to have the ability to respond to rapid changes of pressure, such as a pulsatile artery, damping must be 'critical', that is, reduced to a minimum required to remove noise from the signal without overdamping and losing the peaks and troughs of the pressure wave. This requires the total exclusion of bubbles of air from the manometer and connecting tubing, and the intravascular cannula must be unobstructed. Electrical manometry then yields a plot of instantaneous pressure against time (Figure 7.9). Systolic and diastolic pressures are measured from the peaks and troughs of this trace and the mean pressure is derived electronically.

Figure 7.3 shows the sites at which pressure must be measured to obtain the various forms of pulmonary vascular pressure (page 94). Driving pressure, the most useful of these, requires measurement of pulmonary arterial and pulmonary venous (left atrial) pressures.

Pulmonary arterial pressure may be measured using a balloon flotation catheter. Following insertion into the right atrium via a central vein, a balloon of <1 ml volume is inflated to encourage the catheter tip to follow the flow of blood through the right ventricle and pulmonary valve into the pulmonary artery (see Figure 7.9). The most commonly used catheter is the Swan–Ganz, named after the two cardiologists who devised the catheter after Dr Swan watched sailboats being propelled by the wind in 1967.[60]

Left atrial pressure represents pulmonary venous pressure and is measured in humans by one of three possible techniques, of which only the first is commonly used in clinical practice.

- Pulmonary artery occlusion pressure (PAOP).[61] Occlusion pressures are obtained by advancing the Swan–Ganz catheter into a branch of the pulmonary artery, with the balloon inflated, until the arterial pulsation disappears (see Figure 7.9). There should then be no flow in the column of blood between the tip of the catheter and the left atrium, and the manometer will indicate left atrial pressure.
- A left atrial catheter may be sited during cardiac surgery and passed through the chest wall for use postoperatively.
- A catheter may be passed retrogradely from a peripheral systemic artery.

Pulmonary blood flow

The method used for measurement of pulmonary blood flow will affect whether or not the result includes venous admixture, such as the bronchial circulation and intrapulmonary shunts shown in Figure 7.1. Though of minimal relevance in normal subjects, in patients with lung disease venous admixture may be highly significant. In general, methods involving uptake of an inert gas from the alveoli will exclude venous admixture and all other methods include it.

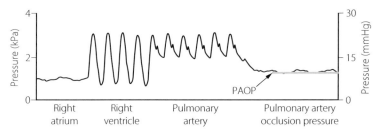

Figure 7.9 Pressure traces obtained when inserting a balloon flotation catheter in a patient receiving intermittent positive-pressure ventilation. With the balloon inflated, the catheter tip follows blood flow through the right atrium, right ventricle and pulmonary artery until it occludes a branch of the pulmonary artery. The pulmonary artery occlusion pressure (PAOP) is the pressure measured distal to the balloon and equates to pulmonary venous and left atrial pressures. Note the respiratory swings in the trace caused by positive-pressure ventilation. PAOP is measured as the mean pressure at end-expiration.

The Fick principle states that the amount of oxygen extracted from the respired gases equals the amount added to the blood which flows through the lungs. Thus the oxygen uptake of the subject must equal the product of pulmonary blood flow and arteriovenous oxygen content difference:

$$\dot{V}_{O_2} = \dot{Q}(Ca_{O_2} - C\bar{v}_{O_2})$$

therefore:

$$\dot{Q} = \frac{V_{O_2}}{(Ca_{O_2} - C\bar{v}_{O_2})}$$

All the quantities on the right-hand side can be measured, although determination of the oxygen content of the mixed venous blood requires catheterisation of the right ventricle or, preferably, the pulmonary artery as described above. Interpretation of the result is less easy. The calculated value includes the intrapulmonary arteriovenous shunt, but the situation is complicated beyond the possibility of easy solution if there is appreciable extrapulmonary admixture of venous blood (see Figure 7.1). The second major problem is that spirometry measures the total oxygen consumption, including that of the lung. The Fick equation excludes the lung (see Figure 11.22), but the difference is negligible with healthy lungs. There is evidence that the oxygen consumption of infected lungs may be very large (page 197) and therefore the Fick method of cardiac output measurement would appear to be invalid under such circumstances.

Methods based on uptake of inert tracer gases.

A modified Fick method of measurement of cardiac output may be employed with any fairly soluble inert gas. The tracer gas is inhaled either continually or for a single breath and the end-tidal partial pressure of tracer gas is then measured. Analysis of volume and composition of expired tracer gas permits measurement of gas uptake. Since the duration of the procedure is short and does not permit recirculation, it may be assumed that the mixed venous concentration of the tracer gas is zero. The Fick equation then simplifies to the following:

Cardiac output =

tracer gas uptake/arterial tracer gas concentration

The arterial tracer gas concentration equals the product of the arterial gas tension (assumed equal to the alveolar [end-tidal] gas tension) and the solubility coefficient of the tracer gas in blood. Thus arterial blood sampling may be avoided, so the method is relatively non-invasive.

All the methods based on the uptake of inert tracer gases have the following characteristics.

- They measure pulmonary capillary blood flow, excluding any flow through shunts. This is in contrast to the Fick and dye methods.

- The assumption that the tension of the tracer gas is the same in end-expiratory gas and arterial blood is invalid in the presence of either alveolar dead space or shunt (see Chapter 8).
- Some of the tracer gas dissolves in the tissues lining the respiratory tract and is carried away by blood perfusing these tissues. The indicated blood flow is therefore greater than the actual pulmonary capillary blood flow.

The tracer gas used has varied over the years, with nitrous oxide and acetylene being used early in the 20th century. In the most recent version of the technique, freon is the tracer gas used. In this case, argon (highly insoluble gas) is added to the gas mixture to ensure complete mixing of the freon with alveolar gas and also to detect subjects with a large respiratory dead space (see Chapter 8), in whom the method is invalid.[62]

Dye or thermal dilution.

Currently the most popular technique for measurement of cardiac output is by dye dilution. An indicator substance is introduced as a bolus into a large vein and its concentration is measured continuously at a sampling site in the systemic arterial tree. Figure 7.10a shows the method as it is applied to continuous non-circulating flow as, for example, of fluids through a pipeline. The downstream concentration of dye is displayed on the y-axis of the graph against time on the x-axis. The dye is injected at time t_1 and is first detected at the sampling point at time t_2. The uppermost curve shows the form of a typical curve. There is a rapid rise to maximum concentration followed by a decay that is an exponential wash-out in form (see Appendix F), reaching insignificant levels at time t_3. The second graph shows the concentration (y-axis) on a logarithmic scale when the exponential part of the decay curve becomes a straight line (see Figure F.5). Between times t_2 and t_3, the mean concentration of dye equals the amount of dye injected, divided by the volume of fluid flowing past the sampling point during the interval $t_2 - t_3$, which is the product of the fluid flow rate and the time interval $t_2 - t_3$. The equation may now be rearranged to indicate the flow rate of the fluid as the following expression:

$$\frac{\text{Amount of dye injected}}{\text{Mean concentration of dye} \times \text{time interval } t_2 - t_3}$$

The amount of dye injected is known and the denominator is the area under the curve.

Figure 7.10b shows the more complicated situation when fluid is flowing round a circuit. Under these conditions, the front of the dye-laden fluid may lap its own tail so that a recirculation peak appears on the graph before the primary peak has decayed to insignificant levels. This commonly occurs when cardiac output is

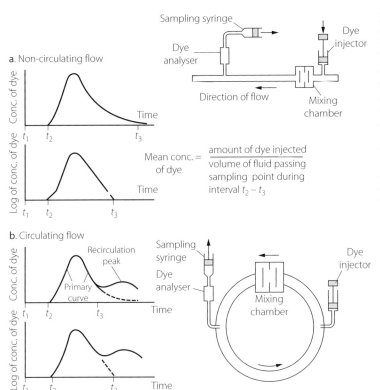

a. Non-circulating flow

Conc. of dye

Time

Log of conc. of dye

t_1 t_2 t_3

Time

t_1 t_2 t_3

$$\text{Mean conc.} = \frac{\text{amount of dye injected}}{\text{volume of fluid passing sampling point during interval } t_2 - t_3}$$

Sampling syringe

Dye analyser

Dye injector

Direction of flow

Mixing chamber

b. Circulating flow

Conc. of dye

Recirculation peak

Primary curve

t_1 t_2 t_3 Time

Log of conc. of dye

t_1 t_2 t_3 Time

Sampling syringe

Dye analyser

Dye injector

Mixing chamber

Figure 7.10 Measurement of flow by dye dilution. **(a)** The measurement of continuous non-circulating flow rate of fluid in a pipeline. The bolus of dye is injected upstream and its concentration is continuously monitored downstream. The relationship of the relevant quantities is shown in the equation. Mean concentration of dye is determined from the area under the curve. **(b)** The more complicated situation when recirculation occurs and the front of the circulating dye laps its own tail, giving a recirculation peak. Reconstruction of the primary curve is based on extrapolation of the primary curve before recirculation occurs. This is facilitated by the fact that the down curve is exponential and therefore a straight line on a logarithmic plot.

determined in humans and steps must be taken to reconstruct the tail of the primary curve as it would have been had recirculation not taken place. This is done by extrapolating the exponential wash-out, which is usually established before the recirculation peak appears. This is shown as the broken lines in the graphs of Figure 7.10b. The calculation of cardiac output then proceeds as described above for non-recirculating flow. This previously laborious procedure is now performed electronically as an integral part of the apparatus for measuring cardiac output.

Many different indicators have been used for the dye dilution technique, but currently the most satisfactory appears to be 'coolth'. A bolus of cold saline is injected and the dip in temperature is recorded downstream with the temperature record corresponding to the dye curve. No blood sampling is required and temperature is measured directly with a thermometer mounted on the catheter. The 'coolth' is dispersed in the systemic circulation and therefore there is no recirculation peak to complicate the calculation. The thermal method is particularly suitable for repeated measurements.

REFERENCES

1. Harris P. The evolution of the pulmonary circulation. *Thorax* 1995; **49**: S5–S8.

2. Deffebach ME, Charan NB, Lakshminarayan S, Butler J. The bronchial circulation: small but a vital attribute to the lung. *Am Rev Respir Dis* 1987; **135**: 463–81.

3. Verloop MC. The arteriae bronchiales and their anastomoses with the arteriae pulmonalis in the human lung: a micro-anatomical study. *Acta Anat* 1948; **5**: 171–205.

4. Hasegawa I, Kobayashi K, Kohda E, Hiramatsu K. Bronchopulmonary arterial anastomosis at the precapillary level in human lung. *Acta Radiol* 1999; **39**: 578–84.

5. Marshall BE, Marshall C. Pulmonary circulation during anaesthesia. In: Stanley TH, Sperry RJ, eds. *Anesthesia and the lung*. Dordrecht: Kluwer, 1992: 31–43.

6. Warrell DA, Evans JW, Clarke RO, Kingaby GP, West JB. Pattern of filling in the pulmonary capillary bed. *J Appl Physiol* 1972; **32**: 346–56.

7. Presson RG, Baumgartner WA, Peterson AJ, Glenny RW, Wagner WW. Pulmonary capillaries are recruited during pulsatile flow. *J Appl Physiol* 2002; **92**: 1183–90.

8. König MF, Lucocq JM, Weibel ER. Demonstration of pulmonary vascular perfusion by electron and light microscopy. *J Appl Physiol* 1993; **75**: 1877–83.

9. Conhaim RL, Harms BA. Perfusion of alveolar septa in isolated rat lungs in zone 1. *J Appl Physiol* 1993; **75**: 704–11.

10. Johnson RL, Hsai CCW. Functional recruitment of pulmonary capillaries. *J Appl Physiol* 1994; **76**: 1405–7.

11. Sobin SS, Fung YC, Tremer HM, Rosenquist TH. Elasticity of the pulmonary alveolar microvascular sheet in the cat. *Circ Res* 1972; **30**: 440–50.

12. Fishman AP. Pulmonary circulation. In: Fishman AP, Fisher AB, Geiger SR, eds. *Handbook of physiology, section 3 – the respiratory system*. Bethesda, MD: American Physiological Society, 1987; 93–7.

13. West JB, Dollery CT, Naimark A. Distribution of blood flow in isolated lung; relation to vascular and alveolar pressures. *J Appl Physiol* 1964; **19**: 713–24.

14. West JB, Dollery CT. Distribution of blood flow and the pressure–flow relations of the whole lung. *J Appl Physiol* 1965; **20**: 175–83.

*15. Cooper CJ, Landzberg MJ, Anderson TJ, *et al*. Role of nitric oxide in the local regulation of pulmonary vascular resistance in humans. *Circulation* 1996; **93**: 266–71.

*16. Barnes PJ, Liu SF. Regulation of pulmonary vascular tone. *Pharmacol Rev* 1995; **47**: 87–131.

17. Kobayashi Y, Amenta F. Neurotransmitter receptors in the pulmonary circulation with particular emphasis on pulmonary endothelium. *J Autonom Pharmacol* 1994; **14**: 137–64.

*18. Wilkins MR, Zhao L, Al-Tubuly R. The regulation of pulmonary vascular tone. *Br J Clin Pharmacol* 1996; **42**: 127–31.

19. Murray KJ. Cyclic AMP and mechanisms of vasodilation. *Pharmacol Ther* 1990; **47**: 329–45.

20. Anggard E. Nitric oxide: mediator, murderer and medicine. *Lancet* 1994; **343**: 1199–206.

21. Moncada S, Palmer R, Higgs E. Nitric oxide: physiology, pathophysiology and pharmacology. *Pharmacol Rev* 1991; **43**: 109–42.

22. Furchgott RF, Zawadzki JV. The obligatory role of endothelial cells in the relaxation of arterial smooth muscle by acetylcholine. *Nature* 1980; **288**: 373–6.

23. Cherry PD, Furchgott RF, Zawadzki JV, Jothianandan D. Role of endothelial cells in relaxation of isolated arteries by bradykinin. *Proc Natl Acad Sci USA* 1982; **79**: 2106–10.

24. Nagao T, Vanhoute PM. Endothelium-derived hyperpolarizing factor and endothelium-dependent relaxations. *Am J Respir Cell Mol Biol* 1993; 8: 1–6.

25. Triggle CR, Ding H. Endothelium-derived hyperpolarizing factor: is there a novel chemical mediator? *Clin Exp Pharmacol Physiol* 2002; **29**: 153–60.

26. Triggle CR, Dong H, Waldron GJ, Cole WC. Endothelium-derived hyperpolarizing factor(s): species and tissue heterogeneity. *Clin Exp Pharmacol Physiol* 1999; **26**: 176–9.

27. Stamler JS, Loh E, Roddy M-A, Currie KE, Craeger MA. Nitric oxide regulated basal systemic and pulmonary vascular resistance in healthy humans. *Circulation* 1994; **89**: 2035–40.

28. Marshall BE, Marshall C, Frasch HF. Control of the pulmonary circulation. In: Stanley TH, Sperry RJ, eds. *Anesthesia and the lung*. Dordrecht: Kluwer, 1992: 9–18.

29. Marshall BE, Marshall C, Magno M, Lilagan P, Pietra GG. Influence of bronchial artery PO_2 on pulmonary vascular resistance. *J Appl Physiol* 1991; **70**: 405–15.

30. Marshall BE, Marshall C. Anesthesia and the pulmonary circulation. In: Covino BG, Fozzard HA, Rehder K, Stricharz G, eds. *Effects of anesthesia*. Bethesda, MD: American Physiological Society, 1983.

31. Anand IS. Hypoxia and the pulmonary circulation. *Thorax* 1994; **49**: S19–S24.

32. Jensen KS, Micco AJ, Czartolomna J, Latham L, Voelkel NF. Rapid onset of hypoxic vasoconstriction in isolated lungs. *J Appl Physiol* 1992; **72**: 2018–23.

33. Morrell NW, Nijran KS, Biggs T, Seed WA. Magnitude and time course of acute hypoxic pulmonary vasoconstriction in man. *Respir Physiol* 1995; **100**: 271–81.

34. Ward JPT, Robertson TP. The role of endothelium in hypoxic pulmonary vasoconstriction. *Exp Physiol* 1995; **80**: 793–801.

35. Archer S, Michelakis E. The mechanism(s) of hypoxic pulmonary vasoconstriction: potassium channels, redox O_2 sensors and controversies. *News Physiol Sci* 2002; **17**: 131–7.

36. Aaronson PI, Robertson TP, Ward JPT. Endothelium-derived mediators and hypoxic pulmonary vasoconstriction. *Respir Physiol Neurobiol* 2002; **132**: 107–20.

*37. Gurney AM. Multiple sites of oxygen sensing and their contributions to hypoxic pulmonary vasoconstriction. *Respir Physiol Neurobiol* 2002; **132**: 43–53.

38. Robin ED, Theodore J, Burke CM, *et al*. Hypoxic pulmonary vasoconstriction persists in the human transplanted lung. *Clin Sci* 1987; **72**: 283–7.

39. Sprague RS, Thiemermann C, Vane JR. Endogenous endothelium-derived relaxing factor opposes hypoxic pulmonary vasoconstriction and supports blood flow to hypoxic alveoli in anaesthetized rabbits. *Proc Natl Acad Sci USA* 1992; **89**: 8711–15.

40. Shimoda LA, Sham JSK, Liu Q, Sylvester JT. Acute and chronic hypoxic pulmonary vasoconstriction: a central role for endothelin-1? *Respir Physiol Neurobiol* 2002; **132**: 93–106.

*41. Coppock EA, Martens JR, Tamkun MM. Molecular basis of hypoxia-induced pulmonary vasoconstriction: role of voltage-gated K^+ channels. *Am J Physiol* 2001; **281**: L1–L12.

42. Waypa GB, Schumacker PT. O_2 sensing in hypoxic pulmonary vasoconstriction: the mitochondrial door re-opens. *Respir Physiol Neurobiol* 2002; **132**: 81–91.

43. Clapp LH, Gurney AM. ATP-sensitive K⁺ channels regulate resting potential of pulmonary arterial smooth muscle cells. *Am J Physiol* 1992; **262**: H916–H920.

44. Suggett AJ, Barer GR, Mohammed FH, Gill GW. The effects of localised hyperventilation on ventilation/perfusion ($\dot{V}/\dot{Q}$) ratios and gas exchange in the dog lung. *Clin Sci* 1982; **63**: 497–503.

45. Rudolph AM, Yuan S. Response of the pulmonary vasculature to hypoxia and H⁺ ion concentration changes. *J Clin Invest* 1966; **45**: 399–411.

46. Benumof JL, Wahrenbrock EA. Blunted hypoxic pulmonary vasoconstriction by increased lung vascular pressures. *J Appl Physiol* 1975; **38**: 846–50.

47. Lloyd TC. Influence of blood pH on hypoxic pulmonary vasoconstriction. *J Appl Physiol* 1966; **21**: 358–64.

48. Pepke-Zaba J, Higgenbottam T, Dinh-Xuan AT, Ridden C, Kealey T. α-Adrenoceptor stimulation of porcine pulmonary arteries. *Eur J Pharmacol* 1993; **235**: 169–75.

49. Reid PG, Fraser A, Watt A, Henderson A, Routledge P. Acute haemodynamic effects of adenosine in conscious man. *Eur Heart J* 1990; **11**: 1018–28.

50. Kalra L, Bone MF. Effect of nifedipine on physiologic shunting and oxygenation in chronic obstructive pulmonary disease. *Am J Med* 1993; **94**: 419–23.

51. Lowson SM. Inhaled alternatives to nitric oxide. *Anesthesiology* 2002; **96**: 1504–13.

52. Bigatello LM, Hurford WE, Hess D. Use of inhaled nitric oxide for ARDS. *Respir Care Clin North Am* 1997; **3**: 437–58.

53. Kavanah BP, Mouchawar A, Goldsmith J, *et al.* Effects of inhaled NO and inhibition of endogenous NO synthesis in oxidant-induced acute lung injury. *J Appl Physiol* 1994; **76**: 1324–9.

54. Cuthbertson BH, Dellinger P, Dyar OJ, *et al.* UK guidelines for the use of inhaled nitric oxide therapy in adult ICUs. *Intens Care Med* 1997; 23: 1212–18.

55. Malarkkan N, Snook NJ, Lumb AB. New aspects of ventilation in acute lung injury. *Anaesthesia* 2003; **58**: 647–67.

56. Fischer LG, van Aken H, Bürkle H. Management of pulmonary hypertension: physiological and pharmacological considerations for anesthesiologists. *Anesth Analg* 2003; **96**: 1603–16.

57. Kiely DG, Cargill RI, Wheeldon NM, Coutie WJ, Lipworth BJ. Haemodynamic and endocrine effects of type 1 angiotensin II receptor blockade in patients with hypoxaemic cor pulmonale. *Cardiovasc Res* 1997; **33**: 201–8.

58. Channick RN, Simonneau G, Sitbon O, *et al.* Effects of the dual endothelin-receptor antagonist bosentan in patients with pulmonary hypertension: a randomised placebo-controlled study. *Lancet* 2001; **358**: 1119–23.

59. Barst RJ, Langleben D, Frost A, *et al.* Sitaxsentan therapy for pulmonary arterial hypertension. *Am J Respir Crit Care Med* 2004; **169**: 441–7.

60. Swan HJC, Ganz W. Hemodynamic monitoring: a personal and historical perspective. *Can Med Assoc J* 1979; **121**: 868–71.

*61. Pinsky MR. Pulmonary artery occlusion pressure. *Intens Care Med* 2003; **29**: 19–22.

62. Winter SM. Clinical non-invasive measurement of effective pulmonary blood flow. *Int J Clin Monit Comput* 1995; **12**: 121–40.

Distribution of pulmonary ventilation and perfusion

The lung may be considered as a simple exchanger with a gas inflow and outflow and a blood inflow and outflow (Figure 8.1). There is near-equilibrium of oxygen and carbon dioxide tensions between the two outflow streams from the exchanger itself. This theoretical model assumes that gas flow in and out of the alveolus and blood flow through the pulmonary capillary are both continuous. This assumption may be true within alveoli, where at normal tidal volumes gas movement is by diffusion (page 17), but pulmonary capillary blood flow is pulsatile. This model has been deliberately drawn without countercurrent flow, which would be far more efficient. Such a system operates in the gills of fishes and brings the PO_2 of arterial blood close to the PO_2 of the environment.

Gas exchange will clearly be optimal if ventilation and perfusion are distributed in the same proportion to one another throughout the lung. Conversely, to take an extreme example, if ventilation were distributed entirely to one lung and perfusion to the other, there could be no gas exchange, although total ventilation and perfusion might each be normal. This chapter begins by considering the spatial and temporal distribution of ventilation, followed by similar treatment for the pulmonary circulation. Distribution of ventilation and perfusion are then considered in relation to one another. Finally the concepts of dead space and shunt are presented.

DISTRIBUTION OF VENTILATION

Spatial and anatomical distribution of inspired gas

Distribution between the two lungs in the normal subject is influenced by posture and by the manner of ventilation. By virtue of its larger size, the right lung normally enjoys a ventilation slightly greater than the left lung in both the upright and the supine position (Table 8.1). In the lateral position, the lower lung is always better ventilated regardless of the side on which the subject is lying, although there still remains a bias in favour of the right side.[1] Fortunately, the preferential ventilation of the lower lung accords with increased perfusion of the same lung, so the ventilation/perfusion ratios of the two lungs are not greatly altered on assuming the lateral position. However, the upper lung tends to be better ventilated in the anaesthetised patient in the lateral position, regardless of the mode of ventilation and particularly with an open chest (see Table 8.1).

Distribution of ventilation to horizontal slices of lung has been studied for many years by inhalation of radioactive isotopes, this technique having the advantage of being easily performed in a variety of postures. In the upright position, with slow vital capacity inspirations, uppermost slices of the lung have a ventilation of around one-third that of slices at the bases.[5] A slow inspiration from functional residual capacity (FRC), as occurs during normal resting ventilation, results in a smaller vertical gradient down the lung, with the ratio of basal to apical ventilation being approximately 1.5/1.[6]

Posture affects distribution, since *inter alia* the vertical height of the lung is reduced by about 30% in the supine position. Therefore the gravitational force generating maldistribution is much less. More modern tech-

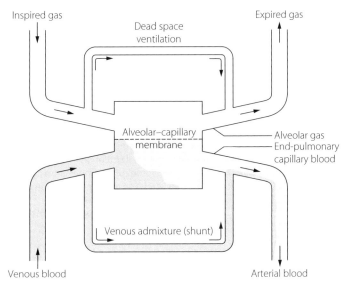

Figure 8.1 In this functional representation of gas exchange in the lungs, the flow of gas and blood is considered as a continuous process with movement from left to right. Under most circumstances equilibrium is obtained between alveolar gas and end-pulmonary capillary blood, the gas tensions in the two phases being almost identical. However, alveolar gas is mixed with dead space gas to give expired gas and end-pulmonary capillary blood is mixed with shunted venous blood to give arterial blood. Thus both expired gas and arterial blood have tensions that differ from those in alveolar gas and end-pulmonary capillary blood.

Table 8.1 Distribution of resting lung volume (FRC) and ventilation between the two lungs in humans

	Supine		Right lateral (left side up)		Left lateral (right side up)	
	Right lung	*Left lung*	*Right lung*	*Left lung*	*Right lung*	*Left lung*
Conscious[1]	1.69	1.39	1.68	2.07	2.19	1.38
	53%	47%	61%	39%	47%	53%
Anaesthetised – spontaneous breathing[2]	1.18	0.91	1.03	1.32	1.71	0.79
	52%	48%	45%	55%	56%	44%
Anaesthetised – artificial ventilation[3]	1.36	1.16	1.33	2.21	2.29	1.12
	52%	48%	44%	56%	60%	40%
Anaesthetised – thoracotomy[4]					–	–
					83%	17%

The first figure is the unilateral FRC (litres) and the second the percentage partition of ventilation. Each study refers to separate subjects or patients.

niques for quantifying regional ventilation include positron emission tomography (PET) and magnetic resonance imaging (MRI), both of which are only possible in supine subjects. These techniques confirm earlier findings that normal tidal breathing in the supine position results in preferential ventilation of the posterior slices of the lungs compared to the anterior slices.[7–9]

Starting from FRC, preferential ventilation of the dependent parts of the lung is only present at inspiratory flow rates below 1.5 l.s^{-1}. At higher flow rates, distribution becomes approximately uniform. Fast inspirations from FRC reverse the distribution of ventilation, with preferential ventilation of the upper parts of the lungs, which is contrary to the distribution of pulmonary blood flow (see below). Normal inspiratory flow rate is, however, much less than 1.5 l.s^{-1} (approximately 0.5 l.s^{-1}), so there will be a small vertical gradient of ventilation during normal breathing.

Overall, the effect of gravity on ventilation seems to be of minor importance in comparison to its effect on perfusion, which will be considered below.

Distribution of inspired gas in relation to the rate of alveolar filling

The rate of inflation of the lung as a whole is a function of inflation pressure, compliance and airway resistance. It is convenient to think in terms of the time constant (explained in Appendix F), which is the product of compliance and resistance and is:

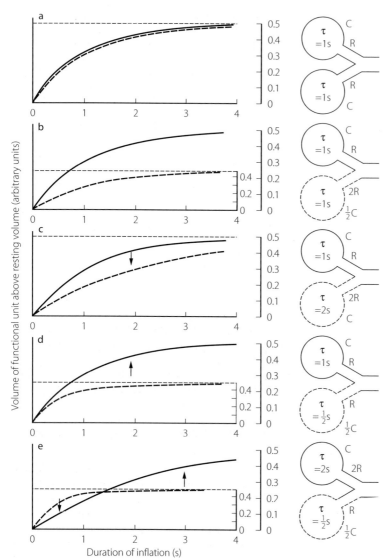

Figure 8.2 The effect of mechanical characteristics on the time course of inflation of different functional units of the lung when exposed to a sustained constant inflation pressure. The *y* coordinate is volume change, but a scale showing intraalveolar pressure is shown on the right. Separate pressure scales are necessary when the compliances are different. In each case the continuous curve relates to the upper unit and the broken curve to the lower unit. Arrows show the direction of gas redistribution if inflow is checked by closure of the upper airway at the times indicated. See text for explanation of the changes. τ = time constant.

- the time required for inflation to 63% of the final volume attained if inflation is prolonged indefinitely

or

- the time that would be required for inflation of the lungs if the initial gas flow rate were maintained throughout inflation (see Appendix F, Figure F.6).

These considerations apply equally to large and small areas of the lungs; Figure 3.6 shows fast and slow alveoli, the former with a short time constant and the latter with a long time constant. Figure 8.2 shows some of the consequences of different *functional units* of the lung having different time constants. For simplicity, Figure 8.2 describes the response to passive inflation of the lungs by development of a constant mouth pressure, but the

considerations are fundamentally similar for both spontaneous respiration and artificial ventilation.

Figure 8.2a shows two functional units of identical compliance and resistance. If the mouth pressure is increased to a constant level, there will be an increase in volume of each unit equal to the mouth pressure multiplied by the compliance of the unit. The time course of inflation will follow the wash-in type of exponential function (Appendix F) and the time constants will be equal to the product of compliance and resistance of each unit and therefore identical. If the inspiratory phase is terminated at any instant, the pressure and volume of each unit will be identical and no redistribution of gas will occur between the two units.

Figure 8.2b shows two functional units, one of which has half the compliance but twice the resistance of the other. The time constants of the two will thus be equal. If a constant inflation pressure is maintained, the one with the lower compliance will increase in volume by half the volume change of the other. Nevertheless, the pressure build-up within each unit will be identical. Thus, as in the previous example, the relative distribution of gas between the two functional units will be independent of the rate or duration of inflation. If the inspiratory phase is terminated at any point, the pressure in each unit will be identical and no redistribution will occur between the different units.

In Figure 8.2c, the compliances of the two units are identical but the resistance of one is twice that of the other. Therefore, its time constant is double that of its fellow and it will fill more slowly, although the volume increase in both units will be the same if inflation is prolonged indefinitely. Relative distribution between the units is thus dependent on the rate and duration of inflation. If inspiration is checked by closure of the upper airway after 2 seconds (for example), the pressure will be higher in the unit with the lower resistance. Gas will then be redistributed from one unit to the other, as shown by the arrow in the diagram.

Figure 8.2d shows a pair of units with identical resistances but the compliance of one being half that of the other. Its time constant is thus half that of its fellow and it has a faster time course of inflation. However, because its compliance is half that of the other, the ultimate volume increase will only be half that of the other unit when the inflation is prolonged indefinitely. The relative distribution of gas between the two units is dependent upon the rate and duration of inflation. Pressure rises more rapidly in the unit with the lower compliance, and if inspiration is checked by closure of the upper airway at 2 seconds (for example), gas will be redistributed from one unit to the other, as shown by the arrow.

An interesting and complex situation occurs when one unit has an increased resistance and the other a reduced compliance (Figure 8.2e). This combination also features in the presentation of the concept of fast and slow alveoli in Figure 3.6. In the present example, the time constant of one unit is four times that of the other, while the ultimate volume changes are determined by the compliance as in Figure 8.2d. When the inflation pressure is sustained, the unit with the lower resistance (the 'fast alveolus') shows the greater volume change at first, but rapidly approaches its equilibrium volume. Thereafter the other unit (the 'slow alveolus') undergoes the major volume changes, the inflation of the two units being out of phase with one another. Throughout inspiration, the pressure build-up in the unit with the shorter time constant is always greater and, if inspiration is checked by closure of the upper airway, gas will be redistributed from one unit to the other, as shown by the arrows in Figure 8.2e.

These complex relationships may be summarised as follows. If the inflation pressure is sustained indefinitely, the volume change in different units of the lungs will depend solely upon their regional compliances. *If their time constants are equal*, the build-up of pressure in the different units will be identical at all times during inflation, and therefore:

- distribution of inspired gas will be independent of the rate, duration or frequency of inspiration
- dynamic compliance (so far as it is influenced by considerations discussed in relation to Figure 3.6) will not be affected by changes in frequency and should not differ greatly from static compliance
- if inspiration is checked by closure of the upper airway, there will be no redistribution of gas within the lungs.

If, however, the time constants of different units are different, it follows that:

- distribution of inspired gas will be dependent on the rate, duration and frequency of inspiration
- dynamic compliance will be decreased as respiratory frequency is increased and should differ significantly from static compliance
- if inspiration is checked by closure of the upper airway, gas will be redistributed within the lungs.

Effect of maldistribution on the alveolar 'plateau'

If different functional units of the lung empty synchronously during expiration, the composition of the expired air will be approximately constant after the gas in the airways (anatomical dead space) has been flushed out. However, this will not occur when there is maldistribution with fast and slow units, as shown in Figure 3.6. The slow units are slow both to fill and to empty and thus are hypoventilated for their volume; therefore they tend to have a high PCO_2 and low PO_2 and are slow to respond to a change in the inspired gas composition. This forms the basis of the single-breath test of maldistribution, in which a single breath of 100% oxygen is used to increase alveolar PO_2 and decrease alveolar PN_2. The greatest increase of PO_2 will clearly occur in the functional units with the best ventilation per unit volume, which will usually have the shortest time constants. The *slow* units will make the predominant contribution to the *latter* part of exhalation, when the mixed exhaled PO_2 will decline and the PN_2 will increase. Thus the expired alveolar plateau of nitrogen will be sloping upwards in patients with maldistribution. It should, however, be stressed that this test will only be positive if maldistribution is accompanied by sequential emptying of units due to differing time constants. For example, Figure 8.2b shows definite maldistribution, due to the different regional compliances that directly influence the regional ventilation. However, because time constants are equal, there will be a constant mix of gas from both units during the course of expiration (i.e. no sequential emptying) and therefore the alveolar plateau would remain flat in spite of PO_2 and PN_2 being different for the two units. However, maldistribution due to the commoner forms of lung disease is usually associated with different time constants and sequential emptying. Routine continuous monitoring of expired carbon dioxide concentration during anaesthesia now allows some assessment of maldistribution of ventilation. As for the single-breath nitrogen test, an upward sloping expiratory plateau of carbon dioxide indicates sequential emptying of alveoli with different time constants (page 162), but a level plateau does not indicate normal distribution of ventilation, just equal time constants of lung units.

DISTRIBUTION OF PERFUSION

Since the pulmonary circulation operates at low pressure, it is rarely distributed evenly to all parts of the lung and the degree of non-uniformity is usually greater than for gas. Maldistribution of pulmonary blood flow is the commonest cause of impaired oxygenation of the arterial blood.

Distribution between the two lungs. Measuring unilateral pulmonary blood flow in humans is difficult, but indirect methods show that unilateral pulmonary blood flow is similar to the distribution of ventilation observed in the supine position (see Table 8.1). In the lateral position, the diameter of the thorax is of the order of 30 cm and so the column of blood in the pulmonary circulation exerts a hydrostatic pressure that is high in relation to the mean pulmonary arterial pressure. A fairly gross maldistribution therefore occurs, with much of the upper lung comprising zone 2 and much of the lower lung comprising zone 3 (see Figure 7.5).[10]

Gravitational effects on regional pulmonary blood flow

In the previous chapter, it was shown how the pulmonary vascular resistance is mainly in the capillary bed and is governed by the relationship between alveolar, pulmonary arterial and pulmonary venous pressures. Early studies with radioactive tracers in the blood took place at total lung capacity and showed flow increasing progressively down the lung in the upright position.[11] However, Hughes *et al.* later found that there was a significant reduction of flow in the most dependent parts of the lung, which was termed zone 4, where the reduction in flow appears to be due to compression of larger blood vessels by increased interstitial pressure.[12] This

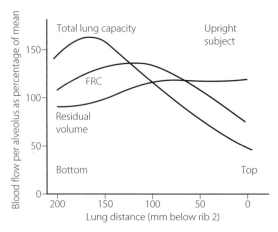

Figure 8.3 Pulmonary perfusion per alveolus as a percentage of that expected if all alveoli were equally perfused (in the upright position). At total lung capacity, perfusion increases down to 150 mm, below which perfusion is slightly decreased (zone 4). At FRC, zone 4 conditions apply below 100 mm and at residual volume the perfusion gradient is actually reversed. It should be noted that perfusion has been calculated *per alveolus*. If shown as perfusion *per unit lung volume*, the non-uniformity at total lung capacity would be the same because alveoli are all the same size at total lung capacity. At FRC there are more but smaller alveoli at the bases and the non-uniformity would be greater. (After reference 12.)

effect becomes progressively more important as lung volume is reduced from total lung capacity towards the residual volume. Figure 8.3 is derived from the work of Hughes' group and shows that pulmonary perfusion *per alveolus* is, in fact, reasonably uniform at the lung volumes relevant to normal tidal exchange. However, the dependent parts of the lung contain larger numbers of smaller alveoli than the apices at FRC, and the perfusion *per unit lung volume* is therefore increased at the bases.[10]

In the supine position the differences in blood flow between apices and bases are replaced by differences between anterior and posterior regions. Supine subjects can be studied using positron emission tomography (PET) scans, which show gradients in alveolar size, ventilation and perfusion which are similar to earlier observations in upright subjects. Blood flow *per unit lung volume* increases by 11% per cm of descent through the lung,[13] whereas ventilation increases but less dramatically (Figure 8.4),[14] resulting in a smaller ventilation to perfusion ratio in dependent areas.[13] These studies also showed that the number of alveoli per cubic centimetre of lung was approximately 30% greater in the posterior than in the anterior lung (see Figure 8.4).[14] Thus the increased perfusion in dependent areas of lung is again mainly caused by an increase in the number of (relatively small) alveoli. Smaller, more numerous alveoli in dependent regions result from the weight of lung tissue

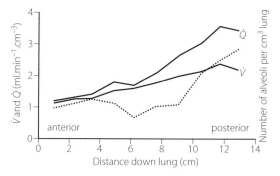

Figure 8.4 Vertical gradients in ventilation and perfusion in the supine position. Data are mean results from PET scans of eight subjects during normal breathing and for each vertical level represent the average value for a horizontal slice of lung. The solid lines relate to the left ordinate and are ventilation ($\dot{V}$) and perfusion ($\dot{Q}$) per cubic centimetre of lung tissue. Ventilation and perfusion both increase on descending through the lung. The dotted line relates to the right ordinate and represents the number of alveoli per unit lung volume, which increases in dependent areas such that the blood flow *per alveolus* remains fairly constant. (After references 13 and 14.)

above, and as blood accounts for two-thirds of the weight of lung tissue, this provides an automatic matching of ventilation and perfusion.

Gravity-independent regional blood flow

Evidence is now accumulating that gravity is not the only cause of the variability of regional pulmonary blood flow. Physiological studies in space have shown that at microgravity regional blood flow becomes more uniform than on Earth but residual non-uniformity still persists (page 280). A variety of methods have been used to study pulmonary blood flow in the prone position.[13-16] These studies have consistently found that although blood flow becomes more uniform, the flow distribution when prone is not simply a reversal of the supine position, as might be expected if gravity were the only influence. Some groups estimate that gravity is responsible for only 10–40% of the regional blood flow variability seen.[15,17] Pulmonary blood flow may vary in a radial fashion, with greater flow to central than to peripheral lung regions in each horizontal slice of lung.[18] Regional flow is also believed to be influenced by vascular structure, with the branching pattern of the pulmonary vasculature being responsible for gravity-independent variation (the fractal hypothesis).[19] Methodological problems continue to impede the study of gravity-independent flow variation and the existence and magnitude of these effects is disputed.[20] However, gravity can no longer be accepted as the sole explanation for variations in regional pulmonary blood flow.

VENTILATION IN RELATION TO PERFUSION[21]

It is convenient to consider the relationship between ventilation and perfusion in terms of the ventilation/perfusion ratio (abbreviated to $\dot{V}/\dot{Q}$). Each quantity is measured in litres per minute and, taking the lungs as a whole, typical resting values might be 4 l.min^{-1} for alveolar ventilation and 5 l.min^{-1} for pulmonary blood flow. Thus the overall ventilation/perfusion ratio would be 0.8. If ventilation and perfusion of all alveoli were uniform then each alveolus would have an individual $\dot{V}/\dot{Q}$ ratio of 0.8. In fact, ventilation and perfusion are not uniformly distributed but may range all the way from unventilated alveoli to unperfused alveoli, with every gradation in between. Unventilated alveoli will have a $\dot{V}/\dot{Q}$ ratio of zero and the unperfused alveoli a $\dot{V}/\dot{Q}$ ratio of infinity.

Alveoli with no ventilation ($\dot{V}/\dot{Q}$ ratio of zero) will have PO_2 and PCO_2 values that are the same as those of mixed venous blood, because the trapped air in the unventilated alveoli will equilibrate with mixed venous blood. Alveoli with no perfusion ($\dot{V}/\dot{Q}$ ratio of infinity) will have PO_2 and PCO_2 values that are the same as those of the inspired gas, because there is no gas exchange to alter the composition of the inspired gas that is drawn into these alveoli. Alveoli with intermediate values of $\dot{V}/\dot{Q}$ ratio will thus have PO_2 and PCO_2 values that are intermediate between those of mixed venous blood and inspired gas. Figure 8.5 is a PO_2/PCO_2 plot with the thick line joining the mixed venous point to the inspired gas point. This line covers all possible combinations of alveolar PO_2 and PCO_2, with an indication of the $\dot{V}/\dot{Q}$ ratios that determine them.

The inhalation of higher than normal partial pressures of oxygen moves the inspired point of the curve to the right. The mixed venous point also moves to the right but only by a small amount, for reasons that are explained on page 348. A new curve must be prepared for each combination of values for mixed venous blood and inspired gas. The curve can then be used to demonstrate the gas tensions in the horizontal strata of the lung according to their different $\dot{V}/\dot{Q}$ ratios (see Figure 8.5).

All the techniques described above that measure regional ventilation and perfusion in horizontal strata of the lung only discriminate between functionally large regions of the lung. This limitation has been overcome by the multiple inert gas elimination technique (MIGET).[22] The methodology, which is outlined on page 128, permits the plotting of the distribution of pulmonary ventilation and perfusion, not in relation to anatomical location but in a large number of compartments defined by their $\dot{V}/\dot{Q}$ ratios, expressed on a logarithmic scale.

Figure 8.6 shows typical plots for healthy subjects.[23] For the young adult (Figure 8.6a), both ventilation and perfusion are mainly confined to alveoli with $\dot{V}/\dot{Q}$ ratios in the range 0.5–2.0. There is no measurable distribution

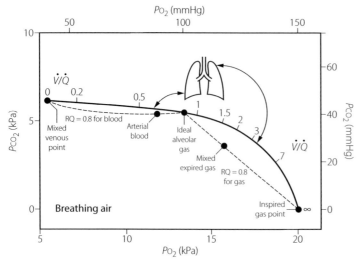

Figure 8.5 The heavy line indicates all possible values for P_{O_2} and P_{CO_2} of alveoli with ventilation perfusion ($\dot{V}/\dot{Q}$) ratios ranging from zero to infinity (subject breathing air). Values for normal alveoli are distributed as shown in accordance with their vertical distance up the lung field. Mixed expired gas may be considered as a mixture of 'ideal' alveolar and inspired gas (dead space). Arterial blood may be considered as a mixture of blood with the same gas tensions as 'ideal' alveolar gas and mixed venous blood (shunt).

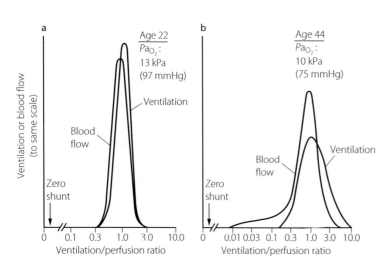

Figure 8.6 The distribution of ventilation and blood flow in relation to ventilation/perfusion ($\dot{V}/\dot{Q}$) ratios in two normal subjects. **(a)** A male aged 22 years with typical narrow spread and no measurable intrapulmonary shunt or alveolar dead space. **(b)** The wider spread of $\dot{V}/\dot{Q}$ ratios in a male aged 44 years. There is still no measurable intrapulmonary shunt or alveolar dead space, but the appreciable distribution of blood flow to underperfused alveoli is sufficient to reduce the arterial P_{O_2} to 10 kPa (75 mmHg) while breathing air. (Reproduced with permission from Wagner PD, Laravuso RB, Uhl RR et al. Continuous distributions of ventilation-perfusion ratios in normal subjects breathing air and 100% O_2. *J Clin Invest* 1974; **54**: 54–68.)

to areas of infinite $\dot{V}/\dot{Q}$ (i.e. alveolar dead space) or zero $\dot{V}/\dot{Q}$ ratio (i.e. intrapulmonary shunt), but the method does not detect extrapulmonary shunt, which must be present to a small extent (page 122). For the older subject (Figure 8.6b), there is a widening of the distribution of $\dot{V}/\dot{Q}$ ratios, with the main part of the curve now in the range of $\dot{V}/\dot{Q}$ ratios 0.3–5.0. In addition, there is the appearance of a 'shelf' of distribution of blood flow to areas of low $\dot{V}/\dot{Q}$ ratio in the range 0.01–0.3. This probably represents gross underventilation of dependent areas of the lung due to airway closure when the closing capacity exceeds the functional residual capacity (see Figure 3.10). The effect of increased spread of $\dot{V}/\dot{Q}$ ratios on gas exchange is considered below (page 125).

The pattern of distribution of $\dot{V}/\dot{Q}$ ratios shows characteristic changes in a number of pathological conditions, such as pulmonary oedema and pulmonary embolus.[24] Some examples are shown in Figure 8.7.

Quantification of spread of $\dot{V}/\dot{Q}$ ratios as if it were due to dead space and shunt

The MIGET method of analysis illustrated in Figures 8.6 and 8.7 is technically complex. A less precise but highly practical approach was described in the 1940s by both Fenn *et al.*[25] and Riley and Cournand.[26] The essence of what has generally become known as the Riley approach is to consider the lung as if it were a three-compartment model (Figure 8.8) comprising:

• ventilated but unperfused alveoli (alveolar dead space)

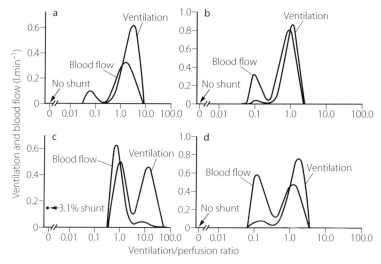

Figure 8.7 Examples of abnormal patterns of maldistribution of ventilation and perfusion, to be compared with the normal curves in Figure 8.6. **(a)** Chronic obstructive pulmonary disease. The blood flow to units of very low $\dot{V}/\dot{Q}$ ratio would cause arterial hypoxaemia and simulate a shunt. **(b)** Asthma, with a more pronounced bimodal distribution of blood flow than the patient shown in (a). **(c)** Bimodal distribution of ventilation in a 60-year-old patient with chronic obstructive pulmonary disease, predominantly emphysema. A similar pattern is seen after pulmonary embolism. **(d)** Pronounced bimodal distribution of perfusion after a bronchodilator was administered to the patient shown in (b). (Reproduced with permission from West JB. *Ventilation: Blood Flow and Gas Exchange*. Oxford: Blackwell Scientific, 1990.)

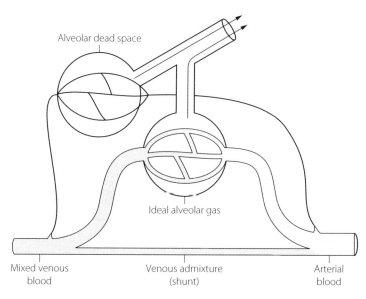

Figure 8.8 Three-compartment (Riley) model of gas exchange. The lung is imagined to consist of three functional units comprising alveolar dead space, 'ideal' alveoli and venous admixture (shunt). Gas exchange occurs only in the 'ideal' alveoli. The measured alveolar dead space consists of true alveolar dead space together with a component caused by $\dot{V}/\dot{Q}$ scatter. The measured venous admixture consists of true venous admixture (shunt) together with a component caused by $\dot{V}/\dot{Q}$ scatter. Note that 'ideal' alveolar gas is exhaled contaminated with alveolar dead space gas, so it is not possible to sample 'ideal' alveolar gas.

- perfused but unventilated alveoli (intrapulmonary shunt)
- ideally perfused and ventilated alveoli.

Gas exchange can only occur in the 'ideal' alveolus. There is no suggestion that this is an accurate description of the actual state of affairs, which is better depicted by the type of plot shown in Figure 8.6, where the analysis would comprise some 50 compartments in contrast to the three compartments of the Riley model. However, the parameters of the three-compartment model may be easily determined and the values obtained are of direct relevance to therapy. Thus an increased dead space can usually be offset by an increased minute

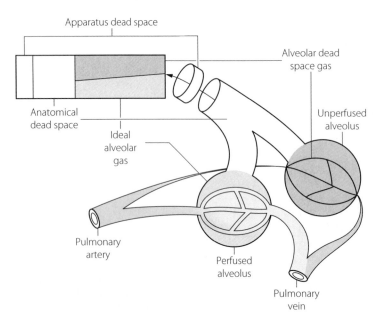

Apparatus dead space

Alveolar dead space gas

Anatomical dead space

Ideal alveolar gas

Unperfused alveolus

Pulmonary artery

Perfused alveolus

Pulmonary vein

Figure 8.9 Components of a single breath of expired gas. The rectangle is an idealised representation of a single expirate. The physiological dead space equals the sum of the anatomical and alveolar dead spaces and is outlined in the heavy black line. The alveolar dead space does not equal the volume of unperfused spaces at alveolar level but only the part of their contents that is exhaled. This varies with tidal volume.

volume and arterial P_{O_2} can be restored to normal with shunts up to about 30% by an appropriate increase in the inspired oxygen concentration (see Figure 8.11 below).

Methods for calculating dead space and shunt for the three-compartment model are described at the end of the chapter, but no analytical techniques are required beyond measurement of blood and gas P_{CO_2} and P_{O_2}. It is then possible to determine what fraction of the inspired tidal volume does not participate in gas exchange and what fraction of the cardiac output constitutes a shunt. However, it is most important to remember that the measured value for 'dead space' will include a fraction representing ventilation of *relatively* underperfused alveoli, and the measured value for 'shunt' will include a fraction representing perfusion of *relatively* underventilated alveoli. Furthermore, although perfusion of relatively underventilated alveoli will reduce arterial P_{O_2}, the pattern of change, in relation to the inspired oxygen concentration, is quite different from that of a true shunt (see Figure 8.12 below).

The concept of 'ideal' alveolar gas is considered below (page 128), but it will be clear from Figure 8.8 that ideal alveolar gas cannot be sampled for analysis. There is a convention that ideal alveolar P_{CO_2} is assumed to be equal to the arterial P_{CO_2} and that the respiratory exchange ratio of ideal alveolar gas is the same as that of expired air.

DEAD SPACE

It was realised in the 19th century that an appreciable part of each inspiration did not penetrate to those regions of the lungs in which gas exchange occurred and

was therefore exhaled unchanged. This fraction of the tidal volume has long been known as the dead space, while the effective part of the minute volume of respiration is known as the alveolar ventilation. The relationship is as follows:

Alveolar ventilation =

respiratory frequency (tidal volume − dead space)
$$\dot{V}_A = f(V_T - V_D)$$

It is often useful to think of two ratios. The first is the dead space/tidal volume ratio (often abbreviated to V_D/V_T and expressed as a percentage). The second useful ratio is the alveolar ventilation/minute volume ratio. The first ratio indicates the wasted part of the breath, and the second gives the utilised portion of the minute volume. The sum of the two ratios is unity, and so one may easily be calculated from the other.

Components of the dead space

The preceding section considers dead space as though it were a single homogeneous component of expired air. The situation is actually more complicated than this and Figure 8.9 shows in diagrammatic form the various components of a single expirate.

The first part to be exhaled will be the *apparatus dead space* if the subject is employing any form of external breathing apparatus. The next component will be from the *anatomical dead space*, which is the volume of the conducting air passages with the qualifications considered below. Thereafter gas is exhaled from the alveolar level and the diagram shows two representative alveoli, corresponding to the two ventilated compartments of the three-compartment lung model shown in Figure 8.8. One alveolus is perfused and, from this, 'ideal' alveolar gas is exhaled. The other alveolus is unperfused and so without gas exchange, and from this alveolus the exhaled gas therefore approximates in composition to inspired gas. This component of the expirate is known as *alveolar dead space* gas, which is important in many pathological conditions. The *physiological dead space* is the sum of the anatomical and alveolar dead spaces and is defined as the sum of all parts of the tidal volume that do not participate in gas exchange.

In Figure 8.9, the final part of the expirate is called an end-tidal or, preferably, an end-expiratory sample and consists of a mixture of ideal alveolar gas and alveolar dead space gas. The proportion of alveolar dead space gas in an end-expiratory sample is variable. In a healthy resting subject the composition of such a sample will be close to that of ideal alveolar gas. However, in many pathological states (and during anaesthesia), an end-expiratory sample may contain a substantial proportion of alveolar dead space gas and thus be unrepresentative of the alveolar (and therefore arterial) gas tensions. For symbols, the small capital A relates to ideal alveolar gas as in PA_{CO_2}, while end-expiratory gas is distinguished by a small capital E, suffixed with a prime (e.g. PE'_{CO_2}) and mixed expired gas a small capital E with a bar ($P\bar{E}_{CO_2}$). The term 'alveolar/arterial PO_2 difference' always refers to ideal alveolar gas. Unqualified, the term 'alveolar' may mean either end-tidal or ideal alveolar, depending on the context. This is a perennial source of confusion and it is better to specify either ideal alveolar gas or end-expiratory gas.

It must again be stressed that Figure 8.9 is only a model to simplify quantification, and there may be an infinite gradation between $\dot{V}/\dot{Q}$ ratios between zero and infinity. However, it is often helpful from the quantitative standpoint, particularly in the clinical field, to consider alveoli *as if* they fell into the three categories shown in Figure 8.8.

Anatomical dead space

The anatomical dead space is now generally defined as the volume of gas exhaled before the CO_2 concentration rises to its alveolar plateau, according to the technique of Fowler[27] outlined at the end of this chapter (see Figure 8.16).

The volume of the anatomical dead space, in spite of its name, is not constant and is influenced by many factors, some of which (listed below) are of considerable clinical importance. Most of these factors influence the anatomical dead space by changing the volume of the conducting airways, except for changes in tidal volume and respiratory rate, which affect the flow pattern of gas passing along the airways.

Factors influencing the anatomical dead space

Size of the subject must clearly influence the dimensions of the conducting air passages and anatomical dead space increases with body size.

Age. In early infancy anatomical dead space is approximately 3.3 ml.kg^{-1}, and by the age of 6 years this has decreased to the adult value of approximately 2 ml.kg^{-1}. Throughout this period of development, intrathoracic anatomical dead space remains constant at 1 ml.kg^{-1} while the volumes of the nose, mouth and pharynx change relative to body weight.[28] From early adulthood, anatomical dead space increases by approximately 1 ml per year.

Posture influences many lung volumes, including the anatomical dead space, with typical mean values for healthy subjects of 150 ml when sitting and 100 ml when supine.[29]

Position of the neck and jaw has a pronounced effect on the anatomical dead space, with mean values in conscious subjects of:[30]

- neck extended, jaw protruded – 143 ml
- normal position – 119 ml
- neck flexed, chin depressed – 73 ml.

It is noteworthy that the first position is the one used by resuscitators and anaesthetists to procure the least possible airway resistance. Unfortunately, it also results in the maximum dead space.

Lung volume at the end of inspiration affects the anatomical dead space, since the volume of the air passages changes in proportion to the lung volume. The increase is of the order of 20 ml additional anatomical dead space for each litre increase in lung volume.[31]

Tracheal intubation, tracheostomy or laryngeal mask airway use will bypass much of the extrathoracic anatomical dead space, which is normally about 70 ml. These methods of airway maintenance bypass approximately half of the total anatomical dead space.[30,32,33] Any advantage gained is usually lost by the addition of further apparatus dead space to the breathing system by, for example, the use of a breathing system filter or a heat-and moisture-exchanging humidifier.[34]

Drugs acting on the bronchiolar musculature will affect the anatomical dead space, with any bronchodilator drug (page 47) causing a small increase in anatomical dead space.

Tidal volume and respiratory rate. A reduction in tidal volume results in a marked reduction of the anatomical dead space as measured by Fowler's method and this limits the fall of alveolar ventilation resulting from small tidal volumes. This is important in the case of comatose or anaesthetised patients who are left to breathe for themselves, often with tidal volumes smaller than the normal anatomical dead space of 150 ml.

Reduced anatomical dead space with small tidal volumes is unlikely to result from changes in the physical dimensions of the airways and arises mostly from changes in the flow patterns and mixing of gases within the airways. First, at low flow rates there is a greater tendency towards laminar flow of gas through the air passages (page 41). Inspired gas advances with a cone front and the tip of the cone penetrates the alveoli before all the gas in the conducting passages has been washed out. In conscious subjects some inspired gas may be detected in the alveoli with tidal volumes as small as 60 ml.[35] Second, with a slow respiratory rate and/or a prolonged inspiratory time, there is more time for mixing of gases between the alveoli and the smaller airways. Mixing will occur by simple diffusion, possibly aided by a mixing effect of the heartbeat, which tends to mix all gas lying below the carina. This effect is negligible at normal rates of ventilation, but becomes marked during hypoventilation. For example, in one hypoventilating patient, Nunn and Hill found alveolar gas at the carina at the beginning of expiration.[32] A similar effect occurs during breath holding when alveolar gas mixes with dead space gas as far up as the glottis.

Alveolar dead space

Alveolar dead space may be defined as the part of the inspired gas that passes through the anatomical dead space to mix with gas at the alveolar level, but which does not take part in gas exchange. The cause of the failure of gas exchange is lack of effective perfusion of the spaces to which the gas is distributed at the alveolar level. Measured alveolar dead space must sometimes contain a component due to the ventilation of *relatively* underperfused alveoli, which have a very high (but not infinite) $\dot{V}/\dot{Q}$ ratio (see Figure 8.7). The alveolar dead space is too small to be measured with confidence in healthy supine humans, but becomes appreciable under some circumstances.

Low cardiac output, regardless of the cause, results in pulmonary hypotension and failure of perfusion of the uppermost parts of the lungs (zone 1, see page 98).

During anaesthesia with controlled ventilation, sudden changes in end-expiratory CO_2 therefore usually indicate changing alveolar dead space secondary to abrupt variations in cardiac output (page 159).

Pulmonary embolism is considered separately in Chapter 29. Apart from its effect on cardiac output, pulmonary embolism is a direct cause of alveolar dead space that may reach massive proportions.

Posture. Changes in position have a significant effect on the distribution of pulmonary blood flow (page 114). Fortunately, during normal breathing there are similar changes in the distribution of ventilation so that $\dot{V}/\dot{Q}$ mismatch is uncommon and there are no significant changes in alveolar dead space. However, if a patient is ventilated artificially in the lateral position, ventilation is distributed in favour of the upper lung (see Table 8.1), particularly in the presence of an open pneumothorax,[4] and under these conditions, part of the ventilation of the upper lung will constitute alveolar dead space.

Physiological dead space

Physiological dead space is the sum of all parts of the tidal volume that do not participate in gaseous exchange. Nowadays it is universally defined by the Bohr mixing equation, with substitution of arterial P_{CO_2} for alveolar P_{CO_2}, as described below.

Physiological dead space remains a fairly constant fraction of the tidal volume over a wide range of tidal volumes. It is, therefore, generally more useful to use the V_D/V_T ratio: the alveolar ventilation will then be $(1-V_D/V_T)$ × the respiratory minute volume. Thus if the physiological dead space is 30% of the tidal volume (i.e. $V_D/V_T = 0.3$), then the alveolar ventilation will be 70% of the minute volume. This approach is radically different from the assumption of a constant 'dead space' which is subtracted from the tidal volume, the difference then being multiplied by the respiratory frequency to indicate the alveolar ventilation.

The Bohr equation

Bohr introduced his equation in 1891[36] when the dead space was considered simply as gas exhaled from the conducting airways (i.e. anatomical dead space only). It may be simply derived as follows. During expiration, all the CO_2 eliminated is contained in the alveolar gas. Therefore:

Volume of CO_2 eliminated in the alveolar gas =

   volume of CO_2 eliminated in the mixed expired gas

that is to say:

Alveolar CO_2 concentration $\times$ alveolar ventilation =

    mixed-expired CO_2 concentration $\times$ minute volume

or, for a single breath:

Alveolar CO_2 concentration $\times$ (tidal volume $-$ dead space)

    = mixed-expired CO_2 concentration $\times$ tidal volume

There are four terms in this equation. There is no serious difficulty in measuring two of them, the tidal volume and the mixed-expired CO_2 concentration. This leaves the alveolar CO_2 concentration and the dead space. Therefore the alveolar CO_2 concentration may be derived if the dead space is known or, alternatively, the dead space may be derived if the alveolar CO_2 concentration is known.

The use of this equation has been expanded to measure various components of the dead space by varying the interpretation of the term 'alveolar'. In the equations above, the word 'alveolar' may be taken to mean end-expiratory gas and therefore this use of the Bohr equation indicates the anatomical dead space. If the 'ideal' alveolar CO_2 concentration were used, then the equation would indicate the physiological dead space comprising the sum of the anatomical and alveolar dead spaces (see Figure 8.9). 'Ideal' alveolar gas cannot be sampled, but arterial P_{CO_2} may be substituted for alveolar P_{CO_2} in the Bohr equation and the value so derived is now widely accepted as the definition of the physiological dead space.

$$\frac{V_D}{V_T} = \frac{(Pa_{CO_2} - P\bar{E}_{CO_2})}{Pa_{CO_2}}$$

In the healthy conscious resting subject, there is no significant difference between the P_{CO_2} of end-expiratory gas and that of arterial blood. The former may therefore be used as a substitute for the latter, as the anatomical and physiological dead spaces should be the same (the normal alveolar dead space being too small to measure). However, the use of the end-expiratory P_{CO_2} in the Bohr equation may cause difficulties in certain situations. In exercise, in acute hyperventilation, or if there is maldistribution of inspired gas with sequential emptying, the alveolar P_{CO_2} rises, often steeply, during expiration of the alveolar gas and the end-tidal P_{CO_2} will depend on the duration of expiration. The dead space so derived will not necessarily correspond to any of the compartments of the dead space shown in Figure 8.9.

Factors influencing the physiological dead space

This section summarises factors that affect physiological dead space in normal subjects, but reasons for the changes have been considered above in the sections on the anatomical and alveolar dead space.

Age and sex.[37] There is a tendency for V_D and also the V_D/V_T ratio to increase with age, as a result of changes in the anatomical component. The volume of V_D in men is around 50 ml greater than in women, but the former have larger tidal volumes and there is little difference between sexes in the V_D/V_T ratios.

Body size. As described above, it is evident that anatomical dead space, and therefore V_D, in common with other pulmonary volumes, will be larger in larger people. Physiological dead space correlates with either weight or height; for example, V_D (in millilitres) approximates to the weight of the subject in pounds (1 pound = 0.45 kg)[38] or increases by 17 ml for every 10 cm increase in height.[37]

Posture. The V_D/V_T ratio decreases from a mean value of 34% in the upright position to 30% in the supine position.[39] This is largely explained by the change in anatomical dead space described above.

Pathology. Changes in dead space are important features of many causes of lung dysfunction, such as pulmonary embolism, smoking, anaesthesia, artificial ventilation etc. These topics are discussed in Part 3 of this book.

Effects of an increased physiological dead space

Regardless of whether an increase in physiological dead space is in the anatomical or the alveolar component, alveolar ventilation is reduced unless there is a compensatory increase in minute volume. Reduction of alveolar ventilation due to an increase in physiological dead space produces changes in the 'ideal' alveolar gas tensions that are identical to those produced when alveolar ventilation is decreased by reduction in respiratory minute volume (see Figure 10.9).

It is usually possible to counteract the effects of an increase in physiological dead space by a corresponding increase in the respiratory minute volume. If, for example, the minute volume is $10\,l.min^{-1}$ and the V_D/V_T ratio 30%, the alveolar ventilation will be 7 $l.min^{-1}$. If the patient were then subjected to pulmonary embolism resulting in an increase of the V_D/V_T ratio to 50%, the minute volume would need to be increased to $14\,l.min^{-1}$ to maintain an alveolar ventilation of $7\,l.min^{-1}$. However, should the V_D/V_T increase to 80%, the minute volume would need to be increased to $35\,l.min^{-1}$. Ventilatory capacity may be a limiting factor with massive increases in dead space and this is a rare cause of ventilatory failure (see Chapter 27).

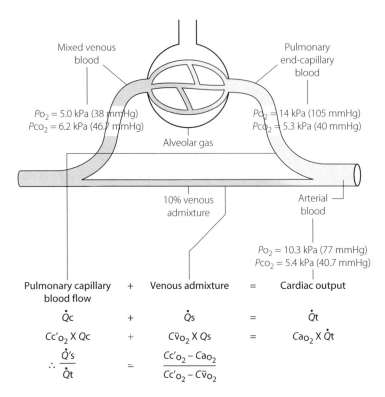

Mixed venous blood

Pulmonary end-capillary blood

$Po_2 = 5.0$ kPa (38 mmHg)
$Pco_2 = 6.2$ kPa (46.7 mmHg)

$Po_2 = 14$ kPa (105 mmHg)
$Pco_2 = 5.3$ kPa (40 mmHg)

Alveolar gas

10% venous admixture

Arterial blood

$Po_2 = 10.3$ kPa (77 mmHg)
$Pco_2 = 5.4$ kPa (40.7 mmHg)

Pulmonary capillary blood flow	+	Venous admixture	=	Cardiac output
$\dot{Q}c$	+	$\dot{Q}s$	=	$\dot{Q}t$
$Cc'_{O_2} \times Qc$	+	$C\bar{v}_{O_2} \times Qs$	=	$Ca_{O_2} \times \dot{Q}t$

$$\therefore \frac{\dot{Q}'s}{\dot{Q}t} = \frac{Cc'_{O_2} - Ca_{O_2}}{Cc'_{O_2} - C\bar{v}_{O_2}}$$

Figure 8.10 A schematic representation of venous admixture. It makes the assumption that all the arterial blood has come either from alveoli with normal $\dot{V}/\dot{Q}$ ratios or from a shunt carrying only mixed venous blood. This is never true, but it forms a convenient method of quantifying venous admixture from whatever cause. The shunt equation is similar to the Bohr equation and is based on the axiomatic relationship that the total amount of oxygen in 1 minute's flow of arterial blood equals the sum of the amount of oxygen in 1 minute's flow through both the pulmonary capillaries and the shunt. Amount of oxygen in 1 minute's flow of blood equals the product of blood flow rate and the oxygen content of the blood. $\dot{Q}t$, total cardiac output; $\dot{Q}c$, pulmonary capillary blood flow; $\dot{Q}s$, blood flow through shunt; Ca_{O_2}, oxygen content of arterial blood; Cc'_{O_2}, oxygen content of pulmonary end-capillary blood; $C\bar{v}_{O_2}$, oxygen content of mixed venous blood.

VENOUS ADMIXTURE OR SHUNT

Admixture of arterial blood with poorly oxygenated or mixed venous blood is a most important cause of arterial hypoxaemia.

Nomenclature of venous admixture

Venous admixture refers to the degree of admixture of mixed venous blood with pulmonary end-capillary blood that would be required to produce the observed difference between the arterial and the pulmonary end-capillary Po_2 (usually taken to equal ideal alveolar Po_2), the principles of the calculation being shown in Figure 8.10. Note that the venous admixture is not the *actual* amount of venous blood that mingles with the arterial blood, but the *calculated* amount that would be required to produce the observed value for the arterial Po_2. Calculated venous admixture and the actual volume of blood mixing differ because of two factors. First, the Thebesian and bronchial venous drainage do not necessarily have the same Po_2 as mixed venous blood. Second, venous admixture includes the contribution to the arterial blood from alveoli having a $\dot{V}/\dot{Q}$ ratio of more than zero but less than the normal value (see Figure 8.6), when again, Po_2 will differ from that of mixed venous blood. Venous admixture is thus a convenient index but defines neither the precise volume nor the anatomical

pathway of the shunt. Nevertheless, it is often loosely termed 'shunt'.

Anatomical (extrapulmonary) shunt refers to the amount of venous blood that mixes with the pulmonary end-capillary blood on the arterial side of the circulation. The term embraces bronchial and Thebesian venous blood flow and also admixture of mixed venous blood caused by atelectasis, bronchial obstruction, congenital heart disease with right-to-left shunting etc. Clearly different components may have different oxygen contents, which will not necessarily equal the mixed venous oxygen content. Anatomical shunt excludes blood draining any alveoli with a $\dot{V}/\dot{Q}$ ratio of more than zero.

Virtual shunt refers to shunt values derived from calculations in which the arterial to mixed-venous oxygen difference is assumed rather than actually measured (see below).

Pathological shunt is sometimes used to describe the forms of anatomical shunt that do not occur in the normal subject.

Physiological shunt. This term is, unfortunately, used in two senses. In the first sense it is used to describe the degree of venous admixture that occurs in a normal healthy subject. Differences between the actual measured venous admixture and the normal value for the 'physiological shunt' thus indicate the amount of venous admixture that results from the disease process. In its alternative sense, physiological shunt is synonymous with venous admixture as derived from the mixing equation (see Figure 8.10). The term is probably best avoided.

Forms of venous admixture

The contribution of $\dot{V}/\dot{Q}$ mismatch to venous admixture is discussed in detail below. Other important sources of venous admixture, both normal and pathological, include the following.

Venae cordis minimae (Thebesian veins). Some small veins of the left heart drain directly into the chambers of the left heart and so mix with the pulmonary venous blood. The oxygen content of this blood is probably very low and therefore the flow (believed to be about 0.3% of cardiac output[40]) causes an appreciable fall in the mixed arterial oxygen tension.

Bronchial veins. Figure 7.1 shows that part of the venous drainage of the bronchial circulation passes by way of the deep true bronchial veins to reach the pulmonary veins. It is uncertain how large this component is in the healthy subject but it is probably less than 1% of cardiac output. In bronchial disease and coarctation of the aorta, the flow through this channel may be greatly increased and in bronchiectasis and emphysema may be as large as 10% of cardiac output. In these circumstances it becomes a major cause of arterial desaturation.

Congenital heart disease. Right-to-left shunting in congenital heart disease is the cause of the worst examples of venous admixture. When there are abnormal communications between right and left heart, shunting will usually be from left to right unless the pressures in the right heart are raised above those of the left heart. This occurs in conditions involving obstruction to the right ventricular ouflow tract (e.g. Fallot's tetralogy) or in prolonged left-to-right shunt when the increased pulmonary blood flow causes pulmonary hypertension and eventually a reversal of the shunt (Eisenmenger's syndrome).

Pulmonary pathology often results in increased venous admixture, thus causing hypoxaemia. Venous drainage from lung tumours constitutes a pathological shunt, but more commonly venous admixture results from pulmonary blood flow past non-ventilated alveoli in conditions such as lobar and bronchopneumonia, pulmonary collapse and acute lung injury. The amount of venous admixture that occurs with lung disease is variable, depending on the balance between hypoxic pulmonary vasoconstriction (page 101) and pathological vasodilation of the pulmonary vessels by inflammatory mediators.

Effect of venous admixture on arterial $P\text{CO}_2$ and $P\text{O}_2$

Qualitatively, it will be clear that venous admixture reduces the overall efficiency of gas exchange and results in arterial blood gas tensions that are closer to those of mixed venous blood than would otherwise be the case. Quantitatively, the effect is simple provided that we consider the *contents* of gases in blood. In the case of the anatomical shunt in Figure 8.10, conservation of mass (oxygen) is the basis of the equations, which simply state that the amount of oxygen flowing in the arterial system equals the sum of the amount of oxygen leaving the pulmonary capillaries and the amount of oxygen flowing through the shunt. For each term in this equation the amount of oxygen flowing may be expressed as the product of the blood flow rate and the oxygen content of blood flowing in the vessel (the symbols are explained in Figure 8.10 and Appendix D). Figure 8.10 shows how the equation may be cleared and solved for the ratio of the venous admixture to the cardiac output. The final equation has a form that is rather similar to that of the Bohr equation for the physiological dead space.

In terms of *content*, the shunt equation is very simple to solve for the effect of venous admixture on arterial oxygen content. If, for example, pulmonary end-capillary oxygen content is 20 ml.dl⁻¹ and mixed venous blood oxygen content is 10 ml.dl⁻¹ then a 50% venous admixture will result in an arterial oxygen content of 15 ml.dl⁻¹, a 25% venous admixture will result in an arterial oxygen content of 17.5 ml.dl⁻¹ and so on. It is then necessary to convert arterial oxygen content to $P\text{O}_2$ by reference to the haemoglobin dissociation curve (see page 177). Since arterial $P\text{O}_2$ is usually on the flat part of the haemoglobin dissociation curve, small changes in content tend to have a very large effect on $P\text{O}_2$, though this effect diminishes at lower arterial $P\text{O}_2$ when the dissociation curve becomes steeper.

The effect of venous admixture on arterial CO_2 *content* is roughly similar in magnitude to that of oxygen content. However, owing to the steepness of the CO_2 dissociation curve near the arterial point (see Figure 10.2), the effect on arterial $P\text{CO}_2$ is very small and far less than the change in arterial $P\text{O}_2$ (Table 8.2).

Two conclusions may be drawn.

- Arterial $P\text{O}_2$ is the most useful blood gas measurement for the detection of venous admixture.
- Venous admixture reduces the arterial $P\text{O}_2$ markedly, but has relatively little effect on arterial $P\text{CO}_2$ or on the content of either CO_2 or O_2 unless the venous admixture is large.

Table 8.2 Effect of 5% venous admixture on the difference between arterial and pulmonary end-capillary blood levels of carbon dioxide and oxygen

	Pulmonary end-capillary blood	Arterial blood
CO_2 content (ml.dl^{-1})	49.7	50.0
PCO_2 (kPa)	5.29	5.33
(mmHg)	39.7	40.0
O_2 content (ml.dl^{-1})	19.9	19.6
O_2 saturation (%)	97.8	96.8
PO_2 (kPa)	14.0	12.0
(mmHg)	105	90

It has been assumed that the arterial/venous oxygen content difference is 4.5 ml.dl^{-1} and that the haemoglobin concentration is 14.9 g.dl^{-1}. Typical changes in PO_2 and PCO_2 have been shown for a 10% venous admixture, as in Figure 8.10.

Elevations of arterial PCO_2 are seldom caused by venous admixture and it is customary to ignore the effect of moderate shunts on PCO_2. In the clinical situation, it is more usual for venous admixture to lower the PCO_2 indirectly, because the decreased PO_2 commonly causes hyperventilation, which more than compensates for the very slight elevation of PCO_2 that would otherwise result from the venous admixture (see Figure 27.1).

Effect of cardiac output on shunt

Cardiac output influences venous admixture, and its consequences, in two opposing ways. First, a reduction of cardiac output leads to a decrease in mixed venous oxygen content, with the result that a given shunt causes a greater reduction in arterial PO_2 *provided the shunt fraction is unaltered*, a relationship that is illustrated in Figure 11.5. Second, it has been observed that, in a very wide range of pathological and physiological circumstances, a reduction in cardiac output causes an approximately proportional reduction in the shunt fraction,[41,42] the only apparent exception being a shunt through regional pulmonary atelectasis.[43] One possible explanation for the reduced shunt fraction is activation of hypoxic pulmonary vasoconstriction as a result of the reduction in PO_2 of the mixed venous blood flowing through the shunt (page 189). It is remarkable that these two effects tend to have approximately equal and opposite effects on arterial PO_2. Thus with a decreased cardiac output there is usually a reduced shunt of a more desaturated mixed venous blood, with the result that the arterial PO_2 is scarcely changed.

The iso-shunt diagram

If we assume normal values for arterial PCO_2, haemoglobin and arterial/mixed venous oxygen content difference, the arterial PO_2 is determined mainly by the inspired oxygen concentration and venous admixture considered in the context of the three-compartment model (see Figure 8.8). The relationship between inspired oxygen concentration and arterial PO_2 is a matter for constant attention in situations such as critical care, and it has been found a matter of practical convenience to prepare a graph of the relationship at different levels of venous admixture (Figure 8.11). The arterial/mixed venous oxygen content difference is often unknown in the clinical situation and therefore the diagram has been prepared for an assumed content difference of 5 ml oxygen per 100 ml of blood. Iso-shunt bands have then been drawn on a plot of arterial PO_2 against inspired oxygen concentration. The bands are sufficiently wide to encompass all values of PCO_2 between 3.3 and 5.3 kPa (25–40 mmHg) and haemoglobin levels between 10 and 14 g.dl^{-1}. Normal barometric pressure is assumed. Since calculation of the venous admixture requires knowledge of the actual arterial/mixed venous oxygen content difference, the iso-shunt lines in Figure 8.11 refer to the *virtual shunt*, which is defined as the shunt calculated on the basis of an assumed value of the arterial/mixed venous oxygen content difference of 5 ml per 100 ml.

In practice, the iso-shunt diagram is useful for adjusting the inspired oxygen concentration to obtain a required level of arterial PO_2. Under stable pathological conditions, changing the inspired oxygen concentration results in changes in arterial PO_2 that are reasonably well predicted by the iso-shunt diagram.[45] In critical care environments, the iso-shunt graph may therefore be used to determine the optimal inspired oxygen concentration to prevent hypoxaemia while avoiding the administration of an unnecessarily high concentration of oxygen.[44] For example, if a patient is found to have an arterial PO_2 of 30 kPa (225 mmHg) while breathing 90% oxygen, he has a virtual shunt of 20%, and if it is required to attain an arterial PO_2 of 10 kPa (75 mmHg), this should be achieved by reducing the inspired oxygen concentration to 45%.

With inspired oxygen concentrations in excess of 35%, perfusion of alveoli with low (but not zero) $\dot{V}/\dot{Q}$ ratios has relatively little effect on arterial PO_2. However, with inspired oxygen concentrations in the range 21–35%, increased scatter of $\dot{V}/\dot{Q}$ ratios has an appreciable effect on arterial PO_2 for reasons that are explained below. Therefore, in these circumstances the standard iso-shunt diagram is not applicable, since arterial PO_2 is less than predicted as the inspired oxygen concentration is reduced towards 21%. A new diagram, which provides a

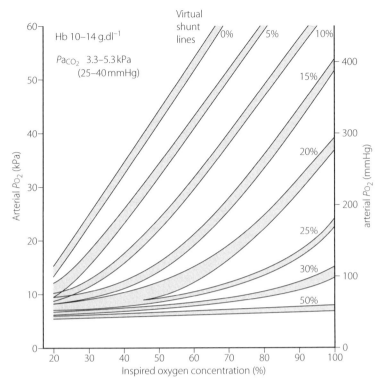

reasonable simulation of scatter of $\dot{V}/\dot{Q}$ ratios *plus* a shunt, is explained below and this diagram (see Figure E.4) appears to be a satisfactory model for a wide variety of patients requiring the administration of oxygen in this range.[46]

THE EFFECT OF SCATTER OF $\dot{V}/\dot{Q}$ RATIOS ON ARTERIAL PO_2

It is usually extremely difficult to say whether reduction of arterial PO_2 is due to true shunt (areas of zero $\dot{V}/\dot{Q}$ ratio) or to an increased scatter of $\dot{V}/\dot{Q}$ ratios with an appreciable contribution to arterial blood from alveoli with very low (but not zero) $\dot{V}/\dot{Q}$ ratios. In the clinical field it is quite usual to ignore scatter of $\dot{V}/\dot{Q}$ ratios (which are difficult to quantify) and to treat blood gas results *as if* the alveolar/arterial PO_2 difference was caused entirely by true shunt. In the example shown in Figure 8.12, it is quite impossible to distinguish between scatter of $\dot{V}/\dot{Q}$ ratios and a shunt on the basis of a single measurement of arterial PO_2. However, the two conditions are quite different in the effect of different inspired oxygen concentrations on the alveolar/arterial PO_2 difference and therefore the apparent shunt.

Figure 8.11 shows that, for a true shunt, with increasing inspired oxygen concentration, the effect on arterial PO_2 increases to reach a plateau value of 2–3 kPa (15–22 mmHg) for each 1% of shunt. This is more precisely shown in terms of alveolar/arterial PO_2 difference, plotted as a function of alveolar PO_2 in Figure 11.4.

It is not intuitively obvious why an increased spread of $\dot{V}/\dot{Q}$ ratios should increase the alveolar/arterial PO_2 difference. There are essentially two reasons. First, there tends to be more blood from the alveoli with low $\dot{V}/\dot{Q}$ ratios. For example, in Figure 8.12, 57% of the arterial blood comes from the alveoli with low $\dot{V}/\dot{Q}$ ratios and low PO_2, whereas only 10% is contributed by the alveoli with high $\dot{V}/\dot{Q}$ ratios and high PO_2. Therefore, the latter cannot compensate for the former, when arterial oxygen levels are determined with due allowance for volume contribution. The second reason is illustrated in Figure 8.13. Alveoli with high $\dot{V}/\dot{Q}$ ratios are on a flatter part of the haemoglobin dissociation curve than are alveoli with low $\dot{V}/\dot{Q}$ ratios. Therefore, the adverse effect on oxygen *content* is greater for alveoli with a low $\dot{V}/\dot{Q}$ and therefore low PO_2 than is the beneficial effect of alveoli with a high $\dot{V}/\dot{Q}$ and therefore high PO_2. Therefore, the greater the spread of $\dot{V}/\dot{Q}$ ratios, the larger the alveolar/arterial PO_2 difference.

Modification of the iso-shunt diagram to include $\dot{V}/\dot{Q}$ scatter. The iso-shunt diagram described above does not take into account $\dot{V}/\dot{Q}$ scatter, and so has bands too wide for practical use below an inspired oxygen concentration of approximately 40% (see Figure 8.11). This problem has been overcome by the development of a two-

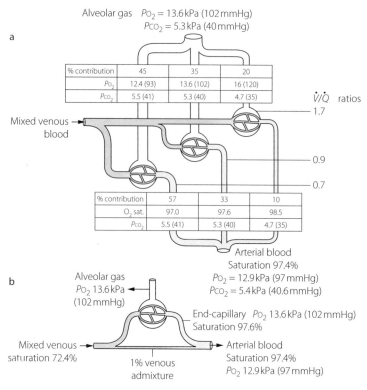

a

% contribution	45	35	20
Po_2	12.4 (93)	13.6 (102)	16 (120)
Pco_2	5.5 (41)	5.3 (40)	4.7 (35)

Alveolar gas $Po_2 = 13.6\,kPa\,(102\,mmHg)$
$Pco_2 = 5.3\,kPa\,(40\,mmHg)$

$\dot{V}/\dot{Q}$ ratios
1.7
0.9
0.7

Mixed venous blood

% contribution	57	33	10
O_2 sat.	97.0	97.6	98.5
Pco_2	5.5 (41)	5.3 (40)	4.7 (35)

Arterial blood
Saturation 97.4%
$Po_2 = 12.9\,kPa\,(97\,mmHg)$
$Pco_2 = 5.4\,kPa\,(40.6\,mmHg)$

b

Alveolar gas
Po_2 13.6 kPa
(102 mmHg)

End-capillary Po_2 13.6 kPa (102 mmHg)
Saturation 97.6%

Mixed venous
saturation 72.4%

1% venous
admixture

Arterial blood
Saturation 97.4%
Po_2 12.9 kPa (97 mmHg)

Figure 8.12 Alveolar to arterial Po_2 difference caused by scatter of $\dot{V}/\dot{Q}$ ratios and its representation by an equivalent degree of venous admixture. **(a)** Scatter of $\dot{V}/\dot{Q}$ ratios corresponding roughly to the three zones of the lung in the normal upright subject. Mixed alveolar gas Po_2 is calculated with allowance for the volume contribution of gas from the three zones. Arterial saturation is similarly determined and the Po_2 derived. There is an alveolar/arterial Po_2 difference of 0.7 kPa (5 mmHg). **(b)** A theoretical situation that would account for the same alveolar to arterial Po_2 difference, caused solely by venous admixture. This is a useful method of quantifying the functional effect of scattered $\dot{V}/\dot{Q}$ ratios, but should be carefully distinguished from the actual situation.

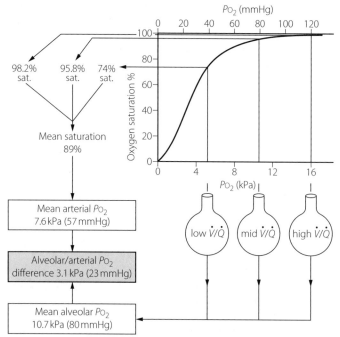

98.2% sat.   95.8% sat.   74% sat.

Mean saturation 89%

Mean arterial Po_2 7.6 kPa (57 mmHg)

Alveolar/arterial Po_2 difference 3.1 kPa (23 mmHg)

Mean alveolar Po_2 10.7 kPa (80 mmHg)

low $\dot{V}/\dot{Q}$ mid $\dot{V}/\dot{Q}$ high $\dot{V}/\dot{Q}$

Figure 8.13 Alveolar/arterial Po_2 difference caused by scatter of $\dot{V}/\dot{Q}$ ratios resulting in oxygen tensions along the upper inflexion of the oxygen dissociation curve. The diagram shows the effect of three groups of alveoli with Po_2 values of 5.3, 10.7 and 16.0 kPa (40, 80 and 120 mmHg). Ignoring the effect of the different volumes of gas and blood contributed by the three groups, the mean alveolar Po_2 is 10.7 kPa. However, owing to the shape of the dissociation curve, the saturations of the blood leaving the three groups are not proportional to their Po_2. The mean arterial saturation is, in fact, 89% and the Po_2 therefore is 7.6 kPa. The alveolar/arterial Po_2 difference is thus 3.1 kPa. The actual difference would be somewhat greater, since gas with a high Po_2 would make a relatively greater contribution to the alveolar gas and blood with a low Po_2 would make a relatively greater contribution to the arterial blood. In this example, a calculated venous admixture of 27% would be required to account for the scatter of $\dot{V}/\dot{Q}$ ratios in terms of the measured alveolar/arterial Po_2 difference, at an alveolar Po_2 of 10.7 kPa.

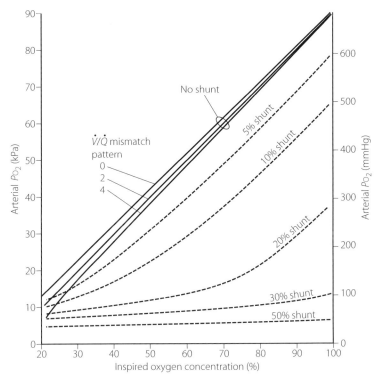

Figure 8.14 The continuous curves show the effect on arterial P_{O_2} of increasing degrees of $\dot{V}/\dot{Q}$ mismatch (using the bimodal two-compartment model of maldistribution[46]) for different values of inspired oxygen concentration in the absence of a true shunt. At lower inspired oxygen the arterial P_{O_2} is progressively decreased below normal for the reasons shown in Figures 8.12 and 8.13. These concave-downward curves may be compared with the concave-upward iso-shunt curves shown as broken lines. $\dot{V}/\dot{Q}$ mismatch patterns 1–4 are combined with the iso-shunt curves in Figure E.4.

compartment model including both true shunt and $\dot{V}/\dot{Q}$ scatter components,[46] which for the latter factor assumes a bimodal distribution of $\dot{V}/\dot{Q}$ scatter and uses five grades of $\dot{V}/\dot{Q}$ mismatch 'severity'. Figure 8.14 shows the effect of $\dot{V}/\dot{Q}$ mismatch on the 0% iso-shunt line, clearly displaying the variation in arterial P_{O_2} with $\dot{V}/\dot{Q}$ scatter at lower inspired oxygen concentrations. Figure E.4 shows further examples of the effect of $\dot{V}/\dot{Q}$ scatter on the inspired to arterial oxygen gradients. This model is clearly an oversimplification of the situation in lung disease (see Figure 8.7). Nevertheless, the second grade of $\dot{V}/\dot{Q}$ mismatch, when combined with a range of shunt values, was found to provide a close simulation of the relationship between arterial P_{O_2} and inspired oxygen concentration for a wide variety of patients with moderate respiratory dysfunction requiring oxygen therapy in the range 25–35% inspired oxygen concentration.[46,47]

PRINCIPLES OF ASSESSMENT OF DISTRIBUTION OF VENTILATION AND PULMONARY BLOOD FLOW

Regional distribution of ventilation and perfusion

Radioactive tracers. Regional distribution of ventilation and perfusion may be conveniently studied with a gamma camera. Ventilation is assessed following inhalation of a suitable radioactive gas that is not too soluble

in blood. Both ^{133}Xe and [81]Kr are suitable for this purpose and the technique has become a routine clinical investigation, usually using [81]Kr because its short half-life (13 s) reduces uptake by the pulmonary circulation. For assessment of regional perfusion, a relatively insoluble gas such as ^{133}Xe or ^{99}Tc may be dissolved in saline and administered intravenously and its distribution within the lung again recorded with a gamma camera. The technique defines both ventilation and perfusion in zones of the lung that can be related to anatomical subdivisions by comparing anteroposterior and lateral scans.

PET scanning is used for research purposes and allows more precise definition of regional ventilation and perfusion, though only in horizontal positions.[7] Once again, radioactive isotopes are inhaled or injected intravenously, for example [13]N₂, and the radioisotopic concentration in a three-dimensional field measured during normal breathing.

MRI scanning is another technique, currently used only for research, which provides unprecedented three-dimensional imaging of ventilation and perfusion. Recent developments in MRI scanning have led to more functionally relevant scans.[9,48] By using non-radioactive tracer gases, such as [3]He that has been magnetically 'hyperpolarised', MRI scans can be greatly enhanced in a similar way to the use of contrast for traditional X-ray radiographs. Hyperpolarised ^{3}He used in this way interacts with the paramagnetic oxygen molecules (page 193) in the lungs, causing oxygen-dependent decay of the hyperpolarisation, and this phenomenon can be used to generate scans showing regional PO_2 in the lung.

Measurement of ventilation and perfusion as a function of $\dot{V}/\dot{Q}$ ratio

The information of the type displayed in Figures 8.6 and 8.7 is obtained by the MIGET,[22,24] which employs six tracer gases with different blood solubilities ranging from very soluble (acetone) to very insoluble (sulphur hexafluoride). Saline is equilibrated with these gases and infused intravenously at a constant rate. After about 20 minutes a steady state is achieved and samples of arterial blood and mixed expired gas are collected. Levels of the tracer gases in the arterial blood are then measured by gas chromatography and levels in the mixed venous blood are derived by use of the Fick principle. It is then possible to calculate the retention of each tracer in the blood passing through the lung and the elimination of each in the expired gas. Retention and elimination are related to the solubility coefficient of each tracer in blood and then, by numerical analysis, it is possible to compute a distribution curve for pulmonary blood flow and alveolar ventilation, respectively, in relation to the spectrum of $\dot{V}/\dot{Q}$ ratios (see Figure 8.6).

The technique is technically demanding and laborious. It has not become widely used, but studies using the technique from a small number of laboratories have made major contributions to our understanding of gas exchange in a variety of circumstances.

Measurement of venous admixture

Venous admixture, according to the Riley three-compartment model (see Figure 8.8), is calculated by solution of the equation shown in Figure 8.10. When the alveolar PO_2 is less than about 30 kPa (225 mmHg), scatter of $\dot{V}/\dot{Q}$ ratios contributes appreciably to the total calculated venous admixture (see Figure 8.14). When the subject breathes 100% oxygen, the component due to scatter of $\dot{V}/\dot{Q}$ ratios is minimal. Nevertheless, the calculated quantity still does not indicate the precise value of shunted blood because some of the shunt consists of blood of which the oxygen content is unknown (e.g. from bronchial veins and venae cordis minimae). The calculated venous admixture is thus at best an index rather than a precise measurement of contamination of arterial blood with venous blood.

To solve the equation shown in Figure 8.10, three quantities are required.

1. **Arterial oxygen content.** Arterial PO_2 or oxygen saturation may be measured on blood drawn from any convenient systemic artery. If arterial PO_2 is measured, this must first be converted to oxygen saturation (page 177 et seq.), before the oxygen content can be calculated (page 188).

2. **Mixed venous oxygen content.** Mixed venous blood must be sampled from the right ventricle or pulmonary artery. Blood from inferior and superior venae cavae and coronary sinus, each with quite different O_2 contents, remain separate in the right atrium. Oxygen content may then be calculated from measured PO_2 as for the arterial sample. An assumed value for arterial/mixed venous blood oxygen content difference is often used if it is not feasible to sample mixed venous blood, and this is inherent in the iso-shunt diagram (see Figure 8.11).

3. **Pulmonary end-capillary oxygen content.** This cannot be measured directly and is assumed to be equal to the alveolar PO_2 (page 138). If Figure 8.8 is studied in conjunction with Figure 8.10, it will be seen that the 'alveolar' PO_2 required is the 'ideal' alveolar PO_2 and not the end-expiratory PO_2, which may be contaminated with alveolar dead space gas. The 'ideal' alveolar PO_2 is derived by solution of one of the alveolar air equations (see below) and again converted to oxygen content.

Non-invasive estimation of venous admixture may be performed without sampling arterial or mixed venous blood, using only measurement of haemoglobin concentration (Hb), end-tidal PCO_2, inspired O_2 concentration and peripheral oxygen saturation (Sp_{O_2}).[49] Arterial O_2 content is calculated from Hb and Sp_{O_2} and alveolar PO_2 from the alveolar air equation described below using inspired O_2 concentration and end-tidal PCO_2 (therefore assuming a normal end-tidal to arterial PCO_2 difference). In a similar fashion to the iso-shunt lines, mixed venous O_2 content is derived from arterial O_2 content using an assumed value for arterial/mixed-venous oxygen difference. Shunt estimated in this way gives results that are ±16% shunt compared to invasive measurements.[49]

The alveolar air equation

The PO_2 of 'ideal' alveolar gas (see Figure 8.8) must be derived by indirect means and was first formulated with some precision by Riley et al. in 1946.[50] The equation exists in several forms that appear very different but give the same result.

Derivation of the ideal alveolar PO_2 is based on the following assumptions.

- Quite large degrees of venous admixture or $\dot{V}/\dot{Q}$ scatter cause relatively little difference between the PCO_2 of ideal alveolar gas (or pulmonary end-capillary blood) and that of arterial blood (see Table 8.2). Therefore ideal alveolar P_{CO_2} is approximately equal to arterial P_{CO_2}.

- The respiratory exchange ratio of ideal alveolar gas (in relation to inspired gas) equals the respiratory exchange ratio of mixed expired gas (again in relation to inspired gas).

From these assumptions it is possible to derive an equation that indicates the ideal alveolar P_{O_2} in terms of arterial P_{CO_2} and inspired gas P_{O_2}. As a very rough approximation, the oxygen and carbon dioxide in the alveolar gas replace the oxygen in the inspired gas. Therefore, very approximately:

$$\text{Alveolar } P_{O_2} \approx \text{inspired } P_{O_2} - \text{arterial } P_{CO_2}$$

This equation is not sufficiently accurate for use, except in the special case when 100% oxygen is breathed. In other situations, three corrections are required to overcome errors due to the following factors.

1. Usually, less carbon dioxide is produced than oxygen is consumed (effect of the respiratory exchange ratio, RQ).
2. The respiratory exchange ratio produces a secondary effect because the expired volume does not equal the inspired volume.
3. The inspired and expired gas volumes may also differ because of inert gas exchange.

The simplest practicable form of the equation makes correction for the principal effect of the respiratory exchange ratio (1), but not the small supplementary error due to the difference between the inspired and expired gas volumes (2):

$$\text{Alveolar } P_{O_2} \approx \text{inspired } P_{O_2} - \text{arterial } P_{CO_2}/RQ$$

This form is suitable for rapid bedside calculations of alveolar P_{O_2}, when great accuracy is not required.

One stage more complicated is an equation that allows for differences in the volume of inspired and expired gas due to the respiratory exchange ratio, but still does not allow for differences due to the exchange of inert gases. This equation exists in various forms, all algebraically identical:[50]

$$\text{Alveolar } P_{O_2} = P_{I_{O_2}} - \frac{Pa_{CO_2}}{RQ}\left(1 - F_{I_{O_2}}(1-RQ)\right)$$

This equation is suitable for use whenever the subject has been breathing the inspired gas mixture long enough for the inert gas to be in equilibrium. It is unsuitable for use when the inspired oxygen concentration has recently been changed, when the ambient pressure has recently been changed (e.g. during hyperbaric oxygen therapy), or when the inert gas concentration has recently been changed (e.g. soon after the start or finish of a period of inhaling nitrous oxide).

Perhaps the most satisfactory form of the alveolar air equation is that which was advanced by Filley, MacIntosh and Wright in 1954.[51] This equation makes no assumption that inert gases are in equilibrium and allows for the difference between inspired and expired gas from whatever cause. It also proves to be very simple in use and does not require the calculation of the respiratory exchange ratio, although it does require sampling of mixed expired gas:

$$\text{Alveolar } P_{O_2} = P_{I_{O_2}} - Pa_{CO_2}\left(\frac{P_{I_{O_2}} - P_{\overline{E}_{O_2}}}{P_{\overline{E}_{CO_2}}}\right)$$

If the alveolar P_{O_2} is calculated separately according to the last two equations, the difference (if any) will be that due to inert gas exchange.

When using these equations in practice it is important to take into account water vapour, as alveolar gas will be saturated with water at body temperature, such that:

$$P_{I_{O_2}} = F_{I_{O_2}} \times (P_B - P_{H_2O})$$

where $F_{I_{O_2}}$ is the fractional inspired oxygen concentration, P_B is barometric pressure and P_{H_2O} is saturated vapour pressure of water at 37°C (6.3 kPa, 47 mmHg).

Distinction between shunt and the effect of $\dot{V}/\dot{Q}$ scatter

Shunt and scatter of $\dot{V}/\dot{Q}$ ratios will each produce an alveolar/arterial P_{O_2} difference from which a value for venous admixture may be calculated. It is usually impossible to say to what extent the calculated venous admixture is due to a true shunt or to perfusion of alveoli with low $\dot{V}/\dot{Q}$ ratios. Three methods are available to distinguish between the two conditions.

If the inspired oxygen concentration is altered, the effect on the arterial P_{O_2} will depend upon the nature of the disorder. If oxygenation is impaired by a shunt, the arterial P_{O_2} will increase as shown in the iso-shunt diagram (see Figure 8.11). If, however, the disorder is due to scatter of $\dot{V}/\dot{Q}$ ratios, the arterial P_{O_2} will approach the normal value for the inspired oxygen concentration as the inspired oxygen concentration is increased (see Figure 8.14). $\dot{V}/\dot{Q}$ scatter has virtually no effect when the subject breathes 100% oxygen. This difference between shunt and $\dot{V}/\dot{Q}$ scatter forms the basis of a non-invasive method for investigating the mechanism of impaired gas exchange in the clinical setting.[52,53] The technique is similar to that already described for assessing venous admixture (page 128). Oxygen saturation is measured at several different inspired oxygen concentrations and an Sp_{O_2} versus $F_{I_{O_2}}$ curve drawn. Mathematical modelling, again using an assumed value

Figure 8.15 Non-invasive evaluation of impaired gas exchange during one-lung anaesthesia and thoracotomy. Oxygen saturation has been measured at nine different inspired oxygen concentrations (dots) and a curve fitted to the points (solid line). Mathematical modelling (broken lines) shows that shunt displaces the curve downwards (0% and 30% shunt shown), whereas $\dot{V}/\dot{Q}$ mismatch displaces the curve to the right. A computer algorithm, using an assumed value for arteriovenous oxygen difference, can compute the virtual shunt and the shift due to $\dot{V}/\dot{Q}$ mismatch from the actual curve obtained from the patient, in this case 30% shunt *and* marked $\dot{V}/\dot{Q}$ mismatch in the patient during one-lung ventilation (page 317). (Reproduced with permission from de Gray L, Rush EM, Jones JG. A noninvasive method for evaluating the effect of thoracotomy on shunt and ventilation perfusion inequality. *Anaesthesia* 1997; **52**: 630–5.)

for arteriovenous oxygen difference, and studies during one-lung anaesthesia have shown that shunt depresses the curve downwards whereas increasing $\dot{V}/\dot{Q}$ mismatch moves the curve to the right (Figure 8.15).[52]

Measurement of the alveolar/arterial P_{N_2} difference is a specific method for quantification of $\dot{V}/\dot{Q}$ scatter, because the P_{N_2} difference is entirely uninfluenced by true shunt.[54] Subjects must be in a state of complete nitrogen equilibrium, which may be difficult to achieve in the clinical environment. The method has not come into general use owing to difficulties in measuring P_{N_2} with adequate precision.

The multiple inert gas elimination technique for analysis of distribution of blood flow in relation to $\dot{V}/\dot{Q}$ ratio is the best method of distinguishing between shunt and areas of low $\dot{V}/\dot{Q}$ ratio (see above).

Measurement of dead space

Anatomical dead space is most conveniently measured by the technique illustrated in Figure 8.16, originally developed for use with a nitrogen analyser by Fowler.[27] The CO_2 concentration at the lips is measured continuously with a rapid gas analyser and then displayed against

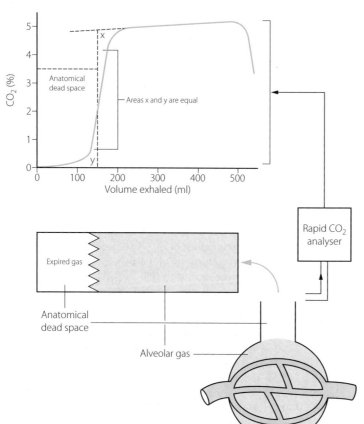

Figure 8.16 Measurement of anatomical dead space using CO_2 as the tracer gas. If the gas passing the patient's lips is continuously analysed for CO_2 concentration, there is a sudden rise to the alveolar plateau level after the expiration of gas from the anatomical dead space. If the instantaneous CO_2 concentration is plotted against the volume exhaled (allowing for delay in the CO_2 analyser), a graph similar to that shown is obtained. A vertical line is constructed so that the two areas x and y are equal. This line will indicate the volume of the anatomical dead space. Note that the abscissa records *volume* rather than *time*, as seen with capnography performed in clinical situations.

the volume actually expired. The 'alveolar plateau' of CO_2 concentration is not flat but slopes gently. Anatomical dead space is easily derived from the graph, as shown in Figure 8.16 or by mathematical solution.[55]

Physiological dead space. Mixed-expired air is collected over a period of 2 or 3 minutes, during which time an arterial blood sample is collected and the PCO_2 of blood and gas are then determined. Provided that the inspired gas is free from carbon dioxide, physiological dead space is indicated by the following form of the Bohr equation:

$$\text{Physiological dead space} = \text{tidal volume} \left(\frac{Pa_{CO_2} - P\overline{E}_{CO_2}}{Pa_{CO_2}} \right)$$

$$- \text{apparatus dead space}$$

Alveolar dead space is measured as the difference between the physiological and anatomical dead space, determined separately but at the same time. When only the physiological dead space is measured, it is often possible to attribute a large increase in physiological dead space to an increase in the alveolar component, since there are few circumstances in which the anatomical dead space is greatly enlarged. Methods are now available for the estimation of anatomical, physiological and therefore alveolar dead spaces from a single-breath recording of expired CO_2 and a single arterial PCO_2 measurement.[56,57] The requirement for an arterial blood sample still makes this an invasive measurement, but the bedside assessment of alveolar dead space is now possible in critical care situations.[57]

The arterial/end-expiratory PCO_2 difference is a convenient and relatively simple method of assessing the magnitude of the alveolar dead space. In Figure 8.9, end-expiratory gas is shown to consist of a mixture of ideal alveolar gas and alveolar dead space gas. If the patient has an appreciable alveolar dead space, the end-expiratory PCO_2 will be less than the arterial PCO_2, which is assumed to be equal to the ideal alveolar PCO_2.

If, for example, ideal alveolar gas has a PCO_2 of 5.3 kPa (40 mmHg) and the end-expiratory PCO_2 is found to be 2.65 kPa (20 mmHg), it follows that the end-expiratory gas consists of equal parts of ideal alveolar gas and alveolar dead space gas. Thus if the tidal volume is 500 ml and the anatomical dead space 100 ml, then alveolar dead space and ideal alveolar gas components would be 200 ml each.

REFERENCES

1. Svanberg L. Influence of posture on lung volumes, ventilation and circulation in normals. *Scand J Clin Lab Invest* 1957; **9**; supp 25.

2. Rehder K, Sessler AD. Function of each lung in spontaneously breathing man anesthetized with thiopental-meperidine. *Anesthesiology* 1973; **38**: 320–7.

3. Rehder K, Hatch DJ, Sessler AD, Fowler WS. The function of each lung of anesthetized and paralyzed man during mechanical ventilation. *Anesthesiology* 1972; **37**: 16–26.

4. Nunn JF. The distribution of inspired gas during thoracic surgery. *Ann Roy Coll Surg Eng* 1961; **28**: 223–37.

5. West JB. Regional differences in gas exchange in the lung of erect man. *J Appl Physiol* 1962; **17**: 893–8.

6. Hughes JMB, Grant BJB, Greene RE, Iliff LD, Milic-Emili J. Inspiratory flow rate and ventilation distribution in normal subjects and in patients with simple chronic bronchitis. *Clin Sci* 1972; **43**: 583–95.

7. Musch G, Layfield JDH, Harris RS, *et al.* Topographical distribution of pulmonary perfusion and ventilation, assessed by PET in supine and prone humans. *J Appl Physiol* 2002; **93**: 1841–51.

8. Rizi RR, Lipson DA, Dimitrov IE, Ishii M, Roberts DA. Operating characteristics of hyperpolarized ^{3}He and arterial spin tagging in MR imaging of ventilation and perfusion in healthy subjects. *Acad Radiol* 2003; **10**: 502–8.

*9. Kauczor HU, Chen XJ, van Beek EJR, Schreiber WG. Pulmonary ventilation imaged by magnetic resonance: at the doorstep of clinical application. *Eur Respir J* 2001; **17**: 1008–23.

10. Kaneko K, Milic-Emili ME, Dolovich MB, Dawson A, Bates DV. Regional distribution of ventilation and perfusion as a function of body position. *J Appl Physiol* 1966; **21**: 767–77.

11. West JB. Distribution of gas and blood in the normal lung. *Br Med Bull* 1963; **19**: 53–8.

12. Hughes JMB, Glazier JB, Maloney JE, West JB. Effect of lung volume on the distribution of pulmonary blood flow in man. *Respir Physiol* 1968; **4**: 58–72.

13. Brudin LH, Rhodes CG, Valind SO, Jones T, Hughes JB. Interrelationship between regional blood flow, blood volume and ventilation in supine humans. *J Appl Physiol* 1994; **76**: 1205–10.

14. Brudin LH, Rhodes CG, Valind SO, Jones T, Jonson B, Hughes JB. Relationship between regional ventilation and vascular and extravascular volume in supine humans. *J Appl Physiol* 1994; **76**: 1195–204.

15. Jones AT, Hansell DM, Evans TW. Pulmonary perfusion in supine and prone positions: an electron-beam computed tomography study. *J Appl Physiol* 2001; **90**: 1342–8.

16. Nyrén S, Mure M, Jacobsson H, Larsson SA, Lindahl SGE. Pulmonary perfusion is more uniform in the prone than in the supine position: scintigraphy in healthy humans. *J Appl Physiol* 1999; **86**: 1135–41.

17. Glenny RW, Bernard S, Robertson HT, Hlastala MP. Gravity is an important but secondary determinant of regional pulmonary blood flow in upright primates. *J Appl Physiol* 1999; **86**: 623–32.

18. Hakim TS, Lisbona R, Dean GW. Gravity-independent inequality in pulmonary blood flow in humans. *J Appl Physiol* 1987; **63**: 1114–21.

*19. Hastala MP, Glenny RW. Vascular structure determines pulmonary blood flow distribution. *News Physiol Sci* 1999; **14**: 182–6.

20. West JB. Importance of gravity in determining the distribution of pulmonary blood flow. *J Appl Physiol* 2002; **93**: 1888–91.

21. Hlastala MP. Ventilation/perfusion: from the bench to the patient. *Cardiologia* 1996; **41**: 405–15.

22. Roca J, Wagner PD. Principles and information content of the multiple inert gas elimination technique. *Thorax* 1993; **49**: 815–24.

23. Wagner PD, Laravuso RB, Uhl RR, West JB. Continuous distributions of ventilation–perfusion ratios in normal subjects breathing air and 100% O_2. *J Clin Invest* 1974; **54**: 54–68.

24. West JB. *Ventilation: blood flow and gas exchange.* Oxford: Blackwell Scientific, 1990.

25. Fenn WO, Rahn H, Otis AB. A theoretical analysis of the composition of alveolar air at altitude. *Am J Physiol* 1946; **146**: 637–53.

26. Riley RL, Cournand A. 'Ideal' alveolar air and the analysis of ventilation perfusion relationships in the lung. *J Appl Physiol* 1949; **1**: 825–49.

27. Fowler WS. Lung function studies. II. The respiratory dead space. *Am J Physiol* 1948; **154**: 405–16.

28. Numa AH, Newth CJL. Anatomic dead space in infants and children. *J Appl Physiol* 1996; **80**: 1485–9.

29. Fowler WS. Lung function studies. IV. Postural changes in respiratory dead space and functional residual capacity. *J Clin Invest* 1950; **29**: 1437–8.

30. Nunn JF, Campbell EJM, Peckett BW. Anatomical subdivisions of the volume of respiratory dead space and effect of position of the jaw. *J Appl Physiol* 1959; **14**: 174–6.

31. Lifshay A, Fast CW, Glazier JB. Effects of changes in respiratory pattern on physiological dead space. *J Appl Physiol* 1971; **31**: 478–83.

32. Nunn JF, Hill DW. Respiratory dead space and arterial to end-tidal CO_2 tension difference in anesthetized man. *J Appl Physiol* 1960; **15**: 383–9.

33. Casati A, Fanelli G, Torri G. Physiological dead space/tidal volume ratio during face mask, laryngeal mask and cuffed oropharyngeal airway spontaneous ventilation. *J Clin Anesth* 1998; **10**: 652–5.

34. Le Bourdellé G, Mier L, Fiquet B, *et al.* Comparison of the effects of heat and moisture exchangers and heated humidifiers on ventilation and gas exchange during weaning trials from mechanical ventilation. *Chest* 1996; **110**: 1294–8.

35. Briscoe WA, Forster RE, Comroe JH. Alveolar ventilation at very low tidal volumes. *J Appl Physiol* 1954; **7**: 27–30.

36. Bohr C. Über die Lungenathmung. *Skand Arch Physiol* 1891; **2**: 236.

37. Harris EA, Hunter ME, Seelye ER, Vedder M, Whitlock RML. Prediction of the physiological dead-space in resting normal subjects. *Clin Sci* 1973; **45**: 375–86.

38. Radford EP. Ventilation standards for use in artificial respiration. *J Appl Physiol* 1955; **7**:451–63.

39. Craig DB, Wahba WM, Don HF, Couture JG, Becklake MR. 'Closing volume' and its relationship to gas exchange in seated and supine positions. *J Appl Physiol* 1971; **31**: 717–21.

40. Ravin MG, Epstein RM, Malm JR. Contribution of thebesian veins to the physiologic shunt in anesthetized man. *J Appl Physiol* 1965; **20**: 1148–52.

41. Dantzker DR, Lynch JP, Weg JG. Depression of cardiac output is a mechanism of shunt reduction in the therapy of acute respiratory failure. *Chest* 1980; **77**: 636–47.

42. Lynch JP, Mhyre JG, Dantzker DR. Influence of cardiac output on intrapulmonary shunt. *J Appl Physiol* 1979; **46**: 315–21.

43. Cheney FW, Colley PS. The effect of cardiac output on arterial blood oxygenation. *Anesthesiology* 1980; **52**: 496–503.

44. Benator SR, Hewlett AM, Nunn JF. The use of iso-shunt lines for control of oxygen therapy. *Br J Anaesth* 1973; **45**: 711–18.

45. Lawler PGP, Nunn JF. A reassessment of the validity of the iso-shunt graph. *Br J Anaesth* 1984; **56**: 1325–35.

46. Petros AJ, Doré CJ, Nunn JF. Modification of the iso-shunt lines for low inspired oxygen concentrations. *Br J Anaesth* 1994; **72**: 515–22.

47. Drummond GB, Wright DJ. Oxygen therapy after abdominal surgery. *Br J Anaesth* 1977; **49**: 789–97.

*48. Mills GH, Wild JM, Eberle B, van Beek EJR. Functional magnetic resonance imaging of the lung. *Br J Anaesth* 2003; **91**: 16–30.

49. Hope DA, Jenkins BJ, Willis N, Maddock H, Mapleson WW. Non-invasive estimation of venous admixture: validation of a new formula. *Br J Anaesth* 1995; **74**: 538–43.

50. Riley RL, Lilienthal JL, Proemmel DD, Franke RE. On the determination of the physiologically effective pressures of oxygen and carbon dioxide in alveolar air. *Am J Physiol* 1946; **147**: 191–8.

51. Filley GF, MacIntosh DJ, Wright GW. Carbon monoxide uptake and pulmonary diffusing capacity in normal subject at rest and during exercise. *J Clin Invest* 1954; **33**: 530–9.

*52. de Gray L, Rush EM, Jones JG. A noninvasive method for evaluating the effect of thoracotomy on shunt and ventilation perfusion inequality. *Anaesthesia* 1997; **52**: 630–5.

53. Kjaergaard S, Rees S, Malczynski J, *et al*. Non-invasive estimation of shunt and ventilation-perfusion mismatch. *Intens Care Med* 2003; **29**: 727–34.

54. Rahn H, Farhi LE. Ventilation, perfusion and gas exchange - VA/Q concept. In: Fenn WO, Rahn H, eds. *Handbook of physiology, section 3 – Respiration*. Washington DC: American Physiological Society, 1964.

55. Heller H, Könen-Bergmann M, Schuster K-D. An algebraic solution to dead space determination according to Fowler's graphical method. *Comput Biomed Res* 1999; **32**: 161–7.

*56. Åström E, Niklason L, Drefeldt B, Bajc M, Jonson B. Partitioning of dead space - a method and reference values in the awake human. *Eur Respir J* 2000; **16**: 659–64.

57. Arnold JH. Measurement of alveolar deadspace: are we there yet ? *Crit Care Med* 2001; **29**: 1287–8.

KEY POINTS

■ For gas to transfer between the alveolus and the haemoglobin in the red blood cell, it must diffuse across the alveolar and capillary walls, through the plasma and across the red cell membrane.

■ The reaction rate for oxygen with haemoglobin also affects the rate at which red blood cells become saturated with oxygen on passing through the pulmonary capillary.

■ Transfer of oxygen and carbon dioxide is very rapid and impairment of this transfer is rarely a cause of impaired gas exchange.

■ Carbon monoxide, because of its high affinity for haemoglobin, is used to assess the diffusing capacity of the lungs.

The preceding chapters described in detail how alveolar gases and pulmonary capillary blood are delivered to their respective sides of the alveolar wall. This chapter deals with the final step of lung function by discussing the transfer of respiratory gases between the alveolus and the blood.

Nomenclature in this field is confusing. In Europe, measurement of the passage of gases between the alveoli and pulmonary capillaries is referred to as lung 'transfer factor' (e.g. TL_{CO} represents lung transfer factor for carbon monoxide). However, the older term 'diffusing capacity' (e.g. DL_{CO} for lung diffusing capacity for carbon monoxide) remains in more common usage, particularly in the USA,[1] in spite of the finding that some of the barrier to oxygen transfer is unrelated to diffusion (see below).

FUNDAMENTALS OF THE DIFFUSION PROCESS

Diffusion of a gas is a process by which a net transfer of molecules takes place from a zone in which the gas exerts a high partial pressure to a zone in which it exerts a lower partial pressure. The mechanism of transfer is the random movement of molecules and the term excludes both active biological transport and transfer by mass movement of gas in response to a *total* pressure difference (i.e. gas flow as occurs during tidal ventilation). The partial pressure (or tension) of a gas in a gas mixture is the pressure which it would exert if it occupied the space alone (equal to total pressure multiplied by fractional concentration). Gas molecules pass in each direction but at a rate proportional to the partial pressure of the gas in the zone they are leaving. The net transfer of the gas is the difference in the number of molecules passing in each direction and is thus proportional to the difference in partial pressure between the two zones. Typical examples of diffusion are shown in Figure 9.1.

In each of the examples shown in Figure 9.1, there is a finite resistance to the transfer of the gas molecules. In Figure 9.1a, the resistance is concentrated at the restriction in the neck of the bottle. Clearly, the narrower the neck, the slower will be the process of equilibration with the outside air. In Figure 9.1b, the site of the resistance to diffusion is less circumscribed but includes gas diffusion within the alveolus, the alveolar/capillary membrane, the diffusion path through the plasma and the delay in combination of oxygen with the reduced haemoglobin in the red blood cell (RBC). In Figure 9.1c, the resistance commences with the delay in the release of oxygen by haemoglobin and includes all the interfaces between the RBC membrane and the site of oxygen consumption in the mitochondria. There may then be an additional component in the rate at which oxygen enters into chemical reactions.

In the living body oxygen is constantly being consumed while carbon dioxide is being produced, so equilibrium cannot be attained, as in the case of the open bottle of oxygen in Figure 9.1a. Instead, a dynamic equilibrium is attained, with diffusion down a gradient between the alveolus and the mitochondria for oxygen and the reverse for carbon dioxide. The maintenance of these tension gradients is, in fact, a characteristic of life.

In the case of gases that are not metabolised to any great extent, such as nitrogen and most inhalational anaesthetic agents, there is always a tendency towards a

a

Net O_2 transfer

100% O_2 (dry)

Air (dry)

P_{O_2} 101 kPa (760 mmHg)

P_{O_2} 21 kPa (160 mmHg)

Partial pressure gradient
for diffusion 80 kPa (600 mmHg)

Figure 9.1 Three examples of diffusion of oxygen. In each case there is a net transfer of oxygen from left to right in accordance with the partial pressure gradient. **(a)** Oxygen passes from one gaseous phase to another. **(b)** Oxygen passes from a gaseous phase to a liquid phase. **(c)** Oxygen passes from one liquid to another.

b

Net O_2 transfer

14.7% O_2 (wet)

Mean pulmonary capillary
P_{O_2} 11.3 kPa (85 mmHg)

Alveolar
P_{O_2} 141 kPa (105 mmHg)

Partial pressure gradient
for diffusion 2.7 kPa (20 mmHg)

c

Net O_2 transfer

Mean systemic capillary
P_{O_2} 6.7 kPa (50 mmHg)

Mean tissue
P_{O_2} 2.7 kPa (20 mmHg)

Partial pressure gradient
for diffusion 4 kPa (30 mmHg)

static equilibrium at which all tissue partial pressures become equal to the partial pressure of the particular gas in the inspired air. This occurs with nitrogen (apart from the small effect of the respiratory exchange ratio) and would also be attained with an inhalational anaesthetic agent if it were administered for a very long time.

Quantification of resistance to diffusion

The propensity of a gas to diffuse as a result of a given pressure gradient is known as its diffusing capacity according to the equation:

$$\text{Diffusing capacity} = \frac{\text{Net rate of gas transfer}}{\text{Partial pressure gradient}}$$

The usual biological unit of diffusing capacity is ml.min^{-1}.mmHg^{-1} or, in SI units, ml.min^{-1}.kPa^{-1}.

Small molecules diffuse more easily than large molecules. Graham's law states that the rate of diffusion of a gas is inversely proportional to the square root of its density. In addition, gases also diffuse more readily at higher temperatures. Apart from these factors, inherent in the gas, the resistance to diffusion is related directly to the length of the diffusion path and inversely to the area of interface that is available for diffusion.

Diffusion of gases in solution

The partial pressure of a gas in solution in a liquid is defined as being equal to the partial pressure of the same gas in a gas mixture that is in equilibrium with the liquid. When a gas is diffusing into or through an aqueous phase, the solubility of the gas in water becomes an important factor and the diffusing capacity under these circumstances is considered to be directly proportional to the solubility. Nitrous oxide would thus be expected to have about 20 times the diffusing capacity of oxygen in crossing a gas–water interface. High solubility does not confer an increased 'agility' of the gas in its negotiation of an aqueous barrier but simply means that, for a given partial pressure, more molecules of the gas are present in the liquid.

Partial pressure versus concentration gradients. Non-gaseous substances in solution diffuse in response to concentration gradients. This is also true for gas mixtures at the same total pressure, when the partial pressure of any component gas is directly proportional to its concentration. This is not the case when a gas in solution in one liquid diffuses into a different liquid in which it has a different solubility coefficient. When gases are in solution, the partial pressure they exert is directly proportional to their concentration in the solvent but inversely to the solubility of the gas in the solvent. Thus, if water and oil have the same concentration of nitrous oxide dissolved in each, the partial pressure of nitrous oxide in the oil will be only one-third of the partial pressure in the water, since the oil/water solubility ratio is about 3/1. If the two liquids are shaken up together, there will be a net transfer of nitrous oxide from the water to the oil until the tension in each phase is the same. At that time the concentration of nitrous oxide in the oil will be about three times the concentration in the water. There is thus a net transfer of nitrous oxide against the concentration gradient, but always with the partial pressure gradient. It is therefore useful to consider partial pressure rather than concentrations in relation to movement of gases and vapours from one compartment of the body to another. The same units of pressure may be used in gas, aqueous and lipid phases.

DIFFUSION OF OXYGEN IN THE LUNGS

It is now widely accepted that oxygen passes from the alveoli into the pulmonary capillary blood by a passive process of diffusion according to physical laws, though for a while it was believed that oxygen was actively secreted into the blood (page 221). It is believed that diffusion equilibrium is very nearly achieved for oxygen during the normal pulmonary capillary transit time in the resting subject. Therefore, in these circumstances, the uptake of oxygen is limited by pulmonary blood flow and not by diffusing capacity. However, when exercising, while breathing gas mixtures deficient in oxygen or at reduced barometric pressure, the diffusing capacity becomes important and may limit oxygen uptake.

Components of the alveolar/capillary diffusion pathway

The gas space within the alveolus. At functional residual capacity, the diameter of the average human alveolus is of the order of 200 μm (page 19) and it is likely that

mixing of normal alveolar gas is almost instantaneous over the small distance from the centre to the periphery. Precise calculations are impossible on account of the complex geometry of the alveolus, but the overall efficiency of gas exchange within the lungs suggests that mixing must be complete within less than 10 ms. Therefore, in practice it is usual to consider alveolar gas of normal composition as uniformly mixed.

This generalisation does not seem to hold when subjects inhale gases of widely different molecular weights. This was first demonstrated in normal subjects inhaling mixtures of sulphur hexafluoride (SF_6) and helium when the SF_6 concentration was found to be higher (relative to helium) earlier in the breath.[2] According to Graham's law, SF_6 (molecular weight 146) would diffuse six times less readily than helium (molecular weight 4) and would therefore tend to remain concentrated at the core of the alveolus. More recently, Landon *et al.* found that a large proportion of the end-expiratory/arterial partial pressure gradient for the anaesthetic isoflurane (molecular weight 184.5) could not be explained by alveolar dead space or shunt and appeared to be due to failure to achieve uniformity within the alveolus.[3] Nevertheless, it seems unlikely that non-uniformity within a single alveolus is an important factor limiting diffusing capacity under normal conditions with gases such as oxygen, nitrogen and carbon dioxide, which have molecular weights that are not greatly different.

Alveolar lining fluid. Alveoli contain a thin layer of surfactant-rich fluid (page 26) through which respiratory gases must diffuse.[4] The depth of this fluid layer, and therefore its impediment to diffusion, is very variable. There are 'pools' of fluid in alveolar corners (see Figure 2.9) and in the depressions between where the capillaries bulge into the alveolus, with only a very thin layer on the surface of the capillary bulges, thus providing the minimal diffusion barrier in the most vital area.

Tissue barrier.[4] Electron microscopy reveals details of the actual path between alveolar gas and pulmonary capillary blood, shown in Figure 2.8. Each alveolus is lined with epithelium which, with its basement membrane, is about 0.2 μm thick, except where epithelial cell nuclei bulge into the alveolar lumen. Beyond the basement membrane is the interstitial space, which is very thin where it overlies the capillaries, particularly on the active side; elsewhere it is thicker and contains collagen and elastic fibres. The pulmonary capillaries are lined with endothelium, also with its own basement membrane, which is approximately the same thickness as the alveolar epithelium, except where it is expanded to enclose the endothelial cell nuclei. The total thickness of the active part of the tissue barrier is thus about 0.5 μm, containing two pairs of lipid bilayers separated by the interstitial space.

Plasma layer. Human pulmonary capillaries are estimated to have a mean diameter of 7 μm, similar to the diameter of an RBC, part of which is therefore forced into contact with the endothelial cell surface (see Figure 2.8). The diffusion path through plasma may therefore be very short indeed, but only a small proportion of the RBC surface will be in such close proximity with the endothelium, much of the RBC passing through the middle of the capillary, up to 3.5 μm from the endothelial cell. Furthermore, since the diameter of the capillary is about 14 times the thickness of the tissue barrier, it is clear that the diffusion path within the capillary is likely to be much longer than the path through the alveolar/capillary membrane. A complex pattern of diffusion gradients is therefore established within the plasma depending on the oxygen tension in the alveolus and the number of RBCs present.[5] This is discussed in more detail below with respect to carbon monoxide.

Diffusion into and within the RBC.[6] Confining haemoglobin within the RBC reduces the oxygen diffusing capacity by 40% in comparison with free haemoglobin solution.[7] There are three possible explanations for this observation. First, there is now good evidence that the rapid uptake of O_2 and CO by RBCs causes depletion of gas in the plasma layer immediately surrounding the RBC.[8] Referred to as the 'unstirred layer', this phenomenon is most likely to occur at low packed cell volume (PCV) when adjacent RBCs in the pulmonary capillary have more plasma between them.[9] Second, oxygen must diffuse across the RBC membrane, though this is not normally believed to be a significant diffusion barrier. Third, once in the cell, oxygen must diffuse through a varying amount of intracellular fluid before combining with haemoglobin, a process that is aided by mass movement of the haemoglobin molecules caused by the deformation of the RBC as it passes through the capillary bed, in effect 'mixing' the oxygen with the haemoglobin.

RBCs change shape as they pass through capillaries (both pulmonary and systemic) and this plays an important role in the uptake and release of oxygen.[6] The dependence of diffusing capacity on RBC shape changes may result from reducing the unstirred layer by 'mixing' the plasma around the RBC, from changes in the cell membrane surface area to RBC volume ratio or from assisting the mass movement of haemoglobin within the cell. This has led to further studies in which the deformability of RBCs is reduced (using chlorpromazine) or increased (using sodium salicylate), which have demonstrated that diffusing capacity is increased with greater RBC deformability.[9] Of more clinical significance are recent studies on the effect of plasma

cholesterol on RBC function.[10] Elevated cholesterol concentration in the plasma causes increased cholesterol in the RBC membrane, a change that is known to make the membrane thicker and less deformable, both of which lead to reduced efficiency of diffusion across the membrane. Oxygen uptake by RBCs in the lung, and its release in the tissues, are both believed to be significantly impaired by hypercholesterolaemia, particularly in tissues with high oxygen extraction ratios such as the heart.

Uptake of oxygen by haemoglobin. The greater part of the oxygen that is taken up in the lungs enters into chemical combination with haemoglobin. This chemical reaction takes a finite time and forms an appreciable part of the total resistance to the transfer of oxygen.[11] This important discovery resulted in an extensive reappraisal of the whole concept of diffusing capacity. In particular, it became clear that measurements of 'diffusing capacity' did not necessarily give an indication of the degree of permeability of the alveolar/capillary membrane.

Quantification of the diffusing capacity for oxygen

The diffusing capacity of oxygen is simply the oxygen uptake divided by the partial pressure gradient from alveolar gas to pulmonary capillary blood, where the relevant tension is the mean pulmonary capillary PO_2:

Oxygen diffusing capacity =

$$\frac{\text{Oxygen uptake}}{\text{Alveolar } PO_2 - \text{mean pulmonary capillary } PO_2}$$

The alveolar PO_2 can be derived with some degree of accuracy (page 128) but there are very serious problems in estimating the mean capillary PO_2.

The mean pulmonary capillary PO_2. It is clearly impossible to make a direct measurement of the mean PO_2 of the pulmonary capillary blood, and therefore attempts have been made to derive this quantity indirectly from the presumed changes of PO_2 that occur as blood passes through the pulmonary capillaries.

The earliest analysis of the problem was made by Bohr in 1909.[12] He made the assumption that, at any point along the pulmonary capillary, the rate of oxygen diffusion was proportional to the PO_2 difference between the alveolar gas and the pulmonary capillary blood at that point. Using this approach, and *assuming a value for the alveolar/pulmonary end-capillary PO_2 gradient*, it seemed possible to construct a graph of capillary PO_2, plotted against the time the blood had been in the pulmonary capillary. A typical curve drawn on this basis is shown as the broken line in Figure 9.2a. Once the curve has been drawn, it is relatively easy to derive the mean

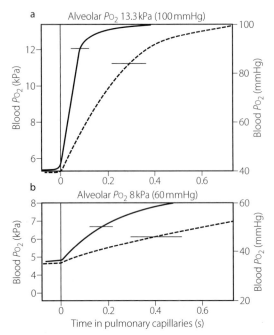

Figure 9.2 Each graph shows the rise in blood P_{O_2} as blood passes along the pulmonary capillaries. The horizontal line at the top of the graph indicates the alveolar P_{O_2} that the blood P_{O_2} is approaching. In **(a)** the subject is breathing air, whereas in **(b)** the subject is breathing about 14% oxygen. The broken curve shows the rise in P_{O_2} calculated according to the Bohr procedure on an assumed value for the alveolar/end-capillary P_{O_2} gradient. The continuous curve shows the values obtained by forward integration.[16] Horizontal bars indicate mean pulmonary capillary P_{O_2} calculated from each curve.

pulmonary capillary P_{O_2}, which then permits calculation of the oxygen diffusing capacity. The validity of the assumption of the alveolar/pulmonary end-capillary P_{O_2} gradient is considered below.

Unfortunately this approach, known as the Bohr integration procedure, was shown to be invalid when it was found that the fundamental assumption was untrue. The rate of oxygen transfer is not proportional to the alveolar/capillary P_{O_2} gradient at any point along the capillary. It would no doubt be true if the transfer of oxygen were a purely physical process, but the rate of transfer is actually limited by the chemical combination of oxygen with haemoglobin, which is sufficiently slow to comprise a major part of the total resistance to transfer of oxygen.

Studies *in vitro* of the rate of combination of oxygen with haemoglobin have shown that this is not directly proportional to the P_{O_2} gradient, for two distinct reasons.

1. The combination of the fourth molecule of oxygen with the haemoglobin molecule ($Hb_4(O_2)_3 + O_2 \rightleftharpoons Hb_4(O_2)_4$) has a much higher velocity constant than

that of the combination of the other three molecules. This is discussed further on page 176.

2. As the capillary oxygen saturation rises, the number of molecules of reduced haemoglobin diminishes and the velocity of the forward reaction must therefore diminish by the law of mass action. This depends upon the haemoglobin dissociation curve and is therefore not a simple exponential function of the actual P_{O_2} of the blood.

When these two factors are combined it is found that the resistance to 'diffusion' due to chemical combination of oxygen within the RBC is fairly constant up to a saturation of about 80% ($P_{O_2} = 6$ kPa or 45 mmHg). Thereafter, it falls very rapidly to become zero at full saturation. In view of these findings the Bohr integration procedure was elaborated to allow for changes in the rate of combination of haemoglobin with oxygen.[13] Assuming traditional values for the alveolar/end-capillary P_{O_2} difference, the resulting curve lies well to the left of the original Bohr curve, as shown by the continuous curve in Figure 9.2a. This indicated a mean pulmonary capillary P_{O_2} greater than had previously been believed, and therefore an oxygen diffusing capacity that was substantially greater than the accepted value. The situation is actually more complicated still, as quick-frozen sections of lung show that the colour of haemoglobin begins to alter to the red colour of oxyhaemoglobin within the pulmonary arterioles before the blood has even entered the pulmonary capillaries. Furthermore, pulmonary capillaries do not cross a single alveolus but may pass over three or more.

Both the classic and the modified Bohr integration procedures for calculation of mean capillary P_{O_2} depended critically on the precise value of the pulmonary end-capillary P_{O_2}. The constructed curve (Figure 9.2a) and therefore the derived mean capillary P_{O_2} were considerably influenced by very small variations in the value that was assumed. The 'ideal' alveolar/arterial P_{O_2} difference could be measured, but the problem was to separate this into its two components: the 'ideal' alveolar/pulmonary end-capillary P_{O_2} difference (due to diffusion block) and the pulmonary end-capillary/arterial P_{O_2} difference (due to venous admixture). Figure 8.8 will make this clear. Ingenious attempts were made to resolve the alveolar/arterial P_{O_2} gradient into its two components,[14] but these failed to produce results that were compatible with observed diffusing capacity, mainly because of the lack of appreciation of the part played by the reaction times of oxygen with haemoglobin.

Forward integration.[15] This involved a new and entirely opposite approach based on the new understanding of the kinetics of the combination of oxygen with haemoglobin (see above) and the pattern of blood flow through

Table 9.1 Values for the alveolar/end-capillary P_{O_2} gradient suggested by the forward integration procedure[15]

Conditions	Capillary transit time (s)	Alveolar/end capillary P_{O_2} gradient (kPa)	(mmHg)
Resting subject ($\dot{V}_{O_2}$ = 270 ml.min^{-1})			
Breathing air	0.760	0.000 000 001	0.000 000 01
($P_{A_{O_2}}$ = 13.3 kPa = 100 mmHg)			
Breathing low oxygen	0.636	0.03	0.2
($P_{A_{O_2}}$ = 6.3 kPa = 47 mmHg)			
Moderate exercise ($\dot{V}_{O_2}$ = 1500 ml.min^{-1})			
Breathing low oxygen	0.476	0.5	4.0
($P_{A_{O_2}}$ = 7.3 kPa = 55 mmHg)			
Heavy exercise ($\dot{V}_{O_2}$ = 3000 ml.min^{1})			
Breathing air	0.496	<0.0001	<0.001
($P_{A_{O_2}}$ = 16 kPa = 120 mmHg)			
Breathing low oxygen	0.304	2.1	16.0
($P_{A_{O_2}}$ = 7.9 kPa = 59 mmHg)			

$P_{A_{O_2}}$, alveolar P_{O_2}; $\dot{V}_{O_2}$, oxygen consumption.

the pulmonary capillaries. Starting at the arterial end of the pulmonary capillaries, the P_{O_2} of the capillary blood is calculated progressively along the capillary until an estimate is obtained of the remaining alveolar/capillary P_{O_2} gradient at the end of the capillary. This procedure of forward integration was thus the reverse of the classic approach which, starting from the alveolar/end-capillary P_{O_2} gradient, worked backwards to see what was happening along the capillary.

Forward integrations gave important results (Table 9.1). They suggested that alveolar/end-capillary P_{O_2} gradients were very much smaller than had previously been thought.

Capillary transit time[16]

Capillary transit time is a most important factor determining both the pulmonary end-capillary P_{O_2} and the diffusing capacity. It will be seen from Figure 9.2a that if the capillary transit time is reduced below 0.25 s, there will be an appreciable gradient between the alveolar and end-capillary P_{O_2}. Because the diffusion gradient from alveolar gas to mean pulmonary capillary blood will be increased, the oxygen diffusing capacity must be decreased.

The mean pulmonary capillary transit time equals the pulmonary capillary blood volume divided by the pulmonary blood flow (approximately equal to cardiac output). This gives a normal time of the order of 0.8 s with a subject at rest. However, because of difficulties measuring pulmonary capillary blood volume and many other methodological problems, there appears to be a wide range of values on either side of the mean and times

as short as 0.1 s[17] or as long as 3 s[18] have been suggested. It is therefore likely that, in a similar fashion to ventilation and perfusion, there is a wide range of normal capillary transit times affected by many factors such as posture, lung volume, cardiac output etc. Blood from capillaries with the shortest time will yield desaturated blood and this will not be compensated by blood from capillaries with longer than average transit times, for the reason shown in Figure 8.13.

DIFFUSION OF CARBON DIOXIDE IN THE LUNGS

Carbon dioxide has a much higher water solubility than oxygen and, although its vapour density is greater, it may be calculated to penetrate an aqueous membrane about 20 times as rapidly as oxygen (Table 9.2). Therefore it was formerly believed that diffusion problems could not exist for carbon dioxide because the patient would have succumbed to hypoxia before hypercapnia could attain measurable proportions. All of this ignored the fact that chemical reactions of the respiratory gases were sufficiently slow to affect the measured 'diffusing capacity' and in fact were generally the limiting factor in gas transfer. The carriage of carbon dioxide in the blood is discussed in Chapter 10, but for the moment it is sufficient to note the essential reactions in the release of chemically combined carbon dioxide.

1. Release of some carbon dioxide from carbamino carriage.
2. Conversion of bicarbonate ions to carbonic acid followed by dehydration to release molecular carbon dioxide.

Table 9.2 The influence of physical properties on the diffusion of gases through a gas–liquid interface

Gas	Density relative to oxygen	Water solubility relative to oxygen	Diffusing capacity relative to oxygen
Oxygen	1.00	1.00	1.00
Carbon dioxide	1.37	24.0	20.5
Nitrogen	0.88	0.515	0.55
Carbon monoxide	0.88	0.75	0.80
Nitrous oxide	1.37	16.3	14.0
Helium	0.125	0.37	1.05
Nitric oxide	0.94	1.70	1.71

The latter reaction involves the movement of bicarbonate ions across the RBC membrane, but its rate is probably limited by the dehydration of carbonic acid. This reaction would be very slow indeed if it were not catalysed by carbonic anhydrase, which is present in abundance in the RBC and also on the endothelium. The important limiting role of the rate of this reaction was elegantly shown in a study of the effect of inhibition of carbonic anhydrase on carbon dioxide transport. This resulted in a large increase in the arterial/alveolar $P\text{CO}_2$ gradient, corresponding to a gross decrease in the apparent 'diffusing capacity' of carbon dioxide.[18]

Equilibrium of carbon dioxide is probably very nearly complete within the normal pulmonary capillary transit time. However, even if it were not so, it would be of little significance since the mixed venous/alveolar $P\text{CO}_2$ difference is itself quite small (about 0.8 kPa or 6 mmHg). Therefore an end-capillary gradient as large as 20% of the initial difference would still be too small to be of any importance and, indeed, could hardly be measured by modern analytical methods.

Hypercapnia is, in fact, never caused by decreased 'diffusing capacity', except when carbonic anhydrase is completely inhibited by drugs such as acetazolamide (page 150). Pathological hypercapnia may always be explained by other causes, usually an alveolar ventilation that is inadequate for the metabolic rate of the patient.

The assumption that there is no measurable difference between the $P\text{CO}_2$ of the alveolar gas and the pulmonary end-capillary blood is used when the alveolar $P\text{CO}_2$ is assumed to be equal to the arterial $P\text{CO}_2$ for the purpose of derivation of the 'ideal' alveolar $P\text{O}_2$ (page 128). The assumption is also made that there is no measurable difference between end-capillary and arterial $P\text{CO}_2$. We have seen in the previous chapter (Table 8.2) that this is not strictly true and a large shunt of 50% will cause an arterial/end-capillary $P\text{CO}_2$ gradient of about 0.4 kPa.

DIFFUSION OF CARBON MONOXIDE IN THE LUNGS

Diffusing capacity is usually measured for carbon monoxide, for the very practical reason that the affinity of carbon monoxide for haemoglobin is so high that the partial pressure of the gas in the pulmonary capillary blood remains effectively zero. The formula for calculation of this quantity then simplifies to the following:

Diffusing capacity for carbon monoxide

$$= \frac{\text{Carbon monoxide uptake}}{\text{Alveolar } P\text{CO}}$$

(compare with corresponding equation for oxygen, page 137).

There are no insuperable difficulties in the measurement of either of the remaining quantities on the right-hand side of the equation and the methods are outlined at the end of the chapter. Traditional units for CO diffusing capacity are ml.min^{-1}.mmHg^{-1}, though in SI units the volume of CO is usually described in molar terms, i.e. mmol.min^{-1}.kPa^{-1}.

Measurement of the carbon monoxide diffusing capacity is firmly established as a valuable routine pulmonary function test, which may show changes in a range of conditions in which other pulmonary function tests yield normal values. It does in fact provide an index that shows that something is wrong, and changes in the index provide a useful indication of progress of the disease. It is also used as an epidemiological tool for assessing lung function in seemingly healthy subjects.[19] However, it is much more difficult to explain a reduced diffusing capacity for carbon monoxide in terms of the underlying pathophysiology (see below).

The diffusion path for carbon monoxide

Diffusion of carbon monoxide within the alveolus, through the alveolar/capillary membrane and through the plasma into the RBC is governed by the same factors that apply to oxygen and these have been outlined above. The quantitative difference is due to the different vapour density and water solubility of the two gases (see Table 9.2). These factors indicate that the rate of diffusion of oxygen up to the point of entry into the RBC is 1.25 times the corresponding rate for carbon monoxide.

Diffusion of CO in plasma. The frequent use of carbon monoxide for measurement of lung diffusing capacity has focused attention on the diffusion pathways for CO which, in spite of the slight differences in the physical properties of CO and oxygen, are likely to be very similar *in vivo*. Clearly, direct measurement of diffusion gradients in a pulmonary capillary is not possible, so attempts to elucidate the diffusion pattern of gases in capillary plasma are based on mathematical models. The first model is known as the morphometric method, in which anatomical sections of rapidly fixed lung tissue were examined microscopically. Capillary dimensions were analysed to calculate the mean distance for gases to diffuse between the endothelial cell and RBC,[4] assuming a linear diffusion path between the two points; that is, respiratory gases take the shortest possible route between the endothelial cell and RBC. A more recent analysis has assumed that there is a gradient of CO concentration within the capillary, with minimal CO in the centre and, using a 'finite element analysis', has shown that diffusion paths for CO are likely to be non-linear.[5] Figure 9.3 shows a theoretical drawing of the CO flux in the capillary at both high and low haematocrit, showing clearly that except in severe anaemia CO uptake is achieved long before diffusion to the centre of the capillary is able to take place. In spite of these detailed models, agreement with observed CO diffusion remains poor under most situations.[5]

Uptake of carbon monoxide by haemoglobin[20]

The affinity of haemoglobin for carbon monoxide is about 250 times as great as for oxygen. Nevertheless, it does not follow that the *rate* of combination of carbon monoxide with haemoglobin is faster than the *rate* of combination of oxygen with haemoglobin: it is, in fact, rather slower.[21] The reaction is slower still when oxygen must first be displaced from haemoglobin according to the equation:

a

b

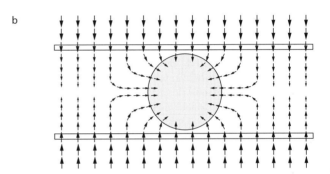

Figure 9.3 Mathematical model of diffusion paths for CO between the alveolus and the red blood cell (RBC). The size and direction of the arrows indicate respectively the magnitude and direction of the CO flux. The RBC is assumed to be an infinite 'sink' for CO. **(a)** Normal. Packed cell volume 66%, under which conditions CO is absorbed by the RBC, mainly at the periphery of the capillary. **(b)** Severe anaemia. Packed cell volume 12%. Diffusion occurs into the centre of the plasma and follows a non-linear path into the RBC. The thickness of the tissue barrier relative to capillary diameter is drawn to scale, showing the relatively small contribution that the alveolar capillary membrane makes to the diffusion barrier in total. (After reference 5.)

$$CO + HbO_2 \rightarrow O_2 + HbCO$$

Therefore, the reaction rate of carbon monoxide with haemoglobin is reduced when the oxygen saturation of the haemoglobin is high. The inhalation of different concentrations of oxygen thus causes changes in the reaction rate of carbon monoxide with the haemoglobin of a patient, an observation that has been utilised to study different components of the resistance to diffusion of carbon monoxide in humans.

Quantification of the components of the resistance to diffusion of carbon monoxide

When two resistances are arranged in series, the total resistance of the pair is equal to the sum of the two individual resistances. Diffusing capacity is analogous to conductance, which is the reciprocal of resistance. Therefore, the reciprocal of the diffusing capacity of the total system equals the sum of the reciprocals of the diffusing capacities of the two components.

$$\frac{1}{\text{total diffusing capacity for CO}} = \frac{1}{\text{diffusing capacity of CO for the alveolar/capillary membrane}} + \frac{1}{\text{'diffusing capacity' of CO in the blood}}$$

In theory, diffusing capacity of carbon monoxide in the blood includes diffusion across the plasma, red cell membrane, diffusion within the red cell and the chemical combination of CO with haemoglobin. However *in vivo*, as in the case of oxygen, the reaction rate of CO with haemoglobin is a significant factor.[21] This 'diffusing capacity' for blood is equal to the product of the pulmonary capillary blood volume (Vc) and the rate of reaction of carbon monoxide with haemoglobin (θ_{CO}), a parameter which varies with the oxygen saturation of the haemoglobin. The equation may now be rewritten:

$$\frac{1}{\text{total diffusing capacity for CO}} = \frac{1}{\text{diffusing capacity of CO for the alveolar / capillary membrane}} + \frac{1}{\text{pulmonary capillary blood volume reaction rate of CO with blood}}$$

The usual symbols for representation of this equation are as follows:

$$\frac{1}{D_{L_{CO}}} = \frac{1}{Dm_{CO}} + \frac{1}{Vc \times \theta_{CO}}$$

The term Dm is often described simply as membrane diffusing capacity. Dm_{CO} equals $0.8\ Dm_{O_2}$ under similar conditions (see Table 9.2).

The total diffusing capacity for carbon monoxide is a routine clinical measurement and is described at the end

of this chapter: θ_{CO} may be determined, at different values of oxygen saturation, by studies *in vitro*.[21] This leaves two unknowns: the diffusing capacity through the alveolar/capillary membrane and the pulmonary capillary blood volume. By repeating the measurement of total diffusing capacity at different arterial oxygen saturations (obtained by inhaling different concentrations of oxygen), it is possible to obtain two simultaneous equations with two unknowns which may then be solved to obtain values for Dm_{CO} and pulmonary capillary blood volume. Measurement of pulmonary capillary blood volume by this technique yields normal values between 60 and 110 ml (depending on subject height),[22] which agrees well with a morphometric estimate of about 100 ml. Normal values are shown in Table 9.3, including the technique of measurement used, which has some influence on the value obtained, probably because of differing lung volumes during the measurement.[22]

FACTORS AFFECTING 'DIFFUSING CAPACITY'

The basic principles of pulmonary diffusion described so far indicate that there are three major mechanisms by which diffusing capacity may alter: changes in the effective surface area of the gas exchange membrane, a change in the physical properties of the membrane, or changes related to the uptake of gases by the RBC. Each of these mechanisms will be discussed individually and then other factors that affect diffusion capacity by either multiple or unknown mechanisms will be described.

Most of the factors outlined in this section will apply equally to oxygen and CO diffusion, though the majority have been studied using CO for the reasons described in the previous section.

Factors influencing diffusing capacity by changes in membrane surface area

Total lung volume, and therefore the number of alveoli available for gas exchange, will clearly affect diffusing capacity. However, only those alveoli that are adequately ventilated and perfused will contribute to gas exchange

Technique of measurement	Total diffusing capacity for CO		Membrane component of diffusing capacity		Pulmonary capillary
	mmol.min⁻¹.kPa⁻¹	*ml.min⁻¹.mmHg⁻¹*	*mmol.min⁻¹.kPa⁻¹*	*ml.min⁻¹.mmHg⁻¹*	Blood volume *(ml)*
Steady state	5.0	15	8.7	26	73
Single breath	10.1	30	19.1	57	79
Rebreathing	9.0	27	13.4	40	110

Table 9.3 Values obtained for diffusing capacity of carbon monoxide by various methods of measurement

and the scatter of ventilation/perfusion therefore has an important influence on the diffusing capacity.

Body size. Stature influences diffusing capacity directly owing to the relationship between height and lung volume. Normal values for total diffusing capacity may be calculated from the formulae:[22]

$$D_{L_{CO}} = 10.9 \times \text{height (m)} - 0.067 \times \text{age (years)} - 5.89$$
(males)

$$D_{L_{CO}} = 7.1 \times \text{height (m)} - 0.054 \times \text{age (years)} - 0.89$$
(females)

A healthy 30-year-old male 1.78 m tall would therefore have a CO diffusing capacity of 11.5 mmol.min^{-1}.kPa^{-1} (34.4 ml.min.$^{-1}$mmHg^{-1}).

Lung volume. Diffusing capacity is directly related to lung volume and so is maximal at total lung capacity.[23] Different techniques for the measurement of diffusing capacity use different lung volumes, so it is now standard practice to simultaneously measure 'alveolar volume' (lung volume at which diffusing capacity was measured) by helium dilution.[1] Diffusing capacity can then be measured as diffusing capacity per litre alveolar volume, with units of mmol.min^{-1}.kPa^{-1}.l^{-1} (ml.min.$^{-1}$mmHg^{-1}.l^{-1}).

Ventilation/perfusion mismatch results in a physiological dysfunction that presents many of the features of a reduction in diffusing capacity. If, for example, most of the ventilation is distributed to the left lung and most of the pulmonary blood flow to the right lung, then the effective interface must be reduced. Minor degrees of maldistribution greatly complicate the interpretation of a reduced diffusing capacity. Both maldistribution and impaired diffusing capacity have a similar effect on the alveolar/arterial P_{O_2} gradient in relation to inspired oxygen concentration (see Figure 8.14) and a distinction cannot be made by simple means.

Posture. Diffusing capacity is substantially increased when the subject is supine rather than standing or sitting, in spite of the fact that lung volume is reduced.[22] This change is probably explained by the increase in pulmonary blood volume and the more uniform distribution of perfusion of the lungs in the supine position.

Pathology. The total area of the alveolar/capillary membrane may be reduced by any disease process or surgery that removes a substantial number of alveoli. For example, emphysema reduces the diffusing capacity mainly by destruction of alveolar septa, such that $D_{L_{CO}}$ correlates with the anatomical degree of emphysematous changes in the lung.[24]

Factors influencing the membrane diffusion barrier

'Alveolar/capillary block' is a term used in the past to describe a syndrome characterised by reduced lung volume, reasonably normal ventilatory capacity, hyperventilation and normal arterial P_{O_2} at rest, but with desaturation on exercise. These patients had reduced diffusing capacity that was believed to be due to an impediment at the alveolar/capillary membrane itself, which might either be thickened or have its permeability to gas transfer reduced by some chemical abnormality. Evidence for such a mechanism was never found and it now seems likely that most of the patients thought to have alveolar/capillary block actually had hypoxaemia as a result of disturbances in distribution of ventilation and/or perfusion.

It will be clear that the oxygen diffusing capacity may be influenced by many factors that are really nothing at all to do with diffusion *per se*. In fact, there is considerable doubt as to whether a true defect of alveolar/capillary membrane diffusion is ever the limiting factor in transfer of oxygen from the inspired gas to the arterial blood.

Chronic heart failure and pulmonary oedema remain the only likely causes of a membrane diffusion barrier. This may occur either via pulmonary capillary congestion increasing the length of the diffusion pathway for oxygen through plasma, by interstitial oedema increasing the thickness of the membrane or by raised capillary pressure damaging the endothelial and epithelial cells, leading to proliferation of type II alveolar cells and thickening of the membrane.[25] Previous work with electron microscopy showed that oedema fluid tends to accumulate on the inactive side of the pulmonary capillary, leaving the active side, and therefore gaseous diffusion, relatively normal. However, the membrane component of diffusing capacity (Dm) is reduced in chronic heart failure and the reduction correlates with symptom severity, whereas capillary volume increases only in severe heart failure.[26] It is therefore possible that despite the negative findings with electron microscopy, heart failure of a suitable severity over a prolonged period does induce a form of 'alveolar/capillary block' described previously.

Factors related to uptake of gases by haemoglobin

Haemoglobin concentration affects diffusing capacity by influencing the rate and amount of oxygen or CO uptake by blood flowing through the pulmonary capillary. Measurements of diffusing capacity are therefore usually mathematically corrected to account for abnormalities in the patient's haemoglobin concentration.[1]

Decreased capillary transit time. In the section above, it has been explained how a reduction in capillary transit time may reduce the diffusing capacity. The mean transit time is reduced when cardiac output is raised and this may increase diffusing capacity substantially, for example during exercise (see below).

Other determinants of diffusing capacity

Age. Even when corrected for changes in lung volume, DL_{CO} declines in a linear fashion with increasing age.[23]

Sex. Women have a reduced total pulmonary diffusing capacity in comparison with men. This difference is almost totally explained by differences in stature and haemoglobin concentration.[19] DL_{CO} in women varies throughout the menstrual cycle, reaching a peak prior to menstruation, and seems to result from changes in θ, the reaction rate of CO with blood. The finding may, however, represent a technical problem with measuring DL_{CO} in that the low value during menstruation could result from a high *endogenous* production of carboxyhaemoglobin during the catabolism of haem compounds.[27]

Exercise. During exercise diffusing capacity may be double the value obtained at rest, as a result of increased cardiac output causing a reduction in capillary transit time and pulmonary capillary recruitment in non-dependent lung zones (page 96). Because of this large effect of cardiac output on the measurement of diffusing capacity, some groups advocate using simultaneous non-invasive measures of cardiac output to aid interpretation of the diffusing capacity result.[28] Paradoxically, hypoxaemia from diffusion limitation during exercise is more common among elite, trained athletes than in the average individual.[16] Physiological changes in exercise are discussed in Chapter 15.

Racial origin. In a US study of over 4000 healthy individuals, DL_{CO} was significantly lower in black subjects than in whites.[19] The reasons for this are not clear.

Smoking history affects diffusing capacity even when most of the other determinants listed in this section are taken into account. DL_{CO} is reduced in proportion to the number of cigarettes per day currently smoked and the total lifetime number of cigarettes ever smoked.[19] The causes of this decline in lung function with smoking are discussed in Chapter 21.

DIFFUSION OF GASES IN THE TISSUES

Oxygen[29,30]

Oxygen leaves the systemic capillaries by the reverse of the process by which it entered the pulmonary capillar-

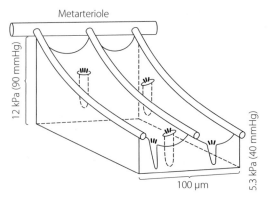

Figure 9.4 Diagrammatic representation of PO_2 within the tissues. The vertical axis represents the actual PO_2; in the horizontal plane is represented the course of three parallel capillaries from the metarteriole to the point of entry into the venule (not shown). The PO_2 falls exponentially along the course of each capillary, with a trough of PO_2 between the capillaries. The pits represent the low spots of PO_2 from about 12 kPa (90 mmHg) in the tissue close to the arterial end of the capillaries down to less than 1 kPa at the mitochondria near the venous end of the capillaries. This is the simplest of many possible models of tissue perfusion.

ies. Chemical release from haemoglobin is followed by diffusion through the capillary wall and thence through the tissues to its site of utilisation in the mitochondria. In an area of tissue supplied by a single capillary there is a longitudinal gradient in tissue PO_2 with an exponential decline between the metarteriole and venule. In addition, around each capillary a radial gradient in tissue PO_2 may be demonstrated, with the rate at which PO_2 declines varying from approximately 0.2 kPa (1.5 mmHg) per µm away from the capillary in neural tissue to 0.013 kPa (0.1 mmHg) per µm in the vitreous humor of the eye. Figure 9.4 shows a model in which an area of tissue is perfused by three parallel capillaries. Vertical height indicates PO_2, which falls exponentially along the line of the capillaries, with troughs lying in between the capillaries. Five 'low spots' corresponding to mitochondria are shown. This diagram makes no pretence to histological accuracy but merely illustrates the difficulty of talking about the 'mean tissue PO_2', which is not an entity like the arterial or mixed venous PO_2.

Diffusion paths are much longer in tissues than in the lung. In well-vascularised tissue, such as brain, each capillary serves a zone of radius about 20 µm, but the corresponding distance is about 200 µm in skeletal muscle and greater still in fat and cartilage, although in muscle tissue myoglobin accelerates the rate of oxygen transfer within the cell.

It is impracticable to talk about mean tissue PO_2 since this varies from one organ to another and must also depend on perfusion in relation to metabolic activity.

Furthermore, within a tissue there must be some cells occupying more favourable sites towards the arterial ends of capillaries, whereas others must accept oxygen from the venous ends of the capillaries, where the P_{O_2} is lower. This is well demonstrated in the liver, where the centrilobular cells must exist at a lower P_{O_2} than those at the periphery of the lobule. Even within a single cell, there can be no uniformity of P_{O_2}. Not only are there 'low spots' around the mitochondria, but those mitochondria in regions of the cell nearest to the capillary presumably enjoy a higher P_{O_2} than those lying further away.

Carbon dioxide

Little is known about the magnitude of carbon dioxide gradients between the mitochondria and the tissue capillaries. It is, however, thought that the tissue/venous P_{CO_2} gradient can be increased by two methods. The first is by inhibition of carbonic anhydrase, which impairs the uptake of carbon dioxide by the blood. The second is by hyperoxygenation of the arterial blood caused by breathing 100% oxygen at high pressures. If the P_{O_2} of the arterial blood exceeds about 300 kPa (2250 mmHg), the dissolved oxygen will be sufficient for the usual tissue requirements. Therefore there will be no significant amount of reduced haemoglobin, which is more effective than oxyhaemoglobin for carbamino carriage of carbon dioxide. The effect of this on tissue P_{CO_2} is likely to be too small to be clinically significant and the alternative method of carbon dioxide carriage as bicarbonate seems to be adequate.

ALVEOLAR/CAPILLARY PERMEABILITY TO NON-VOLATILE SUBSTANCES

The alveolar epithelium and the capillary endothelium have a very high permeability to water, to most gases and to lipophilic substances such as alcohol. However, for many hydrophilic substances of larger molecular diameter and for molecules carrying a charge, there is normally a very effective barrier. Passage of these substances is mainly through the gaps between the cells and must be considered separately for epithelium and endothelium. It was explained in Chapter 2 that the alveolar epithelial type I cells have very tight junctions, effectively limiting the molecular radius to about 0.6 nm. Endothelial junctions are much larger, with gaps of the order of 4–6 nm.

Passage of solutes across the alveolar/capillary membrane is usually described by the clearance of a molecule from the alveoli (i.e. across the epithelium) into the blood and quantified as the half-time of clearance or, alternatively, as the fractional clearance per minute. Clearance bears an approximate inverse relationship to

the molecular weight.[35] Urea (60 daltons, Da) has a fractional clearance of the order of 0.07 per minute, whereas for sucrose (342 Da) the corresponding value is 0.003 per minute and for albumin (64 000 Da) is of the order of 0.0001 per minute. All of these clearances may be greatly increased if the alveolar epithelium is damaged, as in the permeability type of pulmonary oedema (page 391).

A useful tracer molecule for the assessment of permeability is ^{99m}Tc DTPA (diethylene triamine pentaacetate) with a molecular weight of 492 Da.[31] After being aerosolised into the lungs, its concentration can be continuously measured over the lung fields *in vivo* by detection of its gamma emission. In the healthy non-smoker the clearance is very slow, about 0.01 per minute (half-time about 1 hour), but clearance is dramatically increased in many different types of pulmonary damage including, for example, smoking, in which there is a threefold increase.

Electrolytes such as sodium ions can cross the epithelial barrier fairly rapidly, probably by an active process (page 389), but the rate of passage is affected by concentration gradients. Thus, isotonic sodium solutions are cleared from the alveoli more quickly than hypertonic solutions.[32] The normal alveolar epithelium is almost totally impermeable to protein, the half-time for turnover of albumin between plasma and the alveolar compartment being of the order of 36 hours.[33]

The microvascular endothelium, with its larger intercellular gaps, is far more permeable for all molecular sizes and there is normally an appreciable leak of protein. Thus the concentration of albumin in pulmonary lymph is about half the concentration in plasma and may increase to approximate the plasma concentration in conditions of damaged alveolar/capillary permeability. This problem is discussed further in relation to pulmonary oedema in Chapter 29.

PRINCIPLES OF MEASUREMENT OF CARBON MONOXIDE DIFFUSING CAPACITY

All the methods are based on the general equation:

$$D_{CO} = \frac{\dot{V}_{CO}}{P_{A_{CO}} - P_{\overline{C}_{CO}}}$$

In each case it is usual to assume that the mean partial pressure of carbon monoxide in the pulmonary capillary blood ($P_{\overline{C}_{CO}}$) is effectively zero. It is, therefore, only necessary to measure the carbon monoxide uptake ($\dot{V}_{CO}$) and the alveolar carbon monoxide tension ($P_{A_{CO}}$). The diffusing capacity so measured (D_{CO}) is the total diffusing capacity, including that of the alveolar capillary membrane, plasma and the component due to the reaction time of carbon monoxide with haemoglobin.

The steady-state method

The subject breathes a gas mixture containing about 0.3% carbon monoxide for about a minute. After this time, expired gas is collected when the alveolar $P\text{CO}$ is steady but the mixed venous $P\text{CO}$ has not yet reached a level high enough to require consideration in the calculation.

The carbon monoxide uptake ($\dot{V}\text{CO}$) is measured in exactly the same way as oxygen consumption by the open method (page 196): the amount of carbon monoxide expired (expired minute volume × mixed expired CO concentration) is subtracted from the amount of carbon monoxide inspired (inspired minute volume × inspired CO concentration). The alveolar $P\text{CO}$ is calculated from the Filey version of the alveolar air equation (page 129) using carbon monoxide in place of oxygen.

Measurement of inspiratory and expiratory carbon monoxide and expiratory carbon dioxide concentrations presents no serious difficulty, though care must be taken following general anaesthesia when expired nitrous oxide may affect the infrared measurement of carbon dioxide.[34] Alveolar $P\text{CO}_2$ for entry into the alveolar air equation may be determined by sampling arterial blood and assuming that the alveolar $P\text{CO}_2$ is equal to the arterial $P\text{CO}_2$. This is not strictly true in the presence of maldistribution. As an alternative, some workers measure the end-expiratory $P\text{CO}_2$ but neither does this equal the arterial $P\text{CO}_2$ in the presence of alveolar dead space (see Figure 8.9).

The steady-state method requires no special respiratory manoeuvre and is therefore particularly suitable for use in children.[22]

The single-breath method

This method is the most frequently used in clinical practice and has a long history of progressive refinement. There are many variations on the exact method used, which yield broadly similar results,[35] but the multitude of techniques and factors affecting the results have led to attempts to standardise the method between centres.[1,19,36,37]

The patient is first required to exhale maximally. He then draws in a vital-capacity breath of a gas mixture containing about 0.3% carbon monoxide and about 10% helium. The breath is held for 10 seconds and a gas sample is then taken after the exhalation of the first 0.75 l, which is sufficient to wash out the patient's dead space. The breath-holding time is sufficient to overcome maldistribution of the inspired gas.

It is assumed that no significant amount of helium has passed into the blood and, therefore, the ratio of the concentration of helium in the inspired gas to the concentration in the end-expiratory gas, multiplied by the

volume of gas drawn into the alveoli during the maximal inspiration, will indicate the total alveolar volume during the period of breath holding. The alveolar $P\text{CO}$ at the commencement of breath holding is equal to the same ratio multiplied by the $P\text{CO}$ of the inspired gas mixture. The end-expiratory $P\text{CO}$ is measured directly.

From these data, together with the time of breath holding, it is possible to calculate the carbon monoxide uptake and the mean alveolar $P\text{CO}$. Lung diffusing capacity for carbon monoxide can then be calculated and normalised for lung volume using the alveolar volume measured at the same time with helium. These calculations are now usually performed automatically by computer, which will also provide a 'normal' value based on the patient's sex, height, age and smoking status.

The rebreathing method

Somewhat similar to the single-breath method is the rebreathing method, by which gas mixture containing about 0.3% carbon monoxide and 10% helium is rebreathed rapidly from a rubber bag. The bag and the patient's lungs are considered as a single system, with gas exchange occurring in very much the same way as during breath holding. The calculation proceeds in a similar way to that for the single-breath method.

REFERENCES

*1. American Thoracic Society. Single breath carbon monoxide diffusing capacity (transfer factor). Recommendations for a standard technique – 1995 update. *Am J Respir Crit Care Med* 1995; **152**: 2185–98.

2. Georg G, Lassen NA, Mellemgaard K, Vinther A. Diffusion in the gas phase of the lungs in normal and emphysematous subjects. *Clin Sci* 1965; **29**: 525–32.

3. Landon MJ, Matson AM, Royston BD, Hewlett AM, White DC, Nunn JF. Components of the inspiratory–arterial isoflurane partial pressure difference. *Br J Anaesth* 1993; **70**: 605–11.

4. Weibel ER, Federspiel WJ, Fryder-Doffey F, *et al*. Morphometric model for pulmonary diffusing capacity I. Membrane diffusing capacity. *Respir Physiol* 1993; **93**: 125–49.

*5. Hsia CCW, Chuong CJC, Johnson RL. Critique of conceptual basis of diffusing capacity estimates: a finite element analysis. *J Appl Physiol* 1995; **79**: 1039–47.

6. Sarelius I. Invited editorial on 'Effect of RBC shape and deformability on pulmonary O_2 diffusing capacity and resistance to flow in rabbit lungs'. *J Appl Physiol* 1995; **78**: 763–4.

7. Geiser J, Betticher DC. Gas transfer in isolated lungs perfused with red cell suspension or haemoglobin solution. *Respir Physiol* 1989; **77**: 31–40.

8. Yamaguchi K, Nguyen-Phu D, Scheid P, Piper J. Kinetics of O_2 uptake and release by human erythrocyte studied by a stopped-flow technique. *J Appl Physiol* 1985; **58**: 1215–24.

9. Betticher DC, Reinhart WH, Geiser J. Effect of RBC shape and deformability on pulmonary O_2 diffusing capacity and resistance to flow in rabbit lungs. *J Appl Physiol* 1995; **78**: 778–83.

*10. Buchwald H, O'Dea TJ, Menchaca HJ, Michalek VN, Rohde TD. Effect of plasma cholesterol on red blood cell oxygen transport. *Clin Exp Pharmacol Physiol* 2000; **27**: 951–5.

11. Staub NC, Bishop JM, Forster RE. Velocity of O_2 uptake by human red blood cells. *J Appl Physiol* 1961; **16**: 511–16.

12. Bohr C. Über die spezifische Tätigkeit der Lungen bei der respiratorischen Gasaufnahme. *Skand Arch Physiol* 1909; **22**: 221.

13. Staub NC, Bishop JM, Forster RE. Importance of diffusion and chemical reaction rates in O_2 uptake in the lung. *J Appl Physiol* 1962; **17**: 21–7.

14. Riley RL, Lilienthal JL, Proemmel DD, Franke RE. On the determination of the physiologically effective pressures of oxygen and carbon dioxide in alveolar air. *Am J Physiol* 1946; **147**: 191–8.

15. Staub NC. Alveolar-arterial oxygen tension gradient due to diffusion. *J Appl Physiol* 1963; 18: 673–80.

16. Wagner PD. Vascular transit times in the lung. *J Appl Physiol* 1995; **79**: 380–1.

17. McHardy GJR. Diffusing capacity and pulmonary gas exchange. *Br J Dis Chest* 1972; **66**: 1–20.

18. Cain SM, Otis AB. Carbon dioxide transport in anaesthetised dogs during inhibition of carbonic anhydrase. *J Appl Physiol* 1961; **16**: 1023–8.

19. Neas LM, Schwartz J. The determinants of pulmonary diffusing capacity in a national sample of US adults. *Am J Respir Crit Care Med* 1996; **153**: 656–64.

20. Reeves RB, Park HK. CO uptake kinetics of red cells and CO diffusing capacity. *Respir Physiol* 1992; **88**: 1–21.

21. Forster RE. Rate of gas uptake by red cells. In: Fenn WO, Rahn H, eds. *Handbook of physiology, section 3 – Respiration*. Washington DC: American Physiological Society, 1964.

22. Cotes JE. *Lung function. Assessment and application in medicine*, 5th edn. Oxford: Blackwell Scientific Publications, 1993.

23. Stam H, Hrachovina V, Stijnen T, Versprille A. Diffusing capacity dependent on lung volume and age in normal subjects. *J Appl Physiol* 1994; **76**: 2356–63.

24. Cotton DJ, Sparkar GR, Graham BL. Diffusing capacity in the clinical assessment of chronic airflow limitation. *Med Clin North Am* 1996; **80**: 549–64.

25. Kay JM, Edwards FR. Ultra-structure of the alveolar–capillary wall in mitral stenosis. *J Pathol* 1973; **111**: 239–45.

26. Puri S, Baker BL, Dutka DP, Oakley CM, Hughes JMB, Cleland JGF. Reduced alveolar–capillary membrane diffusing capacity in chronic heart failure. *Circulation* 1995; **91**: 2769–74.

27. Sansores RH, Abboud RT, Kennell C, Haynes N. The effect of menstruation on the pulmonary carbon monoxide diffusing capacity. *Am J Respir Crit Care Med* 1995; **152**: 381–4.

28. Hsia CCW. Recruitment of lung diffusing capacity. Update of concept and application. *Chest* 2002; **122**: 1774–83.

*29. Tsai AG, Johnson PC, Intaglietta M. Oxygen gradients in the microcirculation. *Physiol Rev* 2003; **83**: 933–63.

30. Lübbers DW, Baumgärtl H. Heterogeneities and profiles of oxygen pressure in brain and kidney as examples of the pO_2 distribution in living tissue. *Kidney Int* 1997; **51**: 372–80.

31. Jones JG, Royston D, Minty BD. Changes in alveolar–capillary barrier function in animals and humans. *Am Rev Respir Dis* 1983; **127**: S51–S59.

32. Effros RM, Mason GR. Measurements of pulmonary epithelial permeability in vivo. *Am Rev Respir Dis* 1983; **127**: S59–S65.

33. Staub NA. Alveolar flooding and clearance. *Am Rev Respir Dis* 1983; **127**: S44–S51.

34. Gilbert R, Arafat N, Williams L. False-low carbon monoxide diffusing capacity measurement after general anaesthesia. *Chest* 1996; **109**: 592.

35. Beck KC, Offord KP, Scanlon PD. Comparison of four methods for calculating diffusing capacity by the single breath method. *Chest* 1994; **105**: 594–600.

36. British Thoracic Society and Association of Respiratory Technicians and Physiologists. Guidelines for the measurement of respiratory function. *Respir Med* 1994; **88**: 165–94.

37. Punjabi NM, Shade D, Patel AM, Wise RA. Measurement variability in single-breath diffusing capacity of the lung. *Chest* 2003; **123**: 1082–9.

KEY POINTS

- Most of the carbon dioxide carried in blood is in the form of bicarbonate, production of which is catalysed by the enzyme carbonic anhydrase.
- Formation of bicarbonate is enhanced by buffering of hydrogen ions by haemoglobin and by active removal of bicarbonate ions from the red blood cell by band 3 protein.
- Smaller amounts of carbon dioxide are carried in solution in plasma, as carbonic acid, or as carbamino compounds formed with plasma proteins and haemoglobin.
- There is normally a small gradient between arterial and alveolar P_{CO_2} caused by scatter of ventilation/perfusion ratios.

Carbon dioxide is the end-product of aerobic metabolism. It is produced almost entirely in the mitochondria where the P_{CO_2} is highest. From its point of origin, there are a series of partial pressure gradients as carbon dioxide passes through the cytoplasm and the extracellular fluid into the blood. In the lungs, the P_{CO_2} of the blood entering the pulmonary capillaries is normally higher than the alveolar P_{CO_2} and therefore carbon dioxide diffuses from the blood into the alveolar gas, where a dynamic equilibrium is established. The equilibrium concentration equals the ratio between carbon dioxide output and alveolar ventilation. Blood leaving the alveoli has, for practical purposes, the same P_{CO_2} as alveolar gas and arterial blood P_{CO_2} is usually very close to 'ideal' alveolar P_{CO_2}.

Abnormal levels of arterial P_{CO_2} occur in a number of pathological states and have many important physiological effects throughout the body, some as a result of changes in pH, and these are discussed in Chapter 23. Fundamental to all problems relating to P_{CO_2} is the mechanism by which carbon dioxide is carried in the blood.[1]

CARRIAGE OF CARBON DIOXIDE IN BLOOD

In physical solution

Carbon dioxide belongs to the group of gases with moderate solubility in water. According to Henry's law of solubility:

$$P_{CO_2} \times \text{solubility coefficient} = \qquad (1)$$
$$CO_2 \text{ concentration in solution}$$

The solubility coefficient of carbon dioxide (α) is expressed in units of $mmol.l^{-1}.kPa^{-1}$ (or $mmol.l^{-1}.mmHg^{-1}$). The value depends on temperature and examples are listed in Table 10.1. The contribution of dissolved carbon dioxide to the total carriage of the gas in blood is shown in Table 10.2.

As carbonic acid

In solution, carbon dioxide hydrates to form carbonic acid:

$$CO_2 + H_2O \rightleftharpoons H_2CO_3 \qquad (2)$$

The equilibrium of this reaction is far to the left under physiological conditions. Published work shows some disagreement on the value of the equilibrium constant, but it seems likely that less than 1% of the molecules of carbon dioxide are in the form of carbonic acid. There is a very misleading medical convention by which both forms of carbon dioxide in equation (2) are sometimes shown as carbonic acid. Thus the term H_2CO_3 may, in some situations, mean the total concentrations of dissolved CO_2 and H_2CO_3; to avoid confusion it is preferable to use αP_{CO_2} as in equation (7) below. This does not apply to equations (4) and (5) below, where H_2CO_3 has its correct meaning.

Carbonic anhydrase.[4] The reaction of carbon dioxide with water (equation 2) is non-ionic and slow, requiring a period of minutes for equilibrium to be attained. This would be far too slow for the time available for gas exchange in pulmonary and systemic capillaries if the reaction were not catalysed in both directions by the

Table 10.1 Values for solubility of carbon dioxide in plasma and pK' at different temperatures

Temperature (°C)	Solubility of CO_2 in plasma		pK'		
	$mmol.l^{-1}.kPa^{-1}$	$mmol.l^{-1}.mmHg^{-1}$	at pH 7.6	at pH 7.4	at pH 7.2
40	0.216	0.0288	6.07	6.08	6.09
39	0.221	0.0294	6.07	6.08	6.09
38	0.226	0.0301	6.08	6.09	6.10
37	0.231	0.0308	6.08	6.09	6.10
36	0.236	0.0315	6.09	6.10	6.11
35	0.242	0.0322	6.10	6.11	6.12
25	0.310	0.0413	6.15	6.16	6.17
15	0.416	0.0554	6.20	6.21	6.23

Data from references 2 and 3.

Table 10.2 Normal values for carbon dioxide carriage in blood

	Arterial blood (Hb sat. 95%)	Mixed venous blood (Hb sat. 95%)	Arterial/venous difference
Whole blood			
pH	7.40	7.37	−0.033
P_{CO_2} (kPa)	5.3	6.1	+0.8
(mmHg)	40.0	46.0	+6.0
Total CO_2 ($mmol.l^{-1}$)	21.5	23.3	+1.8
($ml.dl^{-1}$)	48.0	52.0	+4.0
Plasma ($mmol.l^{-1}$)			
Dissolved CO_2	1.2	1.4	+0.2
Carbonic acid	0.0017	0.0020	+0.0003
Bicarbonate ion	24.4	26.2	+1.8
Carbamino CO_2	Negligible	Negligible	Negligible
Total	25.6	27.6	+2.0
Red blood cell fraction of 1 litre of blood			
Dissolved CO_2	0.44	0.51	+0.07
Bicarbonate ion	5.88	5.92	+0.04
Carbamino CO_2	1.10	1.70	+0.60
Plasma fraction of 1 litre of blood			
Dissolved CO_2	0.66	0.76	+0.10
Bicarbonate ion	13.42	14.41	+0.99
Total in 1 litre of blood ($mmol.l^{-1}$)	21.50	23.30	+1.80

enzyme carbonic anhydrase (CA). In addition to its role in the respiratory transport of carbon dioxide, CA plays a fundamental role in many body tissues, for example the generation of hydrogen and bicarbonate ions in secretory organs, including the stomach and kidney, and the intracellular transfer of carbon dioxide within both skeletal and cardiac muscle.[4] The enzyme exists as seven isozymes, of which two are involved in blood carbon dioxide transport. Red blood cells (RBCs) contain large amounts of CA II, one of the fastest enzymes known, whereas CA IV is a membrane-bound isozyme present in pulmonary capillaries. There is no CA activity in plasma.

Carbonic anhydrase is a zinc-containing enzyme of low molecular weight and there is now extensive knowledge of the molecular mechanisms of CA.[5,6] First, the zinc atom hydrolyses water to a reactive Zn–OH$^-$ species, while a nearby histidine residue acts as a 'proton shuttle', removing the H$^+$ from the metal-ion centre and transferring it to any buffer molecules near the enzyme. Carbon dioxide then combines with the Zn–OH$^-$ species and the HCO_3^- formed rapidly dissociates from the zinc atom. The maximal rate of catalysis is determined by the buffering power in the vicinity of the enzyme, as the speed of the enzyme reactions is so fast that its kinetics are determined mostly by the ability of the surrounding buffers to provide/remove H^+ ions to/from the enzyme.

Carbonic anhydrase is inhibited by a large number of compounds, including some drugs such as thiazide diuretics and various heterocyclic sulphonamides, of which acetazolamide is the most important. Acetazolamide is non-specific for the different CA isozymes and so inhibits CA in all organs at a dose of 5–20 mg.kg^{-1} and has no other pharmacological effects of importance. Acetazolamide has been used extensively in the study of carbonic anhydrase and has revealed the surprising fact that it is not essential to life. The quantity and efficiency of RBC CA is such that more than 98% of activity must be blocked before there is any discernible change in carbon dioxide transport, though when total inhibition is achieved, $P\text{CO}_2$ gradients between tissues and alveolar gas are increased, pulmonary ventilation is increased and alveolar $P\text{CO}_2$ is decreased.

As bicarbonate ion

The largest fraction of carbon dioxide in the blood is in the form of bicarbonate ion, which is formed by ionisation of carbonic acid thus:

$$H_2CO_3 \rightleftharpoons H^+ + HCO_3^- \rightleftharpoons 2H^+ + CO_3^{2-} \quad (3)$$

The second dissociation occurs only at high pH (above 9) and is not a factor in the carriage of carbon dioxide by the blood. The first dissociation is, however, of the greatest importance within the physiological range. The pK_1' is about 6.1 and carbonic acid is about 96% dissociated under physiological conditions.

According to the law of mass action:

$$\frac{[H^+] \times [HCO_3^-]}{[H_2CO_3]} = K_1' \quad (4)$$

where K_1' is the equilibrium constant of the first dissociation. The subscript 1 indicates that it is the first dissociation and the prime indicates that we are dealing with concentrations rather than the more correct thermodynamic activities.

Rearrangement of equation (4) gives the following:

$$[H^+] = K_1' \frac{[H_2CO_3]}{[HCO_3^-]} \quad (5)$$

The left-hand side is the hydrogen ion concentration and this equation is the non-logarithmic form of the Henderson–Hasselbalch equation.[7] The concentration of carbonic acid cannot be measured and the equation may be modified by replacing this term with the total concentration of dissolved CO_2 and H_2CO_3, most conveniently quantified as $\alpha P\text{CO}_2$ as described above. The equation now takes the form:

$$[H^+] = K_1' \frac{\alpha P\text{CO}_2}{[HCO_3^-]} \quad (6)$$

The new constant K' is the *apparent* first dissociation constant of carbonic acid and includes a factor that allows for the substitution of total dissolved carbon dioxide concentration for carbonic acid.

The equation is now in a useful form and permits the direct relation of plasma hydrogen ion concentration, $P\text{CO}_2$ and bicarbonate concentration, all quantities that can be measured. The value of K' cannot be derived theoretically and is determined experimentally by simultaneous measurements of the three variables. Under normal physiological conditions, if $[H^+]$ is in nmol.l^{-1}, $P\text{CO}_2$ in kPa and HCO_3^- in mmol.l^{-1}, the value of the combined parameter $(\alpha K')$ is about 180. If $P\text{CO}_2$ is in mmHg, the value of the parameter is 24.

Most people prefer to use the pH scale and so follow the approach described by Hasselbalch in 1916 and take logarithms of the reciprocal of each term in equation (6), with the following familiar result:[8]

$$pH = pK' + \log \frac{[HCO_3^-]}{\alpha P\text{CO}_2} = pK' + \log \frac{[CO_2] - \alpha P\text{CO}_2}{\alpha P\text{CO}_2} \quad (7)$$

where pK' has an experimentally derived value of the order of 6.1, but varies with temperature and pH (see Table 10.1). '$[CO_2]$' refers to the total concentration of carbon dioxide in all forms (dissolved CO_2, H_2CO_3 and bicarbonate) in plasma and not in whole blood.

Carbamino carriage

Amino groups in the uncharged $R–NH_2$ form have the ability to combine directly with carbon dioxide to form a carbamic acid. At body pH, the carbamic acid then dissociates almost completely to carbamate:

$$R-N-H + CO_2 \rightleftharpoons R-N-C-OH \rightleftharpoons R-N-C-O^- + H^+$$

In a protein, the amino groups involved in the peptide linkages between amino acid residues cannot combine with carbon dioxide. The potential for carbamino carriage is therefore restricted to the one terminal amino group in each protein chain and to the side chain amino groups that are found in lysine and arginine. Since both hydrogen ions and carbon dioxide compete to react with

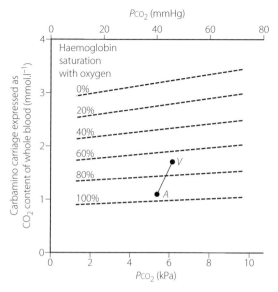

Figure 10.1 The broken lines on the graph indicate the carbamino carriage of carbon dioxide at different levels of oxygen saturation of haemoglobin. It will be seen that oxygen saturation has a far greater influence on carbamino carriage than the actual P_{CO_2} (abscissa). Points A and V represent the saturation and P_{CO_2} of arterial and venous blood, respectively. Note that the arterial/venous difference in carbamino carriage is large in relation to the actual amounts of carbamino carriage.

uncharged amino groups, the ability to combine with carbon dioxide is markedly pH dependent. The terminal α-amino groups are the most effective at physiological pH and one binding site per protein monomer is more than sufficient to account for the quantity of carbon dioxide carried as carbamino compounds.

Carbamino carriage and haemoglobin. Only very small quantities of carbon dioxide are carried in carbamino compounds with plasma protein. Almost all is carried by haemoglobin and reduced haemoglobin is about 3.5 times as effective as oxyhaemoglobin (Figure 10.1), this being a major component of the Haldane effect (see below). Carbon dioxide binds to α-amino groups at the ends of both the α- and β-chains of haemoglobin. Earlier studies of CO_2–haemoglobin reactions using free haemoglobin solution overestimated the magnitude of carbamino binding with haemoglobin, as later work showed that 2,3-diphosphoglycerate (2,3-DPG) present *in vivo* antagonises the binding of CO_2 with haemoglobin. This antagonism results from direct competition between CO_2 and 2,3-DPG for the end-terminal valine of the β-chain of haemoglobin, an effect that is not observed on the α-chains.

The Haldane effect. This is the difference in the quantity of carbon dioxide carried, at constant P_{CO_2}, in oxy-

genated and deoxygenated blood (Figure 10.2). Although the amount of carbon dioxide carried in the blood by carbamino carriage is small, the *difference* between the amount carried in venous and arterial blood is about a third of the total arterial/venous difference (see Table 10.2). This therefore accounts for the major part of the Haldane effect, the remainder being due to the increased buffering capacity of reduced haemoglobin, which is discussed below. When the Haldane effect was described by Christiansen, Douglas and Haldane in 1914, they believed that the whole effect was due to altered buffering capacity:[9] carbamino carriage was not demonstrated until much later (1934).[10]

Formation of carbamino compounds does not require the dissolved carbon dioxide to be hydrated and so is independent of carbonic anhydrase. The reaction is very rapid and would be of particular importance in a patient who had received a carbonic anhydrase inhibitor.

Effect of buffering power of proteins on carbon dioxide carriage

Amino and carboxyl groups concerned in peptide linkages have no buffering power. Neither have most side chain groups (e.g. in lysine and glutamic acid) because their pK values are far removed from the physiological range of pH. In contrast is the imidazole group of the amino acid histidine, which is almost the only amino acid to be an effective buffer in the normal range of pH. Imidazole groups constitute the major part of the considerable buffering power of haemoglobin, each tetramer containing 38 histidine residues. The buffering power of plasma proteins is less and is directly proportional to their histidine content.

The four haem groups of a molecule of haemoglobin are attached to the corresponding four amino acid chains at one of the histidine residues on each chain (page 175) and the dissociation constant of the imidazole groups of these four histidine residues is strongly influenced by the state of oxygenation of the haem. Reduction causes the corresponding imidazole group to become more basic. The converse is also true: in the acidic form of the

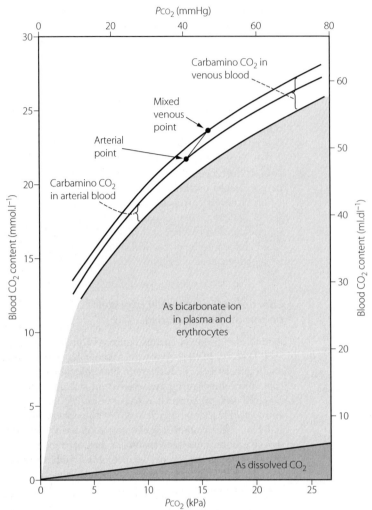

Figure 10.2 Components of the CO_2 dissociation curve for whole blood. Dissolved CO_2 and bicarbonate ion vary with $P\text{CO}_2$ but are little affected by the state of oxygenation of the haemoglobin. (Increased basic properties of reduced haemoglobin cause a slight increase in formation of bicarbonate ion.) Carbamino carriage of CO_2 is strongly influenced by the state of oxygenation of haemoglobin but hardly at all by $P\text{CO}_2$.

imidazole group of the histidine, the strength of the oxygen bond is weakened. Each reaction is of great physiological interest and both effects were noticed many decades before their mechanisms were elucidated.

1. The reduction of haemoglobin causes it to become more basic. This results in increased carriage of carbon dioxide as bicarbonate, since hydrogen ions are removed, permitting increased dissociation of carbonic acid (first dissociation of equation 3). This accounts for part of the Haldane effect, the other and greater part being due to increased carbamino carriage (see above).
2. Conversion to the basic form of histidine causes increased affinity of the corresponding haem group for oxygen. This is, in part, the cause of the Bohr effect (page 177).

Total deoxygenation of the haemoglobin in blood would raise the pH by about 0.03 if the $P\text{CO}_2$ were held con-

stant at 5.3 kPa (40 mmHg), and this would correspond roughly to the addition of 3 mmol of base to 1 l of blood. The normal degree of desaturation in the course of the change from arterial to venous blood is about 25%, corresponding to a pH increase of about 0.007 if $P\text{CO}_2$ remains constant. In fact, $P\text{CO}_2$ rises by about 0.8 kPa (6 mmHg), which would cause a decrease of pH of 0.040 if the oxygen saturation were to remain the same. The combination of an increase of $P\text{CO}_2$ of 0.8 kPa and a decrease of saturation of 25% thus results in a fall in pH of 0.033 (see Table 10.2).

Distribution of carbon dioxide within the blood

Table 10.2 shows the forms in which carbon dioxide is carried in normal arterial and mixed venous blood. Although the amount carried in solution is small, most of the carbon dioxide enters and leaves the blood as CO_2 itself (Figure 10.3). Within the plasma there is little

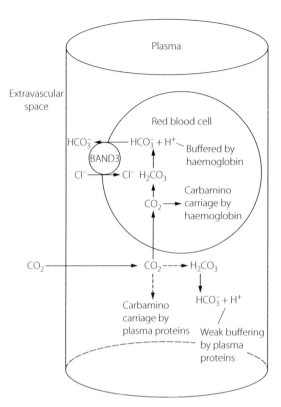

Figure 10.3 How carbon dioxide enters the blood in molecular form. Within the plasma, there is only negligible carbamino carriage by plasma proteins and a slow rate of hydration to carbonic acid owing to the absence of carbonic anhydrase. The greater part of CO_2 diffuses into the red blood cell, where conditions for carbamino carriage (by haemoglobin) are more favourable. In addition, more rapid formation of carbonic acid is facilitated by carbonic anhydrase, the removal of hydrogen ions by haemoglobin buffering and the transfer of bicarbonate out of the red blood cell (in exchange for chloride) by the Hamburger shift.

chemical combination of carbon dioxide, for three reasons. First, there is no carbonic anhydrase in plasma and therefore carbonic acid is formed only very slowly. Second, there is little buffering power in plasma to promote the dissociation of carbonic acid. Third, the formation of carbamino compounds by plasma proteins is not great and must be almost identical for arterial and venous blood.

Carbon dioxide can, however, diffuse freely into the RBC, where two courses are open. First, increasing intracellular PCO_2 will increase carbamino carriage of CO_2 by haemoglobin, an effect greatly enhanced by the fall in oxygen saturation, which is likely to be occurring at the same time (see Figure 10.1). The second course is hydration and dissociation of CO_2 to produce hydrogen and bicarbonate ions, facilitated by the presence of car-

bonic anhydrase in the RBC. However, accumulation of intracellular hydrogen and bicarbonate ions will quickly tip the equilibrium of the reaction against further dissociation of carbonic acid, a situation that is avoided in the RBC by two mechanisms.

Haemoglobin buffering. Hydrogen ions produced by carbonic anhydrase are quickly buffered by the imidazole groups on the histidine residues of the haemoglobin, as described above. Once again, the concomitant fall in haemoglobin saturation enhances this effect by increasing the buffering capacity of the haemoglobin.

Hamburger shift. Hydration of CO_2 and buffering of the hydrogen ions results in the formation of considerable quantities of bicarbonate ion within the RBC. These excess bicarbonate ions are actively transported out of the cell into the plasma in exchange for chloride ions to maintain electrical neutrality across the RBC membrane. This ionic exchange was first suggested by Hamburger in 1918,[11] and believed to be a passive process. It is now known to be facilitated by a complex membrane-bound protein that has been extensively studied and named band 3 after its position on a gel electrophoresis plate.[12–14] Band 3 exchanges bicarbonate and chloride ions by a 'ping-pong' mechanism in which one ion first moves out of the RBC before the other ion moves inwards, in contrast to most other ion pumps, which simultaneously exchange the two ions. Band 3 protein is also intimately related to other proteins in the RBC (Figure 10.4).[13,14]

- RBC cytoskeleton. The cytoplasmic domain of band 3 acts as an anchoring site for many of the proteins involved in the maintenance of cell shape and membrane stability, such as ankyrin and spectrin. A genetically engineered deficiency of band 3 in animals results in small, fragile, spherical RBCs.[12] RBC shape and deformability are now known to be important in oxygen transport in the capillaries (page 137) and it is likely that band 3 is involved in bringing about these shape changes.
- Carbonic anhydrase. Band 3 is also closely associated with carbonic anhydrase and the protein complex formed is believed to act as a metabolon, a term describing the channelling of a substrate directly between proteins that catalyse sequential reactions in a metabolic pathway.[13] In this case the substrate is bicarbonate, which after its formation by CA is transferred directly to band 3, which rapidly exports it from the cell.
- Haemoglobin. Band 3 is also associated with haemoglobin, with which it is believed to form another metabolon system exporting nitric oxide-derived

Figure 10.4 Proteins associated with band 3 in the red blood cell membrane. Band 3 has 12 transmembrane domains forming the bicarbonate/chloride exchange ion channel and four globular cytoplasmic domains (a–d), each of which is associated with different groups of intracellular proteins. (a) Ankyrin and spectrin, to maintain and possibly alter red cell shape. (b) Carbonic anhydrase, with which band 3 acts as a metabolon to directly export bicarbonate ions from the red cell. (c) Haemoglobin, with which band 3 may act as a metabolon to export nitric oxide. (d) Glycolytic enzymes – the functional significance of this association is unknown.

nitrosothiols, possibly to regulate capillary blood flow and oxygen release from haemoglobin (page 181).
- Glycolytic enzymes. Some of the enzymes involved in glycolysis (page 184), including glyceraldehyde-3-phosphate dehydrogenase, phosphofructokinase and aldolase, are bound to band 3; the functional significance of this is unknown.

In the pulmonary capillary, where $P\text{CO}_2$ is low, the series of events described above goes into reverse and the CO_2 released from the RBC diffuses into the alveolus and is excreted.

Dissociation curves of carbon dioxide

Figure 10.2 shows the classic form of the dissociation curve of carbon dioxide relating blood content to tension. For decades there has been great interest in curves that relate any pair of the following: (1) plasma bicarbonate concentration; (2) $P\text{CO}_2$; (3) pH. These three quantities are related by the Henderson–Hasselbalch equation (equation 7) and therefore the third variable can always be derived from the other two. The most famous is the Sigaard-Andersen plot, which relates log $P\text{CO}_2$ to pH (Figure 10.5), though many others have been described. These graphs can be used to explore the effects of changes in respiratory and metabolic acid–base balance, but care must be taken in using these *in vitro* data in intact subjects. For example, if the $P\text{CO}_2$ of an entire patient is altered, the pH changes are not the same as those of a blood sample of which the $P\text{CO}_2$ is altered *in vitro*. This is because the blood of a patient is in continuity with the extracellular fluid (of very low buffering capacity) and also with intracellular fluid (of high buffering capacity). Bicarbonate ions pass rapidly and freely across the various interfaces, and experimental studies have shown the following changes to occur in the arterial blood of an intact subject when the $P\text{CO}_2$ is acutely changed.

- The arterial pH reaches a steady state within minutes of establishment of the new level of $P\text{CO}_2$.
- The change in arterial pH is intermediate between the pH changes obtained *in vitro* with plasma and whole blood after the same change in $P\text{CO}_2$. That is to say, the *in vivo* change in pH is greater than the *in vitro* change in the patient's blood when subjected to the same change in $P\text{CO}_2$.

FACTORS INFLUENCING CARBON DIOXIDE TENSION IN THE STEADY STATE

In common with other catabolites, the level of carbon dioxide in the body fluids depends on the balance between production and elimination. There is a continuous gradient of $P\text{CO}_2$ from the mitochondria to the expired air and thence to ambient air. The $P\text{CO}_2$ in all cells is not identical, but is lowest in tissues with the lowest metabolic activity and the highest perfusion (e.g. skin) and highest in tissues with the highest metabolic activity for their perfusion (e.g. the myocardium). Therefore the $P\text{CO}_2$ of venous blood differs substantially from one tissue to another.

In the pulmonary capillaries, carbon dioxide passes into the alveolar gas and this causes the alveolar $P\text{CO}_2$ to rise steadily during expiration. During inspiration, the inspired gas dilutes the alveolar gas and the $P\text{CO}_2$ falls by about 0.4 kPa, imparting a sawtooth curve to the alveolar $P\text{CO}_2$ when it is plotted against time (Figure 10.6).

Blood leaving the pulmonary capillaries has a $P\text{CO}_2$ that is very close to that of the alveolar gas, and therefore varies with time in the same manner as the alveolar $P\text{CO}_2$. There is also a regional variation, with $P\text{CO}_2$ inversely related to the ventilation/perfusion ratio of dif-

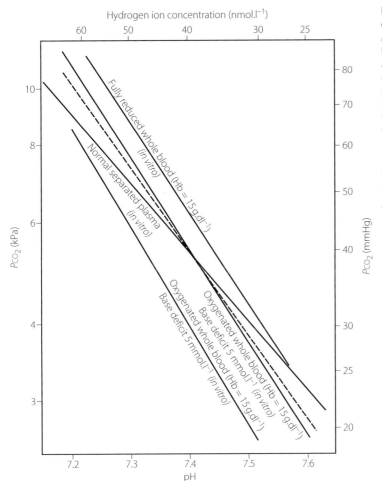

Hydrogen ion concentration (nmol.l^{-1})

P_{CO_2} (kPa)

P_{CO_2} (mmHg)

pH

Fully reduced whole blood (Hb = 15 g.dl^{-1}) (in vitro)

Normal separated plasma (in vitro)

Oxygenated whole blood (Hb = 15 g.dl^{-1}) (in vitro)

Base deficit 5 mmol.l^{-1} (in vitro)

Oxygenated whole blood (Hb = 15 g.dl^{-1})

Base deficit 5 mmol.l^{-1} (in vitro)

Figure 10.5 A number of CO_2 equilibrium curves plotted on the coordinates pH/log P_{CO_2}.[15] For most biological fluids the plot is linear over the physiological range. pH = 7.40 and P_{CO_2} = 5.3 kPa (40 mmHg) are the accepted normal values through which all the curves for normal oxygenated blood or plasma pass. The steepest curve passing through this point is that of normal oxygenated blood; the flattest is that of plasma, both curves being obtained *in vitro*. The uppermost curve is that of reduced but otherwise normal blood equilibrated *in vitro*. The lowermost curve is that of oxygenated blood with a metabolic acidosis (base deficit) of 5 mmol.l^{-1} equilibrated *in vitro*. The broken curve is the only *in vivo* curve, obtained from a normal anaesthetised patient (Hb 15 g.dl^{-1}) whose P_{CO_2} is acutely changed.[16]

ferent parts of the lung (see Figure 8.12). The mixed arterial P_{CO_2} is the integrated mean of blood from different parts of the lung and a sample drawn over several seconds will average out the cyclical variations.

It is more convenient to consider partial pressure than content, because carbon dioxide always moves in accord with partial pressure gradients even if they are in the opposite direction to concentration gradients. Also, the concept of partial pressure may be applied with equal significance to gas and liquid phases, content having a rather different connotation in the two phases. Furthermore, the effects of carbon dioxide (e.g. upon respiration) are a function of partial pressure rather than content. Finally, it is easier to measure blood P_{CO_2} than CO_2 content. Normal values for partial pressure and content are shown in Figure 10.7.

Each factor that influences the P_{CO_2} has already been mentioned in this book and in this chapter they will be drawn together, illustrating their relationship to one another. It is convenient first to summarise the factors

influencing the alveolar P_{CO_2} and then to consider the factors that influence the relationship between the alveolar and the arterial P_{CO_2} (Figure 10.8).

The alveolar P_{CO_2} (PA_{CO_2})

Carbon dioxide is constantly being added to the alveolar gas from the pulmonary arterial blood and removed from it by the alveolar ventilation. Therefore, ignoring inspired carbon dioxide, it follows that:

$$\text{Alveolar } CO_2 \text{ concentration} = \frac{\text{Carbon dioxide output}}{\text{Alveolar ventilation}}$$

This axiomatic relationship is the basis for prediction of the alveolar concentration of any gas that enters or leaves the body. With inclusion of the inspired concentration, it may be written as a form of alveolar air equation (page 128), for which the version for carbon dioxide is as follows:

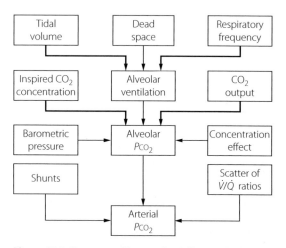

Figure 10.6 Changes in alveolar and mouth P_{CO_2} during the respiratory cycle. The alveolar P_{CO_2} is shown by a continuous curve and the mouth P_{CO_2} by the broken curve. The mouth P_{CO_2} falls at the commencement of inspiration but does not rise during expiration until the anatomical dead space gas is washed out. The alveolar P_{CO_2} rises during expiration and also during the early part of inspiration until fresh gas penetrates the alveoli after the anatomical dead space is washed out. The alveolar P_{CO_2} then falls until expiration commences. This imparts a sawtooth curve to the alveolar P_{CO_2}.

Figure 10.8 Summary of factors that influence P_{CO_2}; the more important ones are indicated with the thicker arrows. In the steady state, the CO_2 output of a resting subject usually lies within the range 150–200 ml.min^{-1} and the alveolar P_{CO_2} is largely governed by the alveolar ventilation, provided that the inspired CO_2 concentration is zero. See text for explanation of the concentration effect.

Figure 10.7 Normal values of CO_2 levels. These normal values are rounded off and ignore the small difference in P_{CO_2} between end-expiratory gas, alveolar gas and arterial blood. Actual values of P_{CO_2} depend mainly on alveolar ventilation but the differences depend on maldistribution; the alveolar/end-tidal expiratory P_{CO_2} difference depends on alveolar dead space and the very small arterial/alveolar P_{CO_2} difference on shunt. Scatter of $\dot{V}/\dot{Q}$ ratios makes a small contribution to both alveolar/end-expiratory and arterial/alveolar P_{CO_2} gradients. The arterial/mixed venous CO_2 content difference is directly proportional to CO_2 output and inversely proportional to cardiac output. Secondary symbols: A, alveolar; a, arterial; Ē, mixed expired; ε', end-expiratory; v̄, mixed venous.

$$\text{Alveolar } P\text{CO}_2 = \underset{\substack{\text{dry} \\ \text{barometric} \\ \text{pressure}}}{} \left(\begin{array}{l} \text{mean inspired CO}_2 \\ \text{concentration} \\ \\ + \dfrac{\text{CO}_2 \text{ output}}{\text{alveolar ventilation}} \end{array} \right)$$

This equation includes all the more important factors influencing $P\text{CO}_2$ (see Figure 10.8), and examples of the hyperbolic relationship between $P\text{CO}_2$ and alveolar ventilation are shown in Figure 10.9. Individual factors will now be considered.

The dry barometric pressure is not a factor of much importance in the determination of alveolar $P\text{CO}_2$ and normal variations of barometric pressure at sea level are unlikely to influence the $P\text{CO}_2$ by more than 0.3 kPa (2 mmHg). At high altitude, the hypoxic drive to ventilation lowers the $P\text{CO}_2$ (see Chapter 17).

The mean inspired CO$_2$ concentration. The effect of inspired carbon dioxide on the alveolar $P\text{CO}_2$ is additive. If, for example, a patient breathes gas containing 4.2% carbon dioxide ($P\text{CO}_2 = 4.0$ kPa or 30 mmHg), the alveolar $P\text{CO}_2$ will be raised 4.0 kPa above the level that it would be if there were no carbon dioxide in the inspired gas and *other factors, including ventilation, remained the same*.

Carbon dioxide output. It is carbon dioxide output and not production that directly influences the alveolar $P\text{CO}_2$. Output equals production in a steady state, but they may be quite different during unsteady states. During acute hypoventilation, much of the carbon dioxide production is diverted into the body stores, so that the output may temporarily fall to very low figures until the alveolar carbon dioxide concentration has risen to its new level. Conversely, acute hyperventilation results in a transient increase in carbon dioxide output. A sudden fall in cardiac output decreases the carbon dioxide output until the carbon dioxide concentration in the mixed venous blood rises. The unsteady state is considered in more detail later in this chapter.

Alveolar ventilation for present purposes means the product of the respiratory frequency and the difference between the tidal volume and the physiological dead space (page 118). It can change over very wide limits and is the most important factor influencing alveolar $P\text{CO}_2$. Factors governing ventilation are considered in Chapter 5 and dead space in Chapter 8.

The concentration effect. Apart from the factors shown in the equation above and in Figure 10.9, the alveolar $P\text{CO}_2$ may be temporarily influenced by net transfer of

Figure 10.9 The effect of CO_2 output, alveolar ventilation and inspired CO_2 concentration on alveolar $P\text{CO}_2$. The lowest curve shows the relationship between ventilation and alveolar $P\text{CO}_2$ for a CO_2 output of 100 ml.min^{-1} (STPD). The blue curve shows the normal relationship when the CO_2 output is 200 ml.min^{-1}. The broken curve represents the relationship when the CO_2 output is 200 ml.min^{-1} and there is an inspired CO_2 concentration of 2%. Two percent CO_2 is equivalent to about 1.9 kPa (14 mmHg) and each point on the broken curve is 1.9 kPa above the upper of the two continuous curves.

soluble inert gases across the alveolar/capillary membrane. Rapid uptake of an inert gas increases the concentration (and partial pressure) of carbon dioxide (and oxygen) in the alveolar gas. This occurs, for example, at the beginning of an anaesthetic, when large quantities of nitrous oxide are passing from the alveolar gas into the body stores and a much smaller quantity of nitrogen is passing from the body into the alveolar gas. The converse occurs during elimination of the inert gas and results in transient reduction of alveolar $P\text{CO}_2$ and $P\text{O}_2$.

The end-expiratory $P\text{CO}_2$ ($P\text{E}'_{\text{CO}_2}$)

In the normal, healthy, conscious subject, the end-expiratory gas is almost entirely alveolar. If, however, appreciable parts of the lung are ventilated but not perfused, they will contribute a significant quantity of CO_2-free gas from the alveolar dead space to the end-expiratory gas (see Figure 8.9). As a result, the end-expiratory $P\text{CO}_2$ will be lower than that of the alveoli which are perfused. Gas cannot be sampled selectively from the perfused alveoli. However, since arterial $P\text{CO}_2$ usually approximates closely to the $P\text{CO}_2$ of the perfused alveoli (see below), it is possible to compare arterial and end-expiratory $P\text{CO}_2$ to demonstrate the existence of an appreciable proportion of underperfused alveoli. Studies during anaesthesia have, for example, shown an arterial/end-tidal $P\text{CO}_2$ gradient between 0.7 and 1.3 kPa (5–10 mmHg).[17,18]

Figure 10.10 A hydrostatic analogy of the elimination of carbon dioxide. See text for full description.

Supply tank

Rapid compartment

Medium compartment

Slow compartment

Waste

The alveolar/arterial P_{CO_2} gradient

For reasons that were discussed in Chapter 9, we may discount the possibility of any significant gradient between the P_{CO_2} of alveolar gas and that of pulmonary end-capillary blood (page 140). Arterial P_{CO_2} may, however, be slightly greater than the mean alveolar P_{CO_2} because of shunting or scatter of ventilation/perfusion ratios. Factors governing the magnitude of the gradient were considered in Chapter 8, where it was shown that a shunt of 10% will cause an alveolar/arterial P_{CO_2} gradient of only about 0.1 kPa (0.7 mmHg) (see Figure 8.10). Because the normal degree of ventilation/perfusion ratio scatter causes a gradient of the same order, neither has much significance for carbon dioxide (in contrast to oxygen) and there is an established convention by which the arterial and 'ideal' alveolar P_{CO_2} values are taken to be identical. It is only in exceptional patients with, for example, a shunt in excess of 30% that the gradient is likely to exceed 0.3 kPa (2 mmHg).

The arterial P_{CO_2} (Pa_{CO_2})

Pooled results for the normal arterial P_{CO_2} reported by various authors show a mean of 5.1 kPa (38.3 mmHg) with 95% limits (2 s.d.) of ±1.0 kPa (7.5 mmHg). Five percent of normal patients will lie outside these limits and it is therefore preferable to call it the reference range rather than the normal range. There is no evidence that P_{CO_2} is influenced by age in the healthy subject.

CARBON DIOXIDE STORES AND THE UNSTEADY STATE

The quantity of carbon dioxide and bicarbonate ion in the body is very large, about 120 l, which is almost 100 times greater than the volume of oxygen. Therefore, when ventilation is altered out of accord with metabolic activity, carbon dioxide levels change only slowly and new equilibrium levels are only attained after about 20–30 minutes. In contrast, corresponding changes in oxygen levels are very rapid.

Figure 10.10 shows a three-compartment hydraulic model in which depth of water represents P_{CO_2} and the volume in the various compartments corresponds to volume of carbon dioxide. The metabolic production of carbon dioxide is represented by the variable flow of water from the supply tank. The outflow corresponds to alveolar ventilation and the controller watching the P_{CO_2} represents the central chemoreceptors. The rapid compartment represents circulating blood, brain, kidneys and other well-perfused tissues. The medium compartment represents skeletal muscle (resting) and other tissues with a moderate blood flow. The slow compartment includes bone, fat and other tissues with a large capacity for carbon dioxide. Each compartment has its own time constant (see Appendix F) and the long time constants of the medium and slow compartments buffer changes in the rapid compartment.

Hyperventilation is represented by a wide opening of the outflow valve with subsequent exponential decline in the levels in all three compartments, the rapid compartment falling most quickly. The rate of P_{CO_2} decrease is governed primarily by ventilation and the capacity of the stores. Hypoventilation is fundamentally different. The rate of P_{CO_2} increase is now limited by the metabolic production of carbon dioxide, which is the *only* factor directly increasing the quantity of carbon dioxide in the body compartments. Therefore, the time course of the P_{CO_2} increase following step decrease of ventilation is not the mirror image of the time course of the P_{CO_2} decrease when ventilation is increased. The rate of rise is much slower than the rate of fall, which is fortunate for patients in asphyxial situations.

Figure 10.11 Time course of changes in end-expiratory P_{CO_2} following step changes in ventilation. The solid circles indicate the changes in end-expiratory P_{CO_2} that follow a change in ventilation from 3.3 to 14 l.min^{-1}. The open circles show the change following a reduction in ventilation from 14 to 3.3 l.min^{-1} in the same patient. During the fall in P_{CO_2}, half the total change is completed in about 3 minutes; during the rise in P_{CO_2}, half-change takes approximately 16 minutes.

When *all* metabolically produced carbon dioxide is retained, the rate of rise of arterial P_{CO_2} is of the order of 0.4–0.8 kPa.min^{-1} (3-mmHg.min^{-1}). This is the result of the rate of carbon dioxide production and the capacity of the body stores for carbon dioxide. During hypoventilation, the rate of increase in P_{CO_2} will be less than this and Figure 10.11 shows typical curves for P_{CO_2} increase and decrease following step changes in ventilation of anaesthetised patients. The time course of P_{CO_2} rise after step reduction of ventilation is faster when the previous level of ventilation has been of short duration.[19]

The difference in the rate of change of P_{CO_2} and P_{O_2} after a step change in ventilation (see Figure 11.19) has two important implications for monitoring and measurement. First, changes in P_{O_2} (or oxygen saturation) will often provide an earlier warning of acute hypoventilation than will the capnogram, provided that the alveolar P_{O_2} is not much above the normal range. However, *in the steady state* P_{CO_2} gives the best indication of the adequacy of ventilation, because oxygenation is so heavily influenced by intrapulmonary shunting and the inspired oxygen concentration. Second, step changes in ventilation are followed by temporary changes in the respiratory exchange ratio because, in the unsteady state, carbon dioxide output changes more than oxygen uptake. However, if the ventilation is held constant at its new level, the respiratory exchange ratio must eventually return to the value determined by the metabolic process of the body.

Cardiac output and CO$_2$ transport. In the normal subject, fluctuations in cardiac output have little effect on arterial, alveolar or end-expiratory P_{CO_2} because of the effi-ciency of the chemical control of breathing. However, with a constant level of artificial ventilation, for example during anaesthesia or cardiopulmonary resuscitation, the situation is quite different. In the extreme circumstance of a total cessation of cardiac output, then alveolar and end-expiratory P_{CO_2} will fall dramatically as the delivery of blood containing carbon dioxide to the lung also ceases. In a similar fashion, a sudden reduction in cardiac output during anaesthesia causes an abrupt reduction in end-expiratory P_{CO_2},[20] an observation first made as long ago as 1957.[21] This almost certainly results from increased alveolar dead space caused by an increase in the number of non-perfused but ventilated alveoli (zone 1, page 97). If low cardiac output is sustained for more than a few minutes, blood P_{CO_2} will rise and the expired P_{CO_2} returns towards normal as the blood passing through perfused lung releases more carbon dioxide into the expired gas.

Apart from being a useful early warning of cardiovascular catastrophe during anaesthesia, the measurement of expired carbon dioxide has also been advocated during cardiopulmonary resuscitation, both as a method of monitoring the efficacy of chest compressions and as an indicator of the return of spontaneous cardiac output.[22]

APNOEA

When a patient becomes apnoeic while breathing air, alveolar gas reaches equilibrium with mixed venous blood within a few minutes. Assuming normal starting conditions and ignoring changes in the composition of the recirculated mixed venous blood, this would entail a rise of alveolar P_{CO_2} from 5.3 to 6.1 kPa (40 to 46 mmHg) and a fall of P_{O_2} from 14 to 5.3 kPa (105 to

40 mmHg). These changes correspond to the uptake of 230 ml of oxygen but the output of only 21 ml of carbon dioxide. Carbon dioxide appears to reach equilibrium within about 10 seconds,[23] whereas oxygen would take about a minute, being limited by the ability of the cardiac output and the arterial/mixed venous oxygen content difference to remove some two-thirds of the oxygen in the alveolar gas (normally about 450 ml).

These calculations assume that alveolar gas is not replenished from outside the patient. What actually happens to the arterial blood gases in apnoea depends upon the patency of the airway and the composition of the ambient gas if the airway is patent.

With airway occlusion. As described above, there is rapid attainment of equilibrium between alveolar and mixed venous P_{CO_2}. Thereafter, arterial, alveolar and mixed venous P_{CO_2} values remain close and, with recirculation of the blood, increase together at the rate of about 0.4–0.8 kPa.min^{-1} (3–6 mmHg.min^{-1}), more than 90% of the metabolically produced carbon dioxide passing into the body stores. Alveolar P_{O_2} decreases close to the mixed venous P_{O_2} within about a minute and then decreases further as recirculation continues. The lung volume falls by the difference between the oxygen uptake and the carbon dioxide output. Initially the rate would be $230 - 21 = 209$ ml.min^{-1}. The change in alveolar P_{O_2} may be calculated, and gross hypoxia supervenes after about 90 seconds if apnoea with airway occlusion follows air breathing at functional residual capacity.

With patent airway and air as ambient gas. The initial changes are as described above. However, instead of the lung volume falling by the net gas exchange rate (initially 209 ml.min^{-1}), this volume of ambient gas is drawn in by mass movement down the trachea. If the ambient gas is air, the oxygen in it will be removed but the nitrogen will accumulate and rise above its normal concentration until gross hypoxia supervenes after about 2 minutes. This is likely to occur when the accumulated nitrogen has reached 90% since the alveolar carbon dioxide concentration will then have reached about 8%. Carbon dioxide elimination cannot occur as there is mass movement of air down the trachea, preventing loss of carbon dioxide by either convection or diffusion.

With patent airway and oxygen as the ambient gas. Oxygen is continuously removed from the alveolar gas as described above, but is replaced by oxygen drawn in by mass movement. No nitrogen is added to the alveolar gas and the alveolar P_{O_2} only falls as fast as the P_{CO_2} rises (about 0.4–0.8 kPa.min^{-1} or 3–6 mmHg.min^{-1}). Therefore the patient will not become seriously hypoxic for several minutes. If the patient has been breathing 100% oxygen prior to the respiratory arrest, the starting

alveolar P_{O_2} would be of the order of 88 kPa (660 mmHg), and therefore the patient could theoretically survive about 100 minutes of apnoea *provided that his airway remained clear and he remained connected to a supply of 100% oxygen.* This does, in fact, happen and has been demonstrated in both animals and man and is referred to as apnoeic mass movement oxygenation or diffusion respiration. The phenomenon enjoyed a brief vogue in anaesthetic practice as a means of maintaining oxygenation during apnoea, particularly for bronchoscopy,[24] and remains a useful technique for short periods during airway surgery such as laryngectomy. However, hypercapnia is an inevitable feature of the technique and arterial P_{CO_2} values as high as 18.7 kPa (140 mmHg) have been reported.[24]

CARBON DIOXIDE CARRIAGE DURING HYPOTHERMIA

Understanding the carriage of CO_2 during hypothermia is of importance both to clinicians involved in the care of hypothermic patients and to the comparative physiologist studying differences between warm-blooded (homeothermic) and cold-blooded (poikilothermic) animals. These two diverse areas of physiology have over recent years converged to produce two alternative theories regarding the optimal system for CO_2 carriage at low temperature.

In common with most gases, carbon dioxide becomes more soluble in water as temperature decreases (see Table 10.1) such that, in plasma, maintenance of the same P_{CO_2} under hypothermic conditions will require a greater total CO_2 content. In addition, decreasing temperature reduces the ionisation of water into H^+ and OH^- ions, so pH increases by approximately 0.016 per degree Celsius fall in temperature.[25] If CO_2 production and excretion remain constant, hypothermia would therefore be expected to result in alkalotic conditions in both the intra- and the extracellular spaces. Different animals are believed to respond to these changes in two ways, as follows.

The pH-stat hypothesis,[26] as the name suggests, involves the animal responding to hypothermia by maintaining the same blood pH regardless of its body temperature. This is achieved by hypoventilation, which increases the P_{CO_2} to maintain pH at close to 7.4 and is seen in hibernating mammals. Indeed, it is thought possible that the high P_{CO_2} and the resulting intracellular acidosis, may contribute to the hypothermic 'sleep' state.

The alphastat hypothesis is more complex.[25,27] In this situation, the pH of the animal is allowed to change in keeping with the physical chemistry laws described above. As temperature falls, the blood pH, again measured at the animal's body temperature, increases. Studies of protein function and acid–base disturbances have revealed the importance of the α-imidazole moiety of histidine in buffering changes in pH, and that the state of dissociation of these α-imidazole groups is crucial to protein function. The pK of α-imidazole is unique among amino acids in that it changes with temperature to a similar degree as the dissociation of water.[27] Thus as temperature decreases, blood and tissue pH rise but the dissociative state of α-imidazole, and thus protein function, remains close to normal. Most poikilothermic animals use an alphastat system and can function well through a broad range of temperatures. Even hibernators, with their pH-stat regulation, maintain an alphastat-type control of some vital tissues such as heart and brain.[28]

There is controversy about whether the blood gases of humans undergoing cardiac surgery during hypothermia should be managed by the alphastat or the pH-stat techniques.[26,29] In the former case, arterial blood drawn from the cold patient is warmed to 37°C before measurement of PCO_2 and the cardiopulmonary bypass adjusted to achieve normal values. For pH-stat control, PCO_2 is again measured at 37°C but mathematically corrected to the patient's temperature and then CO_2 administered to the patient to achieve a pH of 7.4. Increased arterial PCO_2 during pH-stat will in theory improve cerebral perfusion and possibly thereby improve cerebral function.[29] However, there remains little evidence that the two forms of blood gas management result in differences in patient well-being during or after hypothermic surgery, except at very low temperatures, when pH-stat may be superior.[30,31]

OUTLINE OF METHODS OF MEASUREMENT OF CARBON DIOXIDE

Fractional concentration in gas mixtures

Infrared analysis. This is the most widely used method for rapid breath-to-breath analysis and is also very convenient for analysis of discrete gas samples. Most diatomic gases absorb infrared radiation and errors may arise due to overlap of absorption bands and collision broadening.[32] These effects are best overcome by filtering and calibrating with a known concentration of carbon dioxide in a diluent gas mixture that is similar to the gas sample for analysis. Infrared analysers are available with a response time of less than $300\,\mu s$ and will follow the respiratory cycle provided the respiratory frequency is not too high. Breathe-through cells (placed near the patient's airway) have a better frequency response than systems that draw gas from the airway for analysis in a distant machine, as mixing of the inspired and expired gases occurs along the sampling tube. Capnography is described in more detail below.

Mass spectrometry. This powerful technique is established as an alternative method for the rapid analysis of carbon dioxide. The cost is much greater than for infrared analysis, but response times tend to be shorter and there is usually provision for analysis of up to four gases at the same time. In spite of this, mass spectrometry for measurement of respiratory gases remains essentially a research tool.

Blood CO_2 partial pressure

Historically, PCO_2 was measured by allowing blood to equilibrate with gas, in which the CO_2 concentration was then measured. The first practical method, called bubble tonometry, was described as early as 1866 by Pflüger and progressively refined for over 100 years. However, the technique always remained very difficult to master and disappeared from use after 1960. The death knell of these methods was sounded by the development of the interpolation method by Sigaard-Andersen and Astrup in Copenhagen. In their approach, PCO_2 of blood was measured by interpolating the actual pH in a plot of log PCO_2 against pH derived from aliquots of the same blood sample. The plot is linear and the whole operation became a practical proposition following the introduction of the microapparatus described by Sigaard-Andersen *et al*. in 1960.[33]

The Pco_2-sensitive electrode. Both the above methods have given way to the PCO_2-sensitive electrode which, in its automated form, has removed the requirement for technical expertise. Analysis may now be satisfactorily performed by untrained staff on a do-it-yourself basis with results available within 2 minutes. The technique was first described by Severinghaus and Bradley in 1958,[34] and allows the PCO_2 of any gas or liquid to be determined directly. The PCO_2 of a film of bicarbonate solution is allowed to come into equilibrium with the PCO_2 of a sample on the other side of a membrane permeable to carbon dioxide but not to hydrogen ions, usually PTFE. The pH of the bicarbonate solution is constantly monitored by a glass electrode and the log of the PCO_2 is inversely proportional to the recorded pH.

Handling of blood samples.[35,36] It is important that samples be preserved from contact with air, including bubbles and froth in the syringe, to which they may lose carbon dioxide and either lose or gain oxygen depending on the relative PO_2 of the sample and the air. Dilution with excessive volumes of heparin or 'dead space' fluids from indwelling arterial cannulae should be avoided. At very high PO_2 values, oxygen can diffuse across the wall of plastic syringes and glass syringes may therefore be preferable.[36] Analysis should be undertaken quickly, as the PCO_2 of blood *in vitro* rises by about 0.013 kPa per min (0.1 mmHg.min^{-1}) at 37°C, whereas P_{O_2} declines at 0.07–0.3 kPa (0.5–2.3 mmHg) per minute depending on the P_{O_2}. These changes result from metabolic activity, mainly in the white cells.[37] If rapid analysis is not possible (within 10 minutes), the specimen should be stored on ice, which reduces this carbon dioxide production and oxygen consumption by about 90%. Modern blood gas analysers invariably work at 37°C, so for patients with abnormal body temperatures a correction factor should be applied. Nomograms allow correction for both pre-analytic metabolism and patient temperature[38] and examples are shown in Appendix E (Figures E.1 and E.2).

Continuous measurement of arterial P_{CO_2} using indwelling arterial catheters is rapidly becoming a realistic clinical technique.[39] The method uses a 'photochemical optode', which consists of a small optical fibre (140 μm diameter) along which light of a specific wavelength is passed to impinge on a dye incorporated into the tip of the fibre, which lies within the patient's artery.

The dye may either absorb the light or fluoresce (give off light of a different wavelength) in a pH-sensitive fashion and these changes are transmitted back to the analyser via the same or a second optical fibre. For analysis of Pa_{CO_2}, the pH-sensitive optode is again enclosed within a CO_2-permeable PTFE membrane with a bicarbonate buffer as for the P_{CO_2}-sensitive electrode but on a very small scale. The current generation of intraarterial sensors are reasonably accurate, with a precision of 0.4–0.8 kPa (3–6 mmHg).

Capnography[40]

Capnograms consist of plots of CO_2 concentration in airway gas against either time or expired volume. Despite the curves being of similar shape (Figures 8.16 and 10.12) they contain quite different information; for example, time capnography has both inspiratory and expiratory phases, whereas CO_2 against volume plots only involve expiration. Plots of CO_2 and expired volume allow calculation of anatomical dead space (see Figure

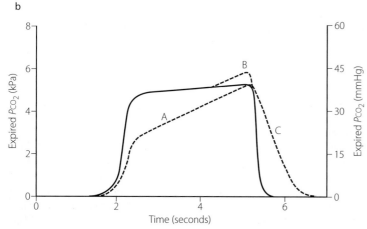

Figure 10.12 Time capnography. **(a)** Normal trace showing the phases of the respiratory cycle and the angles used to quantify the shape of the capnogram. See text for details. **(b)** Dashed lines show abnormalities of the trace, which may occur separately or together. A, varying alveolar time constants (page 113) such as in asthma; B, phase IV terminal upswing seen in pregnancy or obesity; C, rebreathing of expired gases.

8.16), physiological dead space and tidal volume, but this form of capnography is not commonly used clinically.

In the past there has been confusion over the nomenclature of a normal time capnogram, but the most widely accepted terms are shown in Figure 10.12a. There is an inspiratory phase (0) and expiration is divided into three phases: phase I represents CO_2-free gas from the apparatus and anatomical dead space; phase II a rapidly changing mixture of alveolar and dead space gas; phase III the alveolar plateau, the peak of which represents end-expiratory PCO_2 (PE'_{CO_2}). The α and β angles allow quantification of abnormalities of the capnogram. Much information may be obtained from a time capnogram.

- The inspiratory carbon dioxide concentration.
- Respiratory rate.
- The demonstration of the capnogram is a reliable indication of the correct placement of a tracheal tube.
- PE'_{CO_2} is related to arterial PCO_2 (see below).
- Sudden decrease in PE'_{CO_2} at a fixed level of ventilation is a valuable indication of a sudden reduction in cardiac output (page 159) or a pulmonary embolus (see Chapter 29).
- Cardiac arrest during artificial ventilation will cause PE'_{CO_2} to fall to zero.

There are three principal abnormalities of a capnogram,[40] which may occur separately or together and are shown in Figure 10.12b. Line A, with an increased α angle and phase III slope, results from increased ventilation/perfusion mismatch. Almost any lung pathology may result in a sloping phase III and a common clinical cause is acute asthma: line A is typical of a patient with bronchospasm. The gradient of phase III on a capnogram has been proposed as a non-effort-dependent test of the severity of acute asthma.[41] Line B, sometimes referred to as phase IV, is seen in pregnancy or severe obesity. The cause of this appearance is uncertain but may relate to continued evolution of CO_2 from fast alveoli being recorded at the mouth because of the small FRC in which the CO_2 would normally be retained.[40] Line C and an increase in the β angle occur with rebreathing from either excessive apparatus dead space or a malfunctioning anaesthetic breathing system.

Technical considerations should always be borne in mind when considering abnormalities of a capnogram. The response time of the analyser, excessive lengths of sampling tube and inadequate sampling rates will all tend to 'blunt' the normal capnogram trace. This is a particular problem when the tidal volume is low, for example in children or tachypnoeic patients.

Arterial to end-expiratory PCO_2 gradient[18] has already been mentioned above (page 157) and occurs to some extent in almost all subjects, but particularly in elderly patients, smokers, those with lung disease or during anaesthesia.[42,43] The magnitude of the difference is greatest in patients with significant alveolar dead space (page 120)[18] who can be identified from the slope of phase III. Attempts to reduce the gradient by forced or prolonged expiration have generally been unsuccessful.[17] Use of PE'_{CO_2} as a monitor of absolute arterial PCO_2 is therefore unhelpful, but the assessment remains useful for following changes within a subject.

Other indirect measurements of arterial PCO_2

Transcutaneous PCO_2. This technique uses a CO_2-sensitive electrode heated to about 44°C to maximise blood flow to the skin but which is, however, close to the temperature that causes burns. Transcutaneous PCO_2 should be within about 0.5 kPa (3.8 mmHg) of the simultaneous arterial value, but it is necessary to apply a large correction factor for the difference in temperature between body and electrode.[44]

Venous PCO_2. Blood draining skin has a very small arterial/venous PO_2 difference and results are quite acceptable for clinical purposes.[45] However, it is surprisingly difficult to collect a good sample of blood anaerobically from the veins on the back of the hand, and blood from veins draining muscles (e.g. the median cubital vein) has a PCO_2 much higher than the arterial level and is useless as an indication of the arterial PCO_2.

Capillary PCO_2. Blood obtained from a skin prick suffers from the same uncertainties that surround cutaneous venous PCO_2. However, the technique is clearly useful in neonates. The likely error (around 0.6 kPa or 4.5 mmHg) is seldom of much consequence in the management of a patient.

REFERENCES

*1. Geers C, Gros G. Carbon dioxide transport and carbonic anhydrase in blood and muscle. *Physiol Rev* 2000; **80**: 681–715.

2. Severinghaus JW, Stupfel M, Bradley AF. Accuracy of blood pH and PCO_2 determinations. *J Appl Physiol* 1956; **9**: 189–96.

3. Severinghaus JW, Stupfel M, Bradley AF. Variations in serum carbonic acid pK' with pH and temperature. *J Appl Physiol* 1956; **9**: 197–200.

4. Henry RP. Multiple roles of carbonic anhydrase in cellular transport and metabolism. *Annu Rev Physiol* 1996; **58**: 523–38.

5. Henry RP, Swenson ER. The distribution and physiological significance of carbonic anhydrase in vertebrate gas exchange organs. *Respir Physiol* 2000; **121**: 1–12.

*6. Chegwidden WR, Carter ND, Edwards YH, eds. *The carbonic anhydrases. New horizons.* Basel: Birkhäuser Verlag, 2000.

7. Henderson LJ. Das Gleichgewicht zwischen Basen und Säuren im tierischen Organismus. *Ergebn Physiol* 1909; 8: 254.

8. Hasselbalch KA. Die Berechnung der Wasserstoffzahl des Blutes usw. *Biochem Z* 1916; 78: 112–44.

9. Christiansen J, Douglas CG, Haldane JS. The adsorption and dissociation of carbon dioxide by human blood. *J Physiol* 1914; 48: 244–71.

10. Ferguson JKW, Roughton FJW. The direct chemical estimation of carbamino compounds of CO_2 with haemoglobin. *J Physiol* 1934; 83: 68–86.

11. Hamburger HJ. Anionenwanderungen in serum und Blut unter dem Einfluss von CO_2. Säure und Alkali. *Biochem Z* 1918; 86: 309.

*12. Jay DG. Role of band 3 in homeostasis and cell shape. *Cell* 1996; 86: 853–4.

13. Tanner MJA. Band 3 anion exchanger and its involvement in erythrocyte and kidney disorders. *Curr Opin Hematol* 2002; 9: 133–9.

14. Zhang D, Kiyatkin A, Bolin JT, Low PS. Crystallographic structure and functional interpretation of the cytoplasmic domain of erythrocyte membrane band 3. *Blood* 2000; 96: 2925–33.

15. Sigaard-Andersen O. *The acid base status of blood.* Copenhagen: Munksgaard, 1964.

16. Prys-Roberts C, Kelman GR, Nunn JF. Determination of the in vivo carbon dioxide titration curve of anaesthetized man. *Br J Anaesth* 1966; 38: 500–9.

17. Tavernier B, Rey D, Thevenin D, Triboulet J-P, Scherpereel P. Can prolonged expiration manoeuvres improve the prediction of arterial PCO_2 from end-tidal PCO_2? *Br J Anaesth* 1997; 78: 536–40.

18. Nunn JF, Hill DW. Respiratory dead space and arterial to end tidal CO_2 tension difference in anesthetized man. *J Appl Physiol* 1960; 15: 383–9.

19. Ivanov SD, Nunn JF. Influence of the duration of hyperventilation on rise time of PCO_2 after step reduction of ventilation. *Respir Physiol* 1968; 5: 243–9.

20. Shibutani K, Muraoka M, Shirasaki S, Kubal K, Sanchala VT, Gupte P. Do changes in end-tidal PCO_2 quantitatively reflect changes in cardiac output? *Anesth Analg* 1994; 79: 829–33.

21. Leigh MD, Jenkins LC, Belton MK, Lewis GB. Continuous alveolar carbon dioxide analysis as a monitor of pulmonary blood flow. *Anesthesiology* 1957; 18: 878–82.

22. Sanders AB. Capnometry in emergency medicine. *Ann Emerg Med* 1989; 18: 1287–90.

23. Stock MC, Downs JB, McDonald JS, Silver MJ, McSweeney TD, Fairley DS. The carbon dioxide rate of rise in awake apneic humans. *J Clin Anesth* 1988; 1: 96–9.

24. Payne JP. Apnoeic oxygenation in anaesthetised man. *Acta Anaesth Scand* 1962; 6: 129–42.

25. Nattie EE. The alphastat hypothesis in respiratory control and acid-base balance. *J Appl Physiol* 1990; 69: 1201–7.

26. Burrows FA. Con: pH-stat management of blood gases is preferable to alpha-stat in patients undergoing brain cooling for cardiac surgery. *J Cardiothorac Vasc Anesth* 1995; 9: 219–21.

27. Reeves RB. An imidazole alphastat hypothesis for vertebrate acid–base regulation: tissue carbon dioxide content and body temperature in bullfrogs. *Respir Physiol* 1972; 14:219–36.

28. Swain JA, McDonald TJ, Robbins RC, Balaban RS. Relationship of cerebral and myocardial intracellular pH to blood pH during hypothermia. *Am J Physiol* 1991; 260: H1640–4.

29. Kern FH, Greeley WJ. Pro: pH-stat management of blood gases is not preferable to alpha-stat in patients undergoing brain cooling for cardiac surgery. *J Cardiothorac Vasc Anesth* 1995; 9: 215–18.

30. Jonas RA, Bellinger PC, Rappaport LA, *et al.* Relation of pH strategy and developmental outcome after hypothermic circulatory arrest. *J Thorac Cardiovasc Surg* 1993; 106: 362–8.

31. Laussen PC. Optimal blood gas management during deep hypothermic paediatric cardiac surgery: alpha-stat is easier, but pH-stat may be preferable. *Paediatr Anaesth* 2002; 12: 199–204.

32. Cooper EA. Infra-red analysis for the estimation of carbon dioxide in the presence of nitrous oxide. *Br J Anaesth* 1957; 29: 486–90.

33. Sigaard-Anderson O, Engel K, Jorgensen K, Astrup P. A micro-method for determination of pH, carbon dioxide tension, base excess and standard bicarbonate in capillary blood. *Scand J Clin Lab Invest* 1960; 12: 172–6.

34. Severinghaus JW, Bradley AF. Electrodes for blood PO_2 and PCO_2 determination. *J Appl Physiol* 1958; 13: 515–20.

35. Szaflarski NL. Preanalytic error associated with blood gas/pH measurement. *Crit Care Nurse* 1996; 16: 89–100.

36. d'Ortho MP, Delclaux C, Zerah F, Herigault R, Adnot S, Harf A. Use of glass capillaries avoids the time changes in high blood PO_2 observed with plastic syringes. *Chest* 2001; 120: 1651–4.

37. Nunn JF, Sturrock JE, Jones AJ, *et al.* Halothane does not inhibit human neutrophil function in vitro. *Br J Anaesth* 1979; 51: 1101–5.

38. Kelman GR, Nunn JF. Nomograms for correction of blood PO_2, PCO_2, pH and base excess for time and temperature. *J Appl Physiol* 1966; 21: 1484–90.

39. Ganter M, Zollinger A. Continuous intravascular blood gas monitoring: development, current techniques and clinical use of a commercial device. *Br J Anaesth* 2003; **91**: 397–407.

*40. Bhavani-Shankar K, Kumar AY, Moseley HSL, Ahyee-Hallsworth R. Terminology and the current limitations of time capnography: A brief review. *J Clin Monit* 1995; **11**: 175–82.

41. Yaron M, Padyk P, Hutsinpiller M, Cairns CB. Utility of the expiratory capnogram in the assessment of bronchospasm. *Ann Emerg Med* 1996; **28**: 403–7.

42. Wahba RWM, Tessler MJ. Misleading end-tidal CO_2 tensions. *Can J Anaesth* 1996; **43**: 862–6.

43. Fletcher R. Smoking, age and the arterial-end tidal P_{CO_2} difference during anaesthesia and controlled ventilation. *Acta Anaesthesiol Scand* 1987; **31**: 355–6.

44. Severinghaus JW. A combined transcutaneous P_{O_2}-P_{CO_2} electrode with electrochemical HCO_3^- stabilization. *J Appl Physiol* 1981; **51**: 1027–32.

45. Forster HV, Dempsey JA, Thomson J, Vidruk E, Do Pico GA. Estimation of arterial P_{O_2}, P_{CO_2}, pH and lactate from arterialized venous blood. *J Appl Physiol* 1972; **32**: 134–7.

11 Oxygen

KEY POINTS

- Oxygen moves down a partial pressure gradient between the inspired gas and its point of use in the mitochondria, where the oxygen partial pressure may be only 0.13 kPa (1 mmHg).
- Significant barriers to oxygen transfer are between inspired and alveolar gas, between alveolar and arterial oxygen partial pressures, and on diffusion from the capillary to the mitochondria.
- Each 100 ml of arterial blood carries 0.3 ml of oxygen in physical solution and around 20 ml of oxygen bound to haemoglobin, which reduces to around 15 ml in venous blood.
- Oxygen carriage by haemoglobin is influenced by carbon dioxide, pH, temperature and red blood cell 2,3-diphosphoglycerate; the molecular mechanism of haemoglobin is now well elucidated.
- Glucose and other substrates are used to produce energy in the form of adenosine triphosphate (ATP), each glucose molecule yielding 38 molecules of ATP in the presence of oxygen, compared with only two in anaerobic conditions.
- Oxygen delivery is the total amount of oxygen leaving the heart per minute and is around 1000 ml.min^{-1}, compared with oxygen consumption of around 250 ml.min^{-1}.

The appearance of oxygen in the atmosphere of the Earth has played a crucial role in the development of life (see Chapter 1). The whole of the animal kingdom is totally dependent on oxygen, not only for function but also for survival. This is notwithstanding the fact that oxygen is extremely toxic in the absence of elaborate defence mechanisms at a cellular level (see Chapter 26). Before considering the role of oxygen within the cell, it is necessary to bring together many strands from previ-ous chapters and outline the transport of oxygen all the way from the atmosphere to the mitochondria.

THE OXYGEN CASCADE

The P_{O_2} of dry air at sea level is 21.2 kPa (159 mmHg). Oxygen moves down a partial pressure gradient from air through the respiratory tract, the alveolar gas, the arterial blood, the systemic capillaries, the tissues and the cell. It finally reaches its lowest level in the mitochondria, where it is consumed (Figure 11.1). At this point, the P_{O_2} is probably within the range 0.5–3 kPa (3.8–22.5 mmHg), varying from one tissue to another, from one cell to another and from one region of a cell to another.

The steps by which the P_{O_2} decreases from air to the mitochondria are known as the oxygen cascade and are of great practical importance. Any one step in the cascade may be increased under pathological circumstances and this may result in hypoxia. The steps will now be considered *seriatim*.

Dilution of inspired oxygen by water vapour

The normally quoted value for the concentration of atmospheric oxygen (20.94% or 0.2094 fractional concentration) indicates the concentration of oxygen in *dry* gas. As gas is inhaled through the respiratory tract, it becomes humidified at body temperature and the added water vapour dilutes the oxygen and so reduces the P_{O_2} below its level in the ambient air. When dry gas at normal barometric pressure becomes fully saturated with water vapour at 37°C, 100 volumes of the dry gas take up about six volumes of water vapour, giving a total gas volume of 106 units but containing the same number of molecules of oxygen. The P_{O_2} is thus reduced by the fraction 6/106. It follows from Boyle's law that P_{O_2} after humidification is indicated by the following expression:

$$\begin{array}{c} \text{fractional concentration} \\ \text{of oxygen in} \\ \text{the dry gas phase} \end{array} \times \left(\begin{array}{cc} \text{barometric} & \text{saturated water} \\ \text{pressure} & - \text{vapour pressure} \end{array} \right)$$

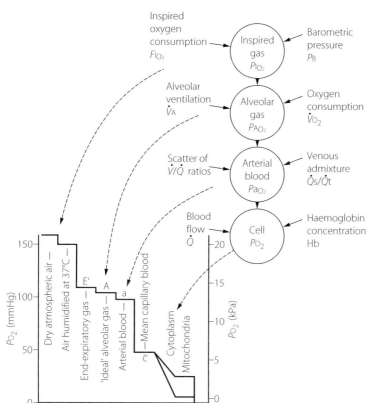

Figure 11.1 On the left is shown the oxygen cascade with PO_2 falling from the level in the ambient air down to the level in mitochondria. On the right is a summary of the factors influencing oxygenation at different levels in the cascade.

(the quantity in parentheses is known as the dry barometric pressure). Therefore the effective PO_2 of inspired air at a body temperature of 37°C is:

$$0.2094 \times (101.3 - 6.3) = 0.2094 \times 95$$
$$= 19.9\,\text{kPa}$$

or, in mmHg:

$$0.2094 \times (760 - 47) = 0.2094 \times 713$$
$$= 149\,\text{mmHg}$$

Primary factors influencing alveolar oxygen tension

Dry barometric pressure. If other factors remain constant, the alveolar PO_2 will be directly proportional to the dry barometric pressure. Thus with increasing altitude, alveolar PO_2 falls progressively to become zero at 19 kilometres, where the actual barometric pressure equals the saturated vapour pressure of water at body temperature (see Table 17.1). The effect of increased pressure is complex (see Chapter 18); for example, a pressure of 10 atmospheres (absolute) increases the alveolar PO_2 by a factor of about 15 if other factors remain constant (see Table 18.1).

Inspired oxygen concentration. The alveolar PO_2 will be raised or lowered by an amount equal to the change in the inspired gas PO_2, provided that other factors remain constant. Because the concentration of oxygen in the inspired gas should always be under control, it is a most important therapeutic tool that may be used to counteract a number of different factors that may impair oxygenation.

Figure 11.2 shows the effect of an increase in the inspired oxygen concentration from 21% to 30% on the relationship between alveolar PO_2 and alveolar ventilation. For any alveolar ventilation, the improvement of alveolar PO_2 will be 8.5 kPa (64 mmHg). This will be of great importance if, for example, hypoventilation while breathing air has reduced the alveolar PO_2 to 4 kPa (30 mmHg), a value that presents a significant threat to life. Oxygen enrichment of inspired gas to 30% will then increase the alveolar PO_2 to 12.5 kPa (94 mmHg), which is almost within the normal range. However, at this level of hypoventilation, arterial PCO_2 would be about 13 kPa (98 mmHg) and might well have risen further on withdrawal of the hypoxic drive to ventilation. In fact, 30% is the maximum concentration of oxygen in the inspired gas that should be required to correct the alveolar PO_2 of a patient breathing air who has become hypoxaemic

Figure 11.2 The effect on alveolar P_{O_2} of increasing the inspired oxygen concentration from 21% (thin curve) to 30% (heavy curve). In this example, the alveolar P_{O_2} is reduced to a dangerously low level when breathing air at an alveolar minute ventilation of 1.5 l.min⁻¹. In this situation, oxygen enrichment of the inspired gas to 30% is sufficient to raise the alveolar P_{O_2} almost to within the normal range. Oxygen consumption is assumed to be 200 ml.min⁻¹ (STPD).

Figure 11.3 The relationship between alveolar ventilation and alveolar P_{O_2} for different values of oxygen consumption for a patient breathing air at normal barometric pressure. The figures on the curves indicate the oxygen consumption in ml.min⁻¹ (STPD). A value of 100 ml.min⁻¹ is typical of a hypothermic patient at 30°C; 200 ml.min⁻¹ a normal subject at rest or during anaesthesia; higher values result from exercise or fever. Note that the alveolar ventilation required to maintain any particular alveolar P_{O_2} is directly proportional to the oxygen consumption. (In calculations of this type it is important to make the correction required by the fact that oxygen consumption and alveolar ventilation values are commonly expressed at different temperatures and pressures – see Appendix C.)

purely as a result of hypoventilation. This problem is discussed further in Chapter 27 (pages 371 *et seq.*).

An entirely different problem is hypoxaemia due to venous admixture. This results in an increased alveolar/arterial P_{O_2} difference which, within limits, can be offset by increasing the alveolar P_{O_2}. Quantitative aspects are quite different from the problem of hypoventilation and are considered later in this chapter.

Oxygen consumption. In the past there has been an unfortunate tendency to consider that all patients consume 250 ml of oxygen per minute under all circumstances. Oxygen consumption must, of course, be raised by exercise but is often well above basal in a patient supposedly 'at rest'. This may be due to restlessness, pain, increased work of breathing, shivering or fever. These factors may well coexist with failure of other factors controlling the arterial P_{O_2}. Thus, for example, a patient may be caught by the pincers of a falling ventilatory capacity and a rising ventilatory requirement (see Figure 27.4).

Figure 11.3 shows the effect of different values for oxygen consumption on the relationship between alveolar ventilation and alveolar P_{O_2} for a patient breathing air and clearly shows the potential for an increase in oxygen consumption to cause hypoxia. Altered oxygen consumption is very common in patients, being substantially increased with sepsis, thyrotoxicosis or convulsions, the first of which may lead to difficulties with weaning patients from artificial ventilation (page 430). Oxygen consumption is reduced with general anaesthesia, hypothyroidism or hypothermia, the last of which causes a marked reduction in oxygen consumption, with values of about 50% of normal at 31°C.

Alveolar ventilation. The alveolar air equation (page 128) implies a hyperbolic relationship between alveolar PO_2 and alveolar ventilation. This relationship, which is considered in Appendix F, is clinically very important. As ventilation is increased, the alveolar PO_2 rises asymptotically towards (but never reaches) the PO_2 of the inspired gas (see Figure 11.2). It will be seen from the shape of the curves that changes in ventilation above the normal level have comparatively little effect on alveolar PO_2. In contrast, changes in ventilation below the normal level may have a very marked effect. At very low levels of ventilation, the alveolar ventilation becomes critical and small changes may precipitate severe hypoxia. Note that there is a finite alveolar ventilation at which alveolar PO_2 becomes zero.

Secondary factors influencing alveolar oxygen tension

Cardiac output. In the short term, cardiac output can influence the alveolar PO_2. For example, if other factors remain constant, a sudden reduction in cardiac output will temporarily increase the alveolar PO_2, because less blood passes through the lungs to remove oxygen from the alveolar gas. However, the reduced cardiac output also causes increased oxygen extraction in the tissues supplied by the systemic circulation and before long the mixed venous oxygen level is decreased. When that has happened, the removal of oxygen from the alveolar gas returns to its original level as the reduction in blood flow rate is compensated by the greater amount of oxygen that is taken up per unit volume of blood flowing through the lungs. Thus, in the long term, cardiac output does not directly influence the alveolar PO_2 and therefore it does not appear in the alveolar air equation.

The 'concentration', third gas or Fink effect. The diagrams and equations above have ignored a factor that influences alveolar PO_2 during exchanges of large quantities of soluble gases such as nitrous oxide. This effect was mentioned briefly in connection with carbon dioxide on page 157, but its effect on oxygen is probably more important. During the early part of the administration of nitrous oxide, large quantities of the more soluble gas

replace smaller quantities of the less soluble nitrogen previously dissolved in body fluids. There is thus a net transfer of 'inert' gas from the alveoli into the body, causing a temporary increase in the alveolar concentration of both oxygen and carbon dioxide, which will thus temporarily exert a higher tension than would otherwise be expected. Conversely, during recovery from nitrous oxide anaesthesia, large quantities of nitrous oxide leave the body to be replaced by smaller quantities of nitrogen. There is thus a net outpouring of 'inert' gas from the body into the alveoli, causing dilution of oxygen and carbon dioxide, both of which will temporarily exert a lower tension than would otherwise be expected. There may then be temporary hypoxia, the direct reduction of alveolar PO_2 sometimes being exacerbated by ventilatory depression due to decreased alveolar PCO_2. Fortunately such effects last only a few minutes, and hypoxia can easily be avoided by small increases in the inspired oxygen concentration when nitrous oxide administration is stopped.

The alveolar/arterial PO_2 difference

The next step in the oxygen cascade is of great clinical relevance. In the healthy young adult breathing air, the alveolar/arterial PO_2 difference does not exceed 2 kPa (15 mmHg) but it may rise to above 5 kPa (37.5 mmHg) in aged but healthy subjects. These values may be exceeded in a patient with any lung disease that causes shunting or mismatching of ventilation to perfusion. An increased alveolar/arterial PO_2 difference is the commonest cause of arterial hypoxaemia in clinical practice and it is therefore a very important step in the oxygen cascade.

Unlike the alveolar PO_2, the alveolar/arterial PO_2 difference cannot be predicted from other more easily measured quantities. There is no simple means of knowing the magnitude of the alveolar/arterial PO_2 difference in a particular patient other than by measurement of the arterial blood gas tensions and calculation of alveolar PO_2. Therefore, it is particularly important to understand the factors that influence the difference, and the principles of restoration of arterial PO_2 by increasing the inspired oxygen concentration when hypoxia is due to an increased alveolar/arterial PO_2 difference.

Factors influencing the magnitude of the alveolar/arterial PO_2 difference

In Chapter 8 it was explained how the alveolar/arterial PO_2 difference results from venous admixture (or physiological shunt), which consists of two components: (1) shunted venous blood that mingles with the oxygenated blood leaving the pulmonary capillaries; (2) a component due to scatter of ventilation/perfusion ratios in different parts of the lungs. Any component due to impaired diffusion across the alveolar/capillary membrane is likely to be very small and in most circumstances can probably be ignored.

Figure 8.10 shows the derivation of the following axiomatic relationship for the first component, shunted venous blood:

$$\frac{\dot{Q}s}{\dot{Q}t} = \frac{Cc'_{O_2} - Ca_{O_2}}{Cc'_{O_2} - C\bar{v}_{O_2}}$$

Two points should be noted.

1. The equation gives a slightly false impression of precision because it assumes that all the shunted blood has the same oxygen content as mixed venous blood. This is not the case, Thebesian and bronchial venous blood being obvious exceptions (see Figure 7.1).
2. Oxygen content of pulmonary end-capillary blood (Cc'_{O_2}) is, in practice, calculated on the basis of the end-capillary oxygen tension (Pc'_{O_2}) being equal to the 'ideal' alveolar P_{O_2} which is derived by means of the alveolar air equation (see page 128).

The equation may be cleared and solved for the pulmonary end-capillary/arterial oxygen content difference as follows:

$$Cc'_{O_2} - Ca_{O_2} = \frac{\dfrac{\dot{Q}s}{\dot{Q}t}(Ca_{O_2} - C\bar{v}_{O_2})}{1 - \dfrac{\dot{Q}s}{\dot{Q}t}} \qquad (1)$$

(Scaling factors are required to correct for the inconsistency of the units which are customarily used for the quantities in this equation.)

$Ca_{O_2} - C\bar{v}_{O_2}$ is the arterial/mixed venous oxygen content difference and is a function of the oxygen consumption and the cardiac output, thus:

$$\dot{Q}t(Ca_{O_2} - C\bar{v}_{O_2}) = \dot{V}_{O_2} \qquad (2)$$

Substituting for $Ca_{O_2} - C\bar{v}_{O_2}$ in equation (1), we have:

$$Cc'_{O_2} - Ca_{O_2} = \frac{\dot{V}_{O_2}\dfrac{\dot{Q}s}{\dot{Q}t}}{\dot{Q}t\left(1 - \dfrac{\dot{Q}s}{\dot{Q}t}\right)} \qquad (3)$$

This equation shows the content difference in terms of oxygen consumption ($\dot{V}_{O_2}$), the venous admixture ($\dot{Q}s/\dot{Q}t$) and the cardiac output ($\dot{Q}t$).

The final stage in the calculation is to convert the end-capillary/arterial oxygen *content* difference to the *tension* difference. The oxygen content of blood is the sum of the oxygen in physical solution and that which is combined with haemoglobin:

Oxygen content of blood $= \alpha P_{O_2} + (S_{O_2} \times [Hb] \times 1.31)$

where α is the solubility coefficient of oxygen in blood (not plasma); S_{O_2} is the haemoglobin saturation and varies with P_{O_2} according to the oxygen dissociation curve, which itself is influenced by temperature, pH and base excess (Bohr effect); [Hb] is the haemoglobin concentration ($g.dl^{-1}$); and 1.31 is the volume of oxygen (ml) that has been found to combine with 1 g of haemoglobin (page 176). Carriage of oxygen in the blood is discussed in detail on pages 174 *et seq.*

Derivation of the oxygen content from the P_{O_2} is laborious if due account is taken of pH, base excess, temperature and haemoglobin concentration. Derivation of P_{O_2} from content is even more laborious, as an iterative approach is required. Tables of tension/content relationships are therefore particularly useful, and Table 11.1 is an extract from one such table to show the format and general influence of the several variables.[1]

The principal factors influencing the magnitude of the alveolar/arterial P_{O_2} difference caused by venous admixture may be summarised as follows.

The magnitude of the venous admixture increases the alveolar/arterial P_{O_2} difference with direct proportionality for small shunts, although this is lost with larger shunts (Figure 11.4). The resultant effect on arterial P_{O_2} is shown in Figure 8.11. Different forms of venous admixture are considered on pages 122 *et seq.*

$\dot{V}/\dot{Q}$ scatter. It was explained in Chapter 8 that scatter in ventilation/perfusion ratios produces an alveolar/arterial P_{O_2} difference for the following reasons.

1. More blood flows through the underventilated overperfused alveoli and the mixed arterial blood is therefore heavily weighted in the direction of the suboxygenated blood from areas of low $\dot{V}/\dot{Q}$ ratio. The smaller amount of blood flowing through areas of high $\dot{V}/\dot{Q}$ ratio cannot compensate for this (see Figure 8.12).
2. Owing to the bend in the dissociation curve around a P_{O_2} of 8 kPa, the fall in saturation of blood from areas of low $\dot{V}/\dot{Q}$ ratio tends to be greater than the rise in saturation of blood from areas of correspondingly high $\dot{V}/\dot{Q}$ (see Figure 8.13).

These two reasons in combination explain why blood from alveoli with a high $\dot{V}/\dot{Q}$ ratio cannot compensate for blood from alveoli with a low $\dot{V}/\dot{Q}$ ratio.

The actual alveolar P_{O_2} has a profound but complex and non-linear effect on the alveolar/arterial P_{O_2} gradient (see Figure 11.4). The alveolar/arterial oxygen *content* difference for a given shunt is uninfluenced by the alveolar P_{O_2} (equation 3) and the effect on the *tension* difference arises entirely in conversion from content to tension: it is thus a function of the slope of the

Table 11.1 Oxygen content of human blood (ml.dl^{-1}) as a function of Po_2 and other variables

	Haemoglobin concentration (g.dl^{-1})		
	10	14	18
Normal			
Po_2 at pH 7.4, 37°C, base excess zero:			
6.7 kPa (50 mmHg)	11.99	16.72	21.45
13.3 kPa (100 mmHg)	13.85	19.27	24.69
26.7 kPa (200 mmHg)	14.41	19.94	25.47
Respiratory acidosis			
Po_2 at pH 7.2, 37°C, base excess zero:			
6.7 kPa (50 mmHg)	10.45	14.57	18.69
13.3 kPa (100 mmHg)	13.62	18.94	24.27
26.7 kPa (200 mmHg)	14.37	19.87	25.38
Hypothermia			
Po_2 at pH 7.4, 34°C, base excess zero:			
6.7 kPa (50 mmHg)	12.81	17.87	22.93
13.3 kPa (100 mmHg)	13.96	19.43	24.89
26.7 kPa (200 mmHg)	14.44	19.98	25.51

Data are from reference 1.

dissociation curve at the Po_2 of the alveolar gas. For example, a loss of 1 ml per 100 ml of oxygen from blood with a Po_2 of 93 kPa (700 mmHg) causes a fall of Po_2 of about 43 kPa (325 mmHg), most of the oxygen being lost from physical solution. However, if the initial Po_2 were 13 kPa (100 mmHg), a loss of 1 ml per 100 ml would cause a fall in Po_2 of only 4.6 kPa (35 mmHg), most of the oxygen being lost from combination with haemoglobin. If the initial Po_2 is only 6.7 kPa (50 mmHg), a loss of 1 ml per 100 ml would cause a very small change in Po_2 of the order of 0.7 kPa (5 mmHg), drawn almost entirely from combination with haemoglobin at a point where the dissociation curve is steep.

The quantitative considerations outlined in the previous paragraph have most important clinical implications. Figure 11.4 clearly shows that, for the same degree of shunt, the alveolar/arterial Po_2 difference will be greatest when the alveolar Po_2 is highest. If the alveolar Po_2 is reduced (e.g. by underventilation), the alveolar/arterial Po_2 gradient will also be diminished if other factors remain the same. The arterial Po_2 thus falls less than the alveolar Po_2. This is fortunate and may be considered as one of the many benefits deriving from the shape of the oxyhaemoglobin dissociation curve. With a 50% venous admixture, changes in the alveolar Po_2 are almost exactly equal to the resultant changes in the alveolar/arterial Po_2 difference (see Figure 11.4). Therefore the arterial Po_2 is almost independent of changes in alveolar

Po_2, and administration of oxygen will do little to relieve hypoxia (see Figure 8.11).

Cardiac output changes have extremely complex effects on the alveolar/arterial Po_2 difference. The Fick relationship (equation 2, page 170) tells us that a reduced cardiac output *per se* must increase the arterial/mixed venous oxygen content difference if the oxygen consumption remains the same. This means that the shunted blood will be more desaturated and will therefore cause a greater decrease in the arterial oxygen level than would less desaturated blood flowing through a shunt of the same magnitude. Equation (3) shows an inverse relationship between the cardiac output and the alveolar/arterial oxygen content difference if the venous admixture is constant (Figure 11.5b). However, when the content difference is converted to tension difference, the relationship to cardiac output is no longer truly inverse but assumes a complex non-linear form in consequence of the shape of the oxyhaemoglobin dissociation curve. An example of the relationship between cardiac output and alveolar/arterial Po_2 difference is shown in Figure 11.5a, but this applies only to the conditions specified, with an alveolar Po_2 of 24 kPa (180 mmHg).

Unfortunately, the influence of cardiac output is even more complicated because it has been observed that a reduction in cardiac output is almost always associated

Figure 11.4 Influence of shunt on alveolar/arterial P_{O_2} difference at different levels of alveolar P_{O_2}. Figures in the graph indicate shunt as percentage of total pulmonary blood flow. For small shunts, the difference (at constant alveolar P_{O_2}) is roughly proportional to the magnitude of the shunt. For a given shunt, the alveolar/arterial P_{O_2} difference increases with alveolar P_{O_2} in a non-linear manner governed by the oxygen dissociation curve. At high alveolar P_{O_2}, a plateau of alveolar/arterial P_{O_2} difference is reached, but the alveolar P_{O_2} at which the plateau is reached is higher with larger shunts. Note that with a 50% shunt, an increase in alveolar P_{O_2} produces an almost equal increase in alveolar/arterial P_{O_2} difference. Therefore, the arterial P_{O_2} is virtually independent of changes in alveolar P_{O_2}, if other factors remain constant. Constants incorporated into the diagram: arterial/venous oxygen content difference, 5 ml.dl⁻¹; Hb concentration 14 g.dl⁻¹; temperature of blood, 37°C; pH of blood, 7.40; base excess, zero.

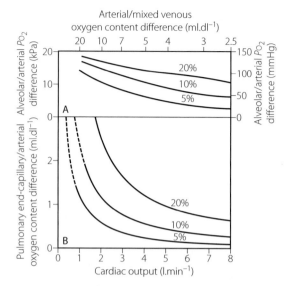

Figure 11.5 Influence of cardiac output on the alveolar/arterial P_{O_2} difference in the presence of shunts (values indicated for each curve). In this example it is assumed that the patient has an oxygen consumption of 200 ml.min⁻¹ and an alveolar P_{O_2} of 24 kPa (180 mmHg). Changes in cardiac output produce an inverse change in the pulmonary end-capillary/arterial oxygen content difference (graph b). When converted to tension differences, the inverse relationship is distorted by the effect of the oxygen dissociation curve in a manner that is applicable only to the particular alveolar P_{O_2} of the patient (graph a). (Alveolar P_{O_2} is assumed to equal pulmonary end-capillary P_{O_2}.)

with a reduction in the shunt fraction. Conversely, an increase in cardiac output usually results in an increased shunt fraction. This approximately counteracts the effect on mixed venous desaturation, so that arterial P_{O_2} tends to be relatively little influenced by changes in cardiac output (see Chapter 8, page 124). Nevertheless, it must be remembered that, even if the arterial P_{O_2} is unchanged, the oxygen delivery (flux) will be reduced in proportion to the change in cardiac output.

Temperature, pH and base excess of the patient's blood influence the oxyhaemoglobin dissociation curve (page 177). In addition, temperature affects the solubility coefficient of oxygen in blood. Thus all three factors influence the relationship between partial pressure and content (see Table 11.1) and hence the effect of venous admixture on the alveolar/arterial P_{O_2} differ-

ence, although the effect is not usually important except in extreme deviations from normal.

Haemoglobin concentration influences the partition of oxygen between physical solution and chemical combination. Although the haemoglobin concentration does not influence the pulmonary end-capillary/arterial oxygen *content* difference (equation 3), it does alter the *tension* difference. An increased haemoglobin concentration causes a small decrease in the alveolar/arterial P_{O_2} difference. Table 11.2 shows an example with a cardiac output of 5 l.min⁻¹, oxygen consumption of 200 ml.min⁻¹ and a venous admixture of 20%. This would result in a pulmonary end-capillary/arterial oxygen content difference of 0.5 ml per 100 ml. Assuming an alveolar P_{O_2} of 24 kPa (180 mmHg), the alveolar/arterial P_{O_2} difference is influenced by haemoglobin concentration, as shown in Table 11.2. (Different figures would be obtained by selection of a different value for alveolar P_{O_2}.)

Alveolar ventilation. The overall effect of changes in alveolar ventilation on the arterial P_{O_2} presents an interesting problem and serves to illustrate the integration of

Table 11.2 Effect of different haemoglobin concentrations on the arterial P_{O_2} under venous admixture conditions defined in the text

Haemoglobin concentration $g.dl^{-1}$	Alveolar/arterial P_{O_2} difference		Arterial P_{O_2}	
	kPa	mmHg	kPa	mmHg
8	15.0	113	9.0	67
10	14.5	109	9.5	71
12	14.0	105	10.0	75
14	13.5	101	10.5	79
16	13.0	98	11.0	82

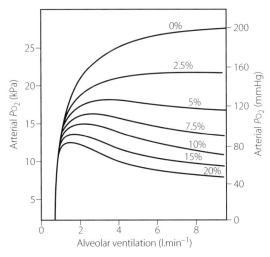

Figure 11.6 The effect of alveolar ventilation on arterial P_{O_2} is the algebraic sum of the effect upon the alveolar P_{O_2} (see Figure 11.2) and the consequent change in alveolar/arterial P_{O_2} difference (see Figure 11.4). When the increase in the latter exceeds the increase in the former, the arterial P_{O_2} will be diminished. The figures in the diagram indicate the percentage venous admixture. The curve corresponding to 0% venous admixture will indicate alveolar P_{O_2}. Constants incorporated in the design of this figure: inspired O_2 concentration, 30%; O_2 consumption, 200 ml.min^{-1}; respiratory exchange ratio, 0.8. It has been assumed that the cardiac output is influenced by the P_{CO_2} according to the equation $\dot{Q} = 0.039 \times P_{CO_2} + 2.23$ (mmHg). (Kelman GR, Nunn JF, Prys-Roberts C, Greenbaum R. The influence of cardiac output on arterial oxygenation. *Br J Anaesth* 1967; **39**: 450-8. © The Board of Management and Trustees of the British Journal of Anaesthesia. Reproduced by permission of Oxford University Press/British Journal of Anaesthesia.)

the separate aspects of the factors discussed above. An increase in the alveolar ventilation may be expected to have the following results.

1. The alveolar P_{O_2} must be raised provided the barometric pressure, inspired oxygen concentration and oxygen consumption remain the same (see Figure 11.2).
2. The alveolar/arterial P_{O_2} difference is increased for the following reasons.
   - The increase in the alveolar P_{O_2} will increase the alveolar/arterial P_{O_2} difference by the same proportion if other factors remain the same (see Figure 11.4).
   - Under many conditions it has been demonstrated that a fall of P_{CO_2} (resulting from an increase in alveolar ventilation) reduces the cardiac output, with the consequent changes that have been outlined above.
   - The change in arterial pH resulting from the reduction in P_{CO_2} causes a small, unimportant increase in alveolar/arterial P_{O_2} difference.

Thus an increase in alveolar ventilation may be expected to increase both the alveolar P_{O_2} and the alveolar/arterial P_{O_2} difference. The resultant change in arterial P_{O_2} will depend upon the relative magnitude of the two changes. Figure 11.6 shows the changes in arterial P_{O_2} caused by variations of alveolar ventilation at an inspired oxygen concentration of 30% in the presence of varying degrees of venous admixture, assuming that cardiac output is influenced by P_{CO_2} as described in the legend. Up to an alveolar ventilation of 1.5 l.min^{-1}, an increase in ventilation will always raise the arterial P_{O_2}. Beyond that, in the example cited, further increases in alveolar ventilation will increase the arterial P_{O_2} only if the venous admixture is less than 3%. For larger values of venous admixture, the increase in the alveolar/arterial P_{O_2} difference exceeds the increase in the alveolar P_{O_2} and the arterial P_{O_2} is thus decreased.

Compensation for increased alveolar/arterial P_{O_2} difference by raising the inspired oxygen concentration

Many patients with severe respiratory dysfunction are hypoxaemic while breathing air. The main objective of treatment is clearly to remove the cause of the hypoxaemia but, when this is not immediately possible, it is often possible to relieve the hypoxaemia by increasing the inspired oxygen concentration. The principles for doing so depend upon the cause of the hypoxaemia. As a broad classification, hypoxaemia may be due to hypoventilation or to venous admixture or to a combination of the two. When hypoxaemia is primarily due to hypoventilation, and when it is not appropriate or possible to restore normal alveolar ventilation, the arterial P_{O_2} can usually be restored by elevation of the inspired oxygen within the range 21–30%, as explained above (page 167 and Figure 11.2) and also in Chapter 27.

Quantitatively, the situation is entirely different when hypoxaemia is primarily due to venous admixture. It is then only possible to restore the arterial PO_2 by oxygen enrichment of the inspired gas when the venous admixture does not exceed the equivalent of a shunt of 30% of the cardiac output, and at this level may require up to 100% inspired oxygen (page 125). The quantitative aspects of the relationship are best considered in relation to the iso-shunt diagram (see Figure 8.11).

THE CARRIAGE OF OXYGEN IN THE BLOOD

The preceding section has considered in detail the factors that influence the PO_2 of the arterial blood. It is now necessary to consider how oxygen is carried in the blood and, in particular, the relationship between the PO_2 and the quantity of oxygen that is carried. The latter is crucially important to the delivery of oxygen and is no less important than the partial pressure at which it becomes available to the tissue.

Oxygen is carried in the blood in two forms. Much the greater part is in reversible chemical combination with haemoglobin, while a smaller part is in physical solution in plasma and intracellular fluid. The ability to carry large quantities of oxygen in the blood is of great importance to the organism. Without haemoglobin the amount carried would be so small that the cardiac output would need to be increased by a factor of about 20 to give an adequate delivery of oxygen. Under such a handicap, animals could not have developed to their present extent. The biological significance of the haemoglobin-like compounds is thus immense. It is interesting that the tetrapyrrole ring, which contains iron in haemoglobin, is also a constituent of chlorophyll (which has magnesium in place of iron) and the cytochromes responsible for cellular oxygen metabolism. This chemical structure is thus concerned with production, transport and utilisation of oxygen.

Physical solution of oxygen in blood

Oxygen is carried in physical solution in both red blood cells (RBCs) and plasma. There appears to have been no recent determination of the solubility coefficient, and we tend to rely on earlier studies indicating that the amount carried in normal blood in solution at 37°C is about 0.0225 ml.dl^{-1}.kPa^{-1} or 0.003 ml.dl^{-1}.mmHg^{-1}. At normal arterial PO_2, the oxygen in physical solution is thus about 0.25–0.3 ml.dl^{-1} or rather more than 1% of the total oxygen carried in all forms. However, when breathing 100% oxygen, the level rises to about 2 ml.dl^{-1}. Breathing 100% oxygen at 3 atmospheres pressure absolute (303 kPa), the amount of oxygen in physical solution rises to about 6 ml.dl^{-1}, which is sufficient for the normal resting arteriovenous extraction. The amount of oxygen in physical solution rises with decreasing temperature for the same PO_2.

Haemoglobin[3]

The haemoglobin molecule consists of four protein chains, each of which carries a haem group (Figure 11.7a), the total molecular weight being 64 458. In the commonest type of adult human haemoglobin (HbA) there are two types of chain, two of each occurring in each molecule. The two α-chains each have 141 amino acid residues, with the haem attached to a histidine residue occupying position 87. The two β-chains each have 146 amino acid residues, with the haem attached to a histidine residue occupying position 92. Figure 11.7b shows details of the point of attachment of the haem in the α-chain.

Molecular mechanisms of oxygen binding[3-5]

The four chains of the haemoglobin molecule lie in a ball like a crumpled necklace. However, the form is not random and the actual shape (the quaternary structure) is of critical importance and governs the reaction with oxygen. The shape is maintained by loose (electrostatic) bonds between specific amino acids on different chains and also between some amino acids on the same chain. One consequence of these bonds is that the haem groups lie in crevices formed by electrostatic bonds between the haem groups and histidine residues, other than those to which they are attached by normal valency linkages. For example, Figure 11.7c shows a section of an α-chain with the haem group attached to the iron atom, which is bound to the histidine residue in position 87. However, the haem group is also attached by an electrostatic bond to the histidine residue in position 58 and also by non-polar bonds to many other amino acids. This forms a loop and places the haem group in a crevice, the shape of which controls the ease of access for oxygen molecules.

In deoxyhaemoglobin, the electrostatic bonds within and between the protein chains are strong, holding the haemoglobin molecule in a tense (T) conformation, in which the molecule has a relatively low affinity for oxygen. In oxyhaemoglobin the electrostatic bonds are weaker and the haemoglobin adopts its relaxed (R) state, in which the crevices containing the haem groups can open and bind oxygen and the molecule's affinity for oxygen becomes 500 times greater than in the T state. Binding of oxygen to just one of the four protein chains induces a conformational change in the whole haemoglobin molecule, which increases the affinity of the other protein chains for oxygen. This 'cooperativity' between oxygen binding sites is fundamental to the physiological role of haemoglobin and affects the kinetics of the

a

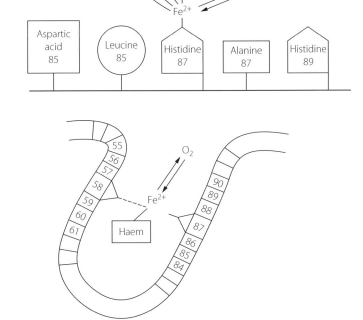

b

Figure 11.7 The haemoglobin molecule consists of four amino acid chains, each carrying a haem group. **(a)** There are two pairs of identical chains: α-chains each with 141 amino acid residues and β-chains each with 146 amino acid residues. **(b)** The attachment of the haem group to the α-chain. **(c)** The crevice that contains the haem group.

reaction between haemoglobin and oxygen, which are described below. The conformational state (R or T) of the haemoglobin molecule is also altered by other factors that influence the strength of the electrostatic bonds; such factors include carbon dioxide, pH and temperature.

The Bohr effect describes the alteration in haemoglobin oxygen affinity that arises from changes in hydrogen ion or carbon dioxide concentrations and is generally considered in terms of its influence upon the dissociation curve (see Figure 11.10 below). Changes in pH affect the numerous electrostatic bonds that maintain the quaternary structure of haemoglobin and so stabilise the molecule in the T conformation, reducing its affinity for oxygen. Similarly, carbon dioxide binds to the N-terminal amino acid residues of the α-chain to form carbaminohaemoglobin (page 151) and this small alteration in the function of the protein chains stabilises the T conformation and facilitates release of the oxygen molecule from haemoglobin.

Conversely, the Haldane effect describes the smaller amount of carbon dioxide that can be carried in oxygenated blood compared with deoxygenated blood (page 151). Crystallographic studies have shown that in deoxyhaemoglobin the histidine in position 146 of the β-chain is loosely bonded to the aspartine residue at position 94, and that when haemoglobin binds oxygen and changes to the R conformation the histidine 146 moves 10 Å further away from the aspartine, which is sufficient distance to change its pK value.[4,6] Once again, this small change in one area of the β-chains has widespread effects on electrostatic bonds throughout the molecule, changing the quaternary structure of the entire molecule and altering its ability to buffer hydrogen ions and form carbamino compounds with carbon dioxide.

Oxygen-combining capacity of haemoglobin. Until 1963, the oxygen-combining capacity of haemoglobin was taken to be 1.34 ml.g^{-1}. Following the precise determination of the molecular weight of haemoglobin, the theoretical value of 1.39 ml.g^{-1} was derived and passed into general use. However, it gradually became clear that this value was not obtained when direct measurements of haemoglobin concentration and oxygen capacity were compared. After an exhaustive study of the subject, Gregory in1974 proposed the values of 1.306 ml.g^{-1} for human adult blood and 1.312 ml.g^{-1} for foetal blood,[7] and these values are now generally accepted for clinical use.[8] Haemoglobin concentrations are ultimately compared with the International Cyan-methaemoglobin Standard, which is based on iron content and not on oxygen-combining capacity. Since some of the iron is likely to be in the form of haemochromogens, it is not surprising that the observed oxygen-combining capacity is less than the theoretical value of 1.39.

Kinetics of the reaction of oxygen with haemoglobin

Over 70 years ago Adair first proposed that the binding of oxygen to haemoglobin proceeds in four separate stages:[9]

$$Hb + 4O_2 \underset{}{\overset{K_1}{\rightleftharpoons}} HbO_2 + 3O_2 \underset{}{\overset{K_2}{\rightleftharpoons}} Hb(O_2)_2 + 2O_2$$

$$\underset{}{\overset{K_3}{\rightleftharpoons}} Hb(O_2)_3 + O_2 \underset{}{\overset{K_4}{\rightleftharpoons}} Hb(O_2)_4$$

For each of the four reactions there are two velocity constants, with small k indicating the reverse reaction (towards deoxyhaemoglobin) and small k prime (k') indicating the forward reaction. Large K is used to represent the ratio of the forward and reverse reactions, thus for example $K_1 = k'_1 / k_1$. In this way, the dissociation between deoxy- and oxyhaemoglobin may be represented by the four velocity constants K_1–K_4.

The Adair equation described assumes that the α- and β-chains of haemoglobin behave identically in their chemical reactions with oxygen, which is unlikely *in vivo*. When α- and β-chains are taken into account there are many different reaction routes that may be followed between deoxy- and oxyhaemoglobin, in theory giving rise to 16 different reversible reactions (Figure 11.8).[10] However, the multiple separate forward and reverse reactions can again be combined to give a single value for K, which does not differ significantly from those obtained using the simpler Adair equation.

In both cases, the separate velocity constants have been measured[10] and values for K_1–K_4 are shown in Figure 11.8. It can be seen that the last reaction has a forward velocity that is many times higher than that of the other reactions. During the oxygenation of the last 25% of deoxyhaemoglobin, the last reaction will predominate and the high velocity constant counteracts the effect of the ever-diminishing number of oxygen-binding sites that would otherwise slow the reaction rate by the law of mass action. The magnitude of the forward reaction for K_4 also explains why the dissociation of oxyhaemoglobin is somewhat slower than its formation.

The velocity constant of the combination of carbon monoxide with haemoglobin is of the same order, but the rate of dissociation of carboxyhaemoglobin is extremely slow by comparison.

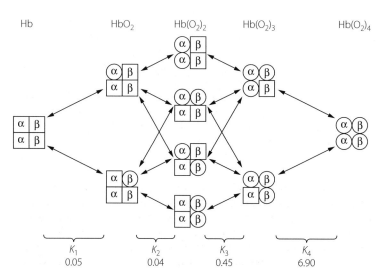

Figure 11.8 Oxygenation of tetrameric haemoglobin. If chemical interactions with oxygen differ between α- and β-chains then the transition from deoxyhaemoglobin to fully oxygenated haemoglobin can take a variety of routes, as shown. Arrows indicate the 16 possible separate dissociation equilibria, which must be combined to derive the four Adair constants K_1–K_4, the values of which are indicated. It can be clearly seen that the final stage of oxygenation is considerably faster than the previous three.[10]

K_1	K_2	K_3	K_4
0.05	0.04	0.45	6.90

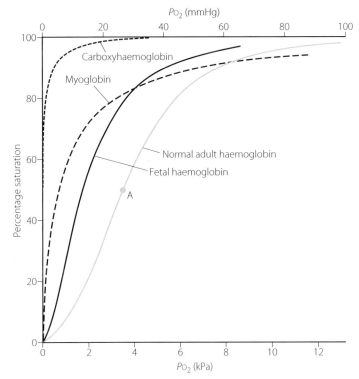

Figure 11.9 Dissociation curves of normal adult and fetal haemoglobins. Curves for myoglobin and carboxyhaemoglobin are shown for comparison. Point A is the P_{50} for this curve and shows the oxygen tension at which the Hb saturation is 50%. Notes: (1) Foetal haemoglobin is adapted to operate at a lower Po_2 than adult blood. (2) Myoglobin approaches full saturation at Po_2 levels normally found in voluntary muscle (2–4 kPa, 15–30 mmHg); the bulk of its oxygen can only be released at very low Po_2 during exercise. (3) Carboxyhaemoglobin can be dissociated only by the maintenance of very low levels of Pco.

The oxyhaemoglobin dissociation curve

As a result of the complex kinetics of the chemical reaction between oxygen and haemoglobin, the relationship between Po_2 and percentage saturation of haemoglobin is non-linear and the precise form of the non-linearity is of fundamental biological importance. It is shown, under standard conditions, in graphical form for adult and fetal haemoglobin and also for myoglobin and carboxyhaemoglobin in Figure 11.9.

Equations to represent the dissociation curve. An 'S' shaped oxyhaemoglobin dissociation curve was first described by Bohr in 1904 (page 221 and Figure 13.11). Adair[9] and Kelman[11] subsequently developed equations that would reproduce the observed oxygen dissociation curve, using a variety of coefficients. Kelman's equation, which uses seven coefficients, generates a curve indistinguishable from the true curve above a Po_2 of about 1 kPa (7.5 mmHg) and this has remained the standard. Calculation of Po_2 from saturation requires an iterative approach, but saturation may be conveniently determined from Po_2 by computer, a calculation that is automatically carried out by most blood gas analysers in clinical use, many of which do not actually measure oxygen saturation. The following simplified version of the Kelman equation is convenient to use and yields similar results at Po_2 values above 4 kPa (30 mmHg):[12]

$$SO_2 = \frac{100(PO_2^3 + 2.667 \times PO_2)}{PO_2^3 + 2.667 \times PO_2 + 55.47}$$

(Po_2 values here are in kilopascals; SO_2 is percentage).

This equation takes no account of the position of the dissociation curve as described in the next section, so must be used with caution in clinical situations.

Factors causing displacement of the dissociation curve

Several physiological and pathological changes to blood chemistry cause the normal dissociation curve to be displaced in either direction along its X axis. A convenient approach to quantifying a shift of the dissociation curve is to indicate the Po_2 required for 50% saturation and, under the standard conditions shown in Figure 11.9, this is 3.5 kPa (26.3 mmHg). Referred to as the P_{50}, this is the usual method of reporting shift of the dissociation curve.

The Bohr effect, as a result of changes in blood pH, is shown in Figure 11.10. Shifts may be defined as the ratio of the Po_2 that produces a particular saturation under standard conditions, to the Po_2 which produces the same saturation with a particular shift of the curve. Standard conditions include pH 7.4, temperature 37°C and

Figure 11.10 The Bohr effect and its effect upon oxygen tension. The centre curve is the normal curve under standard conditions; the other two curves show the displacement caused by differing blood pH as indicated, other factors remaining constant. The venous points have been determined on the basis of a fixed arterial/mixed venous oxygen saturation difference of 25%. They are thus 25% saturation less than the corresponding arterial saturation, which is equivalent to a P_{O_2} of 13.3 kPa (100 mmHg) in each case. Under the conditions shown, alkalosis lowers venous P_{O_2} and acidosis raises venous P_{O_2}. Temperature, 37°C; base excess, zero.

zero base excess. In Figure 11.10, a saturation of 80% is produced by P_{O_2} 6 kPa (45 mmHg) at pH 7.4 (standard). At pH 7.0 the P_{O_2} required for 80% saturation is 9.4 kPa (70.5 mmHg). The ratio is 0.64 and this applies to all saturations at pH 7.0.

Temperature has a large influence on the dissociation curve with a left shift in hypothermia and vice versa.

Base excess is a parameter derived from blood pH and P_{CO_2} to quantify the metabolic (as opposed to respiratory) component of an observed change in blood pH. Compared with pH itself, alterations in base excess have only a small effect on the position of the dissociation curve but must be taken into account for accurate results.

Quantifying displacement of the haemoglobin dissociation curve.

Estimation of haemoglobin saturation from P_{O_2} using the modified Kelman equation has been shown above. However, this equation assumes a normal P_{50}, so will yield erroneous results in all but the most 'normal' physiological circumstances. In clinical practice, the type of patient who requires blood gas measurement invariably also has abnormalities of pH, temperature and base excess. Nomograms may be used to determine the required correction factors before using the modified

Kelman equation above.[13] Alternatively, automated calculation of saturation from P_{O_2} by blood gas analysers routinely takes these factors into account, using a variety of equations to correct for dissociation curve displacement, of which one example is:[14,15]

$$\text{Corrected } P_{O_2} = P_{O_2} \times 10^{[0.48(pH-7.4)-0.024(T-37)-0.0013\times base\ excess]}$$

where P_{O_2} is in kPa and temperature (T) in °C. The corrected P_{O_2} may then be entered into any version of the haemoglobin dissociation curve equation as shown above (page 177).[15]

Clinical significance of displacement of the haemoglobin dissociation curve.

The important effect is on tissue P_{O_2} and the consequences of a shift in the dissociation curve are not intuitively obvious. It is essential to think quantitatively. For example, a shift to the right (caused by low pH or high temperature) impairs oxygenation in the lungs but aids release of oxygen in the tissues. Do these effects in combination increase or decrease tissue P_{O_2}? An illustrative example is set out in Figure 11.10. The arterial P_{O_2} is assumed to be 13.3 kPa (100 mmHg) and there is a decrease in arterial saturation with a reduction of pH. At normal arterial P_{O_2} the effect on arterial saturation is relatively small, but at the venous point the position is quite different and the examples in Figure 11.10 show the venous oxygen tensions to be very markedly affected. Assuming that the arterial/venous oxygen saturation difference is constant at 25% it will be seen that at low pH the venous P_{O_2} is raised to 6.9 kPa (52 mmHg), whereas at high pH the venous P_{O_2} is reduced to 3.5 kPa (26 mmHg). This is important, as the tissue P_{O_2} equates more closely to the venous P_{O_2} than to the arterial P_{O_2}. Thus, in the example shown, the shift to the right is beneficial for tissue oxygenation.

It is a general rule that a shift to the right (increased P_{50}) will benefit venous P_{O_2}, provided that the arterial P_{O_2} is not critically reduced. Below an arterial P_{O_2} of about 5 kPa (38 mmHg), the arterial point is on the steep part of the dissociation curve and the deficiency in oxygenation of the arterial blood would outweigh the improved off-loading of oxygen in the tissues. Thus, with severe arterial hypoxaemia, the venous P_{O_2} would tend to be reduced by a shift to the right and a *leftward* shift would then be advantageous. It is therefore of great interest that a spontaneous leftward shift occurs at extreme altitude when arterial P_{O_2} is critically reduced (see below).

2,3-Diphosphoglycerate

For many years it has been known that the presence of certain organic phosphates in the RBC has a pronounced effect on the P_{50}. The most important of these compounds is 2,3-diphosphoglycerate (DPG),[16] one mole-

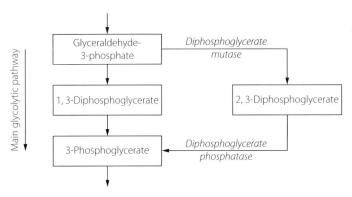

Figure 11.11 Rapoport-Luebering shunt for synthesis of 2,3-diphosphoglycerate.

cule of which becomes bound by electrostatic bonds between the two β-chains, stabilising the T conformation of haemoglobin,[3] reducing its oxygen affinity and so displacing the dissociation curve to the right. The percentage of haemoglobin molecules containing a DPG molecule governs the overall P_{50} of a blood sample within the range 2–4.5 kPa (15–34 mmHg).

DPG is formed in the Rapoport-Luebering shunt off the glycolytic pathway and its level is determined by the balance between synthesis and degradation (Figure 11.11). Activity of DPG mutase is enhanced and DPG phosphatase diminished at high pH, which thus increases the level of DPG.

The relationship between DPG levels and P_{50} suggested that DPG levels would have a most important bearing on clinical practice. Much research effort was devoted to investigating those conditions that might result in substantial changes in DPG levels and possible therapeutic avenues involving the manipulation of DPG levels.[17] In general it may be said that this research failed to substantiate the theoretical importance of DPG for oxygen delivery. In fact, the likely effects of changes in P_{50} mediated by DPG seem to be of marginal significance in comparison with changes in arterial PO_2, acid–base balance and tissue perfusion.[18]

DPG levels with blood storage and transfusion remains the only area where red cell DPG levels may have significant effects in clinical practice. Storage of blood for transfusion at below 6°C reduces glycolysis to less than 5% of normal rates and so reduces DPG production by a similar amount. Thus, after 1–2 weeks of storage, red cell DPG levels are effectively zero. Blood preservation solutions have evolved through the years to include the addition of dextrose to encourage glycolytic activity, citrate to buffer the resulting lactic acid and adenine or phosphate to help maintain ATP levels. Thus storage of blood with citrate-phosphate-dextrose (CPD) reduces the rate of DPG depletion compared with older preservation solutions,[19] but levels still become negligible within 2 weeks.

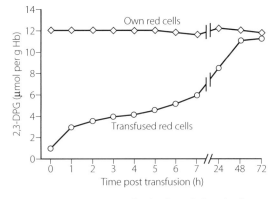

Figure 11.12 Restoration of red cell 2,3-diphosphoglycerate (DPG) levels following blood transfusion. The type O transfused red cells were stored for 35 days in CPD-A preservative solution before being given to type A volunteers. Red cells were subsequently separated into the transfused cells and the volunteer's own cells before analysis. The clinical implications of this slow return to normal DPG levels are unclear; see text for details. (Reproduced with permission from Heaton A, Keegan T, Holme S. In vivo regeneration of red cell 2,3-diphosphoglycerate following transfusion of DPG-depleted AS-1, AS-3 and CPDA-1 red cells. *Br J Haematol* 1989; **71**: 131–136.)

Once transfused, the red blood cells are quickly warmed and provided with all required metabolites, and the limiting factor for return to normal DPG levels will be reactivation of DPG mutase (see Figure 11.11). *In vivo* studies in healthy volunteers indicate that DPG levels in transfused red cells are approximately 50% of normal 7 hours after transfusion, and pretransfusion levels are not achieved until 48 hours (Figure 11.12).[20] This ingenious study involved the administration of 35-day-old CPD-adenine preserved type O blood to type A volunteers, and then in repeated venous samples red cells were separated according to their blood group before measuring DPG levels. In this way, DPG levels of both the recipients' own cells and the transfused cells could be monitored separately (see Figure 11.12).

The clinical significance of the slow return to normal DPG levels is uncertain and in most cases likely to be minimal, as the proportion of the patient's haemoglobin that consists of transfused blood will usually be small. However, rapid transfusion of large volumes of DPG depleted blood does result in a reduced P_{50}, which will in theory impair tissue oxygenation (page 178). However, in humans, little evidence has been found of tissue hypoxia under these circumstances, with no changes in cardiac output or oxygen consumption following transfusion with DPG-depleted blood.[21,22] Changes in the P_{50} of a patient do not usually exceed 0.5 kPa (3.8 mmHg), and it is possible that changes in the haemoglobin dissociation curve are compensated for by changes in blood flow at a capillary level.[23]

Other causes of altered DPG levels. Anaemia results in a raised DPG level, with P_{50} of the order of 0.5 kPa (3.8 mmHg) higher than control levels.[24] The problem of oxygen delivery in anaemia is considered in Chapter 25.

Altitude causes an increased red cell concentration of DPG. However, there is a progressive respiratory alkalosis with increasing altitude, which has an opposite and much more pronounced effect on displacement of the dissociation curve. There is now a firm consensus that there is a *leftward* displacement of the haemoglobin dissociation curve at high altitude (see Chapter 17).

Normal arterial P_{O_2}

In contrast to the arterial P_{CO_2}, the arterial P_{O_2} shows a progressive decrease with age. Using the pooled results from 12 studies of healthy subjects, one review suggested the following relationship in subjects breathing air:[25]

Arterial P_{O_2} = 13.6 − 0.044 × age in years (kPa)
or   = 102 − 0.33 × age in years (mmHg)

About this regression line there are 95% confidence limits of ±1.33 kPa (10 mmHg) (Table 11.3). Five

percent of normal patients will lie outside these limits and it is therefore preferable to refer to this as the reference range rather than the normal range.

It seems likely that some of the scatter of values for P_{O_2} is due to transient changes in ventilation, perhaps associated with arterial puncture. Because of the meagre body oxygen stores, such changes have a greater effect on P_{O_2} than on P_{CO_2}. When breathing oxygen the scatter of normal values for arterial P_{O_2} becomes even greater, usually because of technical problems with delivering an accurate concentration of oxygen (see below). Prediction of a 'normal' value against which to compare a measured arterial P_{O_2} is therefore difficult for different inspired oxygen concentrations, and 'abnormalities' of oxygenation must be interpreted against the high degree of scatter in normal subjects under normal conditions.

Nitric oxide and haemoglobin[26,27]

The enormous interest over recent years in both endogenous and exogenous nitric oxide (NO) has inevitably led to intensive research into its interaction with haemoglobin. It has been known for some time that NO binds to haemoglobin very rapidly,[28] and this observation is fundamental to its therapeutic use when inhaled NO exerts its effects in the pulmonary vasculature but is inactivated by binding to haemoglobin before it reaches the systemic circulation (page 104). There are two quite separate chemical reactions between NO and the haemoglobin molecule.[29]

1. NO binds to the haem moiety of each haemoglobin chain, but the resulting reaction differs with the state of oxygenation. For deoxyhaemoglobin, in the T conformation, a fairly stable Hb–NO complex is rapidly formed, which has little vasodilator activity, whereas for oxyhaemoglobin, in the R conformation, the oxygen is displaced by NO and in doing so the iron atom is oxidised to methaemoglobin and a nitrate ion produced:

$$Hb[Fe^{2+}] + NO \rightarrow Hb[Fe^{2+}]NO$$
$$\text{or} \quad Hb[Fe^{2+}]O_2 + NO \rightarrow Hb[Fe^{3+}] + NO_3^-$$

These reactions are so rapid that there is doubt that endogenous NO itself can exert any effects within blood (e.g. on platelets) before being bound by haemoglobin and must therefore act via an intermediate substance.

2. Nitric oxide is also known to form stable compounds with sulphydryl groups termed *S*-nitrosothiols, with the general formula R-S-NO, where the R group may be glutathione or sulphur containing amino acid residues within proteins.[30] Nitrosothiols retain biological activity as vasodilators[31] and can survive for

	Mean (95% confidence intervals)	
Age (years)	kPa	mmHg
20–29	12.5 (11.2–13.8)	94 (84–104)
30–39	12.1 (10.7–13.4)	90 (80–100)
40–49	11.6 (10.3–13.0)	87 (77–97)
50–59	11.2 (9.9–12.5)	84 (74–94)
60–69	10.7 (9.4–12.1)	81 (71–91)
70–79	10.3 (9.0–11.6)	77 (67–87)
80–89	9.9 (8.5–11.2)	74 (64–84)

Table 11.3 Normal values for arterial P_{O_2}

Figures derived from reference 25.

longer than free NO within the blood vessels. NO forms a nitrosothiol group with the cysteine residue at position 93 on the β-chains, producing *S*-nitrosohaemoglobin (SNO-Hb). As a result of conformational changes in haemoglobin the reaction is faster with R-state oxyhaemoglobin and under alkaline conditions.[29]

Thus *in vivo* NO in arterial blood is predominantly in the form of SNO-Hb, whereas in venous blood haem-bound HbNO predominates.[29] It has been proposed that as haemoglobin passes through the pulmonary capillary, changes in oxygenation, Pco_2 and pH drive the change from the deoxygenated T conformation to the oxygenated R conformation, and this change in quaternary structure of haemoglobin causes the intramolecular transfer of NO from the haem to cysteine-bound positions. In the peripheral capillaries, the opposite sequence of events occurs, which encourages release of NO from the RSNO group, where it may again bind to the haem group or be released from the RBC to act as a local vasodilator, effectively improving flow to vessels with the greatest demand for oxygen.[31,32] Export of NO activity from the RBC is believed to occur via a complex mechanism. Deoxygenated T conformation haemoglobin binds to one of the cytoplasmic domains of the RBC transmembrane band 3 protein (see Figure 10.4),[33] which may act as a metabolon (page 153) and directly transfer the NO, via a series of nitrosothiol reactions, to the outside of the cell membrane where it can exert its vasodilator activity. The vasodilator action of NO in peripheral capillaries is the same as in pulmonary capillaries and is described on page 100. The biological implications of this series of events are yet to be determined. The suggestion that haemoglobin is acting as a nitric oxide carrier to regulate capillary blood flow and oxygen release from the RBC represents a fundamental advance in our understanding of the delivery of oxygen to tissues.[27] Further evidence for this new role for haemoglobin, particularly *in vivo*, is eagerly awaited.[26,30]

Abnormal forms of haemoglobin

There are a large number of alternative amino acid sequences in the haemoglobin molecule. Most animal species have their own peculiar haemoglobins, and in humans, γ- and δ-chains occur in addition to the α- and β-monomers already described. γ- and δ-chains occur normally in combination with α-chains. The combination of two γ-chains with two α-chains constitutes foetal haemoglobin (HbF), which has a dissociation curve well to the left of adult haemoglobin (see Figure 11.9). The combination of two δ-chains with two α-chains constitutes A2 haemoglobin (HbA2), which forms 2% of the total haemoglobin in normal adults. Other variations in the amino acid chains can be considered abnormal, and, although over 600 have been reported and named, only one-third of these have any clinical effects.[34] Some abnormal haemoglobins (such as San Diego and Chesapeake) have a high P_{50} but it is more common for the P_{50} to be lower than normal (such as sickle and Kansas). In the long term, a reduced P_{50} results in excessive production of RBCs (erythrocytosis), presumed to result from cellular hypoxia in the kidney leading to erythropoietin production.[35] However, many abnormal haemoglobins also have a deranged quaternary protein structure and so are unstable, a situation that leads to haemoglobin chains becoming free within the RBC cytoplasm and membrane, causing cell lysis.[35] These patients therefore have a higher than normal rate of RBC production but are generally anaemic because of even greater degrees of RBC destruction. This combination of abnormalities results in severe long-term problems with body iron metabolism.

Sickle cell anaemia is caused by the presence of HbS in which valine replaces glutamic acid in position 6 on the β-chains. This apparently trivial substitution is sufficient to cause critical loss of solubility of reduced haemoglobin, resulting in polymerisation of HbS within the RBC, causing red cells to take on the characteristic 'sickle' shape. It is a hereditary condition and in the homozygous state is a grave abnormality, with sickling occurring at an arterial Po_2 of less than 5.5 kPa (40 mmHg), which is close to the normal venous Po_2. Thus any condition that increases the arteriovenous oxygen difference, such as infection, risks precipitating a sickle 'crisis'. Patients with sickle cell disease have varying degrees of compensatory production of HbF and the amount of HbF found in RBCs is inversely related to the severity of clinical symptoms of sickle cell disease. Thus most therapies in recent years have focused on increasing HbF synthesis by the bone marrow.[36] Heterozygous carriers of the disease only sickle below an arterial Po_2 of 2.7 kPa (20 mmHg) and so are usually asymptomatic.

Thalassaemia is another hereditary disorder of haemoglobin. It consists of a suppression of formation of HbA, again with a compensatory production of HbF, which persists throughout life instead of falling to low levels after birth. The functional disorder thus includes a shift of the dissociation curve to the left (see Figure 11.9).

Methaemoglobin[37] is haemoglobin in which the iron has been oxidised and assumes the trivalent ferric form. One way in which methaemoglobin forms is when oxyhaemoglobin acts as a nitric oxide scavenger, a process that occurs physiologically to limit the biological activity of endogenous NO or pharmacologically during treatment with inhaled NO. Other drugs may cause methaemoglobinaemia, most notably some local anaesthetics (prilocaine, benzocaine) but also nitrites and dapsone.[38] Methaemoglobin is unable to combine with oxygen but is slowly reconverted to haemoglobin in the normal subject by the action of four different systems.

1. NADH–methaemoglobin reductase system of enzymes, which is present in RBCs and uses NADH generated by glycolysis (see Figure 11.13) to reduce methaemoglobin. This system is by far the most important in normal subjects, accounting for over two-thirds of methaemoglobin-reducing activity, and is deficient in familial methaemoglobinaemia.
2. Ascorbic acid may also bring about the reduction of methaemoglobin by a direct chemical effect, though the rate of this reaction is slow and normally only accounts for 16% of total red cell methaemoglobin reduction.[37]
3. Glutathione-based reductive enzymes have a small amount of methaemoglobin reductase activity.
4. NADPH–dehydrogenase enzyme in RBCs can reduce methaemoglobin using NADPH generated from the pentose phosphate pathway. Under physiological conditions, this system has almost no effect and is regarded as the 'reserve' methaemoglobin reductase.

Elevated methaemoglobin levels of whatever cause may be treated by the administration of either ascorbic acid or methylene blue.[37,38] The latter is extremely effective and brings about methaemoglobin reduction by activation of NADPH-dehydrogenase.

Abnormal ligands

The iron in haemoglobin is able to combine with other inorganic molecules apart from oxygen. Compounds so formed are, in general, more stable than oxyhaemoglobin and therefore block the combination of haemoglobin with oxygen. The most important of these abnormal compounds is carboxyhaemoglobin, but ligands may also be formed with nitric oxide (see above), cyanide, sulphur, ammonia and a number of other substances. In addition to the loss of oxygen-carrying power, there is also often a shift of the dissociation curve to the left.

Carboxyhaemoglobin. Carbon monoxide is well known to displace oxygen from combination with haemoglobin, its affinity being approximately 300 times greater than the affinity for oxygen. Thus in a subject with 20% of their haemoglobin bound to carbon monoxide, blood oxygen content will be reduced by a similar amount (the small contribution from dissolved oxygen will be unchanged). However, the presence of carboxyhaemoglobin also causes a leftward shift of the dissociation curve of the remaining oxyhaemoglobin, partly mediated by a reduction in DPG levels. Tissue oxygenation is

therefore impaired to an even greater extent than simply reducing the amount of haemoglobin available for oxygen carriage. This situation contrasts with that of anaemia, where P_{50} is increased so the reduced oxygen carrying capacity is partially alleviated by an improved unloading of oxygen in the tissues (page 178). Exposure to atmospheric carbon monoxide is considered in Chapter 20.

Blood substitutes[39,40]

There are obvious advantages in the provision of an artificial oxygen-carrying solution that would avoid the infectious and antigenic complications seen with transfusion of another individual's red cells. The search for a blood substitute has followed two quite different parallel paths.

Perfluorocarbons.[41] Oxygen is highly soluble in these hydrophobic compounds, which with an 8–10 carbon chain are above the critical molecular size to act as anaesthetics. Perfluorooctyl bromide (Perflubron) is a 60% emulsion, which will carry about 50 ml of oxygen per 100 ml on equilibration with 100% oxygen at normal atmospheric pressure. Since oxygen is in physical solution in fluorocarbons, its 'dissociation curve' is a straight line, with the quantity of dissolved oxygen being directly proportional to PO_2. Because of the requirement to maintain adequate blood constituents apart from red cells (e.g. platelets, clotting factors, blood chemistry and oncotic pressure) the proportion of blood that may be replaced by Perflubron is small, so that even when breathing 100% oxygen the additional oxygen-carrying capacity is limited. Even so, clinical trials of intravenous Perflubron are now taking place[40] and some groups have demonstrated that Perflubron administration may delay the need for blood transfusion.[42]

Droplet size in the emulsion is of the order of 0.2 µm, compared with the 5 µm diameter of an RBC. The flow resistance is considerably less than that of blood, and as it is virtually unaffected by shear rate, the rheological properties are particularly favourable at low flow rates. Fluorocarbons may therefore be useful in partial obstruction of the circulation, for example in myocardial infarction and during percutaneous transluminal coronary angioplasty.[43] Successful use of Perflubron in the lungs for liquid or partial liquid ventilation is now widely reported in premature babies (page 235), children and adults (page 416), with some benefits described.[44]

Perfluorocarbons are cleared from the circulation into the reticuloendothelial system, where they reside for varying lengths of time before being excreted unchanged from the lungs.

Modified haemoglobin solutions.[45–47] Early attempts at using RBC haemolysates resulted in acute renal failure due to the stroma from the RBC rather than the free haemoglobin. Development of stroma-free haemoglobin solutions failed to solve the problem because although relatively stable *in vitro*, the haemoglobin tetramer dissociates in the body into dimers, which are excreted in the urine. This results in a half-life of only 2–4 hours. Other problems include the absence of DPG, resulting in a low P_{50} and a high colloid oncotic pressure, limiting their use to a maximum oncentration of 7 g.dl^{-1}.[39] The short half-life and high oncotic pressure can be improved by either polymerisation of haemoglobin molecules or encapsulation within liposomes or artificial cell membranes.[47] In addition, the haemoglobin molecules used may include recombinant human haemoglobin prepared by expression in genetically modified *E. coli*, such that both the α- and the β-chains are produced to form stable tetramers with a full complement of haem groups.[48] Clearly this approach opens possibilities for producing large quantities of blood without using donors and also modifying the properties of the haemoglobin. An example of this is the deliberate production of a specific variant of human haemoglobin (Presbyterian Hb) which has a naturally higher P_{50}.[49] Bovine haemoglobin has attracted interest due to its unique property of not needing DPG to lower oxygen affinity, having a P_{50} of 3.7 kPa (28 mmHg) in conditions found in the human circulation.[39]

Clinical trials in man of various modified haemoglobin solutions are advanced and side effects seem to be mostly minor.[39,40] Some solutions have been found to produce pulmonary and systemic vasoconstriction, which is believed to result from the free haemoglobin, particularly in the tetrameric form, acting as an NO scavenger.[43,46] This problem is likely to be overcome in the future by genetic manipulation of recombinant haemoglobin, which can alter the quaternary structure of human haemoglobin in order to impair NO binding and provide a haemoglobin molecule with a normal P_{50} in the absence of 2,3-DPG.[47]

Bubbles.[50,51] The intriguing possibility of transporting oxygen in the form of microbubbles has been proposed, but has not yet been explored *in vivo*. Bubbles that are permeable to gases and less than 5 μm in diameter would in theory be able to transport oxygen through the circulation in sufficient quantities to sustain life. Such bubbles can be produced using small amounts of intravenous lipid, in effect forming a gaseous emulsion. Intravenous bubbles can exist for up to 30 minutes, but currently are used only as radiological contrast media in ultrasound investigations.

THE ROLE OF OXYGEN IN THE CELL

Dissolved molecular oxygen (dioxygen) enters into many metabolic processes in the mammalian body. Quantita-

tively much the most important is the cytochrome c oxidase system, which is responsible for about 90% of the total oxygen consumption of the body. However, cytochrome c oxidase is but one of more than 200 oxidases, which may be classified as follows.

Electron transfer oxidases. As a group, these oxidases involve the reduction of oxygen to superoxide anion, hydrogen peroxide or water, the last being the fully reduced state (see Chapter 26, Figure 26.2). The most familiar of this group of enzymes is cytochrome c oxidase. It is located in the mitochondria and is concerned in the production of the high-energy phosphate bond in adenosine triphosphate (ATP), which is the main source of biological energy. This process is described in greater detail below under the heading 'Oxidative phosphorylation'. Another member of this group of oxidases is NADPH oxidase, which is concerned in the generation of superoxide anion in phagocytes. Although the superoxide anion and its derivatives are potentially toxic, they play a major role in bacterial killing (see Chapter 26).

Oxygen transferases (dioxygenases). This group of oxygenases incorporates oxygen into substrates without the formation of any reduced oxygen product. Familiar examples are cyclooxygenase and lipoxygenase, which are concerned in the first stage of conversion of arachidonic acid into prostaglandins and leukotrienes (see Chapter 12).

Mixed function oxidases. These oxidases result in oxidation of both a substrate and a co-substrate, which is most commonly NADPH. Well-known examples are the cytochrome P-450 hydroxylases, which play an important role in detoxification. Mixed function oxidases are also concerned in the conversion of phenylalanine to tyrosine and of dopamine to noradrenaline, the co-substrate being NADPH for the former and ascorbate for the latter.

Energy production

Most of the energy deployed in the mammalian body is derived from the oxidation of food fuels, of which the most important is glucose.

$$C_6H_{12}O_6 + 6O_2 \rightarrow 6CO_2 + 6H_2O + energy$$

The equation accurately describes the combustion of glucose *in vitro*, but is only a crude, overall representation of the oxidation of glucose in the body. The direct reaction would not produce energy in a form in which it could be utilised by the body, so biological oxidation proceeds by a large number of stages with phased production of energy. This energy is not released immediately but is stored mainly by means of the reaction of adenosine diphosphate (ADP) with inorganic phosphate ion to form ATP. The third phosphate group in ATP is held by a high-energy bond that releases its energy when ATP is split back into ADP and inorganic phosphate ion during any of the myriad biological reactions requiring energy input. ADP is thus recycled indefinitely, with ATP acting as a short-term store of energy, available in a form that may be used directly for work such as muscle contraction, ion pumping, protein synthesis and secretion.

There is no large store of ATP in the body and it must be synthesised continuously as it is being used. The ATP/ADP ratio is an indication of the level of energy that is currently carried in the ADP/ATP system and the ratio is normally related to the state of oxidation of the cell. The ADP/ATP system is not the only short-term energy store in the body but it is the most important.

The uses of ATP in the body lie outside the scope of this book, but its production from ADP is highly relevant to this chapter as the most efficient methods of production of ATP require the consumption of oxygen. Complete oxidation of glucose requires a three-stage process, the first of which, glycolysis, is independent of oxygen supply.

Glycolysis and anaerobic energy production

Figure 11.13 shows detail of the glycolytic (Embden–Meyerhof) pathway for the conversion of glucose to lactic acid. Glycolysis occurs entirely within the cytoplasm and under normal conditions proceeds only as far as pyruvic acid, which then enters the citric acid cycle (see below). In RBCs, where there is an absence of the respiratory enzymes located in the mitochondria, or in other cells when cellular PO_2 falls below its critical level, lactic acid is produced. Figure 11.13 shows that, overall, four molecules of ATP are produced, but two of these are consumed in the priming stages prior to the formation of fructose-1,6-diphosphate, 6-phosphofructokinase being the rate-limiting enzyme. The conversion of glyceraldehyde-3-phosphate to 3-phosphoglyceric acid produces a hydrogen ion, which becomes bound to extramitochondrial nicotinamide adenine dinucleotide (NAD). This hydrogen cannot enter the mitochondria for further oxidative metabolism and so is taken up lower down the pathway by the reduction of pyruvic acid to lactic acid.

This series of changes is therefore associated with the net formation of only two molecules of ATP from one of glucose.

$$\text{Glucose} + 2Pi + 2ADP \rightarrow 2\text{Lactic acid} + 2ATP + 2H_2O$$

(Pi = inorganic phosphate.)

However, considerable chemical energy remains in the lactic acid which, in the presence of oxygen, can be reconverted to pyruvic acid and then oxidised in the citric acid cycle (see below), producing a further 36 molecules of ATP. Alternatively, lactic acid may be converted into liver glycogen to await more favourable conditions for oxidation. Conversion of glucose to ethyl alcohol (fermentation) provides energy without the consumption of oxygen in certain organisms but not in animals. This pathway also yields two molecules of ATP for one of glucose.

In spite of its inefficiency for ATP production, anaerobic metabolism is of great biological importance and was universal before the atmospheric PO_2 was sufficiently high for aerobic pathways (see Chapter 1). Anaerobic metabolism is still the rule in anaerobic bacteria and also in the mammalian body when energy requirements outstrip oxygen supply as, for example, during severe exercise or during hypoxia.

Aerobic energy production

The aerobic pathway permits the release of far greater quantities of energy from the same amount of substrate and is therefore used whenever possible. Under aerobic conditions, most reactions of the glycolytic pathway remain unchanged, with two very important exceptions. The conversion of glyceraldehyde-3-phosphate to 3-phosphoglyceric acid occurs in the mitochondrion, when the two NADH molecules formed may enter oxidative phosphorylation (see below) rather than producing lactic acid. Similarly, pyruvate does not continue along the pathway to lactic acid but diffuses into the mitochondria and enters the next stage of oxidative metabolism.

The citric acid (Krebs') cycle occurs within the mitochondria as shown in Figure 11.14. It consists of a series of reactions to reduce the length of the carbon chain of the molecules before adding a new 2-carbon chain (acetyl CoA) derived from glycolysis. During these reactions, six molecules of carbon dioxide are produced (for each molecule of glucose) along with a further eight molecules of NADH and one molecule of $FADH_2$. Therefore in total, each glucose molecule yields 12 hydrogen ions bound to either NAD or FAD carrier molecules.

The scheme shown in Figure 11.14 also accounts for the consumption of oxygen in the metabolism of fat. After hydrolysis, glycerol is converted into pyruvic acid while the fatty acids shed a series of 2-carbon molecules in the form of acetyl CoA. Pyruvic acid and acetyl CoA enter the citric acid cycle and are then degraded in the same manner as though they had been derived from glucose. Amino acids are dealt with in similar manner after deamination.

Oxidative phosphorylation is the final stage of energy production and again occurs in the mitochondria. The hydrogen ions from NADH or $FADH_2$ are passed along

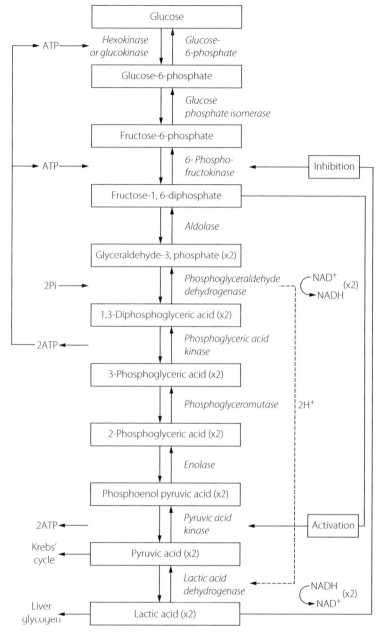

Figure 11.13 The glycolytic (Embden–Meyerhof) pathway for anaerobic metabolism of glucose. From glyceraldehyde-3-phosphate downwards, two molecules of each intermediate are formed from one of glucose. Note the consumption of two molecules of ATP in the first three steps. These must be set against the total production of four molecules of ATP, leaving a net gain of only two molecules of ATP from each molecule of glucose. All the acids are largely ionised at tissue pH.

a chain of hydrogen carriers to combine with oxygen at cytochrome a_3, which is the end of the chain. Figure 11.15 shows the transport of hydrogen along the chain, which consists of structural entities just visible under the electron microscope and arranged in rows along the cristae of the mitochondria. Three molecules of ATP are formed at various stages of the chain during the transfer of each hydrogen ion. The process is not associated directly with the production of carbon dioxide, which is formed only in the citric acid cycle.

Cytochromes have a structure similar to haemoglobin with an iron-containing haem complex bound within a large protein. Their activity is controlled by the availability of oxygen and hydrogen molecules, the local concentration of ADP, and by some unidentified cytosolic factors.[52] Different cytochromes have different values for P_{50} and so may act as oxygen sensors in several areas of the body (page 65). There is evidence for an interaction between NO and several cytochromes, with NO forming nitrosyl complexes in a similar fashion to its

Figure 11.14 Oxidative metabolic pathway of glucose by the citric acid cycle. The shaded area represents the mitochondrion and indicates the reactions that can take place only within them. The names of substances that straddle the shaded area show those that are capable of diffusion across the mitochondrial membrane. Many stages of the glycolytic pathway (see Figure 11.13) have been omitted for clarity. Note that one molecule of glucose will produce two molecules of all the other intermediate substances. Only two molecules of ATP are produced, along with 12 molecules of $NADPH_2$, each of which enters oxidative phosphorylation within the mitochondria, producing three molecules of ATP (see Figure 11.15).

reaction with haemoglobin (page 180).[32] It is postulated that NO, or NO-derived nitrosyl compounds, may play an important role in controlling oxygen consumption at a mitochondrial level. High levels of endogenous NO, for example during sepsis, may produce sufficient inhibition of cytochrome activity and therefore oxygen consumption to contribute to the impaired tissue function seen in vital organs such as the heart.[32] The reduction of oxygen to water by cytochrome a_3 is inhibited by cyanide.

Significance of aerobic metabolism. Glycolysis under aerobic conditions and the citric acid cycle yields a total of 12 hydrogen molecules for each glucose molecule used. In turn, each hydrogen molecule enters oxidative phosphorylation to yield three ATP molecules. These, along with the two produced during glycolysis (see Figure 11.13), result in a total production of 38 ATP molecules.

In simplified form, the contrasting pathways can be shown as follows.

<table>
<tr><td align="center">ANAEROBIC PATHWAY</td><td align="center">AEROBIC PATHWAY</td></tr>
<tr><td align="center">Glucose</td><td align="center">Glucose</td></tr>
<tr><td align="center">↓</td><td align="center">↓</td></tr>
<tr><td align="center">Pyruvic acid</td><td align="center">Pyruvic acid</td></tr>
<tr><td align="center">↓</td><td align="center">↓</td></tr>
<tr><td align="center">Lactic acid + 2 ATP</td><td align="center">$CO_2 + H_2O$ + 38 ATP</td></tr>
<tr><td align="center">(67 kJ of energy)</td><td align="center">(1270 kJ of energy)</td></tr>
</table>

In vitro combustion of glucose liberates 2820 kJ.mol^{-1} as heat. Thus, under conditions of oxidative metabolism, 45% of the total energy is made available for biological work, which compares favourably with most machines.

Use of anaerobic pathways must therefore either consume very much larger quantities of glucose or, alternatively, yield less ATP. In high energy-consuming organs such as brain, kidney and liver it is not, in fact, possible to transfer the increased quantities of glucose, and therefore these organs suffer ATP depletion under hypoxic conditions. In contrast, voluntary muscle is able to function satisfactorily on anaerobic metabolism for short periods, and this is normal in the diving mammals.

The critical oxygen tension for aerobic metabolism. When the mitochondrial PO_2 is reduced, oxidative phosphorylation continues normally down to a level of about 0.3 kPa (2 mmHg). Below this level, oxygen consumption falls and the various members of the electron transport chain tend to revert to the reduced state. $NADH/NAD^+$ and lactate/pyruvate ratios rise and the ATP/ADP ratio falls. The critical PO_2 varies between different organs and different species but, as an approximation, a mitochondrial PO_2 of about 0.13 kPa (1 mmHg) may be taken as the level below which there is serious impairment of oxidative phosphorylation and a switch to anaerobic metabolism. This level is, of course, far below the critical arterial PO_2, because there normally exists a large gradient of PO_2 between arterial blood and the site of utilisation of oxygen in the mitochondria, as part of the oxygen cascade (see Figure 11.1). Tissue hypoxia is discussed further on page 338. The critical PO_2 for oxidative phosphorylation is also known as the Pasteur point and has applications beyond the pathophysiology of hypoxia in man. In particular, it has a powerful bearing on putrefaction, many forms of which are anaerobic metabolism resulting from a fall of PO_2 below the Pasteur point in, for example, polluted rivers.

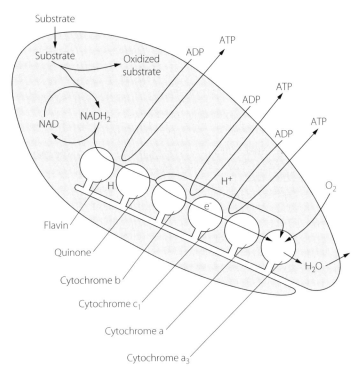

Figure 11.15 Diagrammatic representation of oxidative phosphorylation within the mitochondrion. Intramitochondrial $NADH_2$ produced from glycolysis and the citric acid cycle provides hydrogen to the first of a chain of hydrogen carriers that are attached to the cristae of the mitochondria. When the hydrogen reaches the cytochromes, ionisation occurs; the proton passes into the lumen of the mitochondrion while the electron is passed along the cytochromes, where it converts ferric iron to the ferrous form. The final stage is at cytochrome a_3, where the proton and the electron combine with oxygen to form water. Three molecules of ADP are converted to ATP at the stages shown in the diagram. ADP and ATP can cross the mitochondrial membrane freely, but there are separate pools of intra- and extramitochondrial NAD that cannot interchange.

Tissue PO_2

It is almost impossible to quantify tissue PO_2. It is evident that there are differences between different organs, with the tissue PO_2 influenced not only by arterial PO_2 but also by the ratio of tissue oxygen consumption to perfusion. However, even greater difficulties arise from the regional variations in tissue PO_2 in different parts of the same organ, which are again presumably caused by regional variations in tissue perfusion and oxygen consumption. Nor is this the whole story. As described on page 144, movement of oxygen from capillaries into the tissue is by simple diffusion, with complex radial and longitudinal gradients in PO_2 around individual capillaries (see Figure 9.4). For a single cell, the capillary PO_2 will be that of the nearest section of capillary, and so anywhere between the local arterial and venous values and the final tissue PO_2 will also depend on the distance between the capillary and the cell, which may be up to $200\,\mu m$. These factors explain why the largest drop in PO_2 of the oxygen cascade is the final stage between capillary and mitochondrial PO_2 (see Figure 11.1). In spite of this sometimes long diffusion path and low value for mitochondrial PO_2, oxygen supply is extremely efficient and it is believed to be the supply of metabolic substrates (fatty acids and glucose) that normally limit cellular energy production.[53] Tissue PO_2 is thus an unsatisfactory quantitative index of the state of oxygenation of an organ, and indirect assessments must be made (page 195).

TRANSPORT OF OXYGEN FROM THE LUNGS TO THE CELL

The concept of oxygen delivery

The most important function of the respiratory and circulatory systems is the supply of oxygen to the cells of the body in adequate quantity and at a satisfactory partial pressure. The quantity of oxygen made available to the body in one minute is known as oxygen delivery ($\dot{D}O_2$) or oxygen flux and is equal to cardiac output × arterial oxygen content.

At rest, the numerical values are approximately:

5000 ml blood per min × 20 ml O_2 per 100 ml blood

 (cardiac output) (arterial oxygen content)

        = 1000 ml O_2 per min

         (oxygen delivery)

Of this 1000 ml.min^{-1}, approximately 250 ml.min^{-1} are used by the conscious resting subject. The circulating blood thus loses 25% of its oxygen and the mixed venous blood is approximately 70% saturated (i.e. 95 – 25). The 70% of unextracted oxygen forms an important reserve that may be drawn upon under the stress of such conditions as exercise, to which additional extraction forms one of the integrated adaptations (see Figure 15.3).

Oxygen consumption must clearly depend upon delivery but the relationship is non-linear. Modest reduction of oxygen delivery is well tolerated by the body which is, within limits, able to draw on the reserve of unextracted venous oxygen without reduction of oxygen consumption. However, below a critical value for delivery, consumption is decreased and the subject shows signs of hypoxia. The important quantitative aspects of the relationship between oxygen consumption and delivery are considered below.

Quantification of oxygen delivery

The arterial oxygen content consists predominantly of oxygen in combination with haemoglobin and this fraction is given by the following expression:

$$Ca_{O_2} = Sa_{O_2} \times [Hb] \times 1.31$$

where Ca_{O_2} is the arterial oxygen content, Sa_{O_2} is the arterial oxygen saturation (as a fraction) and [Hb] is the haemoglobin concentration of the blood; 1.31 is the volume of oxygen (ml) which has been found to combine with 1 g of haemoglobin (page 176).

To the combined oxygen must be added the oxygen in physical solution, which will be of the order of 0.3 ml. dl^{-1} and the expression for total arterial oxygen concentration may now be expanded thus:

$$
\begin{array}{cccccc}
Ca_{O_2} = & (Sa_{O_2} & \times & [Hb] & \times & 1.31) + 0.3 \\
ml.dl^{-1} & \%/100 & & g.dl^{-1} & & ml.g^{-1} \quad ml.dl^{-1}
\end{array}
$$

$$\text{e.g.} \quad 19 = (0.97 \times 14.7 \times 1.31) + 0.3 \tag{4}$$

Since oxygen delivery is the product of cardiac output and arterial oxygen content:

$$
\begin{array}{ccccc}
\dot{D}_{O_2} & = & \dot{Q} & \times & Ca_{O_2} \\
ml.min^{-1} & & l.min^{-1} & & ml.dl^{-1}
\end{array}
$$

$$\text{e.g.} \quad 1000 = 5.25 \times 19 \tag{5}$$

$\dot{Q}$ is cardiac output (right-hand side is multiplied by a scaling factor of 10).

By combining equations (4) and (5) the full expression for oxygen delivery is as follows:

$$
\begin{array}{ccc}
\dot{D}_{O_2} & = & \dot{Q} \quad \times \{(Sa_{O_2} \times [Hb] \times 1.31) + 0.3\} \\
ml.min^{-1} & l.min^{-1} & \%/100 \quad g.dl^{-1} \quad ml.g^{-1} \quad ml.dl^{-1}
\end{array}
$$

$$\text{e.g. } 1000 = 5.25 \times \{(0.97 \times 14.7 \times 1.31) + 0.3\} \tag{6}$$

(right-hand side is multiplied by a scaling factor of 10).

For comparison between subjects, values for oxygen delivery must be related to body size, which is done by relating the value to body surface area. Oxygen delivery divided by surface area is known as the oxygen delivery index and has units of $ml.min^{-1}.m^{-2}$.

Interaction of the variable factors governing oxygen delivery

Equation (6) contains, on the right-hand side, three variable factors that govern oxygen delivery.

1. Cardiac output (or, for a particular organ, the regional blood flow). Failure of this factor has been termed 'stagnant anoxia'.
2. Arterial oxygen saturation. Failure of this (for whatever reason) has been termed 'anoxic anoxia'.
3. Haemoglobin concentration. Reduced haemoglobin as a cause of tissue hypoxia has been termed 'anaemic anoxia'.

The classification of 'anoxia' into stagnant, anoxic and anaemic was proposed by Barcroft in 1920[54] and has stood the test of time. The three types of 'anoxia' may be conveniently displayed on a Venn diagram (Figure 11.16), which shows the possibility of combinations of any two types of anoxia or all three together. For example, the combination of anaemia and low cardiac output that occurs in untreated haemorrhage would be indicated by the overlapping area of the stagnant and anaemic circles (indicated by X). If the patient also suffered from lung injury, he might then move into the central area, indicating the addition of anoxic anoxia. On a more cheerful note, compensations are more usual. Patients with anaemia normally have a high cardiac output; subjects resident at altitude have polycythaemia, and so on.

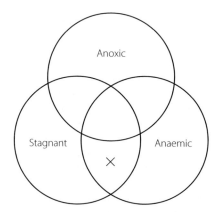

Figure 11.16 Barcroft's classification of causes of hypoxia displayed on a Venn diagram to illustrate the possibility of combinations of more than one type of hypoxia. The lowest overlap, marked with a cross, shows coexistent anaemia and low cardiac output. The central area illustrates a combination of all three types of hypoxia (e.g. a patient with sepsis resulting in anaemia, circulatory failure and lung injury).

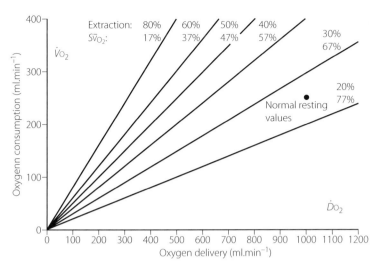

Figure 11.17 Grid relating oxygen delivery and consumption to extraction and mixed venous oxygen saturation, on the assumption of 97% saturation for arterial blood. The spot marks the normal resting values.

It is important to note that oxygen delivery equals the product of three variables and one constant. If one variable is halved, delivery is halved, but if all three variables are simultaneously halved then delivery is reduced to one-eighth of the original value. One-eighth of 1000 is 125 ml.min^{-1} and this is a value that, if maintained for any length of time, is incompatible with life, although the reduction of each individual variable is not in itself lethal.

The relationship between oxygen delivery and consumption

The relationship between $\dot{D}O_2$ and oxygen consumption ($\dot{V}O_2$) is best illustrated on the coordinates shown in Figure 11.17. The abscissa shows oxygen delivery as defined above, while consumption is shown on the ordinate. The fan of lines originating from the zero point indicate different values for oxygen extraction ($\dot{V}O_2/\dot{D}O_2$) expressed as a percentage. Because the mixed venous oxygen saturation is the arterial saturation minus the extraction, it is a simple matter to indicate the mixed venous saturation, which corresponds to a particular value for extraction. The black dot indicates a typical normal resting point, with $\dot{D}O_2$ of 1000 ml.min^{-1}, $\dot{V}O_2$ of 250 ml.min^{-1} and extraction 25%. With an arterial saturation of 95%, the mixed venous saturation will therefore be about 70%.

When oxygen delivery is moderately reduced, for whatever reason, oxygen consumption tends to be maintained at its normal value by increasing oxygen extraction and therefore decreasing mixed venous saturation. There should be no evidence of additional anaerobic metabolism, such as increased lactate production. This is termed 'supply-independent oxygenation', a condition

that applies provided that delivery remains above a critical value. This is shown by the horizontal line in Figure 11.18. Below the critical level of oxygen delivery, oxygen consumption decreases as a linear function of delivery. This is termed 'supply-dependent oxygenation' and is usually accompanied by evidence of hypoxia, such as increased blood lactate and organ failure.

Pathological supply dependency of oxygen consumption has been a source of controversy for many years.[55] In critically ill patients, the transition between supply-dependent and supply-independent oxygen consumption (critical oxygen delivery, see Figure 11.18) was thought to move to the right, such that increasing oxygen delivery continued to increase oxygen consumption even at levels greater than those seen in normal healthy subjects.[56,57] Early work in critical care units claimed better survival in patients in whom oxygen delivery, and therefore consumption, was increased above normal values.[55,58] Unfortunately, much larger randomised studies failed to confirm the benefits of this aggressive management of oxygen delivery.[59,60] Furthermore, a value for critical oxygen delivery in ill patients remained elusive,[61] mostly due to the considerable difficulties in assessing the relationship between oxygen consumption and delivery in this group. It is therefore possible that the value for critical oxygen delivery is unchanged in critically ill patients and that pathological supply dependency may not exist at all, with much of the earlier data resulting from methodological problems and mathematical coupling of the variables being measured. Outcome benefits to patients from deliberately increasing $\dot{D}O_2$ now seem to be minimal or non-existent,[59,60] and current advice is to concentrate more closely on achieving normal values for cardiac output, haemoglobin and blood volume,[55] rather than pursuing supranormal targets.

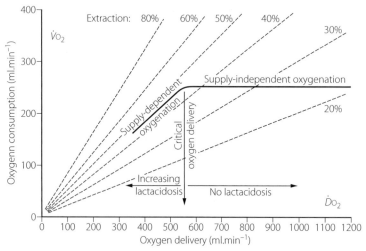

Figure 11.18 This diagram is based on the grid shown in Figure 11.17. For an otherwise healthy subject, the thick horizontal line shows the extent to which oxygen delivery can be reduced without reducing oxygen consumption and causing signs of cellular hypoxia (supply-independent oxygenation). Below the postulated critical delivery, oxygen consumption becomes supply dependent and there are signs of hypoxia. There is uncertainty about the exact values for critical delivery in otherwise healthy subjects.

Table 11.4 Principal stores of body oxygen		
	While breathing air (ml)	While breathing 100% oxygen (ml)
In the lungs (FRC)	450	3000
In the blood	850	950
Dissolved in tissue fluids	50	?100
Combined with myoglobin	? 200	?200
Total	1550	4250

FRC, functional residual capacity.

OXYGEN STORES

In spite of its great biological importance, oxygen is a very difficult gas to store in a biological system. There is no satisfactory method of physical storage in the body. Haemoglobin is the most efficient chemical carrier, but more than 0.5 kg is required to carry 1g of oxygen. The concentration of haemoglobin in blood far exceeds the concentration of any other protein in any body fluid. Even so, the quantity of oxygen in the blood is barely sufficient for 3 minutes' metabolism in the resting state. It is a fact of great clinical importance that the body oxygen stores are so small and, if replenishment ceases, they are normally insufficient to sustain life for more than a few minutes. The principal stores are shown in Table 11.4.

While breathing air, not only are the total oxygen stores very small but also, to make matters worse, only part of the stores can be released without an unaccept-

able reduction in P_{O_2}. Half of the oxygen in blood is still retained when the P_{O_2} is reduced to 3.5 kPa (26 mmHg). Myoglobin is even more reluctant to part with its oxygen and very little can be released above a P_{O_2} of 2.7 kPa (20 mmHg).

Breathing oxygen causes a substantial increase in total oxygen stores. Most of the additional oxygen is accommodated in the alveolar gas, from which 80% may be withdrawn without causing the P_{O_2} to fall below the normal value. With 2400 ml of easily available oxygen after breathing oxygen, there is no difficulty in breath holding for several minutes without becoming hypoxic.

The small size of the oxygen stores means that changes in factors affecting the alveolar or arterial P_{O_2} will produce their full effects very quickly after the change. This is in contrast to carbon dioxide, where the size of the stores buffers the body against rapid changes (page 158). Figure 11.19 compares the time course of changes in P_{O_2} and P_{CO_2} produced by the same changes in ventilation. Figure 10.11 showed how the time course of changes of P_{CO_2} is different for falling and rising P_{CO_2}.

Factors that reduce the P_{O_2} always act rapidly, but two examples of changes that produce anoxia illustrate different degrees of 'rapid'.

Circulatory arrest. When the circulation is arrested, hypoxia supervenes as soon as the oxygen in the tissues and stagnant capillaries has been exhausted. In the case of the brain, with its high rate of oxygen consumption, there is only about 10 seconds before consciousness is lost. Circulatory arrest also differs from other forms of hypoxia in the failure of clearance of products of anaerobic metabolism (e.g. lactic acid), which should not occur in arterial hypoxaemia.

Apnoea. The rate of onset of anoxia depends on the initial alveolar P_{O_2}, the lung volume and the rate of

Figure 11.19 The upper pair of curves indicate the rate of change of arterial PO_2 following a step change in ventilation. Half of the total change occurs in about 30 seconds. The rising curve could be produced by an increase of alveolar ventilation from 2 to 4 l.min^{-1} while breathing air (see Figure 11.2). The falling curve could result from the corresponding reduction of alveolar ventilation from 4 to 2 l.min^{-1}. The lower pair of broken curves indicate the time course of changes in PCO_2, which are much slower than for oxygen (these changes are shown in greater detail in Figure 10.11).

oxygen consumption. It is, for example, more rapid while swimming underwater than while breath holding at rest in the laboratory. Generally speaking, after breathing air, 90 seconds of apnoea results in a substantial fall of PO_2 to a level that threatens loss of consciousness. If a patient has previously inhaled a few breaths of oxygen, the arterial PO_2 should remain above 13.3 kPa (100 mmHg) for at least 3 minutes of apnoea, and this is the basis of the usual method of protection against hypoxia during any deliberate interference with ventilation, as for example during tracheal intubation.

In view of the rapid changes shown in Figure 11.19, it follows that, for a patient breathing air, a pulse oximeter will probably give an earlier indication of underventilation than will a carbon dioxide analyser. However, if the patient is protected from hypoxia by the inhalation of a gas mixture enriched with oxygen, then the carbon dioxide will give the earlier indication of hypoventilation. It should be remembered that oxygen levels change quickly and are potentially much more dangerous. Carbon dioxide levels change only slowly (in response to a change in ventilation) and are usually less dangerous.

CONTROL OF THE INSPIRED OXYGEN CONCENTRATION

Much of this chapter has been concerned with the theoretical basis for selection of the optimal inspired oxygen concentration for a particular pathophysiological state. It now remains to be considered how this should be put into effect.

Fixed performance systems

These allow the delivery of a known concentration of oxygen, independent of the patient's respiratory system; that is, the oxygen concentration delivered is unaffected by respiratory rate, tidal volume and inspiratory flow rate. Methods may be divided into low-flow (closed) or high-flow (open) delivery systems.

Closed delivery systems. A crucial factor in oxygen therapy is the nature of the seal between the patient's airway and the external breathing apparatus. Airtight seals may be obtained with cuffed tracheal or tracheostomy tubes or, at low airway pressures, with a tight-fitting facemask or laryngeal mask airway. These devices should give complete control over the composition of the inspired gas. Any closed delivery system requires the use of a breathing system that provides suitable separation of inspired and expired gases to prevent rebreathing and does not present significant resistance to breathing.

Open delivery systems. Most disposable oxygen masks do not attempt to provide an airtight fit. An alternative solution to the problem of the airtight seal is to provide a high flow of gas, which can vent to atmosphere between the mask and the face, thus preventing the inflow of air. The required flow of air/oxygen mixture needs to be in excess of the peak inspiratory flow rate. For normal resting ventilation this is approximately 30 l.min^{-1} but in patients with respiratory distress may be considerably greater.

Oxygen may be passed through the jet of a Venturi to entrain air. Venturi-based devices are a convenient and highly economical method of preparing high flows of oxygen mixtures in the range 25–40% concentration. For example, 3 l.min^{-1} of oxygen passed through the jet of a Venturi with an entrainment ratio of 8/1 will deliver 27 l.min^{-1} of 30% oxygen. Higher oxygen concentrations require a lower entrainment ratio and therefore a higher oxygen flow in order to maintain an adequate total delivered flow rate. Commercially available Venturi masks now have a variety of colour-coded Venturi attachments that indicate the required oxygen flow rate, the inspired oxygen concentration achieved and the total gas flow rate. With an adequate flow rate of the air/oxygen mixture, the Venturi mask need not fit the face with an airtight seal. The high flow rate escapes round the cheeks as well as through the holes in the mask and room air is effectively excluded. Numerous studies have indicated that the Venturi mask gives excellent control over the inspired oxygen concentration, with an accuracy of ±1% unaffected by variations in the ventilation of the patient.[62] There is no doubt that this is the most satisfactory method of controlling the inspired oxygen concentration of a patient who is breathing spontaneously without tracheal intubation.

Control of the patient's gaseous environment. The popularity of oxygen tents declined because of their large volume and high rate of leakage, which made it difficult to attain and maintain a high oxygen concentration unless the volume was reduced and a high gas flow rate used. In addition, the fire hazard cannot be ignored. These problems are minimised when the patient is an infant and oxygen control within an incubator is a satisfactory method of administering a precise oxygen concentration.

Hyperbaric oxygenation. Two systems are in use. One-man chambers are filled with 100% oxygen and the patient is entirely exposed to 100% oxygen at high pressure, no mask being required. Larger chambers are pressurised with air that is breathed by staff, whereas 100% oxygen is made available to the patient by means of a tight-fitting facemask.

Variable-performance devices

Simple disposable oxygen masks and nasal catheters aim to blow oxygen at or into the air passages. The oxygen is mixed with inspired air to give an inspired oxygen concentration that is a complex function of the geometry of the device, the oxygen flow rate, the patient's ventilation and whether the patient is breathing through his mouth or nose. The effective inspired oxygen concentration is impossible to predict and may vary between very wide limits.[62] These devices cannot be used for oxygen therapy when the exact inspired oxygen concentration is critical (e.g. ventilatory failure), but are useful in less critical situations such as recovery from routine anaesthesia. With simple oxygen masks a small inspiratory reservoir will store fresh gas during expiration for use during inspiration, which will tend to increase the inspired oxygen concentration but, again, in a somewhat unpredictable fashion.

With a device such as a nasal catheter or prongs, the lower the ventilation, the greater will be the fractional contribution of the fixed flow of oxygen to the inspired gas mixture. There is thus an approximate compensation for hypoventilation, with greater oxygen concentrations being delivered at lower levels of ventilation. Arterial P_{O_2} may then be maintained in spite of a progressively falling ventilation. However, this will do nothing to prevent the rise in P_{CO_2}, which may reach a dangerous level without the appearance of cyanosis to warn that all is not well.[63]

CYANOSIS

Cyanosis is a blue discoloration of a subject's skin and mucous membranes and is almost universally caused by arterial hypoxaemia. Though now regarded as a sign of rather advanced hypoxia, there must have been countless occasions in which the appearance of cyanosis has given warning of hypoventilation, pulmonary shunting, stagnant circulation or decreased oxygen concentration of inspired gas. Indeed, it is interesting to speculate on the additional hazards to life if gross arterial hypoxaemia could occur without overt changes in the colour of the blood.

Central and peripheral cyanosis

If shed arterial blood is seen to be purple, this is a reliable indication of arterial desaturation. However, when skin or mucous membrane is inspected, most of the blood that colours the tissue is lying in veins (i.e. sub-papillary venous plexuses) and its oxygen content is related to the arterial oxygen content as follows:

$$\frac{\text{venous oxygen}}{\text{content}} = \frac{\text{arterial oxygen}}{\text{content}} - \frac{\text{arterial/venous}}{\text{oxygen content}} \\ \text{difference}$$

The last term may be expanded in terms of the tissue metabolism and perfusion:

$$\frac{\text{venous}}{\text{oxygen}} = \frac{\text{arterial}}{\text{oxygen}} - \frac{\text{tissue oxygen consumption}}{\text{tissue blood flow}} \\ \text{content} \quad \text{content}$$

In normal circumstances, the oxygen consumption by the skin is usually low in relation to its circulation, so the second term on the right-hand side of the second equation is generally small. Therefore, the cutaneous venous oxygen content is close to that of the arterial blood and inspection of the skin usually gives a reasonable indication of arterial oxygen content. However, when circulation is reduced in relation to skin oxygen consumption, cyanosis may occur in the presence of normal arterial oxygen levels. This occurs typically in patients with low cardiac output or in cold weather. Vigorous coughing, particularly when lying flat, or placing a patient in the Trendelenburg position, causes the skin capillaries of the upper body to become engorged with venous blood, once again causing the appearance of cyanosis with normal arterial oxygen content.

Sensitivity of cyanosis as an indication of hypoxaemia

Two factors may affect the ability to detect cyanosis.

Anaemia. A reduced amount of haemoglobin in blood will inevitably make cyanosis less likely to occur, and for many years it was believed that 5 g.dl^{-1} of reduced haemoglobin were necessary for the detection of cyanosis. The evidence for this was poor and it is now generally found that cyanosis can be detected when *arterial* blood contains more than 1.5 g.dl^{-1} of reduced haemoglobin[64] or at an arterial oxygen saturation of 85–90%, although there is much variation. Such levels would probably correspond to a 'capillary' reduced haemoglobin concentration of about 3 g.dl^{-1}.

The importance of the source of illumination.[65] Different types of fluorescent lighting used in hospitals affect the perceived colour of a patient's skin. Some lamps tend to make the patient look pinker and others impart a bluer tinge. The former gives false negatives (no cyanosis in the presence of hypoxaemia), whereas the latter gives false positives (cyanosis in the absence of hypoxaemia). However, the total number of false results is approximately the same with all tubes. Provided all areas of the same hospital are illuminated with the same type of tube this effect is unlikely to adversely affect the assessment of a patient's colour.

Thus the appearance of cyanosis is considerably influenced by the circulation, patient position, haemoglobin concentration and lighting conditions. Even when all these are optimal, cyanosis is by no means a precise indication of the arterial oxygen level and it should be regarded as a warning sign rather than a measurement. Cyanosis is detected in about half of patients who have an arterial saturation of 93% and about 95% of patients with a saturation of 89%.[65] In other words, cyanosis is not seen in 5% of patients at or below a saturation of 89% (arterial $PO_2 \approx 7.5$ kPa or 56 mmHg). It is quite clear that absence of cyanosis does not necessarily mean normal arterial oxygen levels.

Non-hypoxic cyanosis has several causes, all of which are rare, but worth considering in a patient who appears cyanosed but displays no other evidence of hypoxia. Sulphhaemoglobin and, more importantly, methaemoglobin (at concentrations of 1.5 g.dl^{-1}) cause a blue-grey appearance[37] and chronic use of drugs or remedies that include gold or silver has been reported to cause 'pseudo-cyanosis'.[66]

PRINCIPLES OF MEASUREMENT OF OXYGEN LEVELS

Oxygen concentration in gas samples

Paramagnetic analysers rely on the fact that oxygen will influence an electrically generated magnetic field in direct proportion to its concentration in a mixture of gases.[67] A particularly attractive feature of the method for physiological use is the complete lack of interference by other gases likely to be present, as significant paramagnetic properties are unique to oxygen. Early paramagnetic analysers were cumbersome, delicate, and had slow response times, but technological progress has led to the availability of inexpensive, accurate and robust analysers that are now found in a whole range of anaesthetic and intensive care equipment.

Measurement of breath-to-breath changes in oxygen concentrations of respired gases requires an instrument with a response time of less than about 300 ms. Formerly the only suitable technique for oxygen measurement was the mass spectrometer, but modern paramagnetic analysers have much faster response times and so are easily capable of tracking breath-by-breath oxygen concentration.

Fuel cells have similarities to the polarographic electrode described below. An oxygen-permeable membrane covers a cell made up of a gold cathode and a lead anode separated by potassium hydroxide, which generates a current in proportion to the oxygen concentration. The response time is many seconds, so these analysers are not suitable for measuring inspired and expired oxygen concentrations. No electrical input is needed, the fuel cell acting like a battery generating its own power from the absorption of oxygen. However, the cell therefore also has a limited lifespan, depending on the total amount of oxygen to which it is exposed over time, but in normal clinical use fuel cells last several months.

Blood PO_2

Previous chemical-based analyses have now been completely replaced by a single method.

Polarography. This method, first described by Clark in 1956,[68] is based on a cell formed by a silver anode and a platinum cathode, both in contact with an electrolyte in dilute solution. If a potential difference of about 700 mV is applied to the cell, a current is passed that is directly proportional to the PO_2 of the electrolyte in the region of the cathode. In use, the electrolyte is separated from the sample by a thin membrane that is permeable to oxygen. The electrolyte rapidly attains the same PO_2 as the sample and the current passed by the cell is proportional to the PO_2 of the sample, which may be gas, blood or other liquids. Gas mixtures are normally used for regular calibration and an important source of error is the difference in reading between blood and gas of the same PO_2. Estimates of the ratio very between 1.0 and 1.17 but it may change unexpectedly due to changes in the position of the membrane. This source of error has been greatly reduced in modern microelectrodes, which consume much less oxygen at the cathode. The error may be detected and prevented by calibration with tonometer-equilibrated blood, which is simple to perform. Frequent measurement of PO_2 in blood samples leads to protein deposition on the membrane,

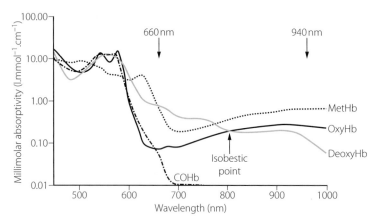

Figure 11.20 Near infrared absorption spectra for the four common types of haemoglobin seen *in vivo*. The isobestic point for oxy- and deoxyhaemoglobin is shown. To measure oxygen saturation, pulse oximeters use two wavelengths at around 660 and 940 nm, where the absorptivities of oxy- and deoxyhaemoglobin differ significantly. If measurement of carboxyhaemoglobin and methaemoglobin is also required, a greater number of wavelengths must be used and current generations of cooximeter use over 100 different wavelengths. (Data from reference 72.)

which over time forms a diffusion barrier between the sample and the electrolyte. Regular cleaning with a proteolytic solution is therefore required.

Polarographic electrodes may now be made small enough to facilitate continuous intraarterial monitoring of PO_2, and more recently a photochemical PO_2 sensor has been developed.[69] Along with pH and PCO_2 sensors (page 162), the intraarterial catheter remains less than 0.5 mm in diameter.

Errors in measuring oxygen levels. Errors arising from the handling of samples for blood gas analysis are considered on page 161. Temperature has a marked effect on PO_2 measurement. If blood PO_2 is measured at a lower temperature than the patient's, the measured PO_2 will be less than the PO_2 of the blood while it was in the patient. It is usual to maintain the measuring apparatus at 37°C, and, if the patient's body temperature differs from this by more than 1°C, then a significant error will result. Correction is possible but the factor is variable depending on the saturation.[70] Automated blood gas machines will perform this correction, provided the patient's temperature is entered; alternatively, a nomogram may be used and is included in Appendix E as Figure E.2.

Transcutaneous PO_2.[71] Cutaneous venous or capillary blood PO_2 may, under ideal conditions, be close to the arterial PO_2, but a modest reduction in skin perfusion will cause a substantial fall in PO_2 since the oxygen is consumed at the flat part of the dissociation curve, where small changes in content correspond to large changes in PO_2. As for transcutaneous PCO_2 (page 163), heating of skin to 44°C minimises differences between arterial and capillary/skin PO_2, which can be measured by a directly applied polarographic electrode. Measurement of PO_2 at this high temperature requires correction for changes in oxygen solubility.

Oxygen saturation

Blood oxygen saturation is measured photometrically. Near infrared absorption spectra for different forms of haemoglobin[72] are shown in Figure 11.20. Methods are based on the fact that the absorption of monochromatic light of certain wavelengths is the same (isobestic) for reduced and oxygenated haemoglobin (800 nm). At other wavelengths there is a marked difference between the absorption of transmitted or reflected light by the two forms of haemoglobin. Use of a greater number of different wavelengths also allows the detection and quantification of other commonly present haemoglobins. For example, current generations of cooximeter measure absorption at 128 different wavelengths and from the spectra obtained can calculate the quantities of oxyhaemoglobin, deoxyhaemoglobin, carboxyhaemoglobin and methaemoglobin.

Saturation may be derived from PO_2, a process which is performed automatically by modern blood gas analysers (page 177). This is reasonably accurate above a PO_2 of about 7.3 kPa (55 mmHg) but is inaccurate at lower tensions because, on the steep part of the curve, the saturation changes by 3% for a PO_2 change of only 0.13 kPa (1 mmHg).

Pulse oximetry.[73] Saturation may be measured photometrically *in vivo* as well as *in vitro*. Light at two different wavelengths is either transmitted through a finger or an ear lobe or else is reflected from the skin, usually on the forehead. The usual wavelengths used are 660 nm, where there is a large difference between the oxy- and deoxyhaemoglobin spectra (see Figure 11.20), and 940 nm, close to the isobestic point. With the original techniques, most of the blood that was visualised was venous or capillary rather than arterial and the result therefore depended on there being a brisk cutaneous blood flow to minimise the arterial/venous oxygen difference. The older techniques have now been completely replaced by pulse oximeters, which relate the optical densities at the two wavelengths to the pulse wave detected by the same sensor. The signal between the pulse waves is subtracted from the signal at the height of the pulse wave, the difference being due to the inflowing arterial blood and so reflecting the saturation of the arterial blood.

Instruments currently available continue to function even in the presence of severe arterial hypotension, although there is usually a delayed indication of changes in saturation.[74] Anaemia tends to exaggerate desaturation readings. At a haemoglobin concentration of 8 g.dl^{-1}, normal saturations were correctly recorded but there was a mean bias of -15% at a true saturation of 53.6%.[75] The problem was only clinically important below a saturation of about 75%. If fingers or toes are used for pulse oximetry then nail polish should be removed. Different coloured polishes cause variable decreases in the oximeter reading, with red/purple colours having very little effect and green/blue colours causing an average of 5.5% decrease in saturation readings.[76]

Pulse oximeters cannot distinguish between carboxy- and oxyhaemoglobin (see Figure 11.20).[73] Methaemoglobin is read as though it were half oxyhaemoglobin and half reduced haemoglobin up to about 20% methaemoglobin. At higher levels of methaemoglobin, pulse oximeter readings tend to become fixed at about 85%.

Calibration of pulse oximeters presents a problem. Optical filters may be used for routine calibration, but the gold standard is calibration against arterial blood PO_2 or saturation, which is seldom undertaken. When oxygenation is critical, there is no substitute for direct measurement of arterial PO_2.

Tissue PO_2

Clearly the tissue PO_2 is of greater significance than the PO_2 at various intermediate stages higher in the oxygen cascade. It would therefore appear logical to attempt the measurement of PO_2 in the tissues, but this has proved difficult both in technique and in interpretation. For experimental procedures needle electrodes may be inserted directly into tissue and PO_2 measured on the tip of a needle. Difficulties of interpretation arise from the fact that PO_2 varies immensely within the tissue and even within a single cell (page 144). Thus direct measurement of tissue PO_2 has no place in clinical monitoring.

Tissue surface electrodes. A miniaturised polarographic electrode may be placed on or attached to the surface of an organ to indicate the PO_2. Interpretation of the reading is subject to many of the same limitations as with the needle electrode. Nevertheless, tissue surface PO_2 may provide the surgeon with useful information regarding perfusion and viability in cases of organ ischaemia. Changes in PO_2 may also provide useful information on the efficacy of surgical techniques to improve circulation.[77]

Near infrared spectroscopy.[78] The biochemical state of tissue oxidation may be determined by the use of transmission spectroscopy in the near infrared (700–1000 nm), where tissues are relatively translucent. The state of relative oxidation of haemoglobin and cytochome a$_3$ may be determined within this waveband. At present it is feasible to study *transmission* spectroscopy over a path length up to about 9 cm, which is sufficient to permit monitoring of the brain of newborn infants. Use in adults requires *reflectance* spectroscopy and does allow assessment of oxygenation in, for example, an area of a few cubic centimetres of brain tissue. This is useful, for example, during surgery on the carotid arteries when changes in oxygenation in the area supplied by the artery concerned can be followed. However, the technique has failed to gain widespread acceptance because of interference from extracranial tissue, particularly scalp blood flow, and difficulties with calibrating the readings and defining any 'normal' values.

Indirect assessment of tissue oxygenation.[79] Such are the difficulties of tissue PO_2 measurements that in clinical practice it is more usual simply to seek evidence of anaerobic tissue metabolism. In the absence of this, tissue perfusion and oxygenation can be assumed to be acceptable. Indirect methods that assess global (i.e. whole-body) tissue perfusion include mixed venous oxygen saturation, measured either by sampling pulmonary arterial blood or by using a fibreoptic catheter to measure oxygen saturation continuously in the pulmonary artery. Blood lactate levels also provide a global indication of tissue perfusion. However, acceptable global tissue oxygenation provides no reassurance about function, either of regions in an individual organ or in an entire organ. Methods of assessing oxygenation in a specific tissue have focused on the gut because of ease of access and the observation that gut blood flow is often the first to be reduced when oxygen delivery is inadequate. Gastric intramucosal pH measurement allows an assessment to be made of cellular pH within the stomach mucosa, which has been shown to correlate with other assessments of tissue oxygenation and patient well-being during critical illness.

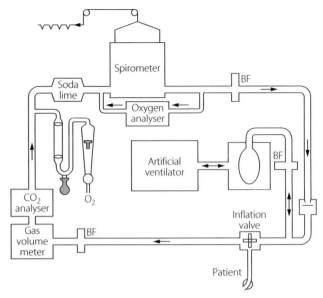

Figure 11.21 A closed-circuit spirometer system for measurement of oxygen consumption by a patient ventilated artificially by means of a box–bag system. When the system is in equilibrium, oxygen consumption is indicated by the oxygen added to the system and carbon dioxide output is measured as the product of expired minute volume and mean carbon dioxide concentration in the expired gas. BF, bacterial filter. (Reproduced with permission from Makita K, Nunn JF, Royston B. Evaluation of metabolic measuring instruments for use in critically ill patients. *Crit Care Med* 1990; **18**: 638–44.)

MEASUREMENT OF OXYGEN CONSUMPTION AND DELIVERY

Oxygen consumption

There are three main methods for the measurement of oxygen consumption:

1. oxygen loss from (or replacement into) a closed breathing system
2. subtraction of the expired from the inspired volume of oxygen
3. multiplication of cardiac output by arterial/mixed venous oxygen content difference.

Oxygen loss from (or replacement into) a closed breathing system. Probably the simplest method of measuring oxygen consumption is by observing the loss of volume from a closed-circuit spirometer, with expired carbon dioxide absorbed by soda lime. It is essential that the spirometer should initially contain an oxygen-enriched mixture so that the inspired oxygen concentration does not fall to a level that is dangerous for the subject or patient. Alternatively, a known flow rate of oxygen may be added to maintain the volume of the spirometer and its oxygen concentration constant: under these conditions, the oxygen inflow rate must equal the oxygen consumption. The technique may be adapted to the conditions of artificial ventilation (Figure 11.21) but the technique, although accurate, is cumbersome.[80]

Subtraction of expired from inspired volume of oxygen. The essence of the technique is subtraction of the volume of oxygen breathed out (expired minute volume × mixed

expired oxygen concentration) from the volume of oxygen breathed in (inspired minute volume × inspired oxygen concentration). The difference between the inspired and expired minute volumes is a very important factor in achieving accuracy with the method, particularly when a high concentration of oxygen is inhaled. Inspired and expired minute volumes differ as a result of the respiratory exchange ratio and also any exchange of inert gas (e.g. nitrogen) that might occur. On the assumption that the patient is in equilibrium for nitrogen and the mass of nitrogen inspired is the same as that expired, it follows that the ratio of inspired/expired minute volumes is inversely proportional to the respective ratios of nitrogen concentrations. Therefore:

Inspired minute volume = expired minute volume

$$\times \frac{\text{Expired nitrogen concentration}}{\text{Inspired nitrogen concentration}}$$

The ratio of the nitrogen concentrations is known as the Haldane transformation factor, which is used to calculate the inspired minute volume from the expired minute volume that is normally measured. Use of Haldane factors is only valid if the subject is in equilibrium with regard to nitrogen.

This is the basis of the classic Douglas bag technique, in which expired gas is measured for volume and analysed for oxygen and carbon dioxide concentrations. The expired nitrogen concentration is determined by subtraction and the inspired minute volume derived. The approach has been automated by several manufacturers and their systems can be used satisfactorily during artificial ventilation.[81] The essential feature is the measurement of gas composition of inspired and expired gas by the same analysers under the same condition of humidity, temperature and pressure, with a very high level of accuracy. The potential for error is theoretically increased when the inspired oxygen concentration and minute volume are increased, but the manufacturers have had considerable success in overcoming the formidable practical problems.

Multiplication of cardiac output by arterial/mixed venous oxygen content difference. This approach is the reverse of using the Fick principle for measurement of cardiac output (see page 106) and is commonly known as the reversed Fick technique.

$$\dot{V}O_2 = \dot{Q}(Ca_{O_2} - C\bar{v}_{O_2})$$

where $\dot{V}O_2$ is the oxygen consumption, $\dot{Q}$ is the cardiac output, Ca_{O_2} is the arterial oxygen content and $C\bar{v}_{O_2}$ is the mixed venous oxygen content.

The technique is essentially invasive, as the cardiac output must be measured by an independent method (usually thermodilution) and it is also necessary to sample arterial and mixed venous blood, the latter preferably from the pulmonary artery. Nevertheless, it is convenient in the critical care situation where the necessary vascular lines are commonly in place.

The method has a larger random error than the gasometric techniques described above,[82] but also has a systematic error as it excludes the oxygen consumption of the lungs (Figure 11.22).[8] In animal studies, the difference is negligible in the case of healthy lungs but is substantial when the lungs are infected.[83] Studies comparing the two methods in humans show wide variations between different patient groups. The necessity for invasive monitoring prevents the study of normal awake subjects, but results from patients in intensive care (with presumed lung pathology) do not seem to differ from patients with normal lungs undergoing cardiac surgery. The contribution of the lungs to total oxygen consumption therefore remains to be fully elucidated, but studies so far indicate that the pulmonary contribution may be very variable, depending on many physiological and pathological factors.[82,84-87]

Validation of methods of measurement of oxygen consumption. Meticulous attention to detail is required if oxygen consumption is to be measured with a satisfactory degree of accuracy. Various metabolic simulators have been described for validation of techniques under different circumstances of use. These include the combustion of known flow rates of an inflammable gas[80,88] and the preparation of a mock 'expired gas' by nitrogen dilution and the addition of carbon dioxide.[89]

Oxygen delivery

Oxygen delivery is measured as the product of cardiac output and arterial oxygen content. This excludes oxygen delivered for consumption within the lung. In the intensive care situation, cardiac output is now commonly measured by thermal dilution and simultaneously an arterial sample is drawn for measurement of oxygen content by any of the methods described above. If oxygen delivery is determined at the same time as oxygen consumption is measured by the reversed Fick technique, it should be remembered that two of the variables (cardiac output and arterial oxygen content) are common to both measurements. This linking of data is a potential source of error in inferring the consequences of changes in one product on the other (see page 189).[90,91]

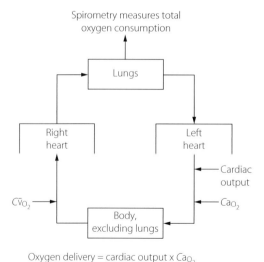

Oxygen delivery = cardiac output x Ca_{O_2}
Oxygen consumption (by reversed Fick technique) = cardiac output $(Ca_{O_2} - C\bar{v}_{O_2})$

Figure 11.22 Schematic representation of the essential differences in measurement of oxygen consumption by spirometry and by the reversed Fick technique, which measures the oxygen consumption of the body *excluding* the lungs.

REFERENCES

1. Kelman GR, Nunn JF. *Computer produced physiological tables*. London: Butterworths, 1968.
2. Kelman GR, Nunn JF, Prys-Roberts C, Greenbaum R. The influence of cardiac output on arterial oxygenation. *Br J Anaesth* 1967; **39**: 450–8.
*3. Hsia CCW. Respiratory function of hemoglobin. *N Engl J Med* 1998; **338**: 239–47.
4. Perutz MF. Stereochemistry of cooperative effects in haemoglobin. *Nature* 1970; **228**: 726–39.
*5. Russo R, Benazzi L, Perrella M. The Bohr effect of hemoglobin intermediates and the role of salt bridges

in the tertiary/quaternary transitions. *J Biol Chem* 2001; **276**: 13628–34.

6. Ho C, Perussi JR. Proton nuclear magnetic resonance studies of haemoglobin. *Meth Enzymol* 1994; **232**: 97–139.

7. Gregory IC. The oxygen and carbon monoxide capacities of foetal and adult blood. *J Physiol* 1974; **236**: 625–34.

8. Nunn JF. Pulmonary oxygen consumption. *Intens Care Med* 1996; **22**: 275–6.

9. Adair GS. The hemoglobin system. VI. The oxygen dissociation curve of hemoglobin. *J Biol Chem* 1925; **63**: 529–45.

10. Imai K. Adair fitting to oxygen equilibration curves of hemoglobin. *Meth Enzymol* 1994; **232**: 559–76.

11. Kelman GR. Digital computer subroutine for the conversion of oxygen tension into saturation. *J Appl Physiol* 1966; **21**: 1375–6.

12. Severinghaus JW, Stafford M, Thunstrom AM. Estimation of skin metabolism and blood flow with $tcPO_2$ and $tcPCO_2$ electrodes by cuff occlusion of the circulation. *Acta Anaesthiol Scand Supp* 1978; **68**: 9–15.

13. Roughton FJW, Severinghaus JW. Accurate determination of O_2 dissociation curve of human blood above 98.7% saturation with data on O_2 solubility in unmodified human blood from 0°C to 37°C. *J Appl Physiol* 1973; **35**: 861–9.

14. Severinghaus JW. Blood gas calculator. *J Appl Physiol* 1966; **21**: 1108–16.

15. Thomas LJ. Algorithms for selected blood acid–base and blood gas calculations. *J Appl Physiol* 1972; **33**: 154–8.

16. MacDonald R. Red cell 2, 3-diphosphoglycerate and oxygen affinity. *Anaesthesia* 1977; **32**: 544–53.

17. Shappell SD, Lenfant CJM. Adaptive, genetic and iatrogenic alterations of the oxyhaemoglobin-dissociation curve. *Anesthesiology* 1972; **37**: 127–39.

18. Morgan TJ, Koch D, Morris D, Clague A, Purdie DM. Reduced red cell 2,3-diphosphoglycerate concentrations in critical illness without decreased in vivo P50. *Anaesth Intens Care* 2001; **29**: 479–83.

19. Shafer AW, Tague LL, Welch MH, Guenter CA. 2, 3-Diphosphoglycerate in red cells stored in acid-citrate-dextrose and citrate-phosphate-dextrose: implications regarding delivery of oxygen. *J Lab Clin Med* 1971; **77**: 430–7.

*20. Heaton A, Keegan T, Holme S. *In vivo* regeneration of red cell 2, 3-diphosphoglycerate following transfusion of DPG-depleted AS-1, AS-3 and CPDA-1 red cells. *Br J Haematol* 1989; **71**: 131–6.

21. Valeri CR, Collins FB. Physiologic effects of 2, 3-DPG-depleted red cells with high affinity for oxygen. *J Appl Physiol* 1971; **31**: 823–7.

22. Sheldon GF. Diphosphoglycerate in massive transfusion and erythrophoresis. *Crit Care Med* 1979; **7**: 407–11.

23. Bowen JC, Fleming WH. Increased oxyhaemoglobin affinity after transfusion of stored blood: evidence for circulatory compensation. *Ann Surg* 1974; **180**: 760–4.

24. Torrance J, Jacobs P, Restrepo A, Eschbach J, Lenfant C, Finch CA. Intraerythrocytic adaptation to anemia. *N Engl J Med* 1970; **283**: 165–9.

25. Marshall BE, Whyche MQ. Hypoxemia during and after anesthesia. *Anesthesiology* 1972; **37**: 178–209.

*26. Hobbs AJ, Gladwin MT, Patel RP, Williams DLH, Butler AR. Haemoglobin: NO transporter, NO inactivator or none the above. *Trends Pharmacol Sci* 2002; **23**: 406–11.

27. Gross SS. Targeted delivery of nitric oxide. *Nature* 2001; **409**: 577–8.

28. Toothill C. The chemistry of the in vivo reaction between haemoglobin and various oxides of nitrogen. *Br J Anaesth* 1967; **39**: 405–12.

*29. Jia L, Bonaventura C, Bonaventura J, Stamler JS. S-nitrosohaemoglobin: a dynamic activity of blood involved in vascular control. *Nature* 1996; **380**: 221–6.

30. Hogg N. The biochemistry and physiology of S-nitrosothiols. *Annu Rev Pharmacol Toxicol* 2002; **42**: 585–600.

31. Stamler JS, Simon DL, Osborne JA, *et al.* S-Nitrosylation of proteins with nitric oxide: synthesis and characterisation of biologically active compounds. *Proc Natl Acad Sci USA* 1992; **89**: 444–8.

32. Shen W, Hintze TH, Wolin MS. Nitric oxide: an important signaling mechanism between vascular endothelium and parenchymal cells in the regulation of oxygen consumption. *Circulation* 1995; **92**: 3505–12.

33. Pawloski JR, Hess DT, Stamler JS. Export by red blood cells of nitric oxide bioactivity. *Nature* 2001; **409**: 622–6.

34. Huisman TH. The structure and function of normal and abnormal haemoglobins. *Baillière's Clin Haematol* 1993; **6**: 1–30.

35. Wajcman H, Galacteros F. Abnormal haemoglobins with high oxygen affinity and erythrocytosis. *Hematol Cell Ther* 1996; **38**: 305–12.

36. Vichinsky E. New therapies in sickle cell disease. *Lancet* 2002; **360**: 629–31.

37. Jaffé ER. Methaemoglobinaemia. *Clin Haematol* 1981; **10**: 99–122.

38. Coleman MD, Coleman NA. Drug-induced methaemoglobinaemia. Treatment issues. *Drug Safery* 1996; **14**: 394–405

39. Mallick A, Bodenham AR. Modified haemoglobins as oxygen transporting blood substitutes. *Br J Hosp Med* 1996; **55**: 443–8.

40. Goodnough LT, Shander A, Brecher ME. Transfusion medicine: looking to the future. *Lancet* 2003; **361**: 161–9.

41. Spiess BD. Perflurocarbon emulsions: one approach to intravenous artificial respiratory gas transport. *Int Anesthesiol Clin* 1995; **33**: 103–13.

42. Spahn DR, van Brempt R, Theilmeier G, *et al*. Perflubron emulsion delays blood transfusions in orthopaedic surgery. European Perflubron Emulsion Study Group. *Anesthesiology* 1999; **91**: 1195–208.

43. Tobias MD, Longnecker DE. Recombinant haemoglobin and other blood substitutes. *Baillière's Clin Anaesth* 1995; **9**: 165–79.

44. Hirschl RB, Pranikoff T, Gauger P, Schreiner RJ, Dechert R, Bartlett RH. Liquid ventilation in adults, children and full-term neonates. *Lancet* 1995; **346**: 1201–2.

45. Ogden JE, Parry ES. The development of hemoglobin solutions as red cell substitutes. *Int Anesthesiol Clin* 1995; **33**: 115–29.

*46. Tremper KK. Hemoglobin-based oxygen carriers: problems and promise. *J Cardiothorac Vasc Anesth* 1997; **11**: 1–2.

*47. Chang TMS. Future generations of red blood cell substitutes. *J Intern Med* 2003; **253**: 527–35.

48. Hoffman SJ, Looker DL, Roehrich JM, *et al*. Expression of fully functional tetrameric human haemoglobin in *Escherichia coli*. *Proc Natl Acad Sci USA* 1990; **87**: 8521–5.

49. Looker D, Abbott-Brown D, Kozart P, *et al*. A human recombinant hemoglobin designed for use as a blood substitute. *Nature* 1992; **356**: 258–60.

50. Burkard ME, Van Liew HD. Oxygen transport to tissues by persistent bubbles: theory and simulations. *J Appl Physiol* 1994; **77**: 2874–8.

51. D'Arrigo JS, Ho S-Y, Simon RH. Detection of experimental rat liver tumors by contrast-assisted ultrasonography. *Invest Radiol* 1993; **28**: 218–22.

52. Korzeniewski B. Theoretical studies on the regulation of oxidative phosphorylation in intact tissues. *Biochim Biophys Acta* 2001; **1504**: 31–45.

53. Weibel ER, Taylor CR, Weber J-M, Vock R, Roberts TJ, Hoppeler H. Design of the oxygen substrate pathways. VII Different structural limits for oxygen and substrate supply to muscle mitochondria. *J Exp Biol* 1996; **199**: 1699–709.

54. Barcroft J. Physiological effects of insufficient oxygen supply. *Nature* 1920; **106**: 125–9.

55. Hinds C, Watson D. Manipulating hemodynamics and oxygen transport in critically ill patients. *N Engl J Med* 1995; **333**: 1074–5.

56. Soni N, Fawcett WJ, Halliday FC. Beyond the lung: oxygen delivery and tissue oxygenation. *Anaesthesia* 1993; **48**: 704–11.

57. Pinsky MR. Beyond global oxygen supply-demand relations: in search of measures of dysoxia. *Intens Care Med* 1994; **20**: 1–3.

58. Shoemaker WC, Bland RD, Apel PL. Therapy of critically ill postoperative patients based on outcome prediction and prospective clinical trials. *Surg Clin North Am* 1985; **65**: 811–33.

59. Gattinoni L, Brazzi L, Pelosi P, *et al*. A trial of goal-oriented hemodynamic therapy in critically ill patients. *N Engl J Med* 1995; **333**: 1025–32.

60. Hayes MA, Timmins AC, Yau EHS, Palazzo M, Hinds CJ, Watson D. Elevation of systemic oxygen delivery in the treatment of critically ill patients. *N Engl J Med* 1994; **330**: 1717–22.

61. Steltzer H, Hiesmayr M, Mayer N, Krafft P, Hammerle AF. The relationship between oxygen delivery and uptake in the critically ill: is there a critical or optimal therapeutic value? A meta-analysis. *Anaesthesia* 1994; **49**: 229–36.

62. Leigh JM. Variation in performance of oxygen therapy devices. *Ann Roy Coll Surg Engl* 1973; **52**: 234–53.

63. Davies RJO, Hopkin JM. Nasal oxygen in exacerbations of ventilatory failure; an underappreciated risk. *Br Med J* 1989; **299**: 43–4.

64. Goss GA, Hayes JA, Burdon JGW. Deoxyhaemoglobin in the detection of central cyanosis. *Thorax* 1988; **43**: 212–13.

65. Kelman GR, Nunn JF. Clinical recognition of hypoxaemia under fluorescent lamps. *Lancet* 1966; **1**: 1400–3.

66. Timmins AC, Morgan GAR. Argyria or cyanosis. *Anaesthesia* 1988; **43**: 755–6.

67. Ellis FR, Nunn JF. The measurement of gaseous oxygen tension utilising paramagnetism: an evaluation of the Servomex OA 150 analyser. *Br J Anaesth* 1968; **40**: 569–78.

68. Clark LC. Monitor and control of tissue oxygen tensions. *Trans Am Soc Artif Intern Organs* 1956; **2**: 41–8.

69. Ganter M, Zollinger A. Continuous intravascular blood gas monitoring: development, current techniques and clinical use of a commercial device. *Br J Anaesth* 2003; **91**: 397–407.

70. Nunn JF, Bergman NA, Bunatyan A, Coleman AJ. Temperature coefficients for P_{CO_2} and P_{O_2} of blood in vitro. *J Appl Physiol* 1965; **20**: 23–6.

71. Severinghaus JW. A combined transcutaneous P_{O_2}-P_{CO_2} electrode with electrochemical HCO_3^- stabilization. *J Appl Physiol* 1981; **51**: 1027–32.

72. Zijlstra WG, Buursma A, Meeuwsen-van der Roest WP. Absorption spectra of human fetal and adult oxyhemoglobin, de-oxyhemoglobin, carboxyhemoglobin and methemoglobin. *Clin Chem* 1991; **37**: 1633–8.

*73. Severinghaus JW, Kelleher JF. Recent developments in pulse oximetry. *Anesthesiology* 1992; **76**: 1018–38.

74. Severinghaus JW, Spellman MJ. Pulse oximeter failure thresholds in hypotension and vasoconstriction. *Anesthesiology* 1990; **73**: 532–7.

75. Severinghaus JW, Koh SO. Effect of anemia on pulse oximeter accuracy at low saturation. *J Clin Monit* 1990; **6**: 85–8.

76. Coté CJ, Goldstein A, Fuchsman WH, Hoaglin DC. The effect of nail polish on pulse oximetry. *Anesth Analg* 1988; **67**: 683–6.

77. Kram HB, Shoemaker WC. Method for intraoperative assessment of organ perfusion and viability using a miniature oxygen sensor. *Am J Surg* 1984; **148**: 404–7.

78. Harris DNF. Near infra-red spectroscopy. *Anaesthesia* 1995; **50**: 1015–16.

79. Vincent JL. Monitoring tissue perfusion. *Can J Anaesth* 1996; **43**: R55–R57.

80. Nunn JF, Makita K, Royston B. Validation of oxygen consumption measurements during artificial ventilation. *J Appl Physiol* 1989; **67**: 2129–34.

81. Makita K, Nunn JF, Royston B. Evaluation of metabolic measuring instruments for use in critically ill patients. *Crit Care Med* 1990; **18**: 638–44.

82. Smithies MN, Royston B, Makita K, Konieczko K, Nunn JF. Comparison of oxygen consumption measurements: indirect calorimetry versus the reversed Fick method. *Crit Care Med* 1991; **19**:1401–6.

83. Light RB. Intrapulmonary oxygen consumption in experimental pneumococcal pneumonia. *J Appl Physiol* 1988; **64**: 2490–5.

84. Hanique G, Dugernier T, Laterre PF, Dougnac A, Roesler J, Reynaert MS. Significance of pathologic oxygen supply dependency in critically ill patients: comparison between measured and calculated methods. *Intens Care Med* 1994; **20**: 12–18.

85. Jolliet P, Thorens JB, Nicod L, Pichard C, Kyle U, Chevrolet JC. Relationship between pulmonary oxygen consumption, lung inflammation and calculated venous admixture in patients with acute lung injury. *Intens Care Med* 1996; **22**:277–85.

86. Oudemans-van Straaten HM, Scheffer GJ, Eysman L, Wildevuur CRH. Oxygen consumption after cardiopulmonary bypass – implications of different measuring methods. *Intens Care Med* 1993; **19**: 105–10.

87. Hanique G, Dugernier T, Laterre PF, Roeseler J, Dougnac A, Reynaert MS. Evaluation of oxygen uptake and delivery in critically ill patients: a statistical reappraisal. *Intens Care Med* 1994; **20**: 19–26.

88. Svensson KL, Sonander HG, Stenqvist O. Validation of a system for measurement of metabolic gas exchange during anaesthesia with controlled ventilation in an oxygen consuming lung model. *Br J Anaesth* 1990; **64**: 311–19.

89. Braun U, Zundel J, Freiboth K, *et al.* Evaluation of methods for indirect calorimetry with a ventilated lung model. *Intens Care Med* 1989; **15**: 196–202.

90. Archie JP. Mathematical coupling of data. A common source of error. *Ann Surg* 1981; **193**: 296–303.

91. Walsh TS, Lee A. Mathematical coupling in medical research: lessons from studies of oxygen kinetics. *Br J Anaesth* 1998; **81**: 118–20.

12 Non-respiratory functions of the lung

KEY POINTS

- The entire cardiac output passes through the pulmonary circulation, so the lungs act as a filter, preventing emboli from passing to the left side of the circulation.
- The lungs constitute a huge interface between the outside environment and the body, requiring the presence of systems for defence against inhaled biological and chemical hazards.
- In the pulmonary circulation there is active uptake and metabolism of many endogenous compounds, including amines, peptides and eicosanoids.

The lungs are primarily adapted for the purpose of gas exchange, and to achieve this with such efficiency almost the entire blood volume passes through the lungs during a single circulation. This characteristic makes the lungs ideally suited to undertake many other important functions. The location of the lungs within the circulatory system is ideal for their role as a filter to protect the systemic circulation, not only from particulate matter but also from a wide range of chemical substances that undergo removal or biotransformation in the pulmonary circulation. The pulmonary arterial tree is well adapted for the reception of emboli without resultant infarction, and the very large area of endothelium gives the lung a metabolic role out of proportion to its total mass. This large interface between the external atmosphere and the circulation is not without its own hazards, and the lung must protect the circulation from many potentially harmful inhaled substances.

FILTRATION

Sitting astride the whole output of the right ventricle, the lung is ideally situated to filter out particulate matter from the systemic venous return. Without such a filter, there would be a constant risk of particulate matter

entering the arterial system, where the coronary and cerebral circulations are particularly vulnerable to damaging emboli. Desirable though this function appears at first sight, it cannot be essential to life, since it is partially bypassed in patients with a right-to-left intracardiac shunt.

Pulmonary capillaries have a diameter of about 7 μm but this does not appear to be the effective pore size of the pulmonary circulation when considered as a filter. There is no clear agreement on the maximal diameter of particles that can traverse the pulmonary circulation. Animal studies have demonstrated the passage through perfused lungs of glass beads up to 500 μm.[1] It is well known that small quantities of gas and fat emboli may gain access to the systemic circulation in patients without intracardiac shunting. Emboli may bypass the alveoli via some of the precapillary anastomoses that are known to exist in the pulmonary circulation (page 92), though the functional role of these anastomoses remains uncertain. More extensive invasion of the systemic arteries may occur in the presence of an overt right-to-left intracardiac shunt, which is now known to be quite common. Post-mortem studies show that over 25% of the population have a 'probe-patent' foramen ovale, usually in the form of a slit-like defect that acts as a valve and which is therefore normally kept closed by the left atrial pressure being slightly greater than the right.[2] In 10% of normal subjects, a simple Valsalva manoeuvre or cough results in easily demonstrable blood flow between the right and left atria.[3] Paradoxical embolism may therefore result from a relative increase in right atrial pressure caused by physiological events or pulmonary embolus (see Chapter 29).

So far as the survival of the lung is concerned, the geometry of the pulmonary microcirculation is particularly well adapted to maintaining alveolar perfusion in the face of quite large degrees of embolisation. However, a significant degree of embolisation inevitably blocks the circulation to parts of the lung, disturbing the balance between ventilation and perfusion. This situation is considered in Chapter 29. Pulmonary microembolism with small clumps of fibrin and/or platelets will not have a direct effect on gas exchange until it is very extensive.

Plugging of pulmonary capillaries by microemboli does, however, initiate neutrophil activation in the area, leading to an increase in endothelial permeability and alveolar oedema,[4] and has been implicated in the aetiology of acute lung injury (see Chapter 31).

Thrombi are cleared more rapidly from the lungs than from other organs. The lung possesses well-developed proteolytic systems not confined to the removal of fibrin. Pulmonary endothelium is known to be rich in plasmin activator, which converts plasminogen into plasmin, which in turn converts fibrin into fibrin degradation products. However, the lung is also rich in thromboplastin, which converts prothrombin to thrombin. To complicate the position further, the lung is a particularly rich source of heparin and bovine lung is used in its commercial preparation. The lung can thus produce high concentrations of substances necessary to promote or delay blood clotting and also for fibrinolysis. Apart from the lung's ability to clear itself of thromboemboli, it may play a role in controlling the overall coagulability of the blood.

DEFENCE AGAINST INHALED SUBSTANCES

The skin, gastrointestinal tract and lungs form the major interfaces between the outside world and the carefully controlled internal body systems. Efficient gas exchange in the lung requires a physically very thin interface between air and blood, which leaves the lung vulnerable to invasion by many airborne hazards, both chemical and biological.

Biological hazards

Inhaled bacteria, viruses, fungi and spores are effectively dealt with by the respiratory mucosa, as described on page 19. Most pathogens are large enough (over 5 μm) to be impacted on the mucous layer in the airways, which allows them to be removed intact. Some will penetrate deeper into the bronchial tree, particularly when the infective load is high during respiratory infections, and must be dealt with by neutrophils, macrophages and other phagocytes.

Protease transport system. Activation of neutrophils in the lung leads to the release of dangerous proteases, particularly elastase and trypsin. These enzymes are highly effective at destroying pathogens but if left unchecked may also damage lung tissues. There are at least two mechanisms to protect against this eventuality. First, the proteases are mostly confined to the mucous layer, which is continually swept towards the larynx by the respiratory epithelium. Second, they are inactivated by conjugation with α_1-antitrypsin, present in plasma. Conjugated proteases are then removed in the pul-

monary circulation or lymph and transferred to conjugation with α_2-macroglobulin, which is finally destroyed in the liver. Inactivation of such powerful protease enzymes presents a significant biochemical challenge and the way that α_1-antitrypsin achieves this has recently been elucidated.[5,6] The α_1-antitrypsin molecule exists in a semistable state, held together by a loop of amino acids that projects from the molecule with a pair of methionine-serine residues at its tip, which acts as a 'bait' for protease enzymes. When a protease binds the peptide loop, the α_1-antitrypsin structure becomes unstable and rapidly flips the bound protease on to the other side of the molecule, an action that has been likened to a mousetrap. Once flipped to the other side of the molecule, the protease becomes bound so tightly within a β-sheet of the α_1-antitrypsin that it is effectively crushed, preventing the conformational changes required for its function.

In 1963 a group of patients were described whose plasma proteins were deficient in α_1-antitrypsin and who had developed emphysema.[7] The enzyme deficiency is inherited as an autosomal recessive gene, with around one in ten people of European descent being carriers for one of the two common mutations of the α_1-antitrypsin gene.[6] Lower plasma levels of α_1-antitrypsin in homozygous patients result not from failed production of α_1-antitrypsin, but from failure to secrete the protein from hepatocytes. The retained α_1-antitrypsin protein polymerises within the cell and leads to hepatic damage.[5] About 1:3000 of the population is believed to be homozygous for the more severe Z mutation of the α_1-antitrypsin gene, though many of these are believed to succumb to pulmonary and liver disease before the α_1-antitrypsin deficiency is ever found.[6,8] Homozygotes do form a higher proportion of patients with emphysema and estimates range from 3% to 26%. These patients tend to have basal emphysema, onset at a younger age and a severe form of the disease. It thus appears that α_1-antitrypsin deficiency is an aetiological factor in a small proportion of patients with emphysema (page 380). Smoking, which increases neutrophil protease production (page 292), is associated with more severe lung disease in patients with a deficiency of α_1-antitrypsin.[8]

Phagocytosis of pathogens. Neutrophils are common in the mucus of the bronchial tree and it is well established that, with more widespread infection, neutrophils, macrophages and other cells can marginate on the pulmonary capillary endothelium (page 403). Following immunological activation, these phagocytic cells are responsible for killing pathogens throughout the lung and do so by the formation of oxygen-derived free radicals. Very substantial quantities of oxygen are consumed in the formation of free radicals and related species derived from molecular oxygen. The mechanism is described elsewhere (page 353) in relation to oxygen toxicity.

Chemical hazards

Many factors will influence the fate of inhaled chemicals.[9]

Particle size, as with biological particles, will affect where in the lung deposition occurs. This is described in more detail below for the delivery of drugs to the lungs.

Water solubility. Once incorporated into the lung tissue, water solubility affects the rate at which chemicals are cleared from the lung, with water-soluble substances taking longer than lipid-soluble ones to be absorbed into the blood for disposal elsewhere.

Concentration of inhaled chemicals is important as metabolic activity within the lung is easily saturated.

Metabolism of inhaled chemicals is poorly understood in the human lung and, though it has been extensively investigated in animals, there are known to be large species differences.[9] Metabolic activity is found in all cell types of the respiratory mucosa, but in animals is particularly well developed in Clara cells and type II alveolar cells (page 21).[9,10] As in the liver, metabolism of toxic chemicals involves two stages.

1. Phase I metabolism, in which the toxic molecule is converted into a different compound, usually by oxidative reactions. This is achieved in the lung by the cytochrome P-450 monooxygenase and, to a much lesser extent, flavin-based monooxygenase systems. The lung is one of the major extrahepatic sites of mixed function oxidation by the cytochrome P-450 systems but, gram for gram, remains considerably less active than the liver.

2. Phase II metabolism involves conjugation of the resulting compounds to 'carrier' molecules, which render them less biologically active, more water soluble and therefore easier to excrete. In the lung, phase II metabolism is normally by conjugation with glucuronide or glutathione.[9]

Metabolic changes to inhaled chemicals may not be beneficial, especially with many synthetic organic compounds and several chemicals in cigarette smoke (page 289). Bio-activation by phase I metabolism converts some quite innocuous compounds into potent carcinogens, whereas slightly different metabolic conversions may do the reverse.[9,11] The balance between activating and inactivating pathways varies between species. What few data are available on human lungs indicate that we are fortunate in having a very favourable ratio, the inactivation of potential carcinogens being 100-fold greater than in rodents.[9] Presumably, without this evolutionary advantage, the history of cigarette smoking would have been considerably different.

PROCESSING OF ENDOGENOUS COMPOUNDS BY THE PULMONARY VASCULATURE[12,13]

Hormones may pass through the lung unchanged, others may be almost entirely removed from the blood during a single pass, and some may be activated during transit (Table 12.1).

Of the many types of cell in the lungs, it is the endothelium that is most active metabolically. The most important location is the pulmonary capillary, but it must be stressed that endothelium from a very wide range of vessels has been shown to possess a similar repertoire of metabolic processes.[14] This is fortunate because it is not

Table 12.1 Summary of metabolic changes to hormones on passing through the pulmonary circulation

| Group | Effect of passing through pulmonary circulation | | |
	Activated	*No change*	*Inactivated*
Amines		Dopamine Adrenaline Histamine	5-Hydroxytryptamine Noradrenaline
Peptides	Angiotensin I	Angiotensin II Oxytocin Vasopressin	Bradykinin Atrial natriuretic peptide Endothelins
Arachidonic acid derivatives	Arachidonic acid	PGI_2 (prostacyclin) PGA_2	PGD_2 PGE_2 $PGF_{2\alpha}$ Leukotrienes
Purine derivatives			Adenosine ATP, ADP, AMP

possible to harvest pulmonary capillary endothelium and so cultures must be prepared from vascular endothelial cells harvested from other sites, such as human umbilical vein. However, there are some important differences in activity between endothelium from different vessels. For example, endothelium grown from various non-pulmonary vessels will not inactivate PGE_2, although this is well known to occur in the pulmonary circulation. The extensive metabolic activity of the pulmonary endothelium takes place in spite of the paucity of organelles that are normally associated with metabolic activity, in particular mitochondria and smooth endoplasmic reticulum or microsomes. Nevertheless, the caveolae result in a major increase in the already extensive surface area of these cells (about 126 m^2),[15] which is particularly advantageous for membrane-bound enzymes.

Catecholamines and acetylcholine

Noradrenaline (norepinephrine). There is a striking difference in the handling of noradrenaline and adrenaline. Although each catecholamine has a half-life of about 20 seconds in blood, some 30% of noradrenaline is removed in a single pass through the lungs,[16] whereas adrenaline (and isoprenaline and dopamine) are unaffected. Monoamine oxidase and catechol-O-methyl transferase within the endothelial cells will metabolise all amine derivatives with equal efficiency. The specificity of pulmonary endothelium for noradrenaline therefore lies with the cell membrane, which selectively takes up only noradrenaline and 5-hydroxytryptamine.[17] Extraneuronal uptake of noradrenaline is not confined to the endothelium of the lungs, but uptake by the pulmonary circulation (uptake 1) differs from extraneuronal uptake (uptake 2) in other tissues, which is less specific for noradrenaline.

5-Hydroxytryptamine (5HT, serotonin) is removed very effectively by the lungs, up to 98% being removed in a single pass. There are considerable similarities to the processing of noradrenaline. 5HT is taken up by the endothelium, mainly in the capillaries, and is then rapidly metabolised by monoamine oxidase. The half-life of 5HT in blood is about 1–2 minutes and pulmonary clearance plays the major role in the prevention of its recirculation. If the uptake of 5HT is inhibited (e.g. by cocaine or tricyclic antidepressant drugs), its pulmonary clearance is greatly reduced.[18]

Histamine, dopamine and adrenaline (epinephrine) are not removed from blood on passing through the pulmonary circulation, in spite of the high concentrations of monoamine oxidase in lung tissue. Their removal from the circulation is limited by the lack of a transport mechanism across the blood–endothelium barrier.

Acetylcholine is rapidly hydrolysed in blood, where it has a half-life of less than 2 seconds. This tends to overshadow any changes attributable to the lung, which nevertheless does contain acetylcholinesterases and pseudocholinesterases.

Peptides

Angiotensin. It has long been known that angiotensin I, a decapeptide formed by the action of renin on a plasma α_2-globulin (angiotensinogen), was converted into the vasoactive octapeptide angiotensin II by incubation with plasma (Figure 12.1). Angiotensin-converting enzyme

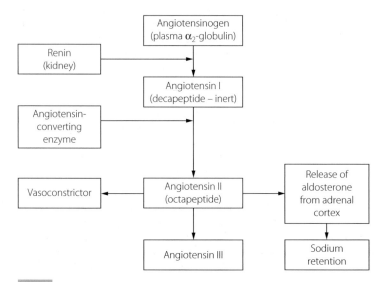

Figure 12.1 Renin–angiotensin–aldosterone axis. Angiotensin-converting enzyme is found in plasma and on systemic vascular endothelium, but is present in much larger quantities on the endothelium of pulmonary vessels.

(ACE) is found free in the plasma, but is also bound to the surface of endothelium. This appears to be a general property of endothelium, but ACE is present in abundance on the vascular surface of pulmonary endothelial cells, also lining the inside of the caveolae and extending on to the projections into the lumen.[14] Some 80% of angiotensin I passing through the lungs is converted to angiotensin II in a single pass. Angiotensin-converting enzyme is a zinc-containing carboxypeptidase with two active sites, each located within a deep groove in the side of the protein.[19] Binding sites in the groove attach the substrate firmly to the protein, and the zinc moiety then cleaves either a phenylalanine–histidine bond (angiotensin I) or a phenylalanine–arginine bond (bradykinin). Drugs that inhibit ACE (see below) do so by becoming buried deep within the protein groove, simply covering the active site.[19]

Bradykinin, a vasoactive nonapeptide, is also very effectively removed during passage through the lung and other vascular beds. The half-life in blood is about 17 seconds but less than 4 seconds in various vascular beds. Like angiotensin I, ACE is the enzyme responsible for metabolism of bradykinin.

By its effects on bradykinin and angiotensin, ACE plays a crucial role in controlling arterial blood pressure. Bradykinin, which promotes blood vessel dilation and a lowering of blood pressure, is inactivated. Conversely, angiotensin II production results in a host of events that increase blood pressure, such as renal sodium retention, vasoconstriction and release of noradrenaline. Drugs that inhibit ACE now have an enormous clinical role in the treatment of cardiovascular disease. However, this also decreases the degradation of bradykinin by ACE, although other enzymes are capable of metabolising bradykinin, so allowing ACE inhibitors to exert their hypotensive effects.

Angiotensin II itself passes through the lung unchanged, as do vasopressin and oxytocin.

Atrial natiuretic peptide (ANP) is largely removed by the lung in many animal species.[20,21] Methodological problems caused by the secretion of ANP from both left and right atria in humans led to uncertainty about the ability of human lungs to metabolise ANP. Studies using radiolabelled ANP have now shown that in humans, ANP is not metabolised by the lung to any significant extent.[21]

Endothelins, a group of 21 amino acid peptides with diverse biological activity (page 99), have a plasma half-life of just a few minutes, being cleared by the kidney, liver and lungs. The pulmonary enzymes responsible are not clearly defined, but there are believed to be several different types in humans.[22]

Arachidonic acid derivatives

The lung is a major site of synthesis, metabolism, uptake and release of arachidonic acid metabolites. The group as a whole are 20-carbon carboxylic acids, generically known as eicosanoids. The initial stages of eicosanoid synthesis involve the conversion, by phospholipase A_2, of membrane phospholipids into arachidonic acid. Metabolism of arachidonic acid involves its oxygenation by two main pathways, for which the enzymes are cyclooxygenase (COX) and lipoxygenase (Figures 12.2 and 4.9, respectively). Oxygenation and cyclisation of arachidonic acid by COX produces the prostaglandin PGG_2 (the subscript 2 indicates two double bonds in the carbon chain). A non-specific peroxidase then converts PGG_2 to PGH_2, which is the parent compound for synthesis of the many important derivatives shown in Figure 12.2.

Eicosanoids are not stored preformed, but are synthesised as required by many cell types in the lung, including endothelium, airway smooth muscle, mast cells, epithelial cells and vascular muscle. Activation of phospholipase initiates the pathway and results from a variety of stimuli such as inflammatory cytokines, complement activation, hormones, allergens or mechanical stimuli. The enzyme for the next step of the pathway, COX, exists in multiple isoforms, including COX-1, which is a constitutive enzyme present at low concentrations, and COX-2, which is induced by inflammatory cytokines. In the normal lung, the physiological role of these COX isoforms is uncertain but in some patients with asthma, inhibition of COX-1 by aspirin induces bronchospasm, whereas inhibition of COX-2 does not (page 378).

$PGF_{2\alpha}$, PGD_2, PGG_2, PGH_2 and thromboxane are bronchial and tracheal constrictors, $PGF_{2\alpha}$ and PGD_2 being much more potent in asthmatic patients than in normal subjects. PGE_1 and PGE_2 are bronchodilators, particularly when administered by aerosol. Prostacyclin (PGI_2) has different effects in different species. In humans, it has no effect on airway calibre in doses that have profound cardiovascular effects.[23] PGI_2 and PGE_1 are pulmonary vasodilators. PGH_2 and $PGF_{2\alpha}$ are pulmonary vasoconstrictors.

Various specific enzymes in the lung are responsible for extensive metabolism of PGE_2, PGE_1 and $PGF_{2\alpha}$ but PGA_2 and PGI_2 pass through the lung unchanged. As for catecholamine metabolism, specificity for pulmonary prostaglandin metabolism is in the uptake pathways rather than with the intracellular enzymes.[13]

Leukotrienes are also eicosanoids derived from arachidonic acid but by the lipoxygenase pathway (see Figure 4.9). The leukotrienes LTC_4 and LTD_4 are mainly responsible for the bronchoconstrictor effects of what was formerly known as slow-reacting substance A or

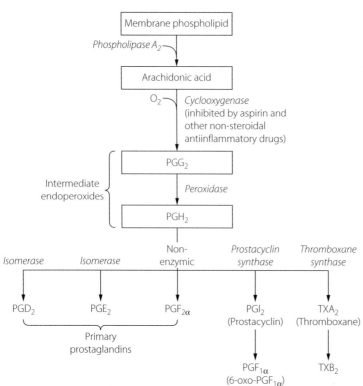

Figure 12.2 The cyclooxygenase pathway for the production of arachidonic acid and its subsequent conversion to form the prostaglandins and thromboxanes. See text for metabolism taking place in the lungs.

SRS-A. SRS-A also contains LTB_4, which is a less powerful bronchoconstrictor but increases vascular permeability. These compounds, which are synthesised by the mast cell, have an important role in asthma and the mechanism of their release is discussed in Chapter 28, whilst drugs that inhibit leukotrienes are described on page 49.

Purine derivatives

Specific enzymes exist on the surface of pulmonary endothelial cells for the degradation of AMP, ADP and ATP to adenosine. Adenosine itself has potent effects on the circulation, but is also inactivated in the lungs by a rapid uptake mechanism into the endothelial cells, where it is either phosphorylated into AMP or deaminated to produce inosine and ultimately uric acid for excretion.

PHARMACOKINETICS AND THE LUNG

Drug delivery[24,25]

Inhalation of drugs to treat lung disease may be considered as topical administration of the drug to the respiratory tract, though systemic absorption is likely to be greater than with other topical routes. Pulmonary administration of a drug that is intended to work sys-temically offers many advantages over other routes, such as very rapid delivery into the circulation and avoidance of first-pass metabolism in the liver. For both these purposes, it is crucial to understand the behaviour of aerosols inhaled into the lung.

Where in the respiratory tract inhaled particles are deposited depends on both their size and the breathing pattern during inhalation. Three mechanisms cause deposition.

1. Inertial impaction occurs with large particles (>3 μm). Large particles (>8 μm) rarely reach further than the pharynx (page 19) before impaction, whereas smaller particles penetrate further into the respiratory tract. Inertial impaction is greatly influenced by the velocity of the particles, so a slower velocity of the aerosol leaving the delivery device or a slower inspiration by the patient will increase the penetration into the lungs of the large particles in an aerosol.
2. Sedimentation with particles of 1–3 μm occurs in the smaller airways or alveoli where slow gas velocity allows the particles to fall out of suspension and be deposited on lung tissue. Breath holding after inhalation of an aerosol encourages sedimentation.
3. Diffusion, caused by Brownian motion of particles, occurs with particles below 0.5–1 μm in size.

For delivery to the alveoli, particles around 3 μm are the optimal size, as larger particles tend to deposit in the airways and smaller particles tend to be inhaled and exhaled without being deposited in lung tissue. Targeted delivery of drugs to specific regions of the respiratory tract should be possible by, for example, modifying the particle size, the timing of its addition to the breath or the breathing pattern during inhalation.[25] In practice, most delivery devices in clinical use produce aerosols containing a wide range of particle sizes, the most commonly used metered-dose inhaler used to treat asthma generating particles between 1 and 35 μm. Use of a spacer device before inhalation allows the largest particles to fall out of the aerosol before inhalation and so reduces their impaction in the pharynx, where they are responsible for many of the side effects of inhaled drugs.

Drug elimination

The wide range of mechanisms present in the lung for the processing of endogenous and inhaled substances makes an effect on drug disposition almost inevitable.

Inhaled drugs will be subjected to the same metabolic activity in the airway and alveolar cells as other toxic chemicals described above. Mixed function oxidase and cytochrome P-450 systems are active in the lung and so are presumed to metabolise drugs in the same way as in hepatocytes. Steroids are known to be metabolised in lung airway tissue, as is isoprenaline.[13] Inhalational anaesthetics, in particular older agents that undergo significant metabolism elsewhere in the body, such as methoxyflurane and halothane, undergo biotransformation in the airways by similar pathways, producing fluoride ions.[26]

Pulmonary circulation.[13,27-29] Many drugs are removed from the circulation on passing through the lungs. However, in the majority of cases this occurs by retention of the drug in lung tissue rather than actual metabolism. This low activity of metabolic enzymes found in the lung occurs for two reasons. First, access to the metabolic enzymes in endothelial cells is closely controlled by highly specific uptake mechanisms that are vital to allow the highly selective metabolism of endogenous compounds. Second, it is possible that the oxidative systems responsible for drug metabolism elsewhere in the body are located mostly in the airways, thus preventing bloodborne drugs gaining access to them. Drugs that are basic (pKa >8) and lipophilic tend to be taken up in the pulmonary circulation, whereas acidic drugs preferentially bind to plasma proteins.[13,29] Drug binding in the pulmonary circulation may act as a first-pass filter for any drug administered intravenously.[28] This drug reservoir within the lung may then be released slowly or even give rise to rapid changes in plasma drug levels when the binding sites become saturated or when one drug is displaced by a different drug with greater affinity for the binding site.

Pulmonary toxicity of drugs. Accumulation of some drugs and other toxic substances in the lung may cause dangerous local toxicity.[30] Paraquat is an outstanding example: it is slowly taken up into alveolar epithelial cells, where it promotes the production of reactive oxygen species (page 351), with resulting lung damage. Some drugs cause pulmonary toxicity by a similar mechanism, including nitrofurantoin and bleomycin, toxicity from the latter being strongly associated with exposure to high oxygen concentrations. Amiodarone, a highly effective and commonly used antiarrhythmic agent, is also associated with pulmonary toxicity, which occurs in 6% of patients given the drug.[31] When toxicity occurs it may be severe and is fatal in up to 10% of cases. The cause is unknown but formation of reactive oxygen species, immunological activation and direct cellular toxicity are all believed to contribute.[31]

THE ENDOCRINE LUNG

To qualify as a true endocrine organ, the lung must secrete a substance into the blood which brings about a useful physiological response in a distant tissue. In spite of its wide-ranging metabolic activities already described, the endocrine functions of the lung remain ill defined. Contenders include the following.

Inflammatory mediators. Histamine, endothelin and eicosanoids are released from the lung following immunological activation by inhaled allergens (see Chapter 28). These mediators are undoubtedly responsible for cardiovascular and other physiological changes in the rest of the body, such as a rash, peripheral vasodilation and a reduction in blood pressure. However, it is doubtful if this can really be regarded as a desirable physiological effect.

Hypoxic endocrine responses.[32] Animal studies have demonstrated the presence of clusters of peptide- and amine-secreting cells in lung tissue. These cells degranulate in the presence of acute hypoxia, but the substances secreted and their effects are not known. The cells belong to the 'diffuse endocrine system' and are present in humans, but their role is extremely unclear.

Nitric oxide (NO) plays an important role in the regulation of airway smooth muscle (page 46) and pulmonary vascular resistance (page 99) and is well known for its effects on platelet function and the systemic vasculature elsewhere in the body. There is no evidence that pulmonary endothelium secretes NO into the blood in order to exert an effect elsewhere, mainly because of the rapid uptake of NO by haemoglobin (page 180). However, this does not rule out an indirect effect of pulmonary NO production in influencing peripheral blood flow, which may be controlled by the balance between different forms of NO–haemoglobin complexes (page 180).

REFERENCES

1. Niden AH, Aviado DM. Effects of pulmonary embolism on the pulmonary circulation with special reference to arteriovenous shunts in the lung. *Circ Res* 1956; **4**: 67–73.

2. Kerut EK, Norfleet WT, Plotnick GD, Giles TD. Patent foramen ovale: a review of associated conditions and the impact of physiological size. *J Am Coll Cardiol* 2001; **38**: 613–23.

3. Fisher DC, Fisher EA, Budd JH, Rosen SE, Goldman ME. The incidence of patent foramen ovale in 1000 consecutive patients. *Chest* 1995; **107**: 1504–9.

4. Malik AB. Pulmonary microembolism and lung vascular injury. *Eur Respir J Suppl* 1990; **11**: 499s–506s.

5. Lomas DA, Mahadeva R. α_1-antitrypsin polymerisation and the serpinopathies: pathobiology and prospects for therapy. *J Clin Invest* 2002; **110**: 1585–90.

*6. Carrell RW, Lomas DA. Alpha$_1$-antitrypsin deficiency – a model for conformational diseases. *N Engl J Med* 2002; **346**: 45–53.

7. Laurell CB, Eriksson S. The electrophoretic α_1-globulin pattern of serum in α_1-antitrypsin deficiency. *Scand J Clin Lab Invest* 1963; **15**: 132–6.

8. Norman MR, Mowat AP, Hutchinson DCS. Molecular basis, clinical consequences and diagnosis of alpha-1 antitrypsin deficiency. *Ann Clin Biochem* 1997; **34**: 230–46.

*9. Bond JA. Metabolism and elimination of inhaled drugs and airborne chemicals from the lungs. *Pharmacol Toxicol* 1993; **72** (Supp 3): 36–47.

10. Dahl AR, Gerde P. Uptake and metabolism of toxicants in the respiratory tract. *Environ Health Perspect* 1994; **102** (Supp 11): 67–70.

11. Kikkawa Y. Diverse role of pulmonary cytochrome P-450 monooxygenase. *Lab Invest* 1992; **67**: 535–9.

12. Davidson JM. Biochemistry and turnover of lung interstitium. *Eur Respir J* 1990; **3**: 1048–68.

13. Bahkle YS. Pharmacokinetic and metabolic properties of the lung. *Br J Anaesth* 1990; **65**: 79–93.

14. Ryan US. Structural basis for metabolic activity. *Annu Rev Physiol* 1982; **44**: 223–39.

15. Weibel ER. How does lung structure affect gas exchange? *Chest* 1983; **83**: 657–65.

16. Sole MJ, Dobrac M, Schwartz L, Hussain MN, Vaughan-Neil EF. The extraction of circulating catecholamines by the lungs in normal man and in patients with pulmonary hypertension. *Circulation* 1979; **60**: 160–3.

17. Gillis CN, Pitt BR. The fate of circulating amines within the pulmonary circulation. *Annu Rev Physiol* 1982; **44**: 269–81.

18. Said SI. Metabolic functions of the pulmonary circulation. *Circ Res* 1982; **50**: 325–33.

19. Brew K. Structure of human ACE gives new insights into inhibitor binding and design. *Trends Pharmacol Sci* 2003; **24**: 391–4.

20. Needleman P, Blaine EH, Greenwald JE, *et al.* The biochemical pharmacology of atrial peptides. *Annu Rev Pharmacol Toxicol* 1989; **29**: 23–54.

21. Iervasi G, Clerico A, Pilo A, *et al.* Atrial natriuretic peptide is not degraded by the lungs in humans. *J Clin Endocrinol Metab* 1998; **83**: 2898–906.

22. Michael JR, Markewitz BA. Endothelins and the lung. *Am J Respir Crit Care Med* 1996; **154**: 555–81.

23. Hardy C, Robinson C, Lewis RA, Tattersfield AE, Holgate ST. Airway and cardiovascular responses to inhaled prostacyclin in normal and asthmatic subjects. *Am Rev Respir Dis* 1985; **131**: 18–21.

*24. Groneberg DA, Witt C, Wagner U, Chung KF, Fischer A. Fundamentals of pulmonary drug delivery. *Respir Med* 2003; **97**: 382–7.

25. Bennett WD, Brown JS, Zeman KL, Hu S-C, Scheuch G, Sommerer K. Targeting delivery of aerosols to different lung regions. *J Aerosol Med* 2002; **15**: 179–88.

26. Blitt CD, Brown BR, Wright BJ, Gandolfi AJ, Sipes G. Pulmonary biotransformation of methoxyflurane: an *in vitro* study in the rabbit. *Anesthesiology* 1979; **51**: 528–31.

27. Bend JR, Serabjit-Singh CJ, Philpot RM. The pulmonary uptake, accumulation and metabolism of xenobiotics. *Annu Rev Pharmacol Toxicol* 1985; **25**: 97–125.

28. Upton RN, Doolette DJ. Kinetic aspects of drug deposition in the lungs. *Clin Exp Pharmacol Physiol* 1999; **26**: 381–391.

*29. Boer F. Drug handling by the lungs. *Br J Anaesth* 2003; **91**: 50–60.

30. Foth H. Role of the lung in accumulation and metabolism of xenobiotic compounds – implications for chemically induced toxicity. *Crit Rev Toxicol* 1995; **25**: 165–205.

31. Reasor MJ, Kacew S. An evaluation of possible mechanisms underlying amiodarone-induced pulmonary toxicity. *Proc Soc Exp Biol Med* 1996; **212**: 297–305.

32. Gosney JR. The endocrine lung and its response to hypoxia. *Thorax* 1994; **49**: S25–S26.

13 The history of respiratory physiology

KEY POINTS

■ That breathing was essential for life was clear to the ancient Egyptian civilisations 5000 years ago, but the reasons for this were unknown.

■ Early explanations for the function of breathing involved the air drawn into the lungs fuelling combustion in the heart and removing 'sooty and fuliginous spirits' from the body.

■ In the Renaissance, advances in knowledge of anatomy led to the discovery of the pulmonary circulation and the observation that blood changed colour on passing through the lungs.

■ Physiology in the 17th century involved more rigorous scientific experimentation and led to several discoveries about the mechanics and function of breathing.

■ Developments in fundamental sciences, particularly chemistry and physics, facilitated the elucidation of current knowledge of breathing and respiration.

The historical path along which we have gained our current knowledge of respiratory physiology is long and varied. There are periods when our understanding leapt forward in just a few years, interspersed by prolonged periods when progress was negligible and even some periods when it was reversed. That breathing is essential for life was clear from the beginnings of history, but the mechanism of breathing and the reasons for it remained elusive for many centuries. Progress usually occurred in parallel with understanding in other scientific disciplines, particularly chemistry, physics and anatomy. Innovative ideas on the physiology of breathing led, in more than one instance, to the premature death of the physiologist, and the history of respiratory physiology includes some of the most famous controversies seen in medical science.

This chapter is of necessity only a brief overview of the subject and ends around 100 years ago, when the explosion of scientific progress makes the subject too large for such a short account. Significant advances in respiratory physiology in the last 100 years are reported in the other chapters of this book and the reader interested in the history of this period is referred to more authoritative accounts.[1–3] For more general information on the history of respiratory physiology, numerous recent sources (by historical standards) are available.[4–6]

ANCIENT CIVILISATIONS

Egyptian physiology[7]

Ancient Egyptian civilisations existed from around 3100BC to 332BC when the Graeco-Roman period began. The most remarkable contribution made to history by the ancient Egyptians is their writings, though knowledge of their language was mostly lost after 500AD. Approximately 1300 years later, 19th-century scholars were able to use the Coptic language to assist in translating the ancient Egyptian writings. This has allowed an insight into medical knowledge from as early as 1820BC, the date of the earliest known medical writings in the Kahun papyrus.

Medical papyri. Many Egyptian papyri are concerned with medical topics, mostly descriptions of pragmatic 'recipes' for the treatment of a multitude of specific conditions.[7]

The longest and best known of the medical papyri is the Ebers papyrus,[8–10] which dates from about 1534BC and is accepted as being a compilation of various earlier works. The Ebers papyrus is unique in containing a section on physiology, including comments on respiration. The overall purpose of respiration is described thus:

'As to the air that penetrates into the nose. It enters into the heart and the lung. They are those which give air to the entire body.'[10]

Further sections include detailed descriptions of specific numbers of *metu* conducting 'moisture and air' to many parts of the body. These *metu* seem to mostly relate to blood vessels but also probably included such structures as tendons, muscles and the ureters. At first, this primitive view of anatomy is surprising considering the embalming abilities of ancient Egyptians, though in practice, embalming was carried out using very small inconspicuous incisions that would have revealed very little internal anatomy. Two *metu* are ascribed to each ear, through which *'the breath of life enters into the right ear and the breath of death enters into the left'*,[10] illustrating the 'magical' aspect of medicine at the time.

Ancient Greece

Greek writers were primarily philosophers, but they were also outstanding physicians, with one of their number, Hippocrates, forming a school that is now widely credited with the foundation of modern medical conduct. Early Greek philosophers such as Anaximenes (570BC–?) clearly stated that *'pneuma'* or air was essential to life,[6] but in contrast to this correct observation, Alcmaeon reportedly claimed that goats breathed through their ears and that some air passed from the nose directly to the brain.[4] Empedocles (495–435BC) disputed many of Alcmaeon's writings, but suggested instead that breathing occurred through the skin and that blood flow from the heart was tidal in nature, ebbing and flowing to and from the heart. Empedocles successfully combined physiology and philosophy in his description of the 'innate heat' in the heart, which was closely related to the soul and which was distributed throughout the body by the heart. This concept of heat generation within the heart gained acceptance throughout the ancient Greek period and was to remain at the centre of respiratory physiological ideas for about 1000 years.

The writings of Plato, Aristotle and the Hippocratic school only rarely directed their attention to respiration, but their contribution to scientific method and thinking was enormous. Subsequent philosopher-physicians adopted a more scientific approach to investigating physiology. At this time, dissection became widely practised, sometimes in public and on both animals and humans. This work was carried out in Alexandria under Ptolemy II in a totally Greek environment freed from the Egyptian embargo on dissection. Animal vivisection also undoubtedly took place and there are even disputed reports of human vivisection of criminals.[4] Herophilus (circa 325BC) distinguished between arteries and veins and, along with Aristotle, asserted that they contained air.

Erasistratus (304–250BC), more widely renowned as the father of philosophy, was the first to apply scientific principles to explain breathing. His view was that air was taken into the lungs and passed to the heart along the pulmonary artery. In the heart, air was converted into a 'vital spirit' that was distributed to all parts of the body by the arteries, while the brain further converted the vital spirit into 'animal spirit' which travelled down the hollow nerves to activate muscles. Erasistratus seemed

to understand that heart valves only allowed flow to occur in one direction, but failed to apply this knowledge to elucidate the transport of vital spirit or blood around the body. After Erasistratus, Greek interest moved away from medicine to philosophy and the physical sciences and the progression of physiological knowledge halted for about 400 years.

Roman medicine and Galen (129–199AD)

By the age of 28 years Claudius Galen was physician to the gladiators of Pergamun and 12 years later became physician to the Roman emperor Marcus Aurelius. He wrote many works on anatomy and physiology, many of which still exist in modern form, including two with much material on respiration: *'On the usefulness of the parts of the body'* and *'On the use of breathing'*.[11,12] Galen's work provides the first direct evidence of experimentation and the application of clinical observations to explain physiology.

Galen's system of physiology and anatomy. In Galen's descriptions, food was processed in the gut before being used by the liver to produce blood, which passed to the right heart. Much of this blood flowed into the pulmonary artery to nourish the lung, while the remainder passed across invisible pores in the interventricular septum, to be combined with *'pneuma'* brought from the lung via the pulmonary vein (Figure 13.1). In the left heart, the pneuma instilled the blood with vital spirit that was circulated to the body and brain, as described by Erasistratus.

Anatomically Galen regarded the lungs as having three types of intertwining vessel: the pulmonary artery, pulmonary vein and the 'rough artery' (trachea) made of membranous ligaments and cartilages, the incomplete cartilaginous rings being essential for voice production. On respiratory mechanics, Galen regards the ribs as primarily providing protection for the intrathoracic organs, particularly the heart, but he also clearly describes the role of the intercostal muscles and diaphragm in effecting both inspiratory and expiratory movements. He understood the potential problems of diaphragmatic splinting, describing respiration as 'little and fast' in such conditions as pregnancy and 'water or phlegm in the liver'.

Experiments on respiration. Galen's experiments provided mixed results.

1. For the first time he proved that arteries contained no air, but only blood, by ligating an animal's artery in two places before opening the vessel under water. He wrote at length about blood flow, realising that tidal blood flow to and from the lungs with each

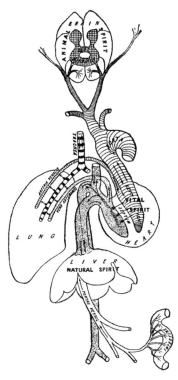

Figure 13.1 Illustration reconstructing Galen's scheme of cardiovascular and respiratory physiology as described in the text. (Galen did not use illustrations in his writings; this diagram is reproduced from Singer C. *A short history of anatomy and physiology from the Greeks to Harvey*. New York: Dover Publications, 1957.)

breath was *'in no way suitable for the blood'*.[11] He suggested the existence of capillaries 1500 years before they were discovered by stating *'All over the body the arteries and veins communicate with one another by common openings and exchange blood and pneuma through certain invisible and extremely narrow passages'*.

2. Galen ligated both carotid arteries of a dog, an intervention that he observed caused the animal no detectable harm. He concluded that the brain could therefore derive pneuma directly from the nose, to make the animal spirit earlier described by the Greeks (termed 'psychic pneuma' by Galen).

3. During his time in the gladiator arena he observed that the level of neck injury sustained by gladiators affected their breathing,[6] so proving that respiration originated in the brain. He did many animal experiments to ascertain more precisely the spinal level at which the nerves responsible for respiration originated and went on to describe the nerve roots and destination of the phrenic nerves.[12]

4. On the necessity for breathing via the mouth and nose Galen was unclear, writing in earlier works that pneuma could enter arteries via the pharynx, heart or skin as well as the lungs. An experiment to attempt to demonstrate this was carried out: *'Covering the mouth and nostrils of a boy with a large ox-bladder, or any such vessel, so that he was unable to draw breath at all outside it, we saw him breathing unhindered through a whole day'*. Galen's conclusion from this study is contradictory: *'Hence it is clear that the arteries all through the animal draw in the outer air very little or not at all'*. Modern views of this experiment are that the ox-bladder was unlikely to be airtight or that Galen's assistants must have removed the bladder to allow the boy to breathe easily when their master was not directly supervising the experiment.[12]

The functions of breathing. Apart from providing pneuma to the heart, Galen described other functions for breathing.

1. *Regulation of heat.* Galen's writings strengthened the analogy between the heart and a flame and several pages of *On the use of breathing* are concerned with the similarities between the two. For example, the observation that flames were extinguished when deprived of air, or that an oil lamp burns out when its sustenance, the oil, is used up, were seen as analogous to humans seen *'perishing when deprived of air'* or who lacked sufficient nourishment. Galen was concerned about the contradictory requirements for the idea of the heart and lungs generating innate heat, realising that a fine balance must be drawn between *'fanning the source of the innate heat and from cooling in due proportion'*, citing examples such as fever, with increased breathing, when the balance was disturbed.

2. *Voice.* Galen described in detail the anatomy of the laryngeal cartilages and muscles and wrote a whole treatise on the voice, clearly recognising the importance of the lungs. The rough artery (trachea) provided preliminary regulation of the voice, which was produced in the larynx and amplified off the roof of the mouth with the uvula acting as a plectrum. The purpose of having such a large volume of air in the lung was to allow continuous use of the voice.

3. *Removal of sooty and fuliginous spirits.* Waste products from the blood were discharged from the lung and this was the function of expiration. Without doing so, the heart would have become stifled by its own 'smoky vapours', once again like a burning flame. Explanations by Galen as to how the body separated the fuliginous spirits from the pneuma have become uncertain with the passage of time, one explanation being that the fuliginous spirits were regurgitated

through the incompetent mitral valve and passed back along the pulmonary vein to the lung.[6]

4. *Physical protection of the heart.* The spongy nature of lung tissue and the position of the heart in the centre of the chest led Galen to suggest that the lung served to cushion the heart from the effects of body movements.

Galen's legacy. Galen was undoubtedly a genius. He was the first physician to apply the Hippocratic methods of scientific thinking to physiology and he ingeniously combined the knowledge of his predecessors with his own thinking to produce an impressive treatise on the workings of the human body. Also, it is from the writings of Galen that we have obtained our knowledge of many of his predecessors: most of what is known of Erasistratus's views on physiology is derived from Galen's comments on them. Galen's work also deserves a place in history as the longest unchallenged scientific work. The physiology described in this section was taught in medical schools throughout the world, and scientifically mostly unchallenged, for around 1400 years.

There was also a darker and more controversial side to Galen. He is widely believed to have been conceited, dogmatic and abusive of those criticising him.[6] *On the usefulness of the parts of the body* contains several prolonged and personal refutations of the ideas of his predecessors, for example accusing '*Asclepiades, wisest of men*' of making errors '*no child would fail to recognise, not to mention a man so full of his own importance*'.

After Galen

When Galen died, the study of physiology and anatomy effectively ceased. The Roman empire was in decline and in 389AD Christian fanatics burned down the library in Alexandria, which contained many writings by the Greek philosopher-physicians.

Preservation of knowledge now fell to scholars of the Byzantine and Arabic empires. The latter embraced Galen's ideas with enthusiasm and translated many Greek works into Arabic, almost certainly adding their own refinements as they did so. The greatest of these Arabic scholars was Avicenna (circa 980–1037), whose canon was an impressive document pulling together and classifying all the available medical knowledge of the time, creating what has been described as a popular medical encyclopaedia of the medieval period. Some years later, Ibn Al Nafis[14] (1210–1288), a prolific Arabic writer on many subjects, studied Avicenna's writings and wrote his own treatise *Sharh Tashirh Al-Qanun* (Commentary on the Anatomy of the Canon of Avicenna). In this he challenged the Galenic view of pores in the interventricular septum through which blood passed and instead suggested that blood passed through the lung

substance, where it permeated with the air.[5,14] This was an early breakthrough in explaining the true nature of the pulmonary circulation, but Ibn Al Nafis' work did not become well known for many more centuries.

THE RENAISSANCE

In the 12th and 13th centuries, scholastic pursuits began again with the foundation of many European universities, first Oxford, Cambridge and Bologna, closely followed by Paris, Naples and Padua. Soon, many of the ancient documents were translated from Greek or Arabic into Latin and human dissection began to be performed after many centuries of interdiction by the Pope. Knowledge of anatomy again began to advance, with publications such as the *Anathomia* by Mondina, a professor of anatomy, at Bologna in 1316. Interest in the function of the body only began again with Leonardo da Vinci in the 15th century.

Leonardo da Vinci (1452–1519)[4]

Leonardo exemplified the Renaissance trend for combining art with science. His anatomical drawings are both extensive and ingenious, being mostly surrounded by extensive explanatory notes.[15–17] These notes are written in Latin and in mirror writing, possibly simply because Leonardo was left-handed and received no formal schooling to correct this, or possibly to make his notes harder to read by uneducated persons described by him as 'bad company'.[4]

Although Leonardo is known to have dissected over 30 human cadavers, most of his drawings of the respiratory system are based on dissections of animals, including Figure 13.2 showing in beautiful detail the structure of the pig lung. In the commentary on this drawing, Leonardo considers the use of the 'substance' of the lung and extends Galen's protective function of the lung parenchyma when he states that '*the substance is interposed between these ramifications* [of the trachea] *and the ribs of the chest to act as a soft covering*'. Structures entering the chest cavity are labelled a–e and their functions described:

a. *trachea, whence the voice passes*
b. *oesophagus, whence the food passes*
c. *apoplectic [carotid] arteries, whence the vital spirit passes*
d. *dorsal spine, whence the ribs arise*
e. *spondyles [spinous processes of the vertebrae], whence the muscles arise which end in the nape of the neck and elevate the face towards the sky.*

Leonardo adhered to other Galenic ideas such as the presence of air in the pleural space, but was unsure how the air entered or left this space, and in his later draw-

Figure 13.2 Leonardo's drawing of the thoracic organs of a pig (*c.* 1508). The organs are labelled in mirror writing in Latin: *polmone,* lung; *feghato,* liver; *milza,* spleen; *stommacco,* stomach; *djaflamma,* diaphragm; *spina,* spine. See text for an explanation of labels a–e above the drawing on the right. (The Royal Collection, © 2005, Her Majesty Queen Elizabeth II.)

Figure 13.3 Leonardo's drawing of the pulmonary circulation in relation to the bronchi (*c.* 1513). Pulmonary vessels arise from several parts of the heart, leading Leonardo to propose a dual blood supply to the lung. Coronary arteries and veins can be clearly seen on the heart. At the lower end of the main drawing, Leonardo has drawn a small circle containing the letter N. The notes describe the structure as having '*a crust, like a nutshell*' containing a '*dust and watery humour*' possibly representing his discovery of a lung cyst[18] or a tuberculous cavity.[16] (The Royal Collection, © 2005, Her Majesty Queen Elizabeth II.)

ings he was clearly beginning to doubt that air was always present. Leonardo's adherence to Galen's ideas was in some areas unshakable, in particular his depiction of the interventricular pores in several drawings of the cardiovascular system.

He did, however, challenge some Galenic ideas by the application of his engineering expertise. For example, he did not accept that the heart generated innate heat, instead writing that heat generation in the heart resulted from mechanical friction between the blood and the walls of the heart.[4] Similarly, his engineering knowledge made him intrigued by the actions of the chest wall and respiratory muscles, including the complexities of defining the different function of internal and external intercostal muscles. For the diaphragm, Leonardo described four functions: dilating the lung for inspiration; pressing the stomach to drive food into the intestine; contracting with the abdominal muscles to drive out abdominal superfluities; and to separate the spiritual (thoracic) organs from the natural (abdominal) ones. Finally, he

considered in detail the movements of the trachea and bronchi on breathing, showing them to dilate and open wider at branches on inspiration, as shown to the right of Figure 13.3.

Leonardo and the bronchial circulation. In Figure 13.3, Leonardo depicts in detail the relationship of the pulmonary circulation to a bronchus. Much of the commentary in the drawing is concerned with the superiority of drawings rather than words to describe such anatomical configurations. The figure clearly shows a dual blood supply to the lung and suggests that the smaller of these two supplies is to '*nourish and vivify the trachea*'. From this drawing, many writers have credited Leonardo with discovering the bronchial circulation, though this claim has recently been disputed.[18,19] The drawing is believed to be based on an ox, a species recently shown to have distinct small pulmonary veins draining directly into the left atrium, which may be those found by Leonardo.

The possibility of artistic licence in his drawings has caused disputes that will never be resolved, such as that of the bronchial circulation. For example, in Figure 13.2 the perfectly branching pattern of the bronchi on the lung surface is clearly not based on true observation of pig lungs. In Figure 13.3 of ox lungs, the right upper lobe bronchus that arises directly from the trachea in this species is absent. However, in spite of these misgivings regarding his drawings, Leonardo's genius in combining art, science and engineering in the study of physiology is undisputed.

Anatomy in the Renaissance

After Leonardo, the pursuit of medical knowledge in the universities continued, with anatomy in particular aided by the continuing resurgence of dissection and vivisection. Andreas Vesalius (1514–1564) is primarily remembered as the founder of modern anatomy, his dissections culminating in the publication in 1543 of *De Humanis Corporis Fabrica*, a book of seven volumes including over 250 anatomical illustrations (Figure 13.4).[20] His ideas

Figure 13.4 Figure from Book VI of Vesalius's *Fabrica*,[20] showing an anterior view of the lungs after removal of the heart. A, oesophagus; B, trachea; C, pulmonary artery; D, pulmonary vein; I, diaphragm. E–H refer to the lobes of the lung – Vesalius's illustrations always showed the lungs as having four lobes.[21] (Reproduced with permission from the Special Collections, Leeds University Library.)

met with resistance from his contemporaries whenever his views were at odds with those of Galen and this eventually forced Vesalius to cease his study of anatomy and to return to work as a physician. Nevertheless, the *Fabrica* continued to gain acceptance and became the foundation for future anatomy texts. Vesalius was also a skilled physiologist. He was the first to describe an experiment reproduced much later, in which a section of the chest wall of an animal was carefully removed without breaching the pleura beneath, so enabling direct observation of lung movements through the transparent pleura.[6]

The pulmonary circulation.[22] Unaware of the earlier writings of Ibn Al Nafis, Servetus (1509–1553), in his religious treatise *Christianismi restitutio*,[23] again challenged the existence of Galen's interventricular pores. He wrote that rather than passing through the middle wall of the heart, '*blood is urged forward by a long course through the lung . . . and is poured from the pulmonary artery to the pulmonary vein*'.[24] He also commented that on passing through the lung the blood changed colour, becoming '*reddish-yellow*', though an explanation for this observation was still two centuries away. Tragically, *Christianismi restitutio* was deemed to be heretical by the Christian church and the book, along with its author, was burned at the stake in 1553. Only three copies of *Christianismi restituto* are believed to exist today,[24] though more recent reprints are available.[25]

Just a few years later, Realdus Colombo (1516–1559) became the third physiologist to apparently independently describe the pulmonary circulation. Colombo, a pupil of Vesalius, posthumously published his account of anatomy, *De Re Anatomicae*, in which he clearly describes blood flowing through the lung while mixing with air.[26] There is a suspicion that Colombo had previously had access to Servetus's *Christianismi restitutio* or that he knew of the writings of Ibn Al Nafis from 300 years earlier, causing confusion as to which of these eminent physiologists should be credited with the discovery of pulmonary blood flow.[5,22]

EXPERIMENTAL PHYSIOLOGY IN THE 17TH CENTURY

At the start of the 17th century the dominance of Italian universities with respect to medicine and anatomy subsided and progress in the understanding of respiration moved to England, where a new approach of experimental philosophy was developing.[4]

Discoveries to assist the respiratory physiologists

Circulation. William Harvey (1578–1657) studied at Cambridge and Padua universities, so was well placed to combine the Italian methods and knowledge of anatomy with the English approach of physiological experimentation engendered by Francis Bacon. The most notable of Harvey's teachers in Padua was Hieronymus Fabricius, who is credited with the discovery of the venous valves, including the simple demonstration in arm veins that valves prevent blood from flowing distally. In 1616 Harvey first presented his ideas of the blood circulating continuously in a lecture to the College of Physicians in London. After a further 12 years of experimentation, Harvey published *De Motu Cordis*, in which he describes the circular motion of the blood in both the lesser (pulmonary) and greater (systemic) circulation.[27,28] Harvey's comments on respiration in *De Motu Cordis* are sparse, and although he refers in several places to a future separate treatise on respiration, it seems this was never written.

Atmospheric pressure.[4] The Italian physicists Berti and Torricelli, both of whom were acquainted with Galileo, accidentally discovered air pressure in their search to create a vacuum. First Berti, with a water barometer built of lead pipe attached to his house in Rome, measured the height of the water column at 27 feet. Torricelli and a mathematician colleague Vivianni then made the first mercury barometer using mercury in a glass tube inverted over a bowl of mercury, and so allowed the height of the column to be visualised. The full implications of their discovery only occurred after Berti and Torricelli died, as the existence of a vacuum was considered by some to be a heresy and fear of persecution resulted in their discoveries not being widely disseminated to the scientific community.

The microscope. Harvey and his numerous predecessors who described blood flowing through the lung tissue were not able to determine by what route this occurred or how the blood and air were mixed. Harvey thought it most likely that the blood and air came into contact through pores in the lung structures. Marcelus Malpighi (1628–1694) used a primitive microscope to observe lung tissue. His original communication in 1661, *De Pulmonibus*,[29,30] consisted of two letters to his friend Borrelli who was a professor of science in Pisa.[5] Malpighi used frogs for his studies and describes in detail the lung preparations used, remarking that he had '*destroyed almost the whole race of frogs*' in the course of his work.[30] He described lung tissue to be '*an aggregate of very light and very thin membranes, which, tense and sinuous, form an almost infinite number of orbicular vesicles and cavities, such as we see in the honeycomb of bees*'. This first description of the alveoli was accompanied by a drawing of his preparation (Figure 13.5) and he went on to describe how the vesicles were all terminations of branches of the bronchi and that under normal circum-

Figure 13.5 Drawing of Malpighi's preparation of frog lungs.[29] I, Seen from the surface of the lungs; II, showing the cut surface of the lung (including blood vessels on the surface of the vesicles [alveoli]); III, a schematic representation of the branching of the bronchi into vesicles. (Reproduced with permission from the Special Collections, Leeds University Library.)

stances the blood and air were separated by them. In his second letter, Malpighi went on to describe the network of capillaries over the surface of the vesicles and even observed the movement of the blood through them.

The mystery of the structure of lung tissue was now solved. Blood flowed from the right heart to the lung, through Malpighi's 'smallest of vessels', past the air-containing vesicles and returned to the left heart. However, scientists were still no closer to discovering the purpose of this elaborate arrangement.

The Oxford physiologists and the 'use of breathing'[1,5,6]

In the mid-17th century a remarkable group of scientists happened upon each other in London, where the group held meetings to exchange ideas and discuss scientific topics, often holding the meetings in their lodgings. The group was initially referred to by its members in London as the 'Invisible College' but later, in Oxford, became the 'Experimental Philosophy Club'. After around 15 years in existence, the club was granted a royal charter by the king and formed the Royal Society of London. Of the numerous notable club members, four are worthy of particular note here in view of their contribution to knowledge of respiration.

Robert Boyle (1627–1691). Assisted by Hooke, Boyle constructed a 'new pneumatical engine' that was capable of pumping air out of closed containers to produce a vacuum. He soon demonstrated that flames were extinguished and animals died in the vacuum and so began to believe there was some vital component present in air that was necessary for both combustion and animal life. Other experiments led Boyle away from the truth about the purpose of respiration. Enclosing a candle and a chick together, he observed that the chick survived much longer than the flame, indicating that combustion and respiration were different. Similarly, using a mercury gauge, observations that the pressure within closed vessels did not change when animals expired led Boyle to believe that the vital component was present in only tiny amounts. For a scientist so dedicated to experimentation, Boyle was often considered to be poor at interpreting their results,[4] often leaving this important task to his close friend Robert Hooke.

Robert Hooke (1635–1702). A crucial partnership between Hooke and Boyle brought about the studies described in the previous paragraph. However, Hooke is best known in the area of respiration for a dramatic demonstration to the Royal Society in 1667.[31] Keeping animals alive by artificial ventilation with bellows had been demonstrated many times before by both Leonardo da Vinci and Vesalius. However, in Hooke's demonstration, he used two pairs of bellows to provide a constant stream of air and ventilated a dog with part of the chest wall removed and with *'numerous small holes pricked in the outer coat of the lungs'* (pleura). With this experiment he achieved successful apnoeic ventilation for well over an hour and so conclusively demonstrated that *'bare motion of the lungs without fresh air contributes nothing to the life of the animal'*.

Richard Lower (1631–1691). Lower performed many animal experiments to investigate the known colour change of blood on exposure to air. First, he proved that the colour change occurred within the lungs, rather than in the heart, demonstrating the colour difference between blood from the pulmonary artery and vein. He then proceeded to show that the colour change occurred only when air was present within the lung by, for example, ceasing artificial respiration of an animal and

observing that blood in the pulmonary vein quickly turned blue.

John Mayow (1641–1679).[4] Mayow was the youngest of the Oxford physiologists, having studied with Lower and worked as Boyle's laboratory assistant. His major work on respiration, *Tractatus Quinque Medico-Physici*,[32] was published in 1674, a few years after Boyle, Lower and Hooke had moved on from their studies of respiration. *Tractatus Quinque* was an impressive treatise, bringing together in a single book the ideas of Mayow's eminent colleagues, supplemented with his own experimental work and ideas on chemistry and the physiology of respiration. His many experiments were illustrated with a single-page drawing containing six figures (Figure 13.6). Mayow again showed that animal respiration and combustion had similar effects on the volume of air within the enclosed glasses. By good fortune, Mayow found a much greater change in volume than Boyle's pressure changes. Mayow's use of water, and observations over a longer time period, allowed the carbon dioxide to be absorbed into the water and the temperature within the vessel to return to ambient. This led him to extend Boyle's ideas that air contained a vital component, which he named nitro-aerial spirit. When breathed in by animals, nitro-aerial spirit combined with salino-sulphureous particles in the blood to produce a 'fermentation', which ultimately gave rise to muscular contraction. This last observation occurred from Mayow's appreciation of increased breathing during exercise.

Tractatus Quinque also contains excellent sections on respiratory mechanics. Mayow clearly understood that lung movement was brought about only by expansion and contraction of the chest wall, with a recognition that expiration was normally a passive process. He demonstrated this by placing a bladder within a pair of bellows fitted with a glass window to allow observation of the bladder inflating and deflating as the bellows were worked (see Figure 13.6). Mayow then applied his knowledge of physiology to pathology, by explaining that difficulty in breathing occurs if the abdominal contents resist the descent of the diaphragm, a situation seen with over-eating, enlarged abdominal viscera, orthopnoea and even in the 'hysteric passion'. He fully understood the problems of pneumothorax, giving advice to his surgical colleagues:

'Here, by the way, surgeons should be warned not to close the wound if the chest has been perforated except when the thorax is contracted to the utmost; for, otherwise, if the opening made by the wound is closed when the chest cavity is expanded it will be impossssible for the chest to contract on account of the resistance of the air inside, or for the lungs

a

b

Figure 13.6 Illustration of Mayow's experiments on respiration.[32] **(a)** Combustible materials, ignited by a magnifying glass and the sun's heat (Fig. 1) or animal respiration (Fig. 6) cause the water to rise within the enclosed glass, or a moistened bladder to be drawn into the glass (Fig. 2). Chemical reactions were instituted within the closed glasses by, for example, adding iron to spirit of nitre (Fig. 4) directly or leaving globules of iron in the base of a glass in contact with diluted spirit of nitre (Fig. 3). Fig. 5 shows Mayow's system for transferring air from one glass to another. **(b)**, drawing of the bladder in the bellows to demonstrate the passive expansion and contraction of the lungs by the chest wall.

to expand, except partially, and, in consequence, suffocation will occur.'

Tractatus Quinque was controversial soon after it was written, with Mayow being accused of failing to acknowledge his use of other people's ideas and '*clogging*

the work with absurd additions of his own'. The work was rarely referred to by his peers and remained obscure for over a century. In particular, it is likely that the chemists of the following century (see below) who discovered oxygen were completely unaware of Mayow's work. More than 250 years after publication, shortly after *Tractatus Quinque* was translated into English,[32] the controversy of Mayow's work was reignited. Patterson, a professor of chemistry, published a vehement attack on Mayow's work, including the comment that '*such views as were sound were not Mayow's, whilst those which were Mayow's were not sound.*'[33] A rebuttal by Partington in 1956 redressed the balance and concluded that Mayow's views were '*a great advance on others of their time*' and that Mayow was '*one of the outstanding experimenters and thinkers of his time*'.[34]

Physiology hibernates

After the death of Mayow, the study of respiratory physiology again halted, this time for about 100 years. The other Oxford scientists had already moved on to different pursuits such as physical chemistry (Boyle), architecture (Hooke) and lucrative private medicine (Lower). The other great centres of learning in Europe did not take up the mantle of respiratory research. The cause of this stagnancy is uncertain:[4] this was another politically turbulent period of history in Europe and conditions may not have been conducive to academic study. There may even have been a sense that respiration was now effectively explained, considering that knowledge of other closely related scientific disciplines, particularly chemistry, was still at a very primitive stage.

CHEMISTRY AND RESPIRATION

Different types of air

Phlogiston.[6] George Ernst Stahl (1660–1734) had begun to investigate the chemistry of combustion in the early 18th century and provided the scientific community with a completely erroneous explanation, which was nevertheless widely accepted. Stahl proposed that all combustible substances were made up of two components: calx, combined with a fiery principle named phlogiston. On burning, the phlogiston was driven off from the substance, leaving just the calx or ash. Substances such as charcoal, which left very little ash, must have contained a greater proportion of phlogiston. Combustion in an enclosed space was extinguished when the air contained within became saturated with phlogiston. Calcination of metals (intense heating in air until oxidation occurs) was explained as driving off the phlogiston contained in the metal, whereas conversion of the metal oxide back to metal by heating with charcoal was achieved by the charcoal donating its phlogiston to recreate the metal. A powerful piece of evidence contradicted the phlogiston theory for metal calcination. Boyle, Mayow and others had all demonstrated that when metals were calcined they gained weight, so could not have lost phlogiston. Stahl provided a very dubious explanation of this by explaining that on calcination the metal also lost some of its 'negative weight'.

Although the phlogiston theory was a complete inversion of what we now know to be true, it fitted with almost all known observations of combustion in the 18th century, with only the single exception already described. Stahl's views therefore became very enduring and are believed to have impeded progress in understanding the chemistry of gases for many decades.

Fixed air and vitiated air. Joseph Black (1728–1799) was a Scottish chemist whose work focused on the chemistry of alkalis, a group of substances widely used at the time for the treatment of kidney complaints. He demonstrated that heating chalk ($CaCO_3$) caused a gas to be liberated and a reduction in weight to occur. To explain the large observed weight loss, Black believed the liberated gas to be air rather than phlogiston. After further experiments Black found that the same gas was produced by fermentation, by burning charcoal, and was present in expired air. From these observations he named it 'fixed air', believing that the gas made up all the non-respirable portion of air. Only a few years later in 1772, the discovery of 'vitiated air' (nitrogen) demonstrated that fixed air was present in only small quantities in air. Black's explanation of the chemical reactions of carbon dioxide did not involve phlogiston at all, which must have been surprising considering the fundamental place phlogiston held in the chemistry of the time, but the phlogiston theory continued unchallenged.

Dephlogisticated air. Two chemists independently demonstrated the concept of oxygen and respiration. Joseph Priestley[35] (1733–1804) in England carried out a range of experiments with respiratory gases. His work was published in '*Experiments and observations on different kinds of air*',[36] which included an illustration of the equipment used (Figure 13.7). Initially described by Priestley as 'pure air', the gas produced by heating mercuric oxide was found to cause a candle to burn with '*a remarkably vigorous flame*' and to allow a mouse to survive much longer than in 'common air'. Priestley tried breathing the pure air himself with no apparent ill effects. His experiments on plants led to the major discovery that vegetation, in particular fast-growing species such as spinach, reversed the gaseous changes caused by respiration, burning candles or putrefaction within his

Figure 13.7 Frontispiece from Priestley's '*Experiments and observations on different kinds of air*',[36] showing the variety of apparatus used in his experiments. Mice can be seen contained within a beer glass (d) which allowed them to breath for 20–30 minutes in 'common air', while others are held in receivers open at the top and bottom for use in later experiments (at the front of the illustration). Plants can be seen growing in the jar on the far right. (Reproduced with permission from the Special Collections, Leeds University Library.)

closed vessels. He fully appreciated the import of this discovery on a global scale by commenting that air in the common atmosphere that has been reduced to a noxious state by respiration or combustion '*has never failed to be perfectly restored by vegetation, so that the growing vegetables with which the surface of the Earth is overspread, may be a cause of the purification of the atmosphere*'. An advocate of phlogiston, Priestley soon renamed his 'pure air' 'dephlogisticated air'. He believed his experiments confirmed the phlogiston theory, i.e. the mercuric oxide removed phlogiston from the air, so allowing candles to burn longer or animals to respire longer, before the air became saturated with phlogiston.

Fire air. Carl Scheele[35] (1742–1786) studied chemistry and pharmacy in Sweden. Unaware of Priestley's work Scheele, using a variety of methods, also produced oxygen, which he named 'fire air'. He too demonstrated its effect on burning candles and animal respiration, but he also failed to use his results to challenge the phlogiston theory.

Oxygen

Antoine-Laurent Lavoisier[35] (1743–1794) was born in Paris and graduated in science before the age of 20, specialising in chemistry soon after. In a very productive few years commencing around 1772, Lavoisier studied combustion and respiration, during which time he was visited by Priestley who discussed his own experiments with 'pure air'. Lavoisier approached chemistry differently, in effect introducing quantitative studies to the qualitative ones of his predecessors.[6] He showed that when metals were calcined in a closed jar the combined weight of apparatus, air and jar remained unchanged, so proving that it was air combining with the metal that increased their weight. In experiments with animals breathing nearly pure oxygen, he observed that the animals died before all the oxygen was used up and this led him to investigate the harmful effects of carbon dioxide in the atmosphere, including in lecture theatres.[4] Respiratory experiments over acidified water allowed the CO_2 produced by respiration to be absorbed and allowed the quantification of oxygen consumption, which in a resting subject was measured by Lavoisier as 1200 cubic inches per hour ($\approx 330 \, ml.min^{-1}$), a result very close to the modern value (page 189). However, it is Lavoisier's discovery that 'eminently respirable air' was a chemical element and his naming of the element as oxygen for which he is most remembered. Once again, the contribution made by the scientists of the time to this seminal discovery is controversial; for example, Priestley was later irritated at Lavoisier's use of the ideas they discussed in 1774 and Mayow's work is never referred to in Lavoisier's writings in spite of his being aware of it at the time.[4] Lavoisier's interests were wider than his study of science and he was closely involved in a French financial institution responsible for generating tax revenues, the Ferme Generale. Income from this clearly provided the resources for Lavoisier's extensive experiments, but also resulted in accusations of financial impropriety, which led to his untimely death at the guillotine in 1794.[6] After Lavoisier's death, his friend Lagrange commented that 'It took but a second to cut off his head; a hundred years will not suffice to produce one like it'.[37]

EARLY DEVELOPMENT OF CURRENT IDEAS OF RESPIRATORY PHYSIOLOGY

Tissue respiration

Ancient ideas of some type of combustion in the heart which generated heat gave way in the 16th century to the suggestion that heat was generated by friction within the ever-moving blood. As chemistry developed, the similarities between combustion and respiration became progressively more compelling, but where this oxidation reaction took place eluded even Lavoisier, who believed it occurred in the bronchi.

The impetus to look beyond the lungs and heart to find the site of combustion in the body came from the discovery of calorimetry by Adair Crawford (1748–1795).[38] Measurements made by Crawford and Lavoisier of the heat generated by the body made it clear to Lavoisier's mathematician friend Lagrange and his colleague Hassenfratz that if all the heat were produced in the lungs, their temperature 'would necessarily be raised so much that one would have reason to fear they would be destroyed'.[39] In Italy, further experiments into where in the body combustion took place were performed by Lazzaro Spallanzani (1729–1799), though his work was only published posthumously in 1803.[40] He studied respiration in a huge variety of creatures, including insects, reptiles, amphibians and mammals, and described how those creatures without lungs exchanged oxygen and carbon dioxide via their integument. That respiration still occurred in the absence of lungs led Spallanzani to his most important respiratory discovery when he showed that a variety of tissues from recently deceased creatures (including humans) continued to respire for some time, so showing that the tissues were the site of oxygen consumption.

In the 19th century, advances in science led to improved techniques for gas and temperature measurement. Heat production was measured in animals and humans and found to correlate with the specific heat capacity of the oxygen consumed and carbon dioxide produced. The respiratory quotient was measured at between 0.6 and 1.0 and found to depend on diet. Finally, with the birth of organic chemistry and the foundation of the laws of conservation of energy, the modern account of energy metabolism was elucidated.[6]

Blood gases

Once it was clear that oxygen metabolism occurred in the tissues, the search was on to find how the blood carried oxygen to and returned carbon dioxide from the tissues in sufficient quantities. However, other fundamental discoveries were needed before this question could be addressed in detail.

Partial pressure. John Dalton (1766–1844), whose law on partial pressures (page 457) is widely used today, first developed the concept that mixtures of gases could exist together irrespective of the pressure and temperature of the mixture. His description stated that the particles of each component gas had no interaction with those of the other gases and so 'arranged themselves just the same as in a void space' while paradoxically occupying the whole space allotted to the mixture of gases. He illustrated this as shown in Figure 13.8.[41]

Paul Bert (1833–1886), most famous for his studies of altitude physiology and medicine, also made a significant contribution to fundamental respiratory physiology by discovering that it was the partial pressure, rather than the concentration, of respiratory gases that affected biological systems.[42,43] In an elegant series of experiments,

Figure 13.8 Dalton's drawing to illustrate a compound atmosphere, made up of a mixture of simple atmospheres.[41] Two centuries after it was drawn, this diagram would be helpful to today's physiology students when first learning Dalton's law of partial pressures. Aqueous vapour, water vapour; oxygenous gas, oxygen; azotic gas, nitrogen; carbonic acid gas, carbon dioxide. (Reproduced by permission of the Wellcome Library of the History of Medicine.)

Figure 13.9 Figure from *La pression barométrique*[42] showing Paul Bert breathing oxygen while sitting in the chamber at progressively subatmospheric pressures. Note the sparrow in the cage above the subject – the bird falls in its cage when the pressure reaches 450 mmHg but Bert persists with the experiment down to 410 mmHg, maintaining consciousness by intermittently breathing oxygen. (Reproduced by permission of the Wellcome Library of the History of Medicine.)

he exposed animals to a variety of atmospheric pressures while maintaining the partial pressure of oxygen constant, with no ill effect on the animals. Whenever inspired PO_2 was reduced below that of air at atmospheric pressure, irrespective of the total pressure, the animal suffered the consequences of hypoxia. He repeated the experiments on humans in a large specially constructed chamber (Figure 13.9) and showed that by breathing supplementary oxygen, the harmful effects of low ambient pressure could be entirely alleviated.

Bert applied his knowledge to the recently discovered pastime of ballooning and assisted his friend Gaston Tissandier to use oxygen to ascend to record new heights in his balloon. However, in his enthusiasm for altitude, M. Tissandier and two friends undertook a balloon flight with the specific aim of reaching 8000 m (26 200 feet) altitude, but in their enthusiasm they did not have time to consult Bert on the likely oxygen requirement. An unusually rapid ascent (Figure 13.10) resulted in confusion in all three balloonists, who were unable to breathe the oxygen and lost consciousness (page 255). Only Tissandier recovered sufficiently to record their altitude as 8600 m (28 200 feet), before battling with hypoxia to intermittently breathe oxygen and facilitate a controlled descent, during which the full tragedy of the flight unfolded and he discovered that his two friends had died some time earlier in the flight.

Haemoglobin and its dissociation curve. Boyle and Mayow had both used a vacuum to extract gases from

Figure 13.10 Diagram of the high-altitude ascent of the balloon *Zenith* on 15 April 1875.[42] The dashed line indicates estimated altitude as the only survivor of the flight, Gaston Tissandier, was too hypoxic to make recordings of the altitude. (Reproduced by permission of the Wellcome Library of the History of Medicine.)

Figure 13.11 The first publication (from 1904) showing the shape of the oxyhaemoglobin dissociation curve.[47] Note the effect of blood P_{CO_2} on the position and shape of the curve (page 177). Pferdeblut, horse blood.

blood and surmised that this may have been air or nitro-aerial spirit (oxygen). In the 19th century the excellence of German chemists led them to dominate this field of research. Gustav Magnus (1802–1870) extracted oxygen and carbon dioxide from blood, showing that the former was more abundant in arterial blood and vice versa.[44] Lothar Meyer did similar experiments in 1857, but showed that the liberation of oxygen as pressure was reduced was not linear, so demonstrating that the oxygen was not simply dissolved in the blood.[45] Meanwhile, the red compound in blood was identified and soon found chemically to be a combination of globulin proteins and an iron containing haematin. The affinity of this new 'haemoglobin' for oxygen was soon understood and Hüfner quantified this binding by showing that 1.34 ml of oxygen combined with 1 g of crystallised haemoglobin, a remarkably accurate measurement (page 176).[46] By 1888, Hüfner had used haemoglobin solutions to record the relationship between the partial pressure of oxygen and haemoglobin saturation and obtained a rectangular hyperbola.[5] Finally in 1904, Christian Bohr and colleagues showed that when fresh whole blood was used to measure the haemoglobin dissociation, an S-shaped curve was found and that the curve altered with varying partial pressures of carbon dioxide (Figure 13.11).[47]

***The oxygen secretion controversy.*[1,48]** Measurement of the partial pressure of oxygen in arterial blood in the 19th century provoked a huge scientific controversy. In 1870, Bohr and colleagues developed a primitive aerotonometer and found arterial P_{O_2} to be around 80 mmHg (10.7 kPa), though in some measurements the arterial

P_{O_2} was found to be slightly higher than the alveolar P_{O_2}. At around this time, physiologists studying other body systems were discovering numerous active membrane transport systems in such places as the kidney and bowel. This led Bohr to suggest that active transport of oxygen may occur in the lung, and he soon had the support for this hypothesis from the eminent respiratory physiologist John Scott Haldane.

In his laboratories in Oxford, Haldane devised a new technique for measuring arterial P_{O_2}. This involved the subject breathing small concentrations of carbon monoxide and then using direct colour matching of the subject's blood with standard samples to ascertain the carboxyhaemoglobin concentration, from which the P_{O_2} could be calculated.[49] To standardise the light used for comparing colours, experiments had to be done during daylight and by today's standards several aspects of the technique seem remarkably subjective, but nevertheless Haldane was an excellent scientist who applied rigorous methodology. Using his technique Haldane found the average arterial P_{O_2} to be 200 mmHg (26.7 kPa), so claiming to have proved that oxygen secretion was occurring in the lung.

A Danish husband and wife team, August and Marie Krogh,[50] became Haldane's adversaries over oxygen secretion. August Krogh, a former pupil of Bohr, continued to refine the technique of aerotonometry, using analysis of smaller volumes of gas from continuously flowing blood samples. His results always showed arterial P_{O_2} to be slightly less than alveolar P_{O_2} even when tested across a variety of inspired oxygen concentrations. Meanwhile, his wife performed extensive investigations of the diffusing capacity of the lung for carbon monoxide to show that, in theory, the lung was easily able to passively absorb sufficient oxygen without the need for active secretion.

Following a bitter exchange of contradictory scientific papers over a period of 20 years, the Kroghs did begin to win the argument. By 1911, Haldane and his team seemed to accept that oxygen secretion might only be occurring when inspired oxygen levels were low. They demonstrated this, using their usual methodology, in an adventurous study of P_{O_2} measurements on the summit of Pike's Peak at an altitude of 4300 m (14100 feet), where they again found arterial P_{O_2} to be higher than alveolar P_{O_2}.[51]

Haldane never abandoned his faith in oxygen secretion, in spite of subsequent investigations in his lifetime by Barcroft, who also found the phenomenon did not exist. Why a physiologist as brilliant as Haldane had such an unshakeable belief in an erroneous hypothesis remains unexplained and for this reason the controversy continues. When a review of these events was published in the *Lancet* in 1987[48] the dispute over Haldane's contribution was reignited.[52,53]

Lung mechanics[54]

Galen knew that inflation of the lungs was a passive phenomenon and occurred as a result of chest movement brought about by the respiratory muscles. However, the way in which this occurred was not understood for many centuries until the discovery of air pressure and therefore the existence of a vacuum, when it soon became clear that chest expansion would draw air into the lungs. Even then there were those who would not accept the scientific explanation; Rene Descartes proposed in 1662 that when the chest expanded, the air outside was pushed away from the chest, compressing adjacent air until the air near the mouth was forced into the lungs.[6] Mayow's elegant demonstration with the bladder within the bellows, described above, provided clear confirmation of the scientific theory.

Around 1500 years after Galen, Vesalius' experiments demonstrated that when the pleura was punchred the lung retracted into the chest cavity. Many of his successors repeated this observation, Mayow commenting that 'the lungs, as if shrinking from observation, cease their movement and collapse at once on the first entrance of light and self-revelation'.[32] It was another 160 years before further investigation of lung elasticity occurred. In 1820 Carson measured the pressure in the trachea (with a closed airway) when the chest was opened and so made the first measurement of lung recoil pressure.[55] A short time later, Ludwig recorded a subatmospheric pressure in the pleura, leading to the proposal by Donders in 1849 that in the intact subject the recoil outwards by the chest wall is equal to the lung recoil inwards[4] (see Chapter 3). Finally, John Hutchinson, whose work on lung volumes is described below, produced the first lung compliance curves in humans, obtained shortly after the subject's death.

Elasticity and surfactant. For some time lung recoil seems to have been adequately explained as resulting simply from the inherent elasticity of lung tissue. At the start of the 20th century the geometry and size of the alveoli were well known and around 100 years had elapsed since Laplace had described the relationship between pressure, surface tension and the radii of curved surfaces (page 26). Yet the inherent instability of lung tissue based on these laws was not recognised until 1929, when Kurt von Neergard first questioned whether tissue elasticity alone was sufficient explanation for the properties of lung tissue.[56] Von Neergard's experiments demonstrated that surface tension in alveoli was indeed lower than expected by Laplace's law, and just a few years later Richard Pattle demonstrated that lung tissue contained an insoluble protein layer that reduced the surface tension of alveoli to almost zero,[57] and surfactant (page 26) was discovered.

Lung volumes. The first measurements of the volume of air contained in the lung were made in the 17th century by Borelli, who also raised the concept of a residual volume.[6] Following this, numerous scientists measured a confusing variety of lung volumes by various methods, such as estimating total lung capacity from plaster casts made in the chest cavity of cadavers. Measurement of lung volumes similar to those in modern use was first made by John Hutchinson in 1846, alongside his description of the first pulmonary spirometer.[58] Hutchinson's spirometer (Figure 13.12) differs little from the water spirometers used until very recently, with a volume measuring chamber over water counterbalanced with weights to offer minimal resistance to the subject's breathing. Hutchinson described the following divisions of the air in the chest, with the modern equivalents (page 35) in parentheses:

Residual air – the quantity of air that remains in the lungs after the most violent muscular effort and over which we have no control (residual volume)

Figure 13.12 The Hutchinson spirometer (1846).[58] This figure shows the operator removing the bung to reset the level of the spirometer before making another measurement. (Reproduced with permission from the Special Collections, Leeds University Library.)

Reserve air – the air in the lungs after a gentle respiratory movement, which may be thrown out if required (expiratory reserve volume)

Breathing air – the portion required to perform ordinary gentle inspiration and expiration (tidal volume)

Complemental air – the volume that can at will be drawn into the lungs by a violent exertion (inspiratory reserve volume)

Vital capacity – the last three divisions combined.

In the same paper,[58] Hutchinson reported his measurements of vital capacity in 1970 healthy subjects to establish normal values. He showed with great accuracy that vital capacity was directly related to subject height and age and obtained measurements comparable with today, e.g. 188 in^3 at 60°F for a 55-year-old male subject 5 feet 4 inches tall (188 in^3 equals 3.31 l BTPS, compared with a modern predicted normal value of 3.64 l). He then measured vital capacity in 60 patients with phthisis (cough) from a variety of causes and compared the results obtained with predicted normal values based on height and weight etc., and was able to use his results to demonstrate declining lung volumes as their respiratory disease progressed.

Control of ventilation

Galen's observations of gladiator injuries had shown that the brain was responsible for respiratory activity and that the phrenic nerves were involved in bringing about this action.

More specific localisation of the respiratory centre did not begin until the 18th century, when the French physiologist Antoine Lorry (1725–1783) showed that in animals all parts of the brain above the brainstem could be removed before respiration ceased.[4] In 1812, the French physiologist Antoine Legallois published reports of similar but more precise experiments showing that rhythmic inspiratory movements ceased only when the medulla was removed.[59] During the next 150 years a long series of distinguished investigators carried out more detailed localisation of the neurones concerned in the control of respiration and studied their interaction.[4] These experiments resulted in the description of anatomical regions which, when isolated in animals, caused a specific respiratory pattern, for example the apneustic and pneumotaxic centres. The complexity of respiratory control in the intact animal is such that this crude anatomical approach to unravelling the various interactions was limited and human studies of function were mostly impossible until recent imaging techniques were developed (page 55).

The origin of rhythmicity in the respiratory centre received much attention from 19th-century physiologists. The role of afferent neural inputs into the respiratory centre, particularly those from the vagus nerve, were clearly demonstrated. In particular, Hering and Breuer described how lung inflation led to inhibition of inspiratory activity, and a 'deflation' reflex was also described (page 60). These observations gave rise to the basis of the *Selbsteuerung* (self-steering) hypothesis whereby rhythm generation was simply two alternating inhibitory reflexes. This concept has played a major role in theories of the control of breathing ever since, and even though its role in man may be questionable, it remains a classic example of a physiological autoregulating mechanism.

Chemical control of breathing. Rapid breathing followed by gasping and death had been observed by the Oxford physiologists in the 17th century in their experiments on animals in closed atmospheres. Around 1850, a similar sequence of events was demonstrated by Kussmaul and Tenner following occlusion of the blood supply to the brain.[60] As the analysis of gases in blood improved, so the chemical control of breathing could be elucidated. In 1868, Pflüger performed a comprehensive study in dogs showing that both oxygen lack and carbon dioxide excess stimulated respiration, and that the former was the stronger stimulant.[61] Soon after, a fellow German physiologist, Miescher-Rusch, investigated the carbon dioxide response in humans to show that the respiratory system exerted very tight control over carbon dioxide concentrations and concluded that this, rather than oxygen, was the predominant chemical stimulus to breathing.[62] Leon Fredericq demonstrated in a series of very elegant experiments that the chemical control of breathing predominated over the vagal reflex control described in the previous paragraph.[63] He managed to cross-connect the blood supply to and from the heads of two animals and, for example, produce apnoea in one dog by hyperventilating the other, the apnoea occurring even though the dog's lungs were not inflated to induce the Hering–Breuer reflex. Finally, at the start of the 20th century, further improvements in analytical chemistry led to the work of Haldane and Priestley, published in 1905, which involved meticulous quantitative analysis of the chemical control of breathing and the interactions between oxygen, carbon dioxide and exercise.[64]

REFERENCES

*1. West JB. *Respiratory physiology: people and ideas.* Oxford: American Physiology Society and Oxford University Press, 1996.

2. West JB. A century of pulmonary gas exchange. *Am J Respir Crit Care Med* 2004; **169**: 897–902.

3. Macklem PT. A century of the mechanics of breathing. *Am J Respir Crit Care Med* 2004; **170**: 10–15.

*4. Proctor DF. *A history of breathing physiology.* New York: Marcel Dekker, 1995.

5. Gottlieb LS. *A history of respiration.* Springfield, IL: Charles C Thomas, 1964.

6. Perkins JF. Historical development of respiratory physiology. In: Fenn WO, Rahn H, eds. *Handbook of physiology – section 3: respiration.* Washington DC: American Physiological Society, 1964.

*7. Nunn JF. *Ancient Egyptian medicine.* London: British Museum Press, 1996.

8. Bryan CP. *Ancient Egyptian medicine: the papyrus Ebers.* Chicago: Ares, 1974.

9. Ebbell B. *The papyrus Ebers: the greatest Egyptian medical document.* London: Humphrey Milford, 1937.

10. Ghalioungui P. *The Ebers papyrus. A new English translation, commentaries and glossaries.* Cairo: Academy of Scientific Research and Technology, 1987.

*11. May MT. *Galen – on the usefulness of the parts of the body.* New York: Cornell University Press, 1968.

12. Furley DJ, Wilkie JS. *Galen on respiration and the arteries.* Princeton, NJ: Princeton University Press, 1984.

13. Singer C. *A short history of anatomy and physiology from the Greeks to Harvey.* New York: Dover Publications, 1957.

14. Bittar EE. A study of Ibn Nafis. *Bull Hist Med* 1955; **29**: 352–68, 429–47.

15. O'Malley CD, Saunders JBM. *Leonardo da Vinci on the human body.* New York: Harry Schuman, 1952.

16. Leonardo da Vinci. *Anatomical drawings from the Royal Collection.* London: Royal Academy of Arts, 1977.

17. Clark K. *The drawings of Leonardo da Vinci in the collection of Her Majesty the Queen at Windsor Castle (volume 3).* London: Phaidon Press, 1969.

18. Mitzner W, Wagner E. On the purported discovery of the bronchial circulation by Leonardo da Vinci. *J Appl Physiol* 1992; **73**: 1196–201.

19. Charan NB, Carvalho P. On the purported discovery of the bronchial circulation by Leonardo da Vinci: a rebuttal. *J Appl Physiol* 1994; **76**: 1836–8.

20. Vesalius A. *De Humani Corporis Fabrica Libri Septem.* Venice: Basel, 1543.

21. Saunders JB, O'Malley CD. *The illustrations from the works of Andreas Vesalius of Brussels.* Cleveland: World Publishing Company, 1950.

22. Coppola ED. The discovery of the pulmonary circulation: a new approach. *Bull Hist Med* 1957; **31**: 44–77.

23. Servetus M. *Christianismi Restitutio.* 1553.

24. O'Malley CD. *Michael Servetus: a translation of his geographical, medical and astrological writings with introductions and notes.* Philadelphia: American Philosophical Society, 1953.

25. Servetus M. *Christianismi Restitutio.* Frankfurt: Minerva, 1966.

26. Colombo R. *De Re Anatomica libri XV.* Paris: Andreum Wechelum, 1572.

27. Harvey W. *De Motu Cordis.* Frankfurt: Wm Fitzeri, 1628.

28. Harvey W. *Movement of the heart and blood in animals.* Oxford: Blackwell Science, 1957.

29. Malpighi M. *De Pulmonibus.* Bologna, 1661.

30. Young J. Malpighi's 'De Pulmonibus'. *Proc Roy Soc Med Lond* 1929; **23**: 1–11.

31. Hooke R. An account of an experiment made by Mr Hook of preserving animals alive by blowing through their lungs with bellows. *Philos Trans Roy Soc Lond* 1667; **2(28)**: 539–40.

*32. Mayow J. *Medico-Physical works: Being a translation of* Tractatus Quinque Medici-Physici. Edinburgh: Alembic Club, 1907.

33. Paterson TS. John Mayow – in contemporary setting. *ISIS* 1931; **15**: 47–96, 504–3.

34. Partington JR. The life and work of John Mayow (1641–1679). *ISIS* 1956; **47**: 217–30, 405–17.

*35. Severinghaus JW. Priestley, the furious free thinker of the enlightenment and Scheele, the taciturn apothecary of Uppsala. *Acta Anesthesiol Scand.* 2002; **46**: 2–9.

36. Priestley J. Experiments and observations on different kinds of air. London: J Johnson, 1775.

37. Lusk G. *Nutrition. Clio medica: a series of primers on the history of medicine, volume 10.* New York: Hoeber, 1933.

38. Crawford A. *Experiments and observations on animal heat and the inflammation of combustible bodies: being an attempt to resolve these phenomena into a general law of nature.* London: J Johnson, 1788.

39. Hassenfratz JH. Mémoire sur la combinaison de l'oxygèn dans le sang et sur la manière dont la calorique se dégage. *Ann Chim Paris* 1791; **9**: 261–74.

40. Spallanzani L. *Mémoire sur la respiration.* Geneva: Paschoud, 1803.

41. Dalton J. Experimental essays on the constitution of mixed gases; on the force of steam or vapour from water and other liquids in different temperatures, both in a Torricellean vacuum and in air; on evaporation; and on the expansion of gases by heat. *Mem Lit Phil Soc, Manchester* 1802; **5**: 535–602.

42. Bert P. *La pression barométrique.* Paris: Masson, 1878.

43. Hitchcock MA, Hitchcock FA. *Paul Bert. Barometric pressure. Researches in experimental physiology.* Columbus, OH: College Book Company, 1943.

44. Magnus H. Ueber die im blute enthalten gase, sauerstoff stickstoff und kohlensäure. *Ann Phys Chem* 1837; **40**: 583–606.

45. Meyer L. Die gase des blutes. *Z Rat Med* 1857; **8**: 256.

46. Hüfner G. Ueber die quantität sauerstoff, welche 1 gramm hämoglobin zu binden vermag. *Z Phys Chem 1877*; **1**(5): 317–29.

47. Bohr C, Hasselbalch K, Krogh A. Ueber einen in biologischer beziehung wichtigen einfluss, den die kohlensäurespannung des blutes auf dessen sauerstoffbindung übt. *Skand Arch Physiol* 1904; **16**: 402–12.

*48. Milledge JS. The great oxygen secretion controversy. *Lancet* 1985; **2**: 1408–11.

49. Haldane JS, Lorrain Smith J. The oxygen tension of arterial blood. *J Physiol* 1891; **20**: 497–520.

50. Schmidt-Nielsen B. August and Marie Krogh and respiratory physiology. *J Appl Physiol* 1984; **57**: 293–303.

51. Douglas CG, Haldane JS, Henderson Y, Schneider EC. Physiological observations made on Pike's Peak, Colorado, with special reference to adaptation to low barometric pressures. *Philos Trans Roy Soc Lond* 1913; **203**: 185–318.

52. Passmore R. Haldane and Barcroft. *Lancet* 1986; **1**: 443.

53. Cunningham DJC. The oxygen secretion controversy. *Lancet* 1986; **1**: 683.

54. Otis AB. History of respiratory mechanics. In: Fishman AP, Macklem PT, Mead JT, Geiger SR, eds. *Handbook of physiology – section 3: the respiratory system.* Bethesda, MD: American Physiological Society, 1986.

55. Carson J. On the elasticity of the lungs. *Philos Trans Roy Soc Lond* 1820; **110**: 29–44.

56. von Neergard K. Neue auffassungen über einen grundbegriff der atemmechanik. Die retraktionkraft der lunge, abhängig von der oberflächenspannung in den alveolen. *Z Ges Exp Med* 1929; **66**: 1–22.

57. Pattle RE. Properties, function and origin of the alveolar lining layer. *Nature* 1955; **175**: 1125–6.

58. Hutchinson J. On the capacity of the lungs and on the respiratory functions, with a view of establishing a precise and easy method of detecting disease by the spirometer. *Med Chir Trans (Series 2)* 1846; **29**: 137–252.

59. Legallois C. *Experiences sur le principe de la vie.* Paris: d'Hautel, 1812.

60. Kussmaul A, Tenner A. Untersuchungen über ursprung und wesen der fallsuchtartigen zuckungen bei der verblutung sowie der fallsucht überhaupt. *Unters Natürl Mensch Tiere* 1857; **3**: 1–124.

61. Pflüger E. Ueber die ursache der athembewegungen, sowie der dyspnoë und apnoë. *Arch Ges Physiol* 1868; **1**: 61–106.

62. Miescher-Rüsch F. Bemerkungen zur lehre von den atembewegungen. *Arch Anat Physiol Leipzig* 1885; **6**: 355–80.

63. Fredericq L. Sur la cause de l'apnée. *Archiv Biol Liége* 1900; **17**: 561–76.

64. Haldane JS, Priestley JG. The regulation of lung ventilation. *J Physiol* 1905; **32**: 225–66.

Part: Two

Applied physiology

Part Two

Chapter

14 Pregnancy, neonates and children

KEY POINTS

- Hormonal changes of pregnancy stimulate breathing, causing an increase in tidal volume and hypocapnia.
- In late pregnancy the enlarged uterus reduces lung volume, particularly in the supine position.
- Human lung development is incomplete at birth, with new alveoli continuing to form until around 3 years of age.
- Compared with adults, the respiratory system of a neonate has a very low compliance and a high resistance.
- In children, most measures of lung function are the same as in adults provided the values are related to lung volume or height.

RESPIRATORY FUNCTION IN PREGNANCY[1]

Several physiological changes occur during pregnancy that affect respiratory function. Fluid retention caused by increasing oestrogen levels causes oedema throughout the airway mucosa and increases blood volume, substantially increasing oxygen delivery. Progesterone levels rise sixfold through pregnancy and have significant effects on the control of respiration and therefore arterial blood gases. Finally, in the last trimester of pregnancy, the enlarging uterus has a direct impact on respiratory mechanics. A summary of the changes for common respiratory measurements is shown in Table 14.1.

Lung volumes. During the last third of pregnancy the diaphragm becomes displaced cephalad by the expansion of the uterus into the abdomen. This reduces both the residual volume (by about 20%) and expiratory reserve volume, such that functional residual capacity is greatly reduced (see Table 14.1). This is particularly true in the supine position and effectively removes one of the largest stores of oxygen available to the body, making pregnant women very susceptible to hypoxia during anaesthesia or with respiratory disease.

Vital capacity, forced expiratory volume in one second and maximal breathing capacity are normally unchanged during pregnancy.[1,4] In the supine position when the diaphragm is high in the chest, inspiratory capacity and maximal breathing capacity may actually exceed non-pregnant values.

Oxygen consumption. Oxygen consumption increases throughout pregnancy, peaking at between 15% and 30% above normal at full term.[2,5] The increase is mainly attributable to the demands of the foetus, uterus and placenta, such that when oxygen consumption is expressed per kg of body weight, there is little change.

Ventilation. Respiratory rate remains unchanged whereas tidal volume, and therefore minute volume of ventilation, increases by up to 40% above normal at full term.[1] The increase in ventilation is beyond the requirements of the enhanced oxygen uptake or carbon dioxide production, so alveolar and arterial P_{CO_2} are reduced to about 4 kPa (30 mmHg).[3] This must facilitate clearance of carbon dioxide by the foetus. There is also an increase in alveolar and arterial P_{O_2} of about 1 kPa (7.5 mmHg).[3] Posture has little effect on oxygenation and in one study mean values for oxygen saturation (by pulse oximetry) in the last 4 weeks of pregnancy were 97.3% sitting and 96.9% supine.[4]

The hyperventilation is attributable to progesterone levels and the mechanism is assumed to be a sensitisation of the central chemoreceptors. Pregnancy gives rise to a threefold increase in the slope of a P_{CO_2}/ventilation response curve.[2] The hypoxic ventilatory response is increased twofold, most of the change occurring before the midpoint of gestation, at which time oxygen consumption has hardly begun to increase.[6]

Dyspnoea occurs in more than half of pregnant women, beginning early in pregnancy, long before the mass effect of the uterus becomes apparent. Dyspnoeic pregnant women, compared with non-dyspnoeic controls, show a greater degree of hyperventilation in spite of having similar plasma progesterone levels.[2] Dyspnoea therefore seems to arise from an increased sensitivity of

Table 14.1 Respiratory function throughout pregnancy

Variable	Non-pregnant	Pregnant		
		1st trimester	2nd trimester	3rd trimester
Tidal volume (l)	0.52	0.60	0.65	0.72
Respiratory rate (breaths per min)	18	18	18	18
Minute volume (l.min^{-1})	9.3	11.0	11.8	13.1
Residual volume (l)	1.37	1.27	1.26	1.01
Functional residual capacity (l)	2.69	2.52	2.48	1.95
Vital capacity (l)	3.50	3.45	3.58	3.0
Oxygen consumption (ml.min^{-1})	194	211	242	258
Arterial P_{O_2} (kPa)	12.6	14.2	13.7	13.6
(mmHg)	95	106	103	102
Arterial P_{CO_2} (kPa)	4.70	3.92	3.93	4.05
(mmHg)	35	29	29	31
CO_2 response slope (l.min^{-1}.kPa^{-1})	11.6	15.0	17.3	19.8
Oxygen saturation response slope (l.min^{-1}.%$^{-1}$)	0.64	1.04	1.13	1.33

Non-pregnant figures refer to normal subjects with an average body weight of 60 kg; pregnant figures refer to the end of each trimester of pregnancy. Derived from references 2 and 3.

the chemoreceptors to the increase in progesterone levels.

THE LUNGS BEFORE BIRTH[7]

Embryology

The lungs develop in four stages.[7-11]

1. Pseudoglandular stage (5–17 weeks of gestation). A ventral outgrowth from the foregut first appears about 24 days after fertilisation, and around week 5 of gestation this begins to form the basic airway and vascular architecture, including the branching patterns of the adult lung. Dividing epithelial cells lengthen the airways and their ability to do this is influenced by physical factors relating to the lung liquid and foetal breathing, described below.

2. Canalicular stage (16–26 weeks gestation). The primitive pulmonary capillaries now become more closely associated with the airway epithelium and the connective tissue architecture of the lung is formed. Fibroblasts and other cells involved in morphogenesis of the lung undergo apoptosis (programmed cell death), so the wall thickness of the embryonic lung structures is reduced.

3. Saccular stage (24 weeks' gestation to term). Distal airways now develop primitive alveoli in their walls to become respiratory bronchi (see Figure 2.5). Saccules form at the termination of airways, these being primitive pulmonary acini.

4. Alveolar stage. Saccules on embryonic bronchioles now expand and septation occurs to form the groups of alveoli seen in adult pulmonary acini. This phase of development begins at 36 weeks' gestation and in humans continues until around 3 years of age. In humans at full term all major elements of the lungs are therefore fully formed, but the number of alveoli present is only about 15% of the adult lung. This postnatal maturation of lung structure is only seen in altricial mammals (human, mouse, rabbit), who have the luxury of being able to remain 'helpless' following birth. Precocial species, such as range animals, are born with a structurally mature lung, ready for immediate activity.[8,12]

The lungs begin to contain surfactant and are first capable of function by approximately 24–26 weeks, this being a major factor in the viability of premature infants.

Lung liquid

Foetal lungs contain 'lung liquid' (LL), which is secreted by the pulmonary epithelial cells and flows out through the developing airway into the amniotic fluid or gastrointestinal tract. The main functions of LL seem to be flushing debris out of the lung and preventing the developing lung tissues from collapsing. It is thought that LL maintains the lung at a slight positive pressure relative to the amniotic fluid, and that this expansion is responsible for stimulating cell division and lung growth. The respiratory tract in late pregnancy contains some 40 ml of LL, but its turnover is rapid, believed to be of the order of 500 ml per day. Its volume corresponds approximately with the functional residual capacity (FRC) after breathing is established.[11]

Foetal breathing movements also contribute to lung development. In humans they begin in the middle trimester of pregnancy and are present for over 20 minutes per hour in the last trimester,[13] normally during periods of general foetal activity. During episodes of breathing, the frequency is about 45 breaths per minute and the diaphragm seems to be the main muscle concerned, producing an estimated fluid shift of about 2 ml at each 'breath'.

Maintenance of a positive pressure in the developing lung requires the upper airway to offer some resistance to the outflow of LL.[11] During apnoea, elastic recoil of the lung tissue and continuous production of LL are both opposed by intrinsic laryngeal resistance and a collapsed

pharynx. Foetal inspiratory activity, as in the adult, includes dilation of the upper airway. With quiet breathing this would allow increased efflux of LL from the airway, but simultaneous diaphragmatic contraction opposes this. During vigorous breathing movements with the mouth open, pharyngeal fluid may be 'sucked' into the airway, thus contributing to the expansion of the lungs. Thus foetal breathing movements are believed to contribute to maintaining lung expansion and their abolition is known to impair lung development.[11]

The foetal circulation

The foetal circulation differs radically from the postnatal circulation (Figure 14.1). Blood from the right heart is deflected away from the lungs, partly through the

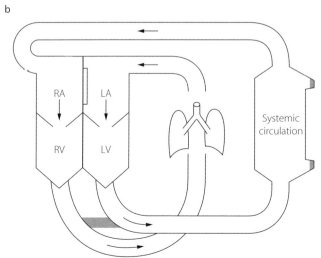

Figure 14.1 Foetal circulation (a) compared with adult circulation (b). The foramen ovale is between right atrium (RA) and left atrium (LA). RV and LV, right and left ventricles.

foramen ovale and partly through the ductus arteriosus. Less than 10% of the output of the right ventricle reaches the lungs, the remainder passing to the systemic circulation and the placenta. Right atrial pressure exceeds left atrial pressure and this maintains the patency of the foramen ovale. Furthermore, because the vascular resistance of the pulmonary circulation exceeds that of the systemic circulation before birth, pressure in the right ventricle exceeds that in the left ventricle and these factors control the direction of flow through the ductus arteriosus. The direction may be reversed in abnormal circumstances if the pressure gradient between the ventricles is reversed.

The umbilical veins drain via the ductus venosus into the inferior vena cava, which therefore contains better oxygenated blood than the superior vena cava. The anatomy of the atria and the foramen ovale is such that the better oxygenated blood from the inferior vena cava passes preferentially into the left atrium and thence to the left ventricle and so to the brain. (This is not shown in Figure 14.1.) Overall gas tensions in the foetus are of the order of 6.4 kPa (48 mmHg) for PCO$_2$ and 4 kPa (30 mmHg) for PO$_2$. The fact that the foetus remains apnoeic for much of the time *in utero* with these blood gas levels is probably in part attributable to central hypoxic ventilatory depression (page 67).

EVENTS AT BIRTH

Oxygen stores in the foetus are small and it is therefore essential that air breathing and oxygen uptake be established within a few minutes of birth. This requires radical changes in the function of both lungs and circulation.

Factors in the initiation of breathing

Most infants take their first breath within 20 seconds of delivery and rhythmic respiration is usually established within 90 seconds. Thoracic compression during vaginal delivery followed by recoil of the ribcage causes air to be drawn passively into the lungs. However, the major stimuli to breathing are probably the cooling of the skin and mechanical stimulation, both acting via the respiratory centre. Without this, babies born via caesarean section would suffer greatly from immediate respiratory difficulties, which is not the case in practice. Hypoxaemia, resulting from apnoea or clamping of the cord, is unlikely to be a reliable respiratory stimulus at this time because of central hypoxic ventilatory depression (see above).

Fate of the foetal lung liquid. The volume of LL decreases just before and during labour. Some of the residual fluid may be expressed during a vaginal delivery but this is not thought to be a major factor. During *in utero* life, the pulmonary epithelium actively secretes LL but at birth this process reverses and the epithelial cells switch to absorption of fluid from the airway.[14] Absorption of fluid from airways and alveoli is an active process facilitated by a sodium channel (page 389). The sodium channels are primed during the third trimester by thyroid and steroid hormones and at birth, foetal adrenaline and oxygen trigger the channels to become active. Aquaporin, a transmembrane protein that facilitates water transport across membranes, is present in lungs at birth but its role remains uncertain.[14,15]

Changes in the circulation

The geometry of the circulation changes radically and quickly at birth. The establishment of spontaneous breathing causes a massive decrease in the vascular resistance of the pulmonary circulation, due partly to mechanical factors and partly to changes in blood gases. Simultaneously there is an increase in the resistance of the systemic circulation, due partly to vasoconstriction and partly to cessation of the placental circulation. As a result, the right atrial pressure falls below the left atrial pressure, to give the relationship that is then maintained throughout life. This normally results in closure of the foramen ovale (see Figure 14.1), which is followed by closure of the ductus arteriosus as a result of active vasoconstriction of its smooth muscle layer in response to increased PO$_2$. The circulation is thus converted from the foetal mode, in which the lungs and the systemic circulation are essentially in parallel, to the adult mode in which they are in series.

Mechanism of reduced pulmonary vascular resistance at birth. Pulmonary vascular resistance declines owing to a combination of ventilation of the lung and changes in blood gases, particularly increasing PO$_2$. Clearly this is a difficult area to study in humans and most work has been performed in other mammals,[11,16] but there is no reason to expect humans to differ significantly.

Removal of LL from the lung establishes an air–liquid interface that is responsible for a rapid increase in lung recoil pressure[11] which, possibly along with changes in chest wall compliance, results in a negative intrapleural pressure as in adult lungs. This creates the transmural pressure gradient between the alveoli and pleura, which physically dilates the pulmonary capillaries (page 97). These mechanical forces leading to a reduction in pulmonary vascular resistance are believed to account for over half of the observed changes at birth.[16]

Further reductions in pulmonary vascular resistance as a result of increased PO$_2$ and decreased PCO$_2$ are believed to be endothelium dependent.[17] Though many mediators may be involved, prostaglandins, endothelin

Table 14.2 The Apgar scoring system

Score	0	1	2
Heart rate	Absent	Less than 100 per min	More than 100 per min
Respiratory effort	Absent	Slow, irregular	Good, crying
Colour	Blue, pale	Body pink, extremities blue	Completely pink
Reflex irritability	Absent	Grimace	Cough, sneeze
Muscle tone	Limp	Some flexion of extremities	Active motion

Add together scores for each section (maximum possible 10). Score at 1 and 5 minutes after delivery. After reference 20.

and nitric oxide are the most widely studied. The first two groups have conflicting effects on the neonatal pulmonary circulation, with *in vitro* studies showing both vasodilating and vasoconstricting effects of different individual mediators. Prostacyclin seems to be involved in the *in vivo* vasodilation of pulmonary blood vessels at birth, but the effect is minor. In animals, inhibition of nitric oxide synthase prior to birth attenuates the reduction in pulmonary vascular resistance on delivery. Nitric oxide is believed to mediate that component of pulmonary vasodilation that occurs in response to oxygen.[18]

Persistent pulmonary hypertension of the newborn (PPHN)[18,19] occurs in about 1 in 1000 births. Pulmonary vascular resistance remains elevated, so right heart pressures remain high and a significant right-to-left shunt continues, with resulting hypoxaemia. Although PPHN may occur with other parenchymal lung problems such as meconium aspiration or respiratory distress syndrome, it also occurs in isolation. Mechanical changes at birth leading to pulmonary vasodilation, as described above, still occur and are probably responsible for bringing about sufficient pulmonary blood flow for immediate survival. However, structural abnormalities of pulmonary vessels are common in PPHN and may limit the vasodilation obtained by mechanical factors. There is undoubtedly an element of abnormal pulmonary vasoconstriction, or at least a failure of oxygen-stimulated vasodilation, in babies with PPHN and abnormalities of both endothelin and nitric oxide activity are implicated.

Treatment is aimed at the correction of any concurrent lung disease and artificial ventilation to try and improve oxygenation. Extracorporeal membrane oxygenation (see Chapter 32) is often required. Inhaled nitric oxide has also had some success in improving hypoxemia but not all babies respond.

The Apgar score

The scoring system devised many years ago by Virginia Apgar is still widely accepted as an assessment of the overall condition of the neonate. This is based on scoring of a scale of 0–2 for five attributes, two of which are related to respiration (Table 14.2).[20] The total score is the sum of each of the five constituent scores and is best undertaken 1 and 5 minutes after delivery. Scores of 8–10 are regarded as normal.

NEONATAL LUNG FUNCTION

Mechanics of breathing. Functional residual capacity is about 30 ml.kg^{-1} and total respiratory compliance 50 ml.kPa^{-1} (5 ml.cmH$_2$O^{-1}). Most of the impedance to expansion is due to the lung and depends primarily on the presence of surfactant in the alveoli. The chest wall of the neonate is highly compliant. This contrasts with the adult, in whom compliances of lung and chest wall are approximately equal. Total respiratory resistance is of the order of 7 kPa.l^{-1}.s (70 cmH$_2$O.l^{-1}.s), most of which is in the bronchial tree. Compliance is about one-twentieth that of an adult and resistance about 15 times greater. At the first breath the infant is capable of generating a subatmospheric intrathoracic pressure of the order of 7 kPa (70 cmH$_2$O).

Ventilation and gas exchange.[21] For a 3 kg neonate, the minute volume is about 0.6 l.min^{-1}, with a high respiratory frequency of 25–40 breaths per minute. Dead space is close to a half of tidal volume, giving a mean alveolar ventilation of about 0.3 l.min^{-1} for a neonate of average size. There is a shunt of about 10% immediately after birth. However, distribution of gas is better than in the adult and there is, of course, a negligible hydrostatic pressure gradient in the vertical axis of the tiny lungs of an infant.

Oxygen consumption is of the order of 20–30 ml.min^{-1}, depending on weight in the range 2–4 kg. Arterial $P\text{CO}_2$ is close to 4.5 kPa (34 mmHg) and $P\text{O}_2$ 9 kPa (68 mmHg). Because of the shunt of 10%, there is an alveolar/arterial $P\text{O}_2$ gradient of about 3.3 kPa (25 mmHg), compared with less than half of this in a young adult. Arterial pH is within the normal adult range.

Control of breathing.[22] Animal studies have shown that, in the foetus, carotid chemoreceptors are active but at a much lower PO_2 than in adults; the ventilatory response curve is displaced far to the left compared with adults. Prolonged periods of apnoea seen *in utero* in spite of this carotid sinus activity occur because of brainstem inhibition of the respiratory centre. In contrast to this, cardiovascular responses to hypoxia are well developed in the foetus, bradycardia and vasoconstriction being well-recognised responses to hypoxia in neonates, as shown by the Apgar score. After birth, there is a very rapid transition towards the adult pattern of respiratory control. Brainstem hypoxic ventilatory depression ceases and the carotid chemoreceptors quickly 'reset' to adult values. Thus hypoxic respiratory stimulation develops and, soon after birth, ventilation is depressed by the inhalation of 100% oxygen, indicating a tonic drive from the peripheral chemoreceptors. Ventilatory response to carbon dioxide appears to be similar to that in the adult if allowance is made for body size, although the response is depressed in REM sleep.[23]

At birth, changes in respiratory pattern must, by necessity, be substantial as the long periods of apnoea seen *in utero* are incompatible with life in the outside world. Although most changes occur shortly after birth, complete transition to 'adult' respiration may take some weeks to complete, particularly in premature and small babies and those with other respiratory problems that cause repeated periods of hypoxia. In the meantime, newborn infants have a variety of breathing patterns. For example, 'periodic breathing' consists of slowly oscillating changes in respiratory rate and tidal volume size; 'periodic apnoea' consists of a series of respiratory pauses of over 4 seconds' duration with a few normal breaths in between. In normal babies aged under 2 months of age, there may be in excess of 200 apnoeic episodes and 50 minutes of periodic breathing per day,[24] and these may be associated with short-lived reductions in saturation.[25] The proportion of time spent with regular breathing increases with age such that, beyond 3 months old, periodic breathing and apnoeas are significantly less.[24] Moderate reductions in inspired oxygen (15%), similar to that seen during flying or at altitude (see Chapter 17), cause a dramatic increase in the amount of time 3-month-old infants spend with periodic apnoea, indicating that adult hypoxic ventilatory responses are not fully developed.[26]

Haemoglobin. Children are normally born polycythaemic with a mean haemoglobin of about 18 g.dl^{-1} and a haematocrit (packed cell volume) of 53%. Some 70% of the haemoglobin is HbF and the resultant P_{50} is well below the normal adult value (see Figure 11.9). Arterial oxygen content is close to the normal adult value in spite of the low arterial PO_2. The haemoglobin con-

centration decreases rapidly to become less than the normal adult value by 3 weeks of life. HbF gradually disappears from the circulation to reach negligible values by 6 months, by which time the P_{50} has already attained the normal adult value.

RESPIRATORY DISTRESS SYNDROME (RDS)[27,28]

The syndrome comprises respiratory distress within a few hours of birth and occurs in 2% of all live births, but with a greatly increased incidence in premature infants. The essential lesion is a deficiency of surfactant, which is first detectable in the foetal lung at 20–24 weeks of gestation, but the concentration increases rapidly after the 30th week. Therefore, prematurity is a major factor in the aetiology of RDS, though male gender, caesarean delivery, perinatal stress or birth asphyxia and maternal diabetes are all additional risk factors for its development. There is believed to be a genetic susceptibility to developing RDS, possibly resulting from inherited variations in surfactant proteins A and B (page 26).

The disease presents with difficulty in inspiration against the decreased compliance due to the high surface tension of the surfactant-deficient alveolar lining fluid. This progresses to ventilatory failure, alveolar collapse, hyaline membrane deposit, pulmonary oedema leading to denaturing of surfactant and ultimately interference with gas exchange, resulting in severe hypoxaemia. Increased pulmonary vascular resistance may raise right atrial pressure and reopen the foramen ovale, so increasing the shunt.

Principles of therapy

The physiological basis of therapy is to supplement surfactant activity and employ artificial ventilation as a temporary expedient to spare the infant the excessive work of breathing against stiff lungs. Overall treatment is very complex and outside the scope of this book, but aspects of treatment with physiological interest are as follows.

Prevention. Amniocentesis allows the measurement of the lecithin (derived from pulmonary surfactant) to sphingomyelin ratio, which is highly predictive of lung maturity.[27] If this ratio is less than 2, then measures may be taken to prolong pregnancy by the administration of tocolytic drugs and steroids may be given to accelerate the rate at which the foetal lungs mature. This, combined with careful obstetric management to prevent perinatal stress, should significantly reduce the incidence and severity of subsequent RDS.

Surfactant replacement therapy.[29–31] Endogenous surfactant is complex, consisting of multiple components divided into phospholipids and proteins (page 26). Currently available synthetic surfactants consist mostly of phospholipids. Alternatively, natural surfactant preparations are obtained from mammalian lungs or human amniotic fluid and contain both phospholipid and some of the surfactant proteins, though not necessarily of the same type and proportion as in humans. Surfactant proteins are important to facilitate spreading of the surfactant around the lung following administration by intratracheal instillation, and there is now evidence that natural surfactants are more effective as therapeutic agents.[29,31] Exogenous surfactant appears to be taken up in type II alveolar cells and recycled and its clearance is fortunately very slow. Surfactant replacement therapy has now been conclusively shown to improve survival and reduce complication rates in many trials in both the USA[29] and Europe.[32] In addition, the importance of surfactant deficiency is now recognised in many other causes of neonatal respiratory failure, such as meconium aspiration and pneumonia, and surfactant replacement seems to be beneficial.[33]

Artificial ventilation. Artificial ventilation is considered in Chapter 32. A high respiratory frequency is required such that inspiratory and expiratory durations may be as little as 0.3 seconds, but inflation pressures are of the same order as those used in adults and do not usually exceed 3 kPa (30 cmH$_2$O). Both the compressible volume of the ventilator circuit and the apparatus dead space tend to be large in relation to the size of very small children, so pressure generators are preferable to volume generators. Bronchopulmonary dysplasia, a relatively common complication of RDS, appears to be a form of pulmonary barotrauma (page 437) in the ventilated infant. Normal humidification and monitoring of airway pressure are important. Improved predelivery care and surfactant replacement therapy have reduced the necessity to ventilate infants with RDS.

Extracorporeal membrane oxygenation (ECMO) is described in Chapter 32. In contrast to its use in adults, ECMO is of proven benefit in infants (page 442), reducing mortality and long-term disability in severe neonatal respiratory failure from a variety of causes,[34] including RDS. Unfortunately, most cases of RDS cannot be treated with ECMO as a result of technical problems in babies of less than 2 kg weight or 35 weeks' gestation.

Partial liquid ventilation with Perflubron, a synthetic oxygen carrier (page 182), has been successfully used in neonates with severe RDS.[35] A volume of Perflubron approximately equal to the infant's FRC is instilled into the lungs and positive-pressure ventilation by conventional methods continued. The liquid improves lung function by replacing the alveolar air–liquid interface, by physically preventing alveolar collapse and by increasing lung compliance, allowing more effective ventilation. Chest radiographs show the extent to which partial liquid ventilation replaces normal gas-filled lung and also shows that clearance of Perflubron by evaporation from the lung takes some time (Figure 14.2).

SUDDEN INFANT DEATH SYNDROME (SIDS)[36,37]

This is defined simply as the sudden death of an infant younger than 1 year of age that remains unexplained after review of the clinical history, examination of the circumstances of the death and a post-mortem examination. The peak incidence is at 2–3 months of age and there remains a multitude of theories regarding the aetiology, though the respiratory system is implicated in most. Some more well-known theories include the following.

The apnoea hypothesis remains popular, mainly because of the frequent periods of apnoea and desaturation observed in almost all babies under 3 months old (see above). The peak incidence of SIDS corresponds to the period of development when the foetal and adult systems for ventilatory control are swapping over, and it is believed that this may make the infant susceptible to respiratory disturbances.[36] Normal patterns of arousal from sleep may be altered in babies who subsequently become SIDS victims.[38] Post-mortem studies have found decreased binding of serotonin in several areas of the brain, including an area which, in adults, is believed to be crucial in controlling arousal from sleep.[37] Despite the popularity of the apnoea hypothesis, evidence that these episodes of periodic breathing or apnoeas contribute to SIDS is lacking. Nevertheless, this hypothesis led to the widespread use of 'apnoea alarms' for babies, though again, evidence that this reduces SIDS has so far not been found.[39]

Temperature regulation may be abnormal in SIDS babies and metabolic rate as a function of body size is particularly high at 3 months of age, leading to the hypothesis that 'heat stress' is responsible.[40]

Infection with common viruses has been implicated in SIDS, possibly mediated via genetic abnormalities of complement components.[37] It is believed that SIDS is more likely to occur during the prodromal phase of an infection before symptoms develop.[36]

Smoking in parents is associated with SIDS, particularly if the infant shares the parent's bed. The mechanism is not clear.

Sleeping position. There is a substantial body of agreement that the prone sleeping position is commoner in

Figure 14.2 Chest radiographs of an infant receiving partial liquid ventilation for severe respiratory distress syndrome. **(a)** Conventional ventilation for respiratory distress syndrome. **(b)** Partial liquid ventilation with Perflubron. **(c)** Forty-eight hours after termination of liquid ventilation, and **(d)** 3 weeks later. (Reproduced with permission from Leach CL, Greenspan JS, Rubenstein SD, *et al*. Partial liquid ventilation with perflubron in premature infants with severe respiratory distress syndrome. The LiquiVent Study Group. *N Engl J Med* 1996; **335**: 761–7. Copyright © 2005 Massachusetts Medical Society. All rights reserved.)

infants dying of SIDS, though the mechanism remains uncertain.[36]

That SIDS is caused by multiple factors is now undisputed. However, its prevention has progressed greatly despite the absence of understanding regarding the aetiology. In the late 1980s and early 1990s many countries introduced national health educational policies to encourage the avoidance of prone sleeping position, parental smoking and overheating in babies. Though these health education measures have had varying degrees of success in different ethnic and socio-economic groups within each country, their overall effect in reducing the incidence of SIDS has been impressive (Figure 14.3).[41]

DEVELOPMENT OF LUNG FUNCTION DURING CHILDHOOD

The lungs continue to develop during childhood. Chest wall compliance, which is very high at birth, decreases rapidly for the first 2 years of life, when it becomes approximately equal to lung compliance as in the adult.[42] Below the age of 8 years, measurement of lung volumes is difficult,[21] but beyond this age many studies of normal

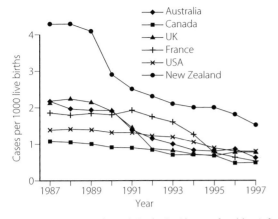

Figure 14.3 National trends in the incidence of sudden infant death syndrome (SIDS) from 1987 to 1997. (Data from reference 41.)

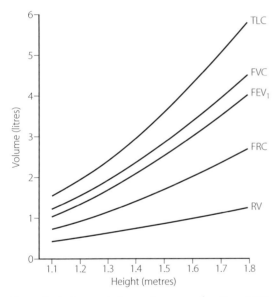

Figure 14.4 Changes in lung volumes as a function of stature. When considering reference values for children, height in metres is used in preference to age to allow for large differences in growth rate. Each graph represents the mean for both boys and girls, though boys generally have greater values at equivalent heights.

lung function are available. Because of large variations in the rate at which children grow, reference values are usually related to height rather than age or weight. Equations relating lung volumes to height are available,[21] and some are shown in graphical form in Figure 14.4.

Various indices of respiratory function are independent of age and body size so that adult values can be used. These include forced expiratory volume (1 second) as a fraction of vital capacity, functional residual capacity and peak expiratory flow rate as a fraction of total lung capacity, *specific* airway conductance and *specific* compliance (page 32), and probably dead space/tidal volume ratio.[21]

Blood gases and the control of breathing. Arterial $P\mathrm{CO}_2$ and alveolar $P\mathrm{O}_2$ do not change appreciably during childhood but arterial $P\mathrm{O}_2$ increases from the neonatal value to reach a maximum of about 13 kPa (98 mmHg) at young adulthood. Much of this increase occurs during the first year of life. There are obvious difficulties in determining the normal arterial $P\mathrm{O}_2$ in children. Ventilatory responses to both hypercapnia and hypoxia are at their highest in early childhood and decrease progressively into adulthood.[43] The changes are small for hypoxic responses, but quite marked for hypercapnia and are believed to relate to the higher metabolic rate in children.

REFERENCES

*1. Elkus R, Popovich J. Respiratory physiology in pregnancy. *Clin Chest Med* 1992; **13**: 555–65.
2. Garcia-Rio F, Pino JM, Gomez L, Alvarez-Sala R, Villasnate C, Villamor J. Regulation of breathing and perception of dyspnoea in healthy pregnant women. *Chest* 1996; **110**: 446–53.
3. Templeton A, Kelman GR. Maternal blood-gases, ($P\mathrm{A}_{\mathrm{O}_2}$-$P\mathrm{a}_{\mathrm{O}_2}$), physiological shunt and $V\mathrm{D}/V\mathrm{T}$ in normal pregnancy. *Br J Anaesth* 1976; **48**: 1001–4.
4. Nørregaard O, Schultz P, Østergaard A, Dahl R. Lung function and postural changes during pregnancy. *Respir Med* 1989; **83**: 467–74.
5. Pernol ML, Metcalfe J, Schlenker TL, Welch JE, Matsumoto JA. Oxygen consumption at rest and during exercise in pregnancy. *Respir Physiol* 1975; **25**: 285–92.
6. Moore LG, McCullough RE, Weil JV. Increased HVR in pregnancy: relationship to hormonal and metabolic changes. *J Appl Physiol* 1987; **62**: 158–63.
7. Merkus PJFM, ten Have-Opbroek AAW, Quanjer PH. Human lung growth: a review. *Pediatr Pulmonol* 1996; **21**: 383–97.
8. Massaro D, Massaro GD. Pulmonary alveoli: formation, the 'call for oxygen' and other regulators. *Am J Physiol Lung Cell Mol Physiol* 2002; **282**: L345–8.
*9. Jeffery PK. The development of large and small airways. *Am J Respir Crit Care Med* 1998; **157**: S174–80.
10. McMurtry IF. Introduction: pre- and postnatal lung development, maturation and plasticity. *Am J Physiol Lung Cell Mol Physiol* 2002; **282**: L341–4.
11. Harding R, Hooper SB. Regulation of lung expansion and lung growth before birth. *J Appl Physiol* 1996; **81**: 209–24.

12. Massaro GD, Massaro D. Formation of pulmonary alveoli and gas-exchange surface area: quantitation and regulation. *Annu Rev Physiol* 1996; **58**: 73–92.

13. Patrick J, Campbell K, Carmichael L, Natale R, Richardson B. Patterns of human foetal breathing during the last 10 weeks of pregnancy. *Obstet Gynecol* 1980; **56**: 24–30.

*14. Barker PM, Olver RE. Clearance of lung liquid during the perinatal period. *J Appl Physiol* 2002; **93**: 1542–8.

15. Verkman AS, Matthay MA, Song Y. Aquaporin water channels and lung physiology. *Am J Physiol Lung Cell Mol Physiol* 2002; **278**: L867–79.

16. Teitel DF, Iwamotot HS, Rudolph AM. Changes in the pulmonary circulation during birth-related events. *Pediatr Res* 1990; **27**: 372–8.

17. Ziegler JW, Ivy DD, Kinsella JP, Abman SH. The role of nitric oxide, endothelin and prostaglandins in the transition of the pulmonary circulation. *Clin Perinatol* 1995; **22**: 387–403.

18. Morin FC, Stenmark KR. Persistent pulmonary hypertension of the newborn. *Am J Respir Crit Care Med* 1995; **151**: 2010–32.

19. Steinhorn RH, Millard SL, Morin FC. Persistent pulmonary hypertension of the newborn. *Clin Perinatol* 1995; **22**: 405–28.

20. McIntosh N. The newborn. In: Campbell AGM, McIntosh N, eds. *Forfar and Arneil's textbook of pediatrics.* Edinburgh: Churchill Livingstone, 1998.

21. Cotes JE. *Lung function: assessment and application in medicine.* Oxford: Blackwell Scientific Publications, 1993.

22. Hanson M, Kumar P. Chemoreceptor function in the foetus and neonate. *Adv Exp Med Biol* 1994; **360**: 99–108.

23. Cohen G, Xu C, Henderson-Smart D. Ventilatory response of the sleeping newborn to CO_2 during normoxic rebreathing. *J Appl Physiol* 1991; **71**: 168–74.

24. Richards JM, Alexander JR, Shinebourne EA, de Swiet M, Wilson AJ, Southall DP. Sequential 22-hour profiles of breathing patterns and heart rate in 110 full-term infants during their first 6 months of life. *Pediatrics* 1984; **74**: 763–77.

25. Stebbens VA, Poets CF, Alexander JR, Arrowsmith WA, Southall DP. Oxygen saturation and breathing patterns in infancy. 1: Full term infants in the second month of life. *Arch Dis Child* 1991; **66**: 569–73.

26. Parkins KJ, Poets CF, O'Brien LM, Stebbens VA, Southall DP. Effect of exposure to 15% oxygen on breathing patterns and oxygen saturation in infants: interventional study. *Br Med J* 1998; **316**: 887–94.

27. Verma R. Respiratory distress syndrome of the newborn infant. *Obstet Gynecol Surv* 1995; **50**: 542–55.

28. Copland IB, Post M. Understanding the mechanisms of infant respiratory distress and chronic lung disease. *Am J Respir Cell Mol Biol* 2002; **26**: 261–5.

29. Soll RF. Surfactant therapy in the USA: trials and current routines. *Biol Neonate* 1997; **71**(Supp 1): 1–7.

30. Enhoring G. From bubbles to babies: the evolution of surfactant replacement therapy. *Biol Neonate* 1997; **71**(Supp 1): 28–31.

31. Merrill JD, Ballard RA. Pulmonary surfactant for neonatal respiratory disorders. *Curr Opin Pediatr* 2003; **15**: 149–54.

32. Halliday HL. Clinical trials of surfactant replacement in Europe. *Biol Neonate* 1997; **71**(Supp 1): 8–12.

33. Barrington KJ, Finer NN. Care of near term infants with respiratory failure. *Br Med J* 1997; **315**: 1215–18.

34. UK Collaborative ECMO Trial Group. UK collaborative trial of neonatal extracorporeal membrane oxygenation. *Lancet* 1996; **348**: 75–82.

35. Leach CL, Greenspan JS, Rubenstein SD, *et al.* Partial liquid ventilation with perflubron in premature infants with severe respiratory distress syndrome.The LiquiVent Study Group. *N Engl J Med* 1996; **335**: 761–7.

36. Sibert J, Fleming PJ. Poisoning, accidents and sudden infant death syndrome. In: Campbell AGM, McIntosh N, eds. *Forfar and Arneil's textbook of pediatrics.* Edinburgh: Churchill Livingstone, 1998.

*37. Hunt CE. Sudden infant death syndrome and other causes of infant mortality. Diagnosis, mechanisms and risk for recurrence in siblings. *Am J Respir Crit Care Med* 2001; **164**: 346–57.

*38. Harper RM. Impaired arousals and sudden infant death syndrome. Pre-existing neuronal injury? *Am J Respir Crit Care Med* 2003; **168**: 1262–3.

39. Keens TG, Ward SL. Apnea spells, sudden deaths and the role of the apnea monitor. *Pediat Clin North Am* 1993; **40**: 897–911.

40. Fleming PJ, Levine MR, Azaz Y, Wigfield R. The development of thermoregulation and interactions with the control of respiration in infants: possible relationship to sudden infant death. *Acta Paediatr Scand* 1993; **389** (Supp): 57–9.

41. Ponsonby A-L, Dwyer T, Cochrane J. Population trends in sudden infant death syndrome. *Semin Perinatol* 2002; **26**: 296–305.

42. Papastamelos C, Panitch HB, England SE, Allen JL. Developmental changes in chest wall compliance in infancy and early childhood. *J Appl Physiol* 1995; **78**: 179–84.

43. Marcus CL, Glomb WB, Basinski DJ, Davidson SL, Keens TG. Developmental pattern of hypercapnic and hypoxic ventilatory responses from childhood to adulthood. *J Appl Physiol* 1994; **76**: 314–20.

15 Exercise

KEY POINTS

- Oxygen consumption increases linearly with the power expended during exercise.
- The extra tissue oxygen requirement is provided by increases in cardiac output and blood oxygen extraction.
- To accommodate these changes ventilation also increases linearly with exercise. This response occurs the moment exercise begins.
- As exercise intensity increases lactate is produced from anaerobic muscle metabolism and blood lactate levels increase, initially reaching a steady state but continuing to rise with severe exercise.

The respiratory response to exercise depends on the level of exercise performed, which can be conveniently divided into three grades.

1. **Moderate exercise** is below the subject's anaerobic threshold (see below) and the arterial blood lactate is not raised. He is able to transport all the oxygen required and remain in a steady state. This would correspond to work (more correctly 'power') levels up to about 100 watts (612 kg.m.min^{-1}).
2. **Heavy exercise** is above the anaerobic threshold. The arterial blood lactate is elevated but remains constant. This too may be regarded as a steady state.
3. **Severe exercise** is well above the anaerobic threshold and the arterial blood lactate continues to rise. This is an unsteady state and the level of work cannot long be sustained.

OXYGEN CONSUMPTION DURING EXERCISE

There is a close relationship between the external power that is produced and the oxygen consumption of the subject (Figure 15.1). The oxygen consumption at rest (the basal metabolic rate) is of the order of 200–250 ml.min^{-1}. As work is done, the oxygen consumption increases by approximately 12 ml.min^{-1} per watt. Exercise intensity is commonly described in terms of *metabolic equivalents* (METs), which refer to the number of multiples of the normal resting oxygen consumption. For example, walking briskly on the level requires an oxygen consumption of about 1 l.min^{-1} or 4 METs, whereas running at 12 km per hour (7.5 miles per hour) requires about 3 l.min^{-1} of oxygen and is rated as 12 METs of activity. Further examples are shown in Figure 15.1.

Time course of the increase in oxygen consumption[2]

Oxygen consumption rises rapidly at the onset of a period of exercise, with an accompanying increase in carbon dioxide production and a small increase in blood lactate. With moderate exercise (Figure 15.2a) a plateau is quickly reached and the lactate level remains well below the normal maximum resting level (<3.5 mmol.l^{-1}). With heavy exercise $\dot{V}O_2$, $\dot{V}CO_2$ and lactate all increase more quickly, again reaching constant levels within a few minutes, the magnitude of which relates to the power generated and the fitness of the subject (Figure 15.2b). If the level of exercise exceeds approximately 60% of the subject's maximal exercise ability (see below), there is usually a secondary 'slow component' to the increase in oxygen consumption, associated with a continuing increase in blood lactate level, which ultimately prevents the exercise from continuing (Figure 15.2c). There have been many explanations proposed for this slow component of $\dot{V}O_2$, including increased temperature, the oxygen cost of breathing,[3] lactic acidosis[2] and changes in muscle metabolism secondary to the use of differing fibre types with prolonged exercise.[4] No consensus has been reached.

Maximal oxygen uptake

Maximal oxygen uptake ($\dot{V}O_{2max}$) refers to the oxygen consumption of a subject when exercising as hard as possible for that subject. A fit and healthy young adult of 70 kg should be able to maintain a $\dot{V}O_{2max}$ of about 3 l.min^{-1}, but this decreases with age to about 2 l.min^{-1} at

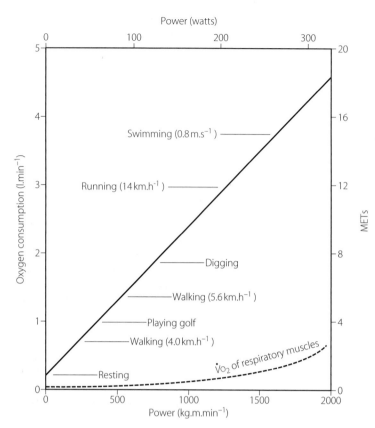

Figure 15.1 Steady-state oxygen consumption with varying degrees of exercise. The continuous straight line denotes whole-body oxygen consumption as a function of the level of power developed. The broken curve is an estimate of the oxygen cost of breathing for the increasing hyperventilation of exercise.[1] MET, metabolic equivalent, which is the number of multiples of basal oxygen consumption required for different activities.

the age of 70. A sedentary existence without exercise can reduce $\dot{V}O_{2max}$ to 50% of the expected value. Conversely, $\dot{V}O_{2max}$ can be increased by regular exercise and athletes commonly achieve values of 5 l.min^{-1}. The highest levels (over 6 l.min^{-1}) are attained in rowers, who utilise a greater muscle mass than other athletes. One study reported an elite group of oarsmen who, for a brief period, attained a mean oxygen consumption of 6.6 l.min^{-1} on the treadmill.[5] This required a minute volume of 200 l.min^{-1} (tidal volume 3.29 l at a frequency of 62 breaths per minute).

$\dot{V}O_{2max}$ is commonly used in exercise physiology as a measure of cardiorespiratory fitness. Subjects undertake a period of graduated exercise while $\dot{V}O_2$ is measured continuously by a spirometric method (page 196). In all but severe exercise, within a few minutes $\dot{V}O_2$ reaches a plateau (Figure 15.2), which is the subject's $\dot{V}O_{2max}$. At higher levels of exercise, as seen in athletes, defining when maximal oxygen uptake is reached may be difficult because of the slow component of oxygen consumption. Many varying definitions of $\dot{V}O_{2max}$ have therefore been used over the years,[6] none of which is universally accepted. Elite athletes rarely reach a satisfactory plateau in $\dot{V}O_2$ and secondary criteria such as high plasma lactate levels or a raised respiratory exchange ratio need to be used to define $\dot{V}O_{2max}$.[6]

At $\dot{V}O_{2max}$ in trained athletes, approximately 80% of the oxygen consumed is used by locomotor muscles. With the high minute volumes seen during exercise, the oxygen consumption of respiratory muscles also becomes significant, being around 5% of total $\dot{V}O_2$ with moderate exercise and 10% at $\dot{V}O_{2max}$ (see Figure 15.1).[1,7]

Response of the oxygen delivery system

A 10- or 20-fold increase in oxygen consumption requires a complex adaptation of both circulatory and respiratory systems.

Oxygen delivery. This is the product of cardiac output and arterial oxygen content (page 187). The latter cannot be significantly increased, so an increase in cardiac output is essential. However, the cardiac output does not, and indeed could not, increase in proportion to the oxygen consumption. For example, an oxygen consumption of 4 l.min^{-1} is a 16-fold increase compared to the resting state. A typical cardiac output at this level of exercise would be only 25 l.min^{-1} (Figure 15.3), which is only five times the resting value. Therefore, there must also be increased extraction of oxygen from the blood. Figure 15.3 shows that the largest relative increase in

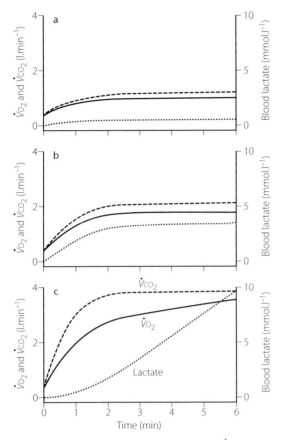

Figure 15.2 Changes in oxygen consumption ($\dot{V}O_2$, solid line), CO_2 production ($\dot{V}CO_2$, dashed line) and blood lactate (dotted line) with the onset of varying levels of exercise. **(a)** Light to moderate exercise with little or no increase in lactate; **(b)** heavy exercise with an increase in lactate to an increased, but steady, level; **(c)** severe exercise, above the anaerobic threshold when levels continue to rise as exercise proceeds. Note that with severe exercise (c), the increase in oxygen consumption is biphasic with a second 'slow' component.

cardiac output occurs at mild levels of exercise. At an oxygen consumption of $1\ \text{l.min}^{-1}$ cardiac output is already close to 50% of its maximal value.

Oxygen extraction. In the resting state, blood returns to the right heart with haemoglobin 70% saturated. This provides a substantial reserve of available oxygen and the arterial/mixed venous oxygen content difference increases progressively as oxygen consumption is increased, particularly in heavy exercise when the mixed venous saturation may be as low as 20% (see Figure 15.3). This decrease in mixed venous saturation covers the steep part of the oxygen dissociation curve (see Figure 11.9) and therefore the decrease in P_{O_2} is relatively less (5 to 2 kPa or 37.5 to 15 mmHg). High levels

of blood lactate seen during heavy exercise may contribute to the increase in oxygen extraction by shifting the dissociation curve to the right at a capillary level.[2]

The additionally desaturated blood returning to the lungs and the greater volume of blood require that the respiratory system transport a larger quantity of oxygen to the alveoli. If there were no increased oxygen transport to the alveoli, the reserve oxygen in the mixed venous blood would be exhausted in one or two circulation times. Fortunately the respiratory system normally responds rapidly to this requirement.

ANAEROBIC METABOLISM

During heavy exercise, the total work exceeds the capacity for aerobic work, which is limited by oxygen transport (see below). The difference is made up by anaerobic metabolism, of which the principal product is lactic acid (see Figure 11.13), which is almost entirely ionised to lactate and hydrogen ions. The anaerobic threshold may be defined as the highest intensity of exercise at which measured oxygen uptake can account for the entire energy requirement.[8] Exercise intensity at the anaerobic threshold depends not only on the power produced but also on many other factors, including environmental temperature, the degree of training undertaken by the subject and altitude. An additional factor is the muscle groups that are used to accomplish the work, as different skeletal muscle fibres, and therefore muscle groups, have different metabolic products.[2]

During severe exercise the lactate level continues to rise (Figure 15.2c) and begins to cause distress at levels above about $11\ \text{mmol.l}^{-1}$, ten times the normal resting level. Lactate accumulation seems to be the limiting factor for sustained heavy work, and the progressive increase in blood lactate results in the level of work being inversely related to the time for which it can be maintained. Thus there is a reciprocal relationship between the record times for various distances and the speed at which they are run.

Oxygen debt

The difference between the total work and the aerobic work is achieved by anaerobic metabolism of carbohydrates to lactate, which is ultimately converted to citrate, enters the citric acid cycle and is then fully oxidised (page 184). Like glucose, lactate has a respiratory quotient of 1.0. Although this process continues during heavy exercise, lactate accumulates and the excess is oxidised in the early stages of recovery. Oxygen consumption remains above the resting level during recovery for this purpose. This constitutes the 'repayment of the oxygen debt' and is related to the lactate level attained by the end of exercise.

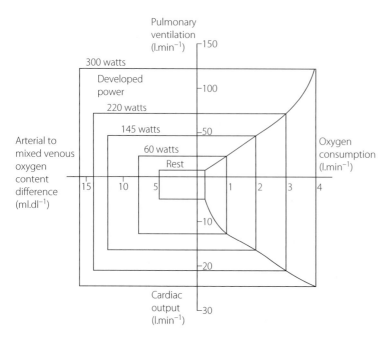

Repayment of the oxygen debt is especially well developed in the diving mammals such as seals and whales. During a dive, their circulation is largely diverted to heart and brain and the metabolism of the skeletal muscles is almost entirely anaerobic (page 271). On regaining the surface, very large quantities of lactate are suddenly released into the circulation and are rapidly metabolised while the animal is on the surface between dives.

Excess postexercise oxygen consumption.[9] Sustained heavy exercise results in an increased $\dot{V}O_2$ even when the subject's blood lactate remains only mildly elevated. Excess oxygen consumption may occur for several hours and is related to both the intensity and duration of exercise undertaken. Previous hypotheses put forward to explain the excess $\dot{V}O_2$ included an increase in body temperature and increased fat metabolism, though proof of these is lacking. Exercise at around 75% of $\dot{V}O_{2max}$ raises levels of catabolic hormones such as cortisol and catecholamines, which may explain the excess $\dot{V}O_2$.[10]

THE VENTILATORY RESPONSE TO EXERCISE

Time course.[11] In the previous section it was seen that exercise without a rapid ventilatory response would be dangerous, if not fatal. In fact, the respiratory system does respond with great rapidity (Figure 15.4). There is an instant increase in ventilation at, if not slightly before, the start of exercise (phase I). During moderate exercise, there is then a further increase (phase II) to reach an equilibrium level of ventilation (phase III) within about 3 minutes.[12] With heavy exercise there is a secondary increase in ventilation that may reach a plateau, but ventilation continues to rise in severe work. At the end of exercise, the minute volume falls to resting levels within a few minutes. After heavy and severe exercise, return to the resting level of ventilation takes longer, as the oxygen debt is repaid and lactate levels return to normal.

The ventilation equivalent for oxygen. The respiratory minute volume is normally very well matched to the increased oxygen consumption and the relationship between minute volume and oxygen consumption is approximately linear up to an oxygen consumption of about 2 l.min^{-1} in the untrained subject and more following training (Figure 15.5). The slope of the linear part is the ventilation equivalent for oxygen and is within the range 20–30 l.min^{-1} ventilation per l.min^{-1} of oxygen consumption.[13] The slope does not appear to change with training.

In heavy exercise, above a critical level of oxygen consumption (Owles point), the ventilation increases above the level predicted by an extrapolation of the linear part of the ventilation/oxygen consumption relationship (see Figure 15.5). This is surplus to the requirement for gas exchange and is accompanied by hypocapnia with arterial P_{CO_2} decreasing by levels of the order of 1 kPa (7.5 mmHg). The excess ventilation is probably driven by lactic acidosis. In the trained athlete, the break from linearity occurs at higher levels of oxygen consumption. This, together with improved tolerance of high minute

Figure 15.4 The time course of changes in ventilation in relation to a short period of moderate exercise. Note the instant increase in ventilation at the start of exercise before the metabolic consequences of exercise have had time to develop.

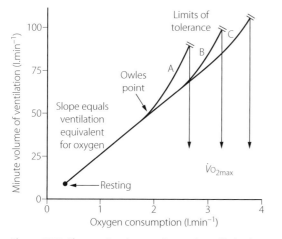

Figure 15.5 Changes in minute volume of ventilation in response to the increased oxygen consumption of exercise. The break from linearity (Owles point) occurs at higher levels of oxygen consumption in trained athletes, who can also tolerate higher minute volumes. A to C shows progressive levels of training. Both mechanisms combine to enable the trained athlete to increase his maximum oxygen consumption.

volumes, allows the trained athlete to increase his $\dot{V}O_{2max}$ as shown in Figure 15.5.

Minute volume and dyspnoea. It is generally believed that the ventilatory system does not limit exercise in normal subjects, although the evidence for this view is elusive.[14] One study[15] found that 50–60% of maximal breathing capacity (MBC) was required for work at 80% of aerobic capacity. However, the breaking point of exercise is usually determined by breathlessness, which occurs when the exercise ventilation utilises a high proportion of the MBC. There is a close correlation between MBC and $\dot{V}O_{2max}$.[13]

Minute volumes as great as 200 l.min^{-1} have been recorded during exercise, although the normal subject cannot maintain a minute volume approaching MBC for more than a very short period. Tidal volume during maximal exercise is about half vital capacity[13] and 70–80% of MBC can normally be maintained, with difficulty, for 15 minutes by fit young subjects.[15] Ventilation approximates to 60% of MBC at maximal oxygen consumption.[12] The usable fraction of the MBC can, however, be increased by training.

Diffusing capacity. Diffusion across the alveolar/capillary membrane does not normally limit the increased oxygen consumption at sea level but this is a limiting factor at altitude (see Chapters 9 and 17). Exercise-induced hypoxia, which is seen fairly commonly in elite endurance athletes, is believed to be caused in part by diffusion limitation along with maldistribution of pulmonary ventilation/perfusion ratios and air flow limitation.[16,17]

Control of ventilation

Elucidation of the mechanisms that underlie the remarkably efficient adaptation of ventilation to the demands of exercise has remained a challenge to generations of physiologists, and a complete explanation remains elusive.[11,12,18]

Neural factors. It has long been evident that neural factors play an important role, particularly as ventilation normally increases at or even before the start of exercise (phase I), when no other physiological variable has changed except cardiac output (see Figure 15.4). There is evidence in humans that the phase I ventilatory response may be in part a 'learned' response to the onset of exercise.[19] Simply imagining exercising in an otherwise relaxed subject causes an increase in ventilation. Under these conditions, positron emission tomography shows activation of several areas of the cerebral cortex, again indicating that the early increase in ventilation with exercise is a behavioural response.[18]

Arterial blood gas tensions and the chemoreceptors. There is a large body of evidence that, during exercise at sea level with oxygen consumption up to about 3 l.min^{-1}, there is no significant change in either PCO$_2$ or PO$_2$ of arterial blood. In one study, even at the point of exhaustion (oxygen consumption 3.5 l.min^{-1}), the arterial PO$_2$ was the same as the resting value and PCO$_2$ was reduced. In healthy subjects, blood gas tensions do not therefore seem at first sight to be the main factor governing the increased minute volume. There is a caveat to this conclusion.

243

Inhalation of 100% oxygen during exercise reduces minute volume for a particular oxygen consumption.[20] The P_{O_2}/ventilation response curve is known to be steeper during exercise (see Figure 5.8), so ventilation will respond to small fluctuations in normal arterial P_{O_2} under these circumstances. Carotid body resection[21] or administration of dopamine to inhibit carotid body activity[22] reduces the ventilatory response to exercise, particularly phase II (see Figure 15.4). Thus it seems likely that the peripheral chemoreceptors do contribute, in a small way, to exercise-induced hyperpnoea, particularly during the non-steady state.[11,23]

In spite of this caveat, it is difficult to avoid the conclusion that arterial blood gas tensions acting on the chemoreceptors cannot be the main factor in the increase of ventilation during exercise. This contrasts sharply with their dominant role in the control of resting ventilation.

Humoral mechanisms. Humoral factors play a comparatively minor role in moderate exercise but are more important in heavy and severe exercise, when metabolic acidosis is an important factor. Lactic acidosis contributes to excess ventilation during heavy and severe exercise (see Figure 15.5), causing a slight reduction in arterial P_{CO_2}. Slight additional respiratory drive may result from hyperthermia.

FITNESS AND TRAINING

The definitions of moderate, heavy and severe exercise at the beginning of this chapter are not transferable between individuals. A given amount of energy expenditure that constitutes severe exercise to a sedentary unfit subject is likely to represent less than moderate exercise to a trained athlete. The linear relationship between power generated and $\dot{V}_{O_2}$ (see Figure 15.1) is remarkably consistent irrespective of fitness and training, but the distance a subject may progress along this line, that is, their $\dot{V}_{O_2max}$, is extremely variable.

In healthy untrained subjects, rapidly increasing lactate levels normally limit exercise tolerance. Intracellular lactic acidosis in muscles gives rise to weakness and cramp, the respiratory stimulation rapidly takes the subject towards an intolerable minute ventilation, and exhaustion occurs. Training changes many aspects of exercise physiology. For example, improved cardiovascular fitness results in improved oxygen delivery, such that the $\dot{V}_{O_2}$ at which lactate rises is greatly increased. Muscle in trained athletes releases less lactate than in untrained subjects (see below), and animal studies indicate that training may improve the ability of the liver to remove circulating lactate.[2] Finally, trained athletes can tolerate much higher blood lactate levels, up to

20 mmol.l^{-1}, or twice that of untrained subjects. There are two respiratory aspects of training that merit further consideration.

Minute volume of ventilation. Maximal expiratory flow rate is limited by flow-dependent airway closure (page 44) and is relatively unaffected by training.[15] However, within the limits of MBC, it is possible to increase the strength and endurance of the respiratory muscles. It is therefore possible to improve the *fraction* of the MBC that can be sustained during exercise. Highly trained athletes may be able to maintain ventilations as much as 90% of their MBC.

Ventilation equivalent for oxygen. There is no evidence that training can alter the slope of the plot of ventilation against oxygen consumption (see Figure 15.5). However, the upward inflection of the curve (Owles point) is further to the right in the trained subject. This permits the attainment of a higher oxygen consumption for the same minute volume. Prolongation of the straight part of the curve is achieved by improving metabolic processes in skeletal muscle to minimise the stimulant effect of lactic acid. There is ample evidence that training can improve the aerobic performance of muscles by many adaptations, including, for example, the increased density of the capillary network in the muscles. The consequent reduction in lactic acidosis and therefore the excess ventilation, together with an increase in the tolerable minute volume, combine to increase the $\dot{V}_{O_2max}$ as shown in Figure 15.5. It would seem that the major factor in increasing the $\dot{V}_{O_2max}$ is improved performance of skeletal muscle and the cardiovascular system, rather than any specific change in respiratory function.

Cardiorespiratory disease[2,4,24,25]

Patients with cardiovascular or respiratory disease have poor exercise tolerance for three main reasons. First, the ventilatory response to exercise is more rapid so a greater minute volume is required to achieve a given $\dot{V}_{O_2}$. Second, the proportion of MBC that a patient can tolerate is reduced and, when combined with the previous observation, this results in an extreme limitation of exercise tolerance before shortness of breath intervenes. Hypoxia or hypercapnia occur more commonly during exercise in patients with respiratory disease. Third, a limited increase in cardiac output in response to exercise means that mixed venous oxygen levels will fall more rapidly, and also causes inadequate muscle blood flow, impairing the function of respiratory and other muscles. Anaerobic metabolism therefore occurs much more quickly, leading to extra ventilatory requirements and exhaustion.

REFERENCES

1. Aaron EA, Seow KC, Johnson BD, Dempsey JA. Oxygen cost of exercise hyperpnea: implications for performance. *J Appl Physiol* 1992; **72**: 1818–25.

*2. Wasserman K. Coupling of external to cellular respiration during exercise: the wisdom of the body revisited. *Am J Physiol* 1994; **266**: E519–E539.

3. Hagberg JM, Mullin JP, Nagle FJ. Oxygen consumption during constant-load exercise. *J Appl Physiol* 1978; **45**: 381–4.

4. Poole DC, Barstow TJ, Gaesser GA, Willis WT, Whipp BJ. $\dot{V}O_2$ slow component: physiological and functional significance. *Med Sci Sports Exerc* 1994; **26**: 1354–8.

5. Clark JM, Hagerman FC, Gelfand R. Breathing patterns during submaximal and maximal exercise in elite oarsmen. *J Appl Physiol* 1983; **55**: 440–6.

6. Howley ET, Bassett DR, Welch HG. Criteria for maximal oxygen uptake: review and commentary. *Med Sci Sports Exerc* 1995; **27**: 1292–301.

7. Dempsey JA, Harms CA, Ainsworth DM. Respiratory muscle perfusion and energetics during exercise. *Med Sci Sports Exerc* 1996; **28**: 1123–9.

8. Svedahl K, MacIntosh BR. Anaerobic threshold: the concepts and methods of measurement. *Can J Appl Physiol* 2003; **28**: 299–323.

9. Gaesser GA, Brooks GA. Metabolic bases of excess post exercise oxygen consumption. *Med Sci Sports Exerc* 1984; **16**: 29–43.

10. Quinn TJ, Vroman NB, Kertzer R. Postexercise oxygen consumption in trained females: effect of exercise duration. *Med Sci Sports Exerc* 1994; **26**: 908–13.

11. Whipp BJ. Peripheral chemoreceptor control of exercise hyperpnea in humans. *Med Sci Sports Exerc* 1994; **26**: 337–47.

12. Wasserman K. Breathing during exercise. *N Engl J Med* 1978; **298**: 780–5.

13. Åstrand P-O, Rodahl K. *Textbook of work physiology*, 3rd edn. New York: McGraw-Hill, 1986.

14. Bye PTP, Farkas GA, Roussos C. Respiratory factors limiting exercise. *Annu Rev Physiol* 1983; **45**: 439–51.

15. Shephard RJ. The maximum sustained voluntary ventilation in exercise. *Clin Sci* 1967; **32**: 167–76.

16. Powers SK, Martin D, Dodd S. Exercise-induced hypoxaemia in elite endurance athletes. *Sports Med* 1993; **16**: 14–22.

17. Dempsey JA, Wagner PD. Exercise-induced arterial hypoxemia. *J Appl Physiol* 1999; **87**: 1997–2006.

18. Thornton JM, Guz A, Murphy K, *et al.* Identification of higher brain centres that may encode the cardiorespiratory response to exercise in humans. *J Physiol* 2001; **533**: 823–36.

*19. Helbling D, Boutellier U, Spengler CM. Modulation of the ventilatory increase at the onset of exercise in humans. *Respir Physiol* 1997; **109**: 219–29.

20. Ward SA, Blesovsky L, Russak S, Ashjian A, Whipp BJ. Chemoreflex modulation of ventilatory dynamics during exercise in humans. *J Appl Physiol* 1988; **63**: 2001–7.

21. Wasserman K, Whipp BJ, Koyal SN, Cleary MG. Effect of carotid body resection on ventilatory and acid-base control during exercise. *J Appl Physiol* 1975; **39**: 354–8.

22. Boetger CL, Ward DS. Effect of dopamine on transient ventilatory response to exercise. *J Appl Physiol* 1986; **61**: 2102–7.

23. Forster HV, Pan LG. The role of carotid chemoreceptors in the control of breathing during exercise. *Med Sci Sports Exerc* 1994; **26**: 328–36.

24. Piña IL, Fitzpatrick JT. Exercise and heart failure. *Chest* 1996; **110**: 1317–27.

*25. Epstein FH. Exercise limitation in health and disease. *N Engl J Med* 2000; **343**: 633–41.

16 Sleep

KEY POINTS

■ During normal sleep tidal volume is reduced, with maximal reduction in ventilation occurring during rapid eye movement sleep when breathing also becomes irregular.

■ Reduction in the speed and strength of pharyngeal muscle reflexes causes increased airways resistance, leading to snoring in many normal individuals.

■ Sleep-disordered breathing describes a continuum of abnormalities ranging from occasional snoring to frequent periods of airway obstruction and hypoxia during sleep.

Sleep-related breathing disorders are now known to be extremely common and their effects present a major public health challenge.[1] This chapter provides a general review of the effects of sleep on respiration in the normal and pathological states.

NORMAL SLEEP

Sleep is classified on the basis of the electroencephalogram (EEG) and electrooculogram (EOG) into rapid eye movement (REM) and non-REM (stages 1–4) sleep.

Stage 1 is dozing, from which arousal easily takes place. The EEG is low voltage and the frequency is mixed but predominantly fast. This progresses to stage 2, in which the background EEG is similar to stage 1 but with episodic sleep spindles (frequency 12–14 Hz) and K complexes (large biphasic waves of characteristic appearance). Slow, large amplitude (δ) waves start to appear in stage 2 but become more dominant in stage 3, in which spindles are less conspicuous and K complexes become difficult to distinguish. In stage 4, which is often referred to as deep sleep, the EEG is mainly high voltage (more than 75 μV) and more than 50% slow (δ) frequency.

REM sleep has quite different characteristics. The EEG pattern is the same as in stage 1 but the EOG shows frequent rapid eye movements that are easily distinguished from the rolling eye movements of non-REM sleep. Dreaming occurs during REM sleep.

The stage of sleep changes frequently during the night and the pattern varies between different individuals and on different nights for the same individual (Figure 16.1). Sleep is entered in stage 1 and usually progresses through stage 2 to 3 and sometimes into 4. Episodes of REM sleep alternate with non-REM sleep throughout the night. On average there are four or five episodes of REM sleep per night, with a tendency for the duration of the episodes to increase towards morning. Conversely, stages 3 and 4 predominate in the early part of the night. The sleeper can pass from any stage to any other stage, but it is unusual to pass from stage 1 or REM into either 3 or 4 or from stage 3 or 4 into REM. However, it is not uncommon for the sleeper to pass from any stage into stage 1 or full consciousness.

Respiratory changes

Ventilation.[2] Tidal volume decreases with deepening levels of non-REM sleep and is minimal in REM sleep, when it is about 25% less than in the awake state. Respiratory frequency is generally unchanged, though breathing is normally irregular during REM sleep. Minute volume is progressively reduced in parallel with the tidal volume. These changes in ventilation are brought about by the same neurochemical changes that cause sleep. Increased activity of GABA-secreting neurones during sleep has a direct depressant effect on the respiratory centre (see Figure 5.4) and activation of cholinergic neurones is thought to be responsible for the respiratory patterns seen during non-REM sleep.[2]

Arterial P_{CO_2} is usually slightly elevated by about 0.4 kPa (3 mmHg). In the young healthy adult, arterial P_{O_2} decreases by about the same amount as the P_{CO_2} is increased and therefore the oxygen saturation remains reasonably normal. Mean value for ribcage contribution to breathing (page 80) was found to be 54% in stages 1–2, decreasing slightly in stages 3–4.[3] However, in REM sleep the value was reduced to 29%, which is close to the normal awake value in the supine position.

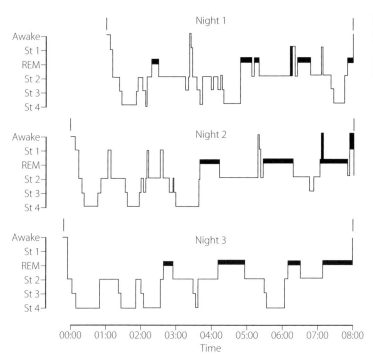

Figure 16.1 Patterns of sleep on three consecutive nights in a young fit man aged 20. The thick horizontal bars indicate rapid eye movement (REM) sleep. (Record kindly supplied by Dr C Thornton.)

Chemosensitivity. In humans, the slopes of the hypercapnic and hypoxic ventilatory responses are markedly reduced during sleep.[4,5] In both cases, the slope is reduced by approximately one-third during non-REM sleep and even further reduced during REM sleep, but fortunately the responses are never abolished completely.

Effect of age. Compared with young subjects, the elderly have more variable ventilatory patterns when awake, which seems to result in more episodes of periodic breathing and apnoea when asleep.[6] Elderly subjects also have significant oscillations in upper airway resistance during sleep (see below),[7] which may contribute to the observed variations in ventilation.[6] Thus as age advances, episodes of transient hypoxaemia occur in subjects who are otherwise healthy, with saturations commonly falling as low as 75% during sleep. Such changes must be regarded as a normal part of the ageing process.

Pharyngeal airway resistance. Air flow through the sharp bends of the upper airway is normally laminar, but is believed to be very close to becoming turbulent even in normal subjects.[8] Pharyngeal muscles may play a crucial role in maintaining the optimum shape of the airway to maintain laminar flow, and the speed at which these control mechanisms can respond to changes in pharyngeal pressure (page 76) may be more critical than previously thought.[9,10] Any condition that attenuates or delays these reflexes even slightly, such as sleep or alcohol ingestion, will then have a major effect on air flow in the pharynx, causing breakdown of the normally laminar flow.

The nasal airway is normally used during sleep and upper airway resistance is consistently increased, especially during inspiration and in REM sleep. The main sites of increase are across the soft palate and in the hypopharynx.[11] Changes in pharyngeal muscle activity with sleep are complex. Muscles with predominantly tonic activity, such as tensor palati, show a progressive decrease in activity with deepening non-REM sleep,[12] reaching only 20–30% of awake activity in stage 4 sleep. This loss of tonic activity correlates very well with increased upper airway resistance.[12] Unlike in the awake state, tensor palati also fails to respond to an inspiratory resistive load. The activity of muscles with predominantly phasic inspiratory activity (e.g. geniohyoid and genioglossus) is influenced little by non-REM sleep.[13] In spite of maintained phasic activity during sleep the tonic activity of geniohyoid is reduced, whereas that of genioglossus is well preserved and responds appropriately to resistive loading.[14] It thus appears that the major effect is upon the tonic activity of nasopharyngeal muscles and the increase in hypopharyngeal resistance seems to be due to secondary downstream collapse. This was clearly shown during application of external resistive loads in normal subjects during non-REM sleep.[15] In one study, pharyngeal collapse occurred at a mean value of 1.3 kPa (13 cmH$_2$O) below atmospheric in normal sleeping subjects.[16]

The ventilatory response to increased airway resistance is important in normal sleep because of the increased pharyngeal resistance and is generally well preserved. There are substantial and rapid increases in both diaphragmatic and genioglossal inspiratory activity following nasal occlusion in normal sleeping adults.[17]

Snoring

Snoring may occur at any age but the incidence is bimodal, peaking in the first and the fifth to sixth decades of life. It is commoner in males than females and linked to obesity. It may occur in any stage of sleep, becoming more pronounced as non-REM sleep deepens, though usually attenuated in REM sleep. Recent work has shown that, as may be expected, snoring is less severe when sleeping in the lateral rather than the supine position.[18] About one-quarter of the population are habitual snorers, but these vary from the occasional snorer (e.g. after alcohol or with an upper respiratory tract infection) to the habitual persistent and heavy snorer.

Snoring originates in the oropharynx and in its mildest form is due to vibration of the soft palate and posterior pillars of the fauces. However, in its more severe forms, during inspiration the walls of the oropharynx collapse and the tongue is drawn back as a result of the subatmospheric pressure generated during inspiration against more upstream airway obstruction. This may be at the level of the palate as described above, or may be the result of nasal polyps, nasal infection or enlarged adenoids, which are the commonest cause of snoring in children.[19] As obstruction develops, the inspiratory muscles greatly augment their action and intrathoracic pressure may fall as low as -7 kPa (-70 cmH$_2$O).

Apart from the annoyance to conjugal partners and others, there are strong associations between snoring and a wide range of pathological conditions, including hypertension, heart and chest disease, rheumatism, diabetes and depression.[20] 'Normal' snoring is not associated with either frequent arousal from sleep or apnoea, but is believed to precede the development of more serious sleep-related breathing disorders.

SLEEP-DISORDERED BREATHING

This term is used to describe a continuum of respiratory abnormalities seen during sleep, which range from simple snoring to life-threatening obstructive sleep apnoea.[1,19,21–23] All are characterised by airway narrowing or obstruction that leads to repeated episodes of arterial hypoxia and arousal as a result of increased respiratory effort. Repeated arousals throughout the night give rise to excessive daytime sleepiness. Three syndromes are described, but there is considerable overlap between them.

Upper airway resistance syndrome[19] in which tidal volume and arterial oxygen saturation (Sa$_{O_2}$) remain normal but at the expense of extensive respiratory effort, which causes over 15 arousals per hour.

Obstructive sleep hypopnoea involving frequent (>15 per hour) episodes of airway obstruction of sufficient severity to reduce tidal volume to less than 50% of normal for over 10 seconds. There may be small decreases in Sa$_{O_2}$.

Obstructive sleep apnoea characterised by more than five episodes per hour of obstructive apnoeas lasting over 10 seconds and associated with severe decreases in Sa$_{O_2}$. In fact, durations of apnoea may be as long as 90 seconds and the frequency of the episodes as high as 160/hour. In severe cases, 50% of sleep time may be spent without tidal exchange.

The last two syndromes are commonly grouped together as sleep apnoea/hypopnoea syndrome (SAHS). Severity is quantified by recording the apnoea/hypopnoea index (AHI), which is simply the number of occurrences per hour of apnoeas or hypopnoeas lasting longer than 10 seconds. Milder forms of sleep-disordered breathing tend to progress to more severe forms as patients grow older and fatter. The prevalence of SAHS, defined as an AHI of over 5, is between 3.5% and 24% in men and between 1.5% and 9% in women, depending on the population studied.[24,25]

Apnoea or hypopnoea may be central or obstructive. Differentiation between central and obstructive apnoea is conveniently made by recording ribcage and abdominal movements continuously during sleep (Figure 16.2). If, as a result of upper airway obstruction, abdominal and ribcage movements become uncoordinated (Figure 16.2c), hypopnoea results. When these movements are equal but opposite in phase, there is obstructive apnoea (Figure 16.2d). Obstructive apnoea may occur in REM or non-REM sleep but the longest periods of apnoea tend to occur in REM sleep. As for snoring, airway obstruction is less frequent when sleeping in the lateral, rather than the supine, position.[18,26] Central apnoeas are more common in elderly patients.

The mechanism of airway obstruction[13,27,28]

Anatomical factors. There is now widespread agreement that, on average, patients with SAHS have anatomically narrower airways than controls, though there is considerable overlap. Anatomical airway narrowing is believed to relate to two main factors.

First, obesity influences pharyngeal airway size. A central pattern of obesity, commonly seen in males, includes extensive fat deposition in the neck tissues. This accounts for the association between SAHS and neck circumference.[29] Adipose tissue is best visualised using

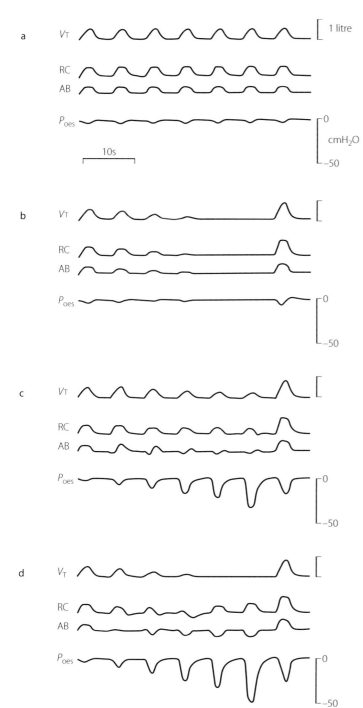

Figure 16.2 Continuous records of breathing during differing types of apnoea and hypopnoea showing tidal volume (V_T), ribcage (RC) and abdominal (AB) contributions to breathing, and oesophageal pressure (P_{oes}). **(a)** normal; **(b)** central apnoea; **(c)** obstructive hypopnoea; **(d)** obstructive apnoea.

magnetic resonance imaging (MRI), and in patients with SAHS collections of fat are invariably seen lateral to the pharynx, between the pterygoid muscles and the carotid artery (Figure 16.3).[30,31] Pharyngeal fat is increased above normal levels even in non-obese patients with SAHS (Figure 16.3c).[32] In addition, the quantity of adipose tissue seen correlates with the AHI and weight loss predictably reduces both.

Second, facial structure may be different in some patients with SAHS, including micrognathia (small mandible) or retrognathia (posterior positioned mandible),[33] both of which will tend to displace the

Masseter m.

Mandible

Pterygoid m.

Oropharynx

Body of C$_2$

Spinal cord

a

b

Parapharyngeal fat

c

Figure 16.3 Magnetic resonance imaging scan of the neck at the level of the oropharynx. In this type of scan fat tissue appears white. **(a)** Normal, non-obese, subject. **(b)** Obese patient with obstructive sleep apnoea, showing deposits of adipose tissue throughout the neck (the uvula is seen in the pharynx). **(c)** Non-obese patient with sleep apnoea, showing fat deposits lateral to the pharynx with normal amounts of adipose tissue elsewhere. (I am indebted to Dr I Mortimore for providing the scans. Parts (a) and (c) reproduced with permission from Mortimore IL, Marshall I, Wraith PK, Sellar RJ, Douglas NJ. Neck and total body fat deposition in nonobese and obese patients with sleep apnea compared with that in control subjects. *Am J Respir Crit Care Med* 1998; **157**: 280–3.)

tongue backwards, requiring extra genioglossus activity to maintain a normal-sized airway. This hypothesis raises the interesting possibility that SAHS may begin in early childhood, when enlarged adenoids and tonsils can influence facial bone development, and may also go some way to explaining familial 'aggregations' of SAHS and snoring.[19]

Pharyngeal dilator muscles are more active in awake subjects with SAHS than in controls, presumably as a physiological response to the anatomically smaller airway. The activity is believed to originate from the usual reflex, stimulated by a negative pharyngeal pressure (page 76), which may be present to a greater extent in SAHS subjects even when awake. This requirement for increased pharyngeal muscle activity to maintain airway size may become impossible to maintain during sleep. Coupled with the normal loss of tonic activity of pharyngeal muscles (see above), sleep quickly results in airway obstruction.

Airway collapse occurs only in obstructive sleep apnoea and normally results from increased upstream resistance behind the soft palate, leading to secondary downstream collapse. The ease with which this collapse occurs is a function of the compliance (collapsibility) of the hypopharyngeal walls, opposed by the action of the pharyngeal dilator muscles. Collapse is more likely to occur when pharyngeal compliance is high and particularly when there is increased submucosal fat in the pharynx,[31] a situation that seems to occur more commonly in men than in women.[34] Severe collapse of the hypopharynx occurs with the combination of enhanced diaphragmatic contraction, depressed pharyngeal dilator muscle activity and upstream obstruction.

Arousal

Apnoea or hypopnoea is terminated when the patient is aroused from sleep, though this arousal is normally subcortical; that is, the patient does not return to full consciousness. Arousal is followed by clearance of the pharyngeal airway, and this is crucially important for survival. In spite of the depressed ventilatory response curves, hypoxia and hypercapnia do contribute to arousal, probably alongside afferent input from pressure-sensitive pharyngeal receptors. Current opinion supports the view that a combination of all these factors results in increased respiratory drive, which brings about arousal.[13] Whatever the mechanism, arousal is accompanied by massive sympathetic discharge.

Medical effects of SAHS[35,36]

The effects of SAHS are not trivial and, over a period of years, mortality in patients with SAHS is considerably higher than controls. However, proving that this excess mortality relates to the SAHS itself has been difficult as most studies have not adequately controlled for the associated risk factors of smoking, obesity and alcohol consumption. There are two main causes of increased mortality.

Arousal. A night's sleep that is disturbed hundreds of times, even subconsciously, leaves the individual with severe daytime somnolence, with decrement of performance in many fields. The ability to drive is impaired, such that patients with SAHS have an odds ratio of 6.3 for having a traffic accident compared with subjects

without SAHS,[37] endangering themselves and other road users.

Cardiovascular effects. Each arousal is associated with significant secretion of catecholamines and repeated episodes of hypoxia and hypercapnia will cause further sympathetic activation. These events, occurring many times each night, cause multiple adverse effects on the cardiovascular system,[38] such as impaired endothelial function and increased platelet aggregation. It is therefore unsurprising that SAHS is strongly implicated in the development of hypertension and believed to contribute to many other cardiovascular diseases.[35,36] Repeated hypoxic episodes may also be responsible for the development of pulmonary hypertension and right-sided heart failure, along with some degree of intellectual deterioration. These effects are considerably worse in patients with other, unrelated, pulmonary diseases.

Principles of therapy[22,23,39]

Conservative treatment. Avoidance of alcohol, sedative drugs and the supine position during sleep will all improve the AHI. Weight loss is effective at reducing the AHI in obese patients with SAHS and is believed to act by reducing peripharyngeal fat, so increasing airway diameter and reducing the tendency of the airway to collapse.[30] There is some evidence that small amounts of weight loss are associated with large reductions in AHI.

Nasal continuous positive airway pressure (nCPAP)[22] aims to avoid the development of a subatmospheric pharyngeal pressure sufficient to cause downstream pharyngeal collapse. It requires a well-fitting nasal mask or soft plastic tubes that fit inside the external nares. Compressed air must then be provided at the requisite gas flow, preferably with humidification. nCPAP serves no useful purpose during expiration and systems have been developed to return airway pressure to atmospheric during expiration. In effect, this provides a low level of intermittent positive-pressure ventilation. Compliance with nCPAP may be poor, but it has proved to be highly effective in the relief of obstructive sleep apnoea, particularly the daytime somnolence that has such a major effect on the patient's life.[40]

Surgical relief of obstruction. For snoring alone, the first approach is the removal of any pathological obstruction such as nasal polyps that cause downstream collapse, though this may not improve patients with SAHS. A more radical approach is uvulo-palato-pharyngoplasty, which reduces the size of the soft palate and so dampens palatal oscillations and reduces pharyngeal collapse at this level. This is usually very effective in the relief of snoring[41] but its value in SAHS is less impressive, with symptoms improving in less than half of patients. Non-obese patients with SAHS who have facial bone abnormalities may benefit from maxillofacial corrective surgery, usually involving advancement of the anterior mandible and/or maxilla. Tracheotomy (opened only at night) has been used in some cases as a last resort.

Oral appliances are available that can be maintained in the mouth at night to move either the tongue or the mandible forward, so increasing the size of the airway. They are effective treatments for moderate SAHS and surprisingly well tolerated by patients.[42]

REFERENCES

1. Fleetham JA. A wake up call for sleep disordered breathing. *Br Med J* 1997; **314**; 839–40.
*2. Joseph V, Pequignot JM, Van Reeth O. Neurochemical perspectives on the control of breathing during sleep. *Respir Physiol Neurobiol* 2002; **130**: 253–63.
3. Millman RP, Knight H, Kline LR, Shore ET, Chung DC, Pack AI. Changes in compartmental ventilation in association with eye movements during REM sleep. *J Appl Physiol* 1988; **65**: 1196–202.
4. Douglas NJ, White DP, Weil JV, Pickett CK, Zwillich CW. Hypercapnic ventilatory response in sleeping adults. *Am Rev Respir Dis* 1982; **126**: 758–62.
5. Douglas NJ, White DP, Weil JV, *et al*. Hypoxic ventilatory response decreases during sleep in normal men. *Am Rev Respir Dis* 1982; **125**: 286–9.
6. Shore ET, Millman RP, Silage DA, Chung DCC, Pack AI. Ventilatory and arousal patterns during sleep in normal young and elderly subjects. *J Appl Physiol* 1985; **59**: 1607–15.
7. Hudgel DW, Devadatta P, Hamilton H. Pattern of breathing and upper airway mechanics during wakefulness and sleep in healthy elderly humans. *J Appl Physiol* 1993; **74**: 2198–204.
*8. Shome B, Wang L-P, Prasad AK, Santere MH, Szeri AZ, Roberts D. Modeling of airflow in the nasopharynx wih applications to sleep apnea. *J Biomech Eng* 1998; **120**: 416–22.
9. Roberts D. Invited editorial on 'Neuromechanical interaction in human snoring and upper airway obstruction'. *J Appl Physiol* 1999; **86**: 1757–8.
10. Huang L, Ffowcs Williams JE. Neuromechanical interaction in human snoring and upper airway obstruction. *J Appl Physiol* 1999; **86**: 1759–63.
11. Hudgel DW, Hendricks C. Palate and hypopharynx – sites of inspiratory narrowing of the upper airway during sleep. *Am Rev Respir Dis* 1988; **138**: 1542–7.
12. Tangel DJ, Mezzanotte WS, White DP. Influence of sleep on tensor palatini EMG and upper airway resistance in normal men. *J Appl Physiol* 1991; **70**: 2574–81.
13. White DP. Pathophysiology of obstructive sleep apnoea. *Thorax* 1995; **50**: 797–804.
14. Henke KG. Upper airway muscle activity and upper airway resistance in young adults during sleep. *J Appl Physiol* 1998; **84**: 486–91.
15. Wiegand DA, Zwillich CW, White DP. Collapsibility of the human upper airway during normal sleep. *J Appl Physiol* 1989; **66**: 1800–8.
16. Schwartz AR, Smith PL, Wise RA, Gold AR, Permutt S. Induction of upper airway occlusion in sleeping individuals with subatmospheric nasal pressure. *J Appl Physiol* 1988; **64**: 535–42.
17. Kuna ST, Smickley J. Response of genioglossus muscle activity to nasal airway occlusion in normal sleeping adults. *J Appl Physiol* 1988; **64**: 347–53.
*18. Nakano H, Ikeda T, Hayashi M, Ohshima E, Onizuka A. Effects of body position on snoring in apneic and nonapneic snorers. *Sleep* 2003; **2**: 169–72.
19. Rappai M, Colop N, Kemp S, deShazo R. The nose and sleep-disordered breathing. What we know and what we do not know. *Chest* 2003; **124**: 2309–23.
20. Norton PG, Dunn EV. Snoring as a risk factor for disease: an epidemiological survey. *Br Med J* 1985; **291**: 630–2.
*21. Stradling JR, Davies RJO. Obstructive sleep apnoea/hypopnoea syndrome: definitions, epidemiology and natural history. *Thorax* 2004; **59**: 73–8.
22. Olson EJ, Moore WR, Morgenthaler TI, Gay PC, Staats BA. Obstructive sleep apnea-hypopnea syndrome. *Mayo Clin Proc* 2003; **78**: 1545–52.
23. Flemons WW. Obstructive sleep apnea. *N Engl J Med* 2002; **347**: 498–504.
24. Strohl KP, Redline S. Recognition of obstructive sleep apnea. *Am J Respir Crit Care Med* 1996; **154**: 279–89.
25. Ohayon MM, Guilleminault C, Priest RG, Caulet M. Snoring and breathing pauses during sleep: telephone interview survey of United Kingdom population sample. *Br Med J* 1997; **314**: 860–3.
26. Akita Y, Kawakatsu K, Hattori C, Hattori H, Suzuki K, Nishimura T. Posture of patients with sleep apnea during sleep. *Acta Otolaryngol Supp* 2003; **550**: 41–5.
*27. Sanders MH. The upper airway and sleep-disordered breathing. Getting the big picture. *Am J Respir Crit Care Med* 2003; **168**: 509–15.
28. Douglas NJ. Pathogenesis of obstructive sleep apnoea/hypopnoea syndrome. *Lancet* 1994; **344**: 653–5.
29. Davies RJO, Stradling JR. The relationship between neck circumference, radiographic pharyngeal anatomy and the obstructive sleep apnoea syndrome. *Eur Respir J* 1990; **3**: 509–14.
30. Shelton KE, Woodson H, Gay S, Suratt PM. Pharyngeal fat in obstructive sleep apnoea. *Am Rev Respir Dis* 1993; **148**: 462–6.

31. Horner RL, Mohiaddin RH, Lowell DG, *et al*. Sites and sizes of fat deposits around the pharynx in obese patients with obstructive sleep apnoea and weight matched controls. *Eur Respir J* 1989; **2**: 613–22.

*32. Mortimore IL, Marshall I, Wraith PK, Sellar RJ, Douglas NJ. Neck and total body fat deposition in nonobese and obese patients with sleep apnea compared with that in control subjects. *Am J Respir Crit Care Med* 1998; **157**: 280–3.

33. Jamieson A, Guilleminault C, Partinen M, Quera-Salva MA. Obstructive sleep apnneic patients have craniomandibular abnormalities. *Sleep* 1986; **9**: 469–78.

34. O'Donnell CP, Schwartz AR, Smith PL. Upper airway collapsibility. The importance of gender and adiposity. *Am J Respir Crit Care Med* 2000; **162**: 1606–7.

35. Wolk R, Kara T, Somers VK. Sleep-disordered breathing and cardiovascular disease. *Circulation* 2003; **108**: 9–12.

36. Shamsuzzaman ASM, Gersh BJ, Somers VK. Obstructive sleep apnea. Implications for cardiac and vascular disease. *JAMA* 2003; **290**: 1906–14.

37. Terán-Santos J, Jiménez-Gómez A, Cordero-Guevara J and the Cooperative Group Burgos-Santander. The association between sleep-apnea and the risk of traffic accidents. *N Engl J Med* 1999; **340**: 847–51.

38. Sin DD. Sleep-disordered breathing. A heart-changing experience? *Chest* 2003; **124**: 778–9.

39. Hudgel DW. Treatment of obstructive sleep apnoea. *Chest* 1996; **109**: 1346–58.

40. Wright J, Johns R, Watt I, Melville A, Sheldon T. Health effects of obstructive sleep apnoea and the effectiveness of continuous positive airway pressure: a systematic review of the research evidence. *Br Med J* 1997; **314**: 851–60.

41. Sharp JF, Jalaludin M, Murray JAM, Maran AGD. The uvulopalatopharyngoplasty operation: the Edinburgh experience. *J Roy Soc Med* 1990; **83**: 569–70.

42. Ferguson KA, Ono T, Lowe AA, Keenan SP, Fleetham JA. A randomised crossover study of an oral appliance vs. nasal continuous positive airway pressure in the treatment of mild-moderate obstructive sleep apnoea. *Chest* 1996; **109**: 1269–75.

KEY POINTS

- The low inspired oxygen partial pressure experienced at altitude causes hyperventilation and hypocapnia, which is partially reversed as acclimatisation occurs over a few days at altitude.
- The rate of ascent and the altitude achieved are determinants of altitude-related illnesses, which vary from mild acute mountain sickness to potentially lethal high-altitude pulmonary oedema.
- Populations who reside at high altitude have adaptations to their environment, such as lesser degrees of hyperventilation compensated for by a greater lung surface area for gas exchange.
- Commercial aircraft cabins are pressurised to an equivalent altitude of below 2400 m (8000 ft) and so represent a level of hypoxia similar to breathing 15% oxygen at sea level.

With increasing altitude, the barometric pressure falls but the fractional concentration of oxygen in the air (0.21) and the saturated vapour pressure of water at body temperature (6.3 kPa or 47 mmHg) remain constant. The PO_2 of the inspired air is related to the barometric pressure as follows:

Inspired gas $PO_2 = 0.21$
$$\times (\text{Barometric pressure} - 6.3) \text{ kPa}$$
or Inspired gas $PO_2 = 0.21 \times (\text{Barometric}$
$$\text{pressure} - 47) \text{ mmHg}$$

The influence of the saturated vapour pressure of water becomes relatively more important until, at an altitude of approximately 19 000 m or 63 000 feet, the barometric pressure equals the water vapour pressure and alveolar PO_2 and PCO_2 become zero.

Table 17.1 is based on the standard table relating altitude and barometric pressure. However, there are important deviations from the predicted barometric pressure under certain circumstances, particularly at low latitudes. At the summit of Everest, the actual baro-metric pressure was found to be 2.4 kPa (18 mmHg) greater than predicted and this was crucial to reaching the summit without oxygen. The uppermost curve in Figure 17.1 shows the expected PO_2 of air as a function of altitude, while the crosses indicate observed values in the Himalayas that have been consistently higher than expected.

Equivalent oxygen concentration

The acute effect of altitude on inspired PO_2 may be simulated by reduction of the oxygen concentration of gas inspired at sea level (see Table 17.1). Conversely, up to 10 000 m (33 000 ft), it is possible to restore the inspired PO_2 to the sea level value by an appropriate increase in the oxygen concentration of the inspired gas (also shown in Table 17.1). Lower inspired PO_2 values may be obtained between 10 000 and 19 000 m, above which body fluids boil.

RESPIRATORY SYSTEM RESPONSES TO ALTITUDE

Ascent to altitude presents three main challenges to the respiratory system, resulting from progressively reduced inspired PO_2, low relative humidity and, in outdoor environments, extreme cold. Hypoxia is by far the most important of these and requires significant physiological changes to allow continuation of normal activities at altitude. The efficiency of these changes depends on many factors, such as the normal altitude at which the subject lives, the rate of ascent, the altitude attained and the health of the subject.

Acute exposure to altitude

Transport technology now permits altitude to be attained quickly and without the exertion of climbing. Within a few hours, rail, air, cable car or motor transport may take a passenger from near sea level to as high as 4000 m (13 100 ft).

Ventilatory changes. At high altitude the decrease in inspired gas PO_2 reduces alveolar and therefore arterial

Table 17.1 Barometric pressure relative to altitude

Altitude		Barometric pressure		Inspired gas PO_2		Equivalent oxygen %	Percentage oxygen required to give sea level value of inspired gas PO_2
feet	metres	kPa	mmHg	kPa	mmHg	at sea level	
0	0	101	760	19.9	149	20.9	20.9
2 000	610	94.3	707	18.4	138	19.4	22.6
4 000	1 220	87.8	659	16.9	127	17.8	24.5
6 000	1 830	81.2	609	15.7	118	16.6	26.5
8 000	2 440	75.2	564	14.4	108	15.1	28.8
10 000	3 050	69.7	523	13.3	100	14.0	31.3
12 000	3 660	64.4	483	12.1	91	12.8	34.2
14 000	4 270	59.5	446	11.1	83	11.6	37.3
16 000	4 880	54.9	412	10.1	76	10.7	40.8
18 000	5 490	50.5	379	9.2	69	9.7	44.8
20 000	6 100	46.5	349	8.4	63	8.8	49.3
22 000	6 710	42.8	321	7.6	57	8.0	54.3
24 000	7 320	39.2	294	6.9	52	7.3	60.3
26 000	7 930	36.0	270	6.3	47	6.6	66.8
28 000	8 540	32.9	247	5.6	42	5.9	74.5
30 000	9 150	30.1	226	4.9	37	5.2	83.2
35 000	10 700	23.7	178	3.7	27	3.8	–
40 000	12 200	18.8	141	2.7	20	2.8	–
45 000	13 700	14.8	111	1.8	13	1.9	–
50 000	15 300	11.6	87	1.1	8	1.1	–
63 000	19 200	6.3	47	0	0	0	–

100% oxygen restores sea level inspired PO_2 at 10 000 m (33 000 ft).

PO_2. The actual decrease in alveolar PO_2 is mitigated by hyperventilation caused by the hypoxic drive to ventilation. However, on acute exposure to altitude, the ventilatory response to hypoxia is very short-lived owing to a combination of the resultant hypocapnia and hypoxic ventilatory decline (page 66 and Figure 5.7). During the first few days at altitude, this disadvantageous negative feedback is reversed by acclimatisation (see below).

Signs and symptoms. Impairment of night vision is the earliest sign of hypoxia and may be detected as low as 1200 m (4000 ft). However, the most serious aspect of acute exposure to altitude is impairment of mental performance, culminating in loss of consciousness, which usually occurs on acute exposure to altitudes in excess of 6000 m (about 20 000 ft). The time to loss of consciousness varies with altitude and is of great practical importance to pilots in the event of loss of pressurisation (Figure 17.2). The shortest possible time to loss of consciousness (about 15 seconds) applies above about 16 000 m (52 000 ft) and is governed by lung-to-brain circulation time and the capacity of high-energy phosphate stores in the brain (page 334).

Acclimatisation to altitude

Acclimatisation is the processes by which tolerance and performance are improved over a period of hours to weeks after an individual who normally lives at relatively low altitude ascends to a much higher area. Everest has been climbed without oxygen by well-acclimatised lowlanders, although without acclimatisation the barometric pressure on the summit would cause rapid loss of consciousness (see Figure 17.2). Adaptation to altitude (described below) refers to physiological differences in permanent residents at high altitude and is quite different from acclimatisation.

Earlier studies of acclimatisation took place in the attractive, though somewhat hostile, environment of high-altitude expeditions in many mountain ranges. Technical limitations in these conditions led, in 1985, to Operation Everest II, in which eight volunteers spent over 32 days in a decompression chamber in which an ascent to the summit of Everest was simulated.[3] These conditions permitted extensive physiological research to be undertaken, including arterial and Swan–Ganz catheterisation at rest and during exercise.

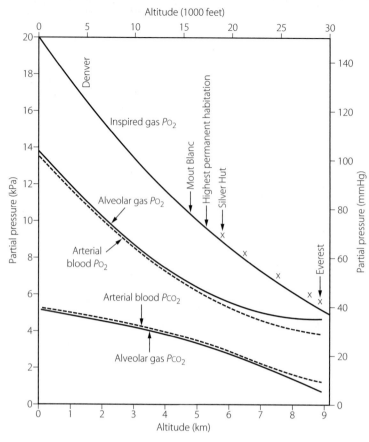

Figure 17.1 Inspired, alveolar and arterial gas partial pressures at rest, as a function of altitude. The curve for inspired P_{O_2} is taken from standard data in Table 17.1, but the crosses show actual measurements in the Himalayas. The alveolar gas data are from reference 1 and agree remarkably well with the arterial blood data from the simulated ascent of Everest.[2]

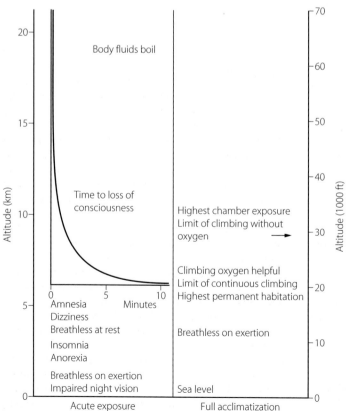

Figure 17.2 Symptoms of acute and chronic exposure to altitude.

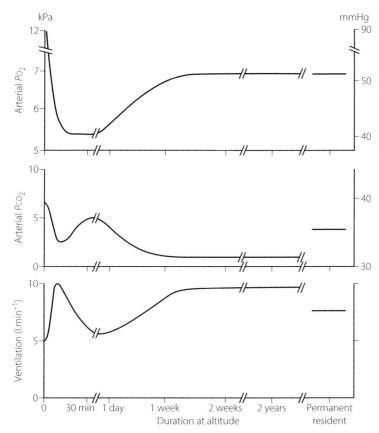

Figure 17.3 Effects of prolonged hypoxia (equivalent to 4300 m, 14 100 ft) on ventilation and blood gases. The first section of the graph shows the acute hypoxic response and hypoxic ventilatory decline described in Chapter 5. Acclimatisation then takes place, partially restoring PO_2 by means of long-term hyperventilation and hypocapnia, a situation that is maintained indefinitely while remaining at altitude. Individuals who reside throughout life at this altitude maintain similar PO_2 values with lesser degrees of hyperventilation, but still have a minute ventilation greater than sea level normal. (After reference 4.)

Ventilatory control. Prolonged hypoxia results in several complex changes in ventilation and arterial blood gases, which are shown in Figure 17.3.[4] The initial hypoxic drive to ventilation on acute exposure is short-lived and after about 30 minutes ventilation returns to only slightly above normoxic levels, with PCO_2 just below control levels (Figure 17.3). This poor ventilatory response causes significant arterial hypoxaemia and results in many of the symptoms seen during the first few hours and days at altitude. Over the next few days ventilation slowly increases, with an accompanying reduction of PCO_2 and increase in arterial PO_2. This increase is relatively small in magnitude and can never correct PO_2 to normal (sea level) values, but it does seem to be enough to ameliorate most of the symptoms of acute exposure to altitude.

There are significant differences between species in the rate at which acclimatisation takes place, being just a few hours in most animals and several days or weeks in humans.[4] Both the rate of ascent and the altitude attained influence the speed at which ventilatory acclimatisation occurs,[5] but in humans, most subjects are fully acclimatised within 1 week.

There are many possible mechanisms to explain the ventilatory changes seen with acclimatisation.[4,6] In spite of the low blood PCO_2, stimulation of the central chemoreceptors almost certainly plays a part in the hyperventilation that occurs with acclimatisation. It was first suggested in 1963 that the restoration of cerebrospinal fluid (CSF) pH, by means of bicarbonate transport, might explain this acclimatisation of ventilation to altitude.[7,8] Shortly afterwards Severinghaus and his colleagues measured their own CSF pH during acclimatisation to altitude and showed that it did indeed tend to return towards its initial value of 7.2.[7] Subsequent work showed that the time course of changes in CSF pH did not match changes in ventilation,[4] with most studies finding a persistent increase in CSF pH during continued exposure to hypoxia.[6] Changes in CSF pH therefore seem unlikely to represent an important mechanism of acclimatisation.[9] Other studies, mainly in animals, indicate that acclimatisation represents an increase in the responsiveness of the respiratory centre to hypoxia from both direct effects of prolonged hypoxia on the central nervous system and prolonged maximal afferent input from the peripheral chemoreceptors. This increased responsiveness may be mediated by alterations in the sensitivity to neurotransmitters involved in respiratory control (see Figure 5.4). For example, increased sensitivity to glutamate will directly increase ventilation, whereas decreasing GABA sensitivity will effectively reduce hypoxic ventilatory decline (page 66).[6]

In addition to changes affecting the central chemoreceptors, there is evidence that peripheral chemoreceptor sensitivity is increased during prolonged hypoxia, so contributing to the progressive hyperventilation seen with acclimatisation. In humans, the acute hypoxic ventilatory response is increased during the first few days at altitude and for several days after return to sea level. The mechanism of this increased sensitivity to hypoxia is not known, but is independent of changes in $P\text{CO}_2$[10] and may reside either with increased sensitivity of the carotid bodies themselves or with the increased responsiveness of the respiratory centre described in the previous paragraph.[4,6]

Respiratory alkalosis at altitude is counteracted, over the course of a few days, by renal excretion of bicarbonate, resulting in a degree of metabolic acidosis that will tend to increase respiratory drive (see Figure 5.5).

This was formerly thought to be the main factor in the ventilatory adaptation to altitude, but it now appears to be of minor importance compared to the changes in the central and peripheral chemoreceptors.

Blood gas tensions. Figure 17.3 shows the time course of blood gas changes during acclimatisation and Figure 17.1 shows changes in alveolar gas tensions with altitude in fully acclimatised mountaineers at rest. Alveolar $P\text{O}_2$ was found to be unexpectedly well preserved at extreme altitude and above 8000 m (26 000 ft) tended to remain close to 4.8 kPa (36 mmHg).[1] Operation Everest II found a mean arterial $P\text{O}_2$ of 4 kPa (30 mmHg) at a pressure equivalent to the summit of Everest (32 kPa or 240 mmHg) (Table 17.2), with an alveolar/arterial $P\text{O}_2$ difference of less than 0.3 kPa (2 mmHg) at rest.[11]

Haemoglobin concentration and oxygen affinity. An increase in haemoglobin concentration was the earliest

Table 17.2 Cardiorespiratory data obtained at rest and during exercise at extreme reduction of ambient pressure during the simulated ascent of Everest in a low-pressure chamber

	Sea-level equivalent		Extreme altitude equivalent	
Ambient pressure (kPa)	101		33.7	
(mmHg)	760		253	
Haemoglobin concentration (g.dl^{-1})	13.5		17.0	
$\dot{V}\text{O}_{2max}$ (ml.min^{-1}, STPD)	3980		1170	

State	Rest	Exercise	Rest	Exercise
Exercise intensity (watts)	0	281	0	90
Ventilation (l.min^{-1}, BTPS)	11	107	42.3	157.5
$\dot{V}\text{O}_2$ (ml.min^{-1}, STPD)	350	3380	386	1002
Ventilation equivalent	31	32	110	157
Arterial $P\text{O}_2$ (kPa)	13.2	12.0	4.0	3.7
(mmHg)	99.3	90.0	30.3	27.7
Arterial $P\text{CO}_2$ (kPa)	4.5	4.7	1.5	1.3
(mmHg)	33.9	35.0	11.2	10.1
Arterial/venous O_2 content difference (ml.dl^{-1})	5.7	15.0	4.6	6.7
Mixed venous $P\text{O}_2$ (kPa)	4.7	2.6	2.9	1.9
(mmHg)	35.1	19.7	22.1	14.3
Cardiac output (l.min^{-1})	6.7	27.2	8.4	15.7
Pulmonary arterial pressure (mean, mmHg)	15	33	33	48

Notes
1. Actual ambient pressure at simulated high altitude was 32 kPa (240 mmHg) but leakage of oxygen from masks worn by investigators had caused the oxygen concentration in the chamber to rise to 22%, the equivalent of 33.7 kPa at 21%, which is equivalent to the summit of Everest.
2. Study 12 reported cardiovascular data for a mean exercise intensity of 90 watts at the highest altitude. Data from other studies have been interpolated to give values corresponding to the same exercise intensity in order to achieve compatibility.
(Data from references 2, 12 and 13.)

adaptation to altitude to be demonstrated. Operation Everest II reported an increase from 13.5 to 17 g.dl^{-1} which, at the resting value of 58% saturation, maintained an arterial oxygen content of 12 ml.dl^{-1}.[2] Plasma erythropoietin levels begin to increase within a few hours at altitude, reaching a maximum at 24–48 hours and then declining.[14] Haemoglobin concentrations may also be influenced by changes in plasma volume. Increases in haemoglobin concentration to above about 18 g.dl^{-1} are probably detrimental because of the increased viscosity of the blood.

The haemoglobin dissociation curve at altitude is affected by changes in both pH and 2,3-diphosphoglycerate (DPG) concentration (page 178). 2,3-DPG concentrations increased from 1.7 to 3.8 mmol.l^{-1} on Operation Everest II.[2] It has been estimated that the resultant effect is a leftward shift at extreme altitude, where oxygen loading in the lung takes priority over maintaining P_{O_2} at the point of release.[14]

Adaptation to altitude[15]

Adaptation refers to physiological and genetic changes that occur over a period of years to generations by those who have taken up permanent residence at high altitude. There are qualitative as well as quantitative differences between acclimatisation and adaptation, but each is remarkably effective. High altitude residents have a remarkable ability to exercise under grossly hypoxic conditions, but their adaptations show many striking differences from those in acclimatised lowlanders. Residents in different high-altitude areas of the world have different adaptations.[16]

Long-term residence at altitude leads to a reduced ventilatory response to hypoxia, the magnitude of which relates to the product of altitude level and years of residence there.[4] This results in a reduction of ventilation compared with an acclimatised lowlander and a rise in P_{CO_2}, though neither of these returns to sea level values (see Figure 17.3). High altitude residents maintain similar arterial P_{O_2} values to acclimatised lowlanders in spite of the reduced ventilation and the lower alveolar P_{O_2}. Pulmonary diffusing capacity must therefore be increased, and depends on anatomical pulmonary adaptations increasing the area available for diffusion by the generation of greater numbers of alveoli and associated capillaries. This adaptation seems not to be inherited, but occurs in children and infants who spend their formative years at altitude. In humans, the development of alveoli by septation of saccules formed *in utero* occurs mostly after birth (page 230) and it is this process that must be stimulated by hypoxia, though the mechanism of this stimulation remains unknown.[17] An adult moving permanently to high altitude will therefore never achieve the same degree of adaptation as a native of the area, so

explaining the ability of high altitude residents to exercise to a much greater degree than their non-resident visitors.

Recent work has found that residents of high-altitude areas of the Andes hyperventilate less than residents at equivalent altitude in Tibet.[16] This higher ventilation in Tibetans may explain their reduced susceptibility, in comparison with populations in the Andes, to chronic mountain sickness (see below) and some complications of pregnancy that are normally associated with high-altitude life.[18] Human occupation of Tibet is believed to have begun earlier than in other high-altitude areas of the world, and these differences in Tibetan physiology could represent a more advanced genetic adaptation to the physiologically hostile environment.

Polycythaemia is normal and the highest levels (haemoglobin concentrations of 22.9 g.dl^{-1}) occur in Andean miners living at 5300 m (17 500 ft). Another major adaptation to altitude by long-term residents appears to be increased vascularity of heart and striated muscles, a change that is also important for the trained athlete. For the high altitude resident, increased perfusion appears to compensate very effectively for the reduced oxygen content of the arterial blood.

Limits for residence and work.[19] The upper limit for sustained work seems to be 5950 m (19 500 ft) at the Aucanquilcha sulphur mine in the Andes. The upper limit for elective permanent habitation is lower and the Andean miners declined to live in accommodation built for them near the mine, preferring to live at 5330 m (17 500 ft) and climb every day to their work. Increased commercial pressure for mining has led to an increase in high-altitude activity and West has suggested the use of oxygen enrichment of sleeping quarters to reduce altitude-induced illness (see below), with each 1% increase in oxygen concentration being equivalent to 300 m (1000 ft) of descent.[20]

Chronic mountain sickness (Monge's disease). A small minority of those who dwell permanently at very high altitude develop this dangerous illness. It is characterised by an exceptionally poor ventilatory response to hypoxia resulting in low arterial P_{O_2} and high P_{CO_2}. There is cyanosis, high haematocrit, finger clubbing, pulmonary hypertension, right heart failure, dyspnoea and lethargy.

Exercise at high altitude[21]

The summit of Everest was attained without the use of oxygen in 1978 by Messner and Habeler and by many other climbers since that date. Studies of exercise have been made at various altitudes up to and including the summit and on the simulated ascent in Operation

Everest II. Of necessity, these observations are largely confined to very fit subjects.

Capacity for work performed. There is a progressive decline in the external work that can be performed as altitude increases. On Operation Everest II, 300–360 watts was attained at sea level, 240–270 watts at 440 mmHg pressure (equivalent to 4300 m, 14 000 ft) and 120 watts at 280 mmHg (Everest summit), very close to the results obtained on Everest.[22] $\dot{V}O_{2max}$ declined in accord with altitude to 1177 ml.min^{-1} at 240 mmHg pressure.[13] Resting cardiac output is unchanged at moderate altitude and only slightly increased at extreme altitude. During exercise, for a given power expenditure the increase in cardiac output at altitude is the same as at sea level.[2]

Ventilation equivalent of oxygen consumption. Figure 15.5 shows that ventilation as a function of $\dot{V}O_2$ is comparatively constant. The length of the line increases with training but the slope of the linear portion remains the same. With increasing altitude, the slope and intercept are both dramatically increased up to four times the sea-level value,[2,13] with maximal ventilation approaching 200 l.min^{-1} (Figure 17.4). This is because ventilation is

reported at body temperature and pressure saturated (BTPS) and oxygen consumption at standard temperature and pressure dry (STPD) – see Appendix C.

Fortunately, the density of air is reduced in proportion to the barometric pressure at altitude. Resistance to turbulent flow is decreased and therefore the work of breathing at a particular minute volume of respiration is less. Even with this mitigation, the extra ventilation needed to deliver the oxygen requirement at altitude means that the energy expenditure upon breathing for a given intensity of exercise is considerably higher than at sea level.

P_{CO_2} and P_{O_2}. During exercise at altitude, alveolar P_{CO_2} falls and alveolar P_{O_2} rises (Figure 17.5).[2,23] Arterial P_{CO_2} falls with alveolar P_{CO_2} but the alveolar/arterial P_{O_2} difference increases more than the alveolar P_{O_2} rises[23] and there is a consistent decrease in arterial P_{O_2} during exercise at altitude, leading to very low values for P_{O_2} (see Figure 17.5). The lower alveolar to pulmonary capillary P_{O_2} gradient, along with a faster pulmonary capillary transit time during exercise, causes diffusion limitation of oxygen uptake. There is also some evidence that ventilation/perfusion inequality occurs during exercise at altitude and adversely affects oxygenation.[21]

ALTITUDE ILLNESS[24–26]

Acute mountain sickness

Acute mountain sickness (AMS) is characterised by headache, nausea, fatigue, anorexia, dyspnoea, difficulty in sleeping (see below) and impaired climbing performance (see Figure 17.2). Symptoms normally begin to occur at above 2000 m (6600 ft), though cases are described at lower altitudes.[27] At 5000 m (16 000 ft), there are feelings of unreality (often enhanced by the environment!), amnesia and dizziness. The unacclimatised person has extreme dyspnoea on exertion at this level and has dyspnoea at rest. Severity varies greatly, from a mild inconvenient headache to a severe life-threatening illness involving cerebral and pulmonary oedema.

The likelihood of developing AMS relates to altitude (particularly sleeping altitude), the rate of ascent and the degree of exertion. The mountaineer is therefore affected by altitude in a manner that differs from that of the aviator because his physical exertion is much greater and the time course of exposure is different. Rate of ascent seldom exceeds 2000 m (6500 ft) per day from sea level, decreasing to only 300 m (1000 ft) per day at very high altitude. Over half of mountaineers develop AMS above 4000 m (13 000 ft),[24] whereas one-quarter of tourists travelling to resorts between 2000 and 3000 m (6300–9700 ft) high develop it.[28]

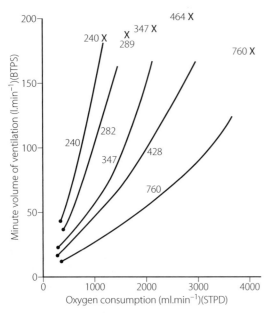

Figure 17.4 The relationship between minute volume of ventilation and oxygen consumption at rest and during exercise at altitude. The relationship is radically changed at altitude, primarily because ventilation is reported at body temperature and pressure (saturated), whereas oxygen consumption is reported at standard temperature and pressure (dry). Numbers in the figure indicate barometric pressure. •, resting points; ×, values at $\dot{V}O_{2max}$ from reference 13. (Data from reference 2.)

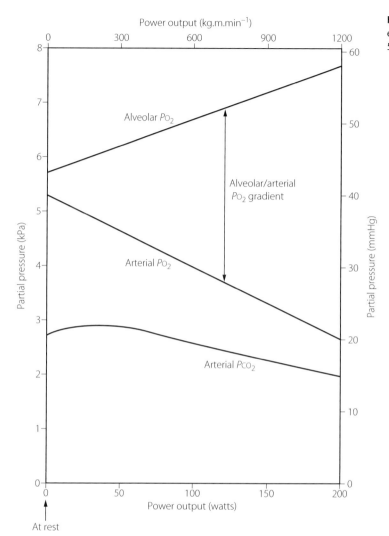

Figure 17.5 Po_2 and Pco_2 changes during exercise in a single subject (Dr John West) at 5800 m (19 000 ft). (Data from reference 25.)

High-altitude pulmonary oedema (HAPE)

About 1% of climbers develop HAPE[24] following acute exposure to altitudes in excess of about 3000 m (10 000 ft), usually following rapid ascent and strenuous exercise. It is most commonly seen in the unacclimatised and overambitious climber. It also occurs in high altitude residents following their return from low-altitude travel. Clinical features include cough, dyspnoea and hypoxia with clinical and radiological signs of pulmonary oedema. Untreated, HAPE has a mortality rate of almost 50%, but with appropriate treatment this is normally less than 3%.

The pathophysiology of HAPE is complex.[25,26,29] Subjects with HAPE have significant pulmonary hypertension secondary to hypoxia and low pulmonary capillary wedge pressures indicating normal left ventricular func-

tion. Subjects who are susceptible to HAPE seem to have an excessive hypoxic pulmonary vasoconstriction response to hypoxia, and this may in part be due to impaired release of endothelial relaxing factors such as nitric oxide (page 102). Compared with subjects who are not susceptible to HAPE, susceptible subjects exhaled lower concentrations of nitric oxide during a high-altitude trip[30] and in another study demonstrated a greater amount of pulmonary vasodilation when inhaling NO at high altitude.[31] In addition, pulmonary vasoconstrictors such as endothelin-1 are found in higher concentrations in HAPE-susceptible subjects, who also have greater sympathetic responses to hypoxia. Pulmonary shadows on chest X-rays with HAPE are typically patchy, indicating that pulmonary vasoconstriction is non-uniform, such that some areas of lung have little blood flow whereas in others blood flow is greatly increased.

High capillary flow in some areas is postulated to lead to 'stress failure' of capillaries. This mechanism would explain the association between exercise and HAPE, with increased cardiac output causing huge blood flows through vasodilated sections of lung. Disruption of endothelial cell architecture will lead to pulmonary oedema either directly or via activation of inflammatory mediators. Although inflammation is not believed to be a primary event in the pathogenesis of HAPE, it does commonly occur in severe cases and explains why coincidental lung inflammation from, for example, lower respiratory tract infections may exacerbate or even cause HAPE.

Other respiratory problems at altitude

Cerebral oedema is also potentially lethal and is manifest in the early stages by ataxia, irritability and irrational behaviour, and may progress to hallucinations, drowsiness and coma. Postmortem studies have shown that cerebral oedema may be accompanied by intracranial thrombosis and haemorrhage.[14] Pulmonary and cerebral forms of severe acute mountain sickness may both be present in the same patient, but a common aetiology has not been found. Mild, or localised, brain swelling is thought to occur in all people ascending to high altitudes, but it is unclear whether this always represents cerebral oedema.[26] The neurological symptoms that develop, varying from mild headache through AMS to lethal cerebral oedema, may simply depend on the individual's ability to compensate for the inevitable brain swelling at high altitude.[25]

Following return to low altitude, cerebral disturbance may persist. Investigations up to 30 days after expeditions to very high altitudes have shown a variety of impairments, including visual long-term memory.[32] Changes were more marked in people with a vigorous hypoxic ventilatory response, perhaps because of hypocapnia-induced decrease in cerebral blood flow.

Cough.[33] Almost half of trekkers in Nepal complain of a cough, which may be severe. Coughing normally develops after a few days at altitude and airway sensitivity to irritants is increased as a result of hyperventilation of low humidity cold air. Development of a cough may, however, be the first manifestation of impending HAPE.

Sleep disturbance. Periodic breathing occurs in most individuals during the first few nights above about 4000 m (13 000 ft). Breathing patterns are similar to those of the sleep apnoea/hypopnoea syndrome (page 248). There are cyclical changes in tidal volume, often associated with central (rather than obstructive) apnoeas, with or without arousal from sleep (see Figure 16.2). Apnoeas may result in considerable additional hypoxaemia at high altitude. Studies at 4500 m (15 000 ft)[34] and at 6300 m (21 000 ft)[19] found nocturnal reductions in saturation of 8% and 10%, respectively; in the former study this reduced median nocturnal saturation to just 50%. The primary problem is an abnormality of respiratory control, with arousal occurring at the end of a period of apnoea, presumably secondary to hypoxia. The severity of periodic breathing is related to the strength of the subject's hypoxic ventilatory drive[24] and is seldom seen in high altitude residents, who have a much attenuated hypoxic drive. The onset of sleep disturbance and severe nocturnal hypoxia may also contribute to the symptoms of AMS, and subjects developing HAPE have lower oxygen saturations during sleep.[34]

Therapy for altitude-induced illness

For any severe form of AMS, administration of oxygen and descent to a lower altitude are the first essentials. Without these simple interventions, patients with cerebral oedema or HAPE will have a high mortality. Nifedipine is now an established treatment for HAPE and when used prophylactically prevents HAPE developing in susceptible individuals.[24–26] It is an effective drug for treating pulmonary hypertension and the convenience of administration by the oral or sublingual routes makes it a popular choice for mountaineers.

People with milder degrees of AMS do not need to be removed from high altitude. With acclimatisation, most symptoms of AMS will resolve but, if time is limited or symptoms interfere with planned activities, acetazolamide may be useful. This carbonic anhydrase inhibitor (page 148) interferes with the transport of carbon dioxide out of cells, causing an intracellular acidosis that includes the cells of the medullary chemoreceptors and so drives respiration.[35] In effect, this accelerates acclimatisation and so may improve the arterial PO_2. Acetazolamide also improves sleep-induced periodic breathing, reducing the number and severity of apnoeas, and thereby alleviates daytime symptoms.

FLYING

Only a very small number of people will ever visit places of high enough altitude to induce any of the respiratory changes described in this chapter so far. However, worldwide, almost 2 billion people per year fly in commercial aircraft, so the final section of this chapter deals with the respiratory effects of aviation.

Altitude exposure[36]

For reasons of fuel economy and avoidance of weather systems, commercial aircraft operate at between 9000 and 12 000 m (30–40 000 ft). The passenger cabin must

Table 17.3 Cabin pressure characteristics of commercial aircraft

Aircraft	Differential pressure kPa	Cabin pressure at 10 700 m (35 000 ft)		Cabin 'altitude' at 10 700 m (35 000 ft)		Equivalent oxygen at sea level
		mmHg	kPa	ft	m	%
Boeing 727	59.3	623	83.0	5400	1650	17.0
Boeing 737	51.4	563	75.1	8000	2440	15.2
Boeing 747	61.4	638	85.1	4700	1430	17.4
Boeing 767	59.3	623	83.0	5400	1650	17.0
Boeing 777	60.5	631	84.2	5000	1520	17.2
DC8	60.5	631	84.2	5000	1520	17.2
DC9	53.5	579	77.2	7300	2220	15.7
DC10	59.3	623	83.0	5400	1650	17.0
Airbus A320	57.2	607	80.9	6000	1830	16.5
Concorde	73.8	731	97.5	1000	300	20.2
Concorde*	73.8	604	80.6	6500	1980	16.4

Differential pressure is the absolute pressure difference between the cabin and outside environments. Atmospheric pressure at 10 700 m (35 000 ft) is 23.7 kPa (178 mmHg). Concorde* data refer to Concorde at its usual cruise height of 18 300 m (60 000 ft) where atmospheric pressure is only 6.8 kPa (51 mmHg). (Data from reference 40 and Dr M Bagshaw, British Airways Medical Services, 1998.)

therefore be pressurised and a typical design aims for a cabin pressure equivalent to less than 2400 m (8000 ft), often referred to as the 'cabin altitude'.[37] Cabin pressure is maintained by indrawing and compression of external air while limiting cabin air outflow to maintain the desired pressure. In practice, a differential pressure is established, which represents the absolute pressure difference between the outside and the inside of the aircraft. Differential pressure is increased as the aircraft climbs, and vice versa. Thus cabin pressure changes in parallel with altitude, but to a much lesser degree than the external pressure. Maximum cabin differential pressures and normal operating cabin altitudes for common commercial aircraft are shown in Table 17.3. Peak cabin altitude measured on commercial aircraft is around 2000–2400 m (6200–7600 ft), with newer aircraft tending to operate with *higher* cabin altitudes than older models.[37,38] Compressed external air is obtained from the compression chamber of the engines, so cabin pressure may vary during flight according to engine performance. For example, when flying over high-altitude terrain such as the Himalayas or South America, cabin altitude will be increased. This occurs partly as a result of increased cruise altitude, but also because compressed air supply from the engine will be reduced to facilitate acceptable engine performance at higher altitude (personal communication, Dr M Bagshaw, British Airways).

Supersonic flight required much higher operating altitude to reduce air resistance, so Concorde's cruise altitude was 18 300 m (60 000 ft). The differential pressure must therefore be greater to sustain a normal cabin environment at this altitude (see Table 17.3), which was facilitated in Concorde by the significantly more powerful engines from which compressed air was drawn. Military aircraft fly prolonged reconnaissance missions at an altitude of 22 400 m (73 500 ft), with the cockpit pressurised to an equivalent altitude of 9000 m (30 000 ft). Pilots must therefore breathe 100% oxygen by mask to maintain an inspired PO_2 close to sea level to facilitate the required mental performance. At this altitude, military pilots are also at risk of altitude decompression sickness, which is discussed on page 273.[39]

In theory, cabin altitudes of below 2400 m (8000 ft) should represent a minimal physiological challenge to healthy individuals, resulting in a drop of only a few percent in oxygen saturation. In practice, a study of healthy cabin crew during normal flight patterns showed that over half had saturation drops to less than 90%.[37] The effects of this degree of hypoxia on performance are controversial, though impaired night vision or colour recognition may occur at this altitude (page 255).[37]

Depressurisation. Loss of cabin pressure at altitude, through either equipment failure or accident, is extremely rare. In the case of slow loss of cabin pressure, oxygen is provided for passengers as an interim measure until the aircraft can descend: 100% oxygen provides adequate protection from loss of consciousness up to an altitude of about 12 000 m (40 000 ft), where the atmospheric pressure is roughly equal to the sea-level atmospheric PO_2.

There are sporadic reports of stowaway passengers undertaking long-haul flights in the wheel well of modern aircraft.[41] This environment affords little protection against the cold and severe hypoxia of altitude levels well above that of Everest. That half of these stowaways die is not surprising, but it is remarkable that half of them survive. Severe hypothermia is believed to protect them against the effects of hypoxia.

Air travel in patients with respiratory disease[42–44]

To patients with respiratory disease flying may present a significant problem, particularly if arterial hypoxaemia already exists at sea level, and careful preflight assessment is required.[36] A variety of preflight clinical evaluations and investigations have been recommended to determine whether an individual patient would require supplemental oxygen during flight. Recent British Thoracic Society guidelines[44] have provided recommendations for assessing patients with respiratory disease, a summary of which is shown in Table 17.4. For patients with an oxygen saturation while breathing air of less than 92%, or in those with Sa_{O_2} of 92–95% with other risk factors (see Table 17.4), then a hypoxic challenge test is recommended. This test involves measurement of

Table 17.4 British Thoracic Society recommendations on assessing the need for in-flight supplemental oxygen in patients with respiratory disease[44]

Assessment result	Action
Screening:	
Sa_{O_2} >95%	Oxygen not required
Sa_{O_2} 92–95% and no risk factor[†]	Oxygen not required
Sa_{O_2} 92–95% and additional risk factor[†]	Hypoxic challenge test
Sa_{O_2} <92%	In-flight oxygen
Hypoxic challenge test:	
Pa_{O_2} >7.4 kPa (>55 mmHg)	Oxygen not required
Pa_{O_2} 6.6–7.4 kPa (50–55 mmHg)	Borderline – walk test may be helpful
Pa_{O_2} <6.6 kPa (<50 mmHg)	In-flight oxygen

Screening test is oxygen saturation while breathing air at sea level. Hypoxic challenge test is arterial oxygen tension after breathing 15% oxygen for 20 minutes.
[†], additional risk factors include hypercapnia; FEV_1 <50% of predicted; lung cancer; restrictive lung disease involving the parenchyma, chest wall (kyphoscoliosis) or respiratory muscles; ventilator support; cerebrovascular or cardiac disease; within 6 weeks of discharge for an exacerbation of chronic lung or cardiac disease.

arterial PO_2 while simulating flying conditions by using a hypoxic gas mixture, usually 15% oxygen. This inspired PO_2 equates to a cabin altitude of 2400 m (8000 ft) and represents the lowest oxygen tension that should be experienced during a commercial flight (see Table 17.1).

Cabin air quality[36,38,45,46]

Aircraft ventilation systems deliver 4–8 $l.s^{-1}$ of air per passenger during flight. However, compression and temperature regulation of fresh air from outside is expensive in energy terms and more recent designs of aircraft incorporate cabin air recirculation systems.[46,47] Total air delivered remains the same, but up to 50% may be recirculated rather than fresh. This recirculation of cabin air has caused concerns about the potential transmission of airborne pathogens between passengers. These fears seem to be unfounded: recirculated air passes through a high-efficiency particulate air filter before reentering the cabin,[45] and studies comparing passengers travelling on aircraft with recirculated rather than 100% fresh air ventilation systems found no difference in the likelihood of developing a common cold after the flight.[47]

Carbon dioxide concentration in aircraft often exceeds the generally accepted 'comfort' level of 1000 ppm and would be expected to be higher in aircraft with greater amounts of recirculation air conditioning. Concentrations observed in aircraft vary between around 700 and 1700 ppm[48,49] and are highest when the aircraft is occupied but on the ground and lowest while flying at cruise altitude. Carbon dioxide itself does not cause respiratory problems at these levels, but is used more as a marker of the adequacy of ventilation.

Humidity is invariably low in aircraft, with most studies finding relative humidity to average 14–19% during flight compared with in excess of 50% in most other sea-level environments.[50] Like carbon dioxide, cabin humidity is maximal when on the ground and minimal at cruise altitude.[49] The low humidity occurring in aircraft is responsible for many minor symptoms, such as irritation of the eyes and upper airway, although such symptoms are unusual with less than 3–4 hours of exposure.[50]

Ozone concentration in atmospheric air increases with greater altitude. At altitudes used by Concorde, outside ozone levels are approximately 4000 ppb, well in excess of thresholds known to cause respiratory problems (page 294). Fortunately, compression of outside air at this altitude involves heating the air to 400°C, which completely removes ozone by its conversion to oxygen, and cabin ozone concentrations remain very low. Atmospheric ozone concentrations are much lower below 12 000 m (40 000 ft) so other aircraft are generally unaffected,[48] though one study did find significant levels in Boeing 747s.[51]

Smoking during flight has now been banned by many airlines worldwide, possibly as a result of reduced fresh air ventilation coupled with the threat of legal challenge for passive smoking-related illness.[36,38] In fact, aircraft ventilation systems are highly effective at preventing the spread of tobacco smoke through the cabin. Nicotine and carbon monoxide levels are higher in the smoking than in non-smoking sections of aircraft, but levels seen in the non-smoking areas are the same as on completely non-smoking flights.[48] On this basis, provided seating areas are separated, passive smoking is minimal.

With the exception of low humidity, there is therefore little evidence that the cabin air of aircraft poses any threat to healthy passengers. Thus the numerous symptoms reported following air travel almost certainly have their origins in other activities associated with air travel, in particular the consumption of alcohol and differing time zones.

REFERENCES

1. West JB, Hackett PH, Maret KH, *et al*. Pulmonary gas exchange on the summit of Mount Everest. *J Appl Physiol* 1983; **55**: 678–87.
2. Sutton JT, Reeves JT, Wagner PD, *et al*. Operation Everest II: oxygen transport during exercise at extreme simulated altitude. *J Appl Physiol* 1988; **64**: 1309–21.
3. Houston CS, Sutton JR, Cymerman A, Reeves JT. Operation Everest II: man at extreme altitude. *J Appl Physiol* 1987; **63**: 877–82.
4. Bisgard GE, Forster HV. Ventilatory responses to acute and chronic hypoxia. In: Fregly MJ, Blatteis CM, eds. *Handbook of physiology – section 4: Environmental physiology*. New York: Oxford University Press, 1996.
5. Purkayastha SS, Ray US, Arora BS, *et al*. Acclimatisation at high altitude in gradual and acute induction. *J Appl Physiol* 1995; **79**: 487–92.
*6. Powell FL, Huey KA, Dwinell MR. Central nervous system mechanisms of ventilatory acclimatisation to hypoxia. *Respir Physiol* 2000; **121**: 223–36.
7. Severinghaus JW, Mitchell RA, Richardson BW, Singer MM. Respiratory control at high altitude suggesting active transport regulation of CSF pH. *J Appl Physiol* 1963; **18**: 1155–66.
8. Michel CC, Milledge JS. Respiratory regulation in man during acclimatisation to high altitude. *J Physiol* 1963; **168**: 631–43.
9. Crawford RD, Severinghaus JW. CSF pH and ventilatory acclimatisation to altitude. *J Appl Physiol* 1978; **45**: 275–83.
10. Tansley JG, Fatemian M, Howard LSGE, Poulin MJ, Robbins PA. Changes in respiratory control during and after 48 h of isocapnic and poikilocapnic hypoxia in humans. *J Appl Physiol* 1998; **85**: 2125–34.
11. Wagner PD, Sutton JT, Reeves JT, Cymerman A, Groves BM, Malconian MK. Operation Everest II: pulmonary gas exchange during a simulated ascent of Mt. Everest. *J Appl Physiol* 1987; **63**: 2348–59.
12. Groves BM, Reeves JT, Sutton JT, *et al*. Operation Everest II: elevated high-altitude pulmonary resistance unresponsive to oxygen. *J Appl Physiol* 1987; **63**: 521–30.
13. Cymerman A, Reeves JT, Sutton JT, *et al*. Operation Everest II: maximal oxygen uptake at extreme altitude. *J Appl Physiol* 1989; **66**: 2446–53.
14. Ward MP, Milledge JS, West JB. *High altitude medicine and physiology*. London: Chapman & Hall, 1995.
*15. Ramirez G, Bittle PA, Rosen R, Rabb H, Pineda D. High altitude living: genetic and environmental adaptation. *Aviat Space Environ Med* 1999; **70**: 73–81.
16. Moore LG. Comparative human ventilatory adaptation to high altitude. *Respir Physiol* 2000; **121**: 257–76.
17. Massaro D, Massaro GD. Pulmonary alveoli: formation, the 'call for oxygen' and other regulators. *Am J Physiol Lung Cell Mol Physiol* 2002; **282**: L345–8.
*18. Moore LG, Armaza F, Villena M, Vargas E. Comparative aspects of high-altitude adaptation in human populations. *Adv Exp Med Biol* 2000; **475**: 45–62.
19. West JB. Highest inhabitants in the world. *Nature* 1986; **324**: 517.
20. West JB. Oxygen enrichment of room air to relieve the hypoxia of high altitude. *Respir Physiol* 1995; **99**: 225–32.
21. Schoene RB. Limits of human lung function at high altitude. *J Exp Biol* 2001; **204**: 3121–7.
22. West JB, Boyer SJ, Graber DJ, *et al*. Maximal exercise at extreme altitudes on Mount Everest. *J Appl Physiol* 1983; **55**: 688–98.
23. Pugh LGCE, Gill MB, Lahiri S, Milledge JS, Ward MP, West JB. Muscular exercise at great altitudes. *J Appl Physiol* 1964; **19**: 431–40.
24. Pollard AJ, Murdoch DR. *The high altitude medicine handbook*. Oxford: Radcliffe Medical Press, 1997.
25. Hackett PH, Roach RC. High-altitude illness. *N Engl J Med* 2001; **345**: 107–14.
*26. Basnyat B, Murdoch DR. High-altitude illness. *Lancet* 2003; **361**: 1967–74.
27. Gabry AL, Ledoux X, Mozziconacci M, Martin C. High-altitude pulmonary edema at moderate altitude (<2400 m; 7870 feet). A series of 52 patients. *Chest* 2003; **123**: 49–53.

28. Honigman B, Theis MK, Koziol-McLain J, *et al.* Acute mountain sickness in a general tourist population at moderate altitudes. *Ann Intern Med* 1993; **118**: 587–92.

29. Jerome EH, Severinghaus JW. High-altitude pulmonary edema. *N Engl J Med* 1996; **334**: 662–3.

30. Duplain H, Sartori C, Lepori M, *et al.* Exhaled nitric oxide in high-altitude pulmonary edema. Role in the regulation of pulmonary vascular tone and evidence for a role against inflammation. *Am J Respir Crit Care Med* 2000; **162**: 221–4.

31. Scherrer U, Vollenweider L, Delabays A, *et al.* Inhaled nitric oxide for high-altitude pulmonary edema. *N Engl J Med* 1996; **334**: 624–9.

32. Hornbein TH, Townes BD, Schoene RB, Sutton JR, Houston CS. The cost to the central nervous system of climbing to extremely high altitude. *N Engl J Med* 1989; **321**: 1714–19.

33. Barry PW, Mason NP, Riordan M, O'Callaghan C. Cough frequency and cough-receptor sensitivity are increased in man at altitude. *Clin Sci* 1997; **93**: 181–6.

34. Eichenberger U, Weiss E, Riemann D, Oelz O, Bärtsch P. Nocturnal periodic breathing and the development of acute high altitude illness. *Am J Respir Crit Care Med* 1996; **154**: 1748–54.

35. Milledge JS. Acute mountain sickness: pulmonary and cerebral oedema of high altitude. *Intens Care Med* 1985; **11**: 110–15.

36. Harding RM, Mills FJ. *Aviation medicine.* London: BMJ Publishing Group, 1993.

37. Cottrell JJ, Lebovitz BL, Fennell RG, Kohn GM. Inflight arterial saturation: continuous monitoring by pulse oximetry. *Aviat Space Environ Med* 1995; **66**: 126–30.

38. Smith T. Smoke free flying. *Br Med J* 1988; **297**: 1001.

39. Bendrick GA, Ainscough MJ, Pilmanis AA, Bisson RU. Prevalence of decompression sickness among U-2 pilots. *Aviat Space Environ Med* 1996; **67**: 199–206.

40. Cottrell JJ. Altitude exposures during aircraft flight. *Chest* 1988; **92**: 81–4.

41. Veronneau SJH, Mohler SR, Pennybaker AL, Wilcox BC, Sahiar F. Survival at high altitudes: wheel-well passengers. *Aviat Space Environ Med* 1996; **67**: 784–6.

42. Johnson AOC. Chronic obstructive pulmonary disease. 11: Fitness to fly with COPD. *Thorax* 2003; **58**: 729–32.

43. Mortazavi A, Eisenberg MJ, Langleben D, Ernst P, Schiff RL. Altitude-related hypoxia: risk assessment and management for passengers on commercial aircraft. *Aviat Space Environ Med* 2003; **74**: 922–7.

44. British Thoracic Society Standards of Care Committee. Managing passengers with respiratory disease planning air travel: British Thoracic Society recommendations. *Thorax* 2002; **57**: 289–304.

*45. Rayman RB. Cabin air quality: An overview. *Aviat Space Environ Med* 2002; **73**: 211–5.

46. Hocking MB. Trends in cabin air quality of commercial aircraft: Industry and passenger perspectives. *Rev Environ Health* 2002; **17**: 1–49.

47. Zitter JN, Mazonson PD, Miller DP, Hulley SB, Balmes JR. Aircraft cabin air recirculation and symptoms of the common cold. *JAMA* 2002; **288**: 483–6.

48. Crawford WA, Holcomb LC. Environmental tobacco smoke (ETS) in airliners – A health hazard evaluation. *Aviat Space Environ Med* 1991; **62**: 580–6.

49. Lindgren T, Norbäck D. Cabin air quality: indoor pollutants and climate during intercontinental flights with and without tobacco smoking. *Indoor Air* 2002; **12**: 263–72.

50. Nagda NL, Hodgson M. Low relative humidity and aircraft cabin air quality. *Indoor Air* 2001; **11**: 200–14.

51. Nastrom GD, Holdeman JD, Perkins PJ. Measurements of cabin and ambient ozone on B747 airplanes. *J Aircraft* 1980; **17**: 246–9.

KEY POINTS

■ When diving in water the increased density of inhaled gases and immersion in water cause an increase in the work of breathing, which can impair gas exchange during exercise.

■ Above about 4 atmospheres absolute pressure, nitrogen has anaesthetic effects and divers must breathe helium, which also overcomes the problem of increased gas density.

■ On ascent from a dive, expansion of gases in closed body spaces and bubble formation in the tissues and blood can cause pulmonary barotrauma and decompression sickness.

Humans have sojourned temporarily in high-pressure environments since the introduction of the diving bell. The origin of this development is lost in antiquity, but Alexander the Great was said to have been lowered to the seabed in a diving bell.

The environment of the diver is often, but not invariably, aqueous. Saturation divers spend most of their time in a gaseous environment in chambers that are held at a pressure close to that of the depth of water at which they will be working. Tunnel and caisson workers may also be at high pressure in a gaseous environment. Those in an aqueous environment also have the additional effect of different gravitational forces applied to their trunks, which influence the mechanics of breathing and other systems of the body. Workers in both environments share the physiological problems associated with increased ambient pressures and partial pressures of respired gases.

In this field, as in others, we cannot escape from the multiplicity of units and some of these are set out in Table 18.1. Note particularly that 'atmosphere gauge' is relative to ambient pressure. Thus 2 atmospheres absolute (ATA) equals 1 atmosphere gauge relative to sea level. Throughout this chapter atmospheres of pressure refer to absolute and not gauge.

EXCHANGE OF OXYGEN AND CARBON DIOXIDE[1]

Effect of pressure on alveolar $P\text{CO}_2$ and $P\text{O}_2$

Pressure has complicated and very important effects on $P\text{CO}_2$ and $P\text{O}_2$. The alveolar concentration of CO_2 equals its rate of production divided by the alveolar ventilation (page 157). However, both gas volumes must be measured under the same conditions of temperature and pressure. Alveolar CO_2 concentration at 10 ATA will be about one-tenth of sea-level values, i.e. 0.56% compared with 5.3% at sea level. When these concentrations are multiplied by pressure to give $P\text{CO}_2$, values are similar at sea level and 10 atmospheres. Thus, as a rough approximation, alveolar CO_2 concentration decreases inversely to the environmental pressure, but the $P\text{CO}_2$ remains near its sea-level value.

Effects on the $P\text{O}_2$ are slightly more complicated but no less important. The difference between the inspired and alveolar oxygen *concentrations* equals the ratio of oxygen uptake to inspired alveolar ventilation. This fraction, like the alveolar CO_2 concentration, decreases inversely with the increased pressure. However, the corresponding *partial pressure* will remain close to the sea level value, as does the alveolar $P\text{CO}_2$. Therefore the difference between the inspired and alveolar $P\text{O}_2$ will remain roughly constant and the alveolar $P\text{O}_2$, to a first approximation, increases by the same amount as the inspired $P\text{O}_2$ (Figure 18.1). However, these considerations only take into account the direct effect of pressure on gas tensions. There are other, more subtle, effects on respiratory mechanics and gas exchange which must now be considered.

Effect on mechanics of breathing[2]

Two main factors must be considered. First, there is the increased density of gases at pressure, although this can be reduced by changing the composition of the inspired gas. The second factor is the pressure of water on the body, which alters the gravitational effects to which the respiratory system is normally exposed.

Table 18.1 Pressures and P_{O_2} values at various depths of sea water

| Depth of sea water | | Pressure (absolute) | | P_{O_2} breathing air | | | | | Percentage oxygen to give sea level inspired P_{O_2} |
| | | | | inspired | | alveolar | | | |
metres	feet	atm.	kPa	kPa	mmHg	kPa	mmHg		
0	0	1	101	19.9	149	13.9	104		20.9
10	32.8	2	203	41.2	309	35.2	264		10.1
20	65.6	3	304	62.3	467	56.3	422		6.69
50	164	6	608	126	945	120	900		3.31
Usual limit for breathing air									
100	328	11	1 110						1.80
200	656	21	2 130						0.94
Usual limit for saturation dives									
Threshold for high-pressure nervous syndrome									
500	1640	51	5 170						0.39
1000	3280	101	10 200						0.20
Depth reached by sperm whale									
2000	6560	201	20 400						0.098
2500	8200	251	25 400						0.078
Pressure reached by non-aquatic mammals with pharmacological amelioration of high-pressure nervous syndrome									

Notes
10 metres sea water = 1 atmosphere (gauge). Alveolar P_{O_2} is assumed to be 6 kPa (45 mmHg) less than inspired P_{O_2}.

Gas density is increased in direct proportion to pressure. Thus air at 10 atmospheres has ten times the density of air at sea level, which increases the resistance to turbulent gas flow (page 40) and limits the maximal breathing capacity (MBC) that can be achieved. In fact, it is usual to breathe a helium/oxygen mixture at pressures in excess of about 6 atmospheres because of nitrogen narcosis (see below). Helium has only one-seventh the density of air and so is easier to breathe. Furthermore, lower inspired oxygen concentrations are both permissible and indeed desirable as the pressure increases (see Table 18.1). Therefore, at 15 atmospheres it would be reasonable to breathe a mixture of 98% helium and 2% oxygen. This would more than double the MBC that the diver could attain while breathing air at that pressure. Hydrogen has even lower density than helium and has been used in gas mixtures for dives to more than 500 metres deep.[3]

The effect of immersion is additional to any change in the density of the respired gases. In open-tube snorkel breathing, the alveolar gas is close to normal atmospheric pressure but the trunk is exposed to a pressure depending on the depth of the subject, which is limited by the length of the snorkel tube. This is equivalent to a standing subatmospheric pressure applied to the mouth and it is difficult to inhale against a 'negative' pressure loading of more than about 5 kPa (50 cmH$_2$O). This corresponds to a mean depth of immersion of only 50 cm and it is therefore virtually impossible to use a snorkel tube at a depth of 1 metre. However, the normal length of a snorkel tube assures that the swimmer is barely more than awash and so these problems should not arise.

'Negative' pressure loading is prevented by supplying gas to the diver's airway at a pressure that is close to the hydrostatic pressure surrounding the diver. This may be achieved by providing an excess flow of gas with a pressure-relief valve controlled by the surrounding water pressure. Such an arrangement was used for the traditional helmeted diver supplied by an air pump on the surface. Free-swimming divers carrying their own compressed gas supply rely on inspiratory demand valves, which are also balanced by the surrounding water pressure.

These arrangements supply gas that is close to the hydrostatic pressure surrounding the trunk. However, the precise 'static lung loading' depends on the location of the pressure-controlling device in relation to the geometry of the chest. Minor differences result from the various postures that the diver may assume. Thus, if he is 'head-up' when using a valve at mouthpiece level, the pressure surrounding the trunk is higher than the airway

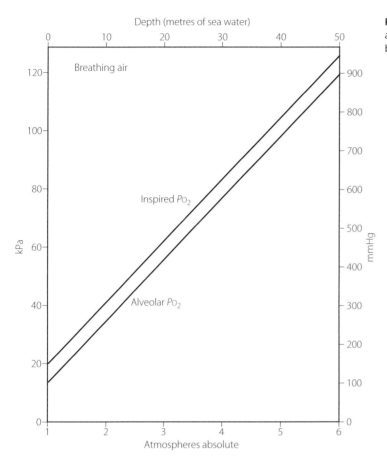

Figure 18.1 Inspired and alveolar Po_2 values as a function of increasing pressure while breathing air at rest.

pressure by a mean value of about 3 kPa (30 cmH$_2$O). If he is 'head-down', airway pressure is greater than the pressure to which the trunk is exposed. The head-down position thus corresponds to positive-pressure breathing and the head-up position to negative-pressure breathing. The latter causes a reduction of functional residual capacity (FRC) of about 20–30%, but breathing is considered to be easier head-up than head-down.[1]

Apart from these considerations, immersion has relatively little effect on respiratory function and the additional respiratory work of moving extracorporeal water does not seem to add appreciably to the work of breathing.

Effect on efficiency of gas exchange

Dead space/tidal volume ratio in divers increases with greater depth.[2,4] Changes are seen at relatively low pressures; for example, in one study dead space/tidal volume ratio increased from 37% at sea level to 42% at 2.8 ATA.[2] During exercise at this pressure, values decreased to around 20%.

The best measure of the efficiency of oxygenation of the arterial blood is the alveolar/arterial Po_2 gradient.

Measurement of arterial blood gas tensions presents formidable technical difficulties at high pressures. However, studies at 2.8, 47 and 66 ATA have reported only small increases in alveolar/arterial Po_2 gradient.[2,4] Since it is customary to supply deep divers with an inspired oxygen tension of at least 0.5 ATA, arterial hypoxaemia is unlikely to occur either from hypoventilation or from maldistribution of pulmonary ventilation and perfusion in healthy subjects.[4] More elderly, unfit or obese divers, faced with a reduced FRC as described above, do however display some degree of hypoxaemia during diving as FRC approaches their closing volume, causing airway closure and pulmonary shunting.[5]

The position as regards arterial Pco_2 is less clear. Hypercapnia is a well-recognised complication of diving and divers are known to have a blunted Pco_2/ventilation response, though the cause of this is unknown.[1] Hypercapnia in divers at rest is uncommon, but during exercise elevated end-tidal and arterial Pco_2 levels are described. Arterial Pco_2 levels during exercise at 2.8 ATA were around 5 kPa (37.4 mmHg),[2] but at pressures of 47 and 66 ATA were in the range 6.2–8.3 kPa (46.7–62.2 mmHg).[4] This is potentially hazardous because 9 kPa is approaching the level at which there may be some clouding of consciousness, and that is potentially dangerous at depth. High gas density at depth causing increased work of breathing is believed to be responsible for the inadequate ventilation during exercise.

Oxygen consumption

The relationship between power output and oxygen consumption at pressures up to 66 ATA, whether under water or dry, is not significantly different from the relationship at normal pressure[4] shown in Figure 15.1. Oxygen consumption is expressed under standard conditions of temperature and pressure, dry (STPD, see Appendix C) and therefore represents an absolute quantity of oxygen. However, this volume, when expressed at the diver's environmental pressure, is inversely related to the pressure. Thus, an oxygen consumption of $1\ l.min^{-1}$ (STPD) at a pressure of 10 atmospheres would be only $100\ ml.min^{-1}$ when expressed at the pressure to which the diver is exposed. Similar considerations apply to carbon dioxide output.

The ventilatory requirement for a given oxygen consumption at increased pressure is also not greatly different from the normal relationship shown in Figure 15.5, provided that the oxygen consumption is expressed at STPD and minute volume is expressed at body temperature, saturated with water vapour and at the pressure to which the diver is exposed (BTPS, see Appendix C). Considerable confusion is possible as a result of the different methods of expressing gas volumes and though the differences are trivial at sea level, they become very important at high pressures.

Exercise.[3] Oxygen consumption may reach very high values during free swimming (see Figure 15.1) and are of the order of $2\text{--}3\ l.min^{-1}$ (STPD) for a swimming speed of only $2\ km.h^{-1}$. Maximal oxygen consumption ($\dot{V}_{O_{2}max}$) during exercise is improved slightly at modest high pressures (<20 ATA), an observation that results from hyperoxia (0.3 ATA oxygen) normally used at this depth. With deeper dives, there is a progressive reduction in exercise capacity, irrespective of the oxygen pressure, as a result of respiratory limitation secondary to higher gas density.

EFFECTS ATTRIBUTABLE TO THE COMPOSITION OF THE INSPIRED GAS

Air

Oxygen. When breathing air at a pressure of 6 ATA, the inspired P_{O_2} will be about 126 kPa (945 mmHg) and the alveolar P_{O_2} about 120 kPa (900 mmHg). This is below the threshold for oxygen convulsions of about 2 ATA, but probably above the threshold for pulmonary oxygen toxicity if exposure is continued for more than a few hours[1] (see Chapter 26).

Nitrogen. It is actually nitrogen that limits the depth to which air may be breathed. It has three separate undesirable effects.

First, nitrogen is an anaesthetic and, in accordance with its lipid solubility, can cause full surgical anaesthesia at a partial pressure of about 30 ATA. The narcotic effect of nitrogen is first detectable when breathing air at about 4 ATA, and there is usually serious impairment of performance at 10 atmospheres.[6] This effect is known as nitrogen narcosis or 'the rapture of the deep'. It is a general rule that nitrogen narcosis precludes the use of air at depths greater than 100 metres of sea water (11 ATA pressure) and, in fact, air is not used today at pressures greater than 6 ATA. Helium is the preferred substitute at higher pressures and has no detectable narcotic properties up to at least 100 ATA.

The second problem attributable to nitrogen at high pressures is its density, which causes greatly increased hindrance to breathing at high pressure (see above). Helium has only one-seventh of the density of nitrogen and this is the second reason for its choice.

The third problem with nitrogen is its solubility in body tissues, with the resultant formation of bubbles on decompression. This is discussed in more detail below. Other inert gases, particularly helium, are less soluble in body tissues and this is the third reason for the use of helium at high pressures.

Helium/oxygen mixtures (Heliox)

For the three reasons outlined in the previous section, helium is the preferred diluent inert gas at pressures above about 6 ATA. The concentration of oxygen required to give the same inspired gas P_{O_2} as at sea level is shown in Table 18.1. In fact, it is usual practice to provide an inspired P_{O_2} of about 0.5 ATA (50 kPa or 375 mmHg) to give a safety margin in the event of error in gas mixing and to provide protection against hypoventilation or defective gas exchange. This level of P_{O_2} appears to be below the threshold for pulmonary oxygen toxicity, even during prolonged saturation dives.

With an inspired P_{O_2} of 0.5 ATA, the *concentration* of oxygen in the gas mixture is very low at high pressures (e.g. 2.5% oxygen at 20 atmospheres pressure). Clearly such a mixture would be lethal if breathed at sea level. Therefore, the inspired oxygen concentration must be very carefully monitored as it is changed during compression and decompression.

A special problem of helium is its very high thermal conductivity, which tends to cause hypothermia unless the diver's environment is heated. Heat loss from radiation and evaporation remains generally unchanged, but convective heat loss from the respiratory tract and skin is greatly increased.[3] It is usual for chambers to be maintained at temperatures as high as 30–32°C during saturation dives on helium/oxygen mixtures.

Helium/oxygen/nitrogen mixtures (Trimix)

The pressure that can be attained while breathing helium/oxygen mixtures is currently limited by the high-pressure nervous syndrome (HPNS).[3,7] This is a hyperexcitable state of the central nervous system which appears to be due to hydrostatic pressure *per se* and not to any changes in gas tensions. It becomes a serious problem for divers at pressures in excess of about 50 atmospheres, but is first apparent at about 20 atmospheres.

Various treatments can mitigate this effect and so increase the depth at which a diver can operate safely. The most practicable is the addition of 5–10% nitrogen to the helium/oxygen mixture. This in effect reverses HPNS with partial nitrogen narcosis, whereas the HPNS reverses the narcosis that would be caused by the nitrogen. Trimix containing 5% nitrogen allows divers to function normally at depths of over 600 metres.[3]

TYPES OF DIVING ACTIVITY AND THEIR RESPIRATORY EFFECTS

Snorkelling is the simplest form of human diving but, as described above, respiratory effects limit the diver to the top 50 cm of water. Many other forms of diving have therefore evolved.

Breath-hold diving[8,9]

The simplest method of diving is by breath holding and this is still used for collecting pearls, sponges and food from the sea bed. After breathing air, breath-holding time is normally limited to 60–75 seconds and the changes in alveolar gas tensions are shown in Figure 5.10. Astonishingly, the depth record is currently 150 metres, requiring 3.5 minutes of submersion. Many remarkable mechanisms interact to make this possible.

Lung volume. As pressure increases lung volume decreases by Boyle's law (page 456). Thus at 10 ATA, an initial lung volume of 6 litres would be reduced to about 600 ml, well below residual volume (RV) and with the loss of 5.4 kg of buoyancy. During descent a point is reached when the body attains neutral buoyancy and will sink below that depth.

Alveolar P_{O_2} increases with greater depth as the alveolar gas is compressed, providing a doubling of P_{O_2} at about

8 metres deep. More of the alveolar oxygen is therefore available at depth. Conversely, during ascent, alveolar P_{O_2} decreases, due partly to oxygen consumption but mainly to decreasing pressure. There is thus danger of hypoxia just before reaching the surface. However, when the alveolar P_{O_2} falls below the mixed venous P_{O_2}, there is a paradoxical transfer of oxygen from mixed venous blood to alveolar gas and the arterial P_{O_2} is maintained above the very low partial pressure that would otherwise occur in the alveoli. This may be an important factor in preventing loss of consciousness in the final stages of ascent.

Alveolar P_{CO_2}. By a similar mechanism, alveolar P_{CO_2} is greater during a breath-hold dive than during a simple breath hold at sea level. At an environmental pressure of only 12 kPa (90 mmHg) gauge, the alveolar P_{CO_2} will be increased above the mixed venous P_{CO_2} and there will be a paradoxical transfer of carbon dioxide from alveolus to arterial blood. Fortunately there is a limited quantity of carbon dioxide in the alveolar gas and the process is reversed during late descent and ascent. Duration of breath hold can be increased by previous hyperventilation, but this carries the danger of syncope from hypoxia before the breaking point is reached. Duration can be more safely increased by preliminary oxygen breathing, resulting in a record surface breath hold of 14 minutes.

Adaptations in the diving mammals.[10] The diving mammals rely on breath holding for dives and have adaptations that permit remarkably long times under water and the attainment of great depths. Sperm whales, for example, can attain depths of 1000 metres.[7] Weddell seals can reach 500 metres and remain submerged for 70 minutes.[11] Such feats depend on a variety of biochemical, cardiovascular and respiratory adaptations. It seems likely that the lungs of the Weddell seal collapse completely at depths between 25 and 50 metres, thus preventing the partial pressure of nitrogen increasing above the level of 320 kPa (2400 mmHg) which has been recorded at depths between 40 and 80 metres.

Many diving mammals are believed to use the spleen as a reservoir for oxygenated blood during dives. In some diving species, the spleen represents over 10% of body mass and contains a much more muscular capsule than in terrestrial animals. Splenic contraction is the probable cause of an increase of haemoglobin concentration from 15 to 25 g.dl^{-1} during long dives.[12] Furthermore, these animals have twice the blood volume per kilogram body weight relative to humans, so oxygen stored in blood for a dive is proportionately about three times that of humans.

Limited-duration dives

Most dives are of relatively brief duration and involve a rapid descent to operating depth, a period spent at depth, followed by an ascent, the rate of which is governed by the requirement to avoid release of inert gas dissolved in the tissues. The profile and the duration of the ascent are governed by the depth attained, the time spent at depth and the nature of the diluent inert gas.

The diving bell. The simplest and oldest technique was the diving bell. Air was trapped on the surface but the internal water level rose as the air was compressed at depth. Useful time at depth was generally no more than 20–30 minutes. Crude though this technology appears, it was used to recover most of the guns from the Wasa in Stockholm harbour in 1663 and 1664 from a depth of 34 metres. At a later date, additional air was introduced into the bell under pressure from the surface.

The helmeted diver. From about 1820 until recent times, the standard method of diving down to 100 metres has been by a helmeted diver supplied with air pumped from the surface into the helmet and escaping from a relief valve controlled by the water pressure. This gave much greater mobility than the old diving bell and permitted the execution of complex tasks.

SCUBA diving.[13] There was for some years a desire to move towards free-swimming divers carrying their own gas supply (SCUBA – self-contained underwater breathing apparatus), first achieved in 1943 by Jacques Cousteau and Emile Gagnon. The system is based on a demand valve that is controlled by both the ambient pressure and the inspiration of the diver. Air-breathing SCUBA dives are usually restricted to depths of 30 metres. Greater depths are possible but special precautions must then be taken to avoid decompression sickness. SCUBA divers are far more mobile than helmeted divers and can work in almost any body position.

Caisson and tunnel working. Since 1839, tunnel and bridge foundations have been constructed by pressurising the work environment to exclude water. The work environment is maintained at pressure, normally of less than 4 ATA, with staff entering and leaving by air locks. Entry is rapid but exit requires adherence to the appropriate decompression schedule if the working pressure is in excess of 2 ATA. Workers can be rapidly transferred from the working pressure to atmosphere and then, within 5 minutes, transferred to a separate chamber where they are rapidly recompressed to the working pressure and then follow the decompression schedule. This process, known as decanting, has obvious logistic advantages.

Free submarine escape. It is possible to escape from a submarine by free ascent from depths down to about 100 metres. The submariner first enters an escape chamber which is then pressurised to equal the external water pressure. He then opens a hatch communicating with the exterior and leaves the chamber. During the ascent, the gas in his lungs expands according to Boyle's law. It is therefore imperative that he keeps his glottis and mouth open, allowing gas to escape in a continuous stream. If gas is not allowed to escape, barotrauma is almost certain to occur (see below). In an uneventful escape, the time spent at pressure is too short for there to be any danger of decompression sickness. Thorough training is necessary and all submariners are trained in a vertical tank of 100 feet depth. The maintenance of an adequate atmosphere in submarines is described on page 277.

Saturation dives

When prolonged and repeated work is required at great depths, it is more convenient to hold the divers in a dry chamber, kept on board a ship or oil rig and held at a pressure close to the pressure of their intended working depth. Divers transfer to a smaller chamber at the same pressure, which is lowered to depth as and when required. The divers then leave the chamber for work, without any major change in pressure, but remaining linked to the chamber by an umbilical. On return to the chamber, they can be raised to the surface where they wait, still at pressure, until they are next required. A normal tour of duty is about 3 weeks, the whole of which is spent at operating pressure, currently up to about 20 atmospheres breathing helium/oxygen mixtures.

During the long period at pressure, tissues are fully saturated with inert gas at the chamber pressure and prolonged decompression is then required, which may last for several days.

RESPIRATORY ASPECTS OF DECOMPRESSION ILLNESS

Returning to the surface following a dive is a hazardous procedure and can give rise to a variety of complications variously known as 'bends', 'chokes' or caisson disease. In its mildest form, subjects have short-lived joint pain, but more serious presentations include pulmonary barotrauma or neurological deficit that can result in permanent disability. In the late 19th century, before decompression illness was understood, the effects on caisson workers were severe. For example, of the 600 men involved in building the underwater foundations of the St Louis Bridge in the USA, 119 had serious decompression illness and 14 died.[14] Nowadays some form of decompression illness is thought to affect 1 in 3500–10 000 recreational dives[15] and one in 500–1000 commercial dives.[14] Nomenclature of the many syndromes associated with decompression is confusing, but there are two main ways in which illness arises.

Barotrauma

Barotrauma as a result of change in pressure will affect any closed body space containing gas and tends to occur during ascent when the gas expands. The ears and sinuses are the most commonly affected areas, but pulmonary barotrauma, although rare, is much more dangerous. Pulmonary barotrauma may occur during rapid ascent in untrained subjects, for example during submarine escape training (see above) when the subject forgets to exhale during ascent.[16] Barotrauma results in disruption of the airway or alveolar wall and air may enter either the pulmonary vessels or the interstitial tissue, from where it spreads to the pleura, mediastinum or subcutaneous tissues. Mediastinal or pleural air pockets continue to expand during ascent, until chest pain or breathing difficulties occur within a few minutes of surfacing. Air entering the pulmonary vessels will produce arterial gas embolism and almost certainly result in decompression sickness.

Some divers develop barotrauma during relatively shallow dives[17] and efforts have been made to identify which divers are at risk.[18] In this case, barotrauma is believed to result from expansion of air trapped in the periphery of the lung by small airway closure. Subjects with reduced expiratory flow rates at low lung volume, including some asthmatics, are therefore at a theoretically greater risk.[18] There is currently only weak evidence that this is a practical problem in asthmatic patients taking part in recreational diving.[19]

Decompression sickness

Tissue bubble formation[1,14] occurs when tissues become 'supersaturated' with an inert gas, usually nitrogen. As decompression occurs, tissue PN_2 becomes greater than the ambient pressure and bubbles form, exactly as occurs when opening a carbonated drink. The increase in tissue PN_2 during descent and the decrease in PN_2 on ascent are both exponential curves. Tissues poorly perfused with blood have the slowest half-time for both uptake and elimination; hence on decompression, tissue PN_2 decreases most slowly in poorly perfused tissues such as cartilage, giving rise to the 'bends'.

Arterial gas embolism. Venous bubbles occur commonly during decompression and the filtration provided by the lung is extremely effective. Overload of the filtration system may result in arterial gas embolism, but this is only believed to be the case in severe decompression sickness. There is an increasing body of evidence that arterial gas embolism follows shunting of blood containing air bubbles from the right to left sides of the heart through an otherwise asymptomatic atrial septal defect (page 201).[15,20] Whatever the origins, arterial gas embolism is believed to be the major factor causing the neurological deficits of decompression sickness and may be contributing to long-term neurological damage in professional divers.[21]

Treatment of decompression sickness is best achieved by avoidance. Detailed and elaborate tables have been prepared to indicate the safe rate of decompression depending on the pressure and time of exposure. Administration of oxygen will reduce the blood PN_2 and so accelerate the resorption of bubbles in both blood and tissue. In severe cases, including all divers with neurological deficits, urgent recompression in a chamber is required, followed by slow decompression with oxygen and other therapeutic interventions.[22]

Altitude decompression sickness[23-25]

Flying at high altitude in military aircraft exposes the pilots to significant degrees of decompression, a cabin altitude of 9000 m (30 000 ft) being equivalent to approximately 0.3 ATA (see Chapter 16). During actual flights, symptoms of decompression sickness tend to be underreported because these elite pilots may fear restrictions on their flying activities. However, during their careers, three-quarters of pilots experience problems and almost 40% of trainee pilots develop symptoms during hypobaric chamber testing to normal cabin altitudes.[25] Joint pain is predictably the most common symptom, and the 'chokes' (substernal pain, cough and dyspnoea) occurs in 1–3% of cases. Breathing oxygen prior to altitude exposure is likely to significantly ameliorate the symptoms seen and is required by the US Air Force. Many pilots who have experienced decompression symptoms when flying are known to voluntarily increase their oxygen prebreathing time before subsequent flights.

Flying in the partially pressurised cabin (page 262) of commercial aircraft shortly after underwater diving increases the risk of decompression sickness. The likelihood of developing symptoms is increased by both greater depth of the last dive and shorter duration of time between the dive and flying. Dives to less than 18.5 m deep and leaving over 24 hours between diving and flying are generally accepted as resulting in a minimal, but not zero, risk of decompression sickness.[26,27]

REFERENCES

1. Lundgren CEG, Harabin A, Bennett PB, Van Liew HD, Thalmann ED. Gas physiology in diving. In: Fregly MJ, Blatteis CM, eds. *Handbook of physiology – section 4: Environmental physiology.* New York: Oxford University Press, 1996.

2. Mummery HJ, Stolp BW, Dear GdeL, *et al.* Effects of age and exercise on physiological dead space during simulated dives at 2.8 ATA. *J Appl Physiol* 2003; **94**: 507–17.

3. Hong SK, Bennett PB, Shiraki K, Lin Y-C, Claybaugh JR. Mixed gas saturation diving. In: Fregly MJ, Blatteis CM, eds. *Handbook of physiology – section 4: Environmental physiology.* New York: Oxford University Press, 1996.

4. Salzano JV, Camporesi EM, Stolp BW, Moon RE. Physiological responses to exercise at 47 and 66 ATA. *J Appl Physiol* 1984; **57**: 1055–68.

5. Prefaut C, Ramonatxo M, Boyer R, Chardon G. Human gas exchange during water immersion. *Respir Physiol* 1978; **34**: 307–18.

6. Bennett PB. Inert gas narcosis. In: Bennett PB, Elliott DH, eds. *The physiology and medicine of diving.* London: Baillière Tindall, 1982.

7. Halsey MJ. The effects of high pressure on the central nervous system. *Physiol Rev* 1982; **62**: 1341–77.

8. Lin Y-C, Hong SK. Hyperbaria: breath-hold diving. In: Fregly MJ, Blatteis CM, eds. *Handbook of physiology – section 4: Environmental physiology.* New York: Oxford University Press, 1996.

*9. Ferretti G. Extreme human breath-hold diving. *Eur J Appl Physiol* 2001; **84**: 254–71.

*10. Butler PJ, Jones DR. Physiology of diving of birds and mammals. *Physiol Rev* 1997; **77**: 837–95.

11. Zapol WM. Diving adaptations of the Weddell seal. *Sci Am* 1987; **256**: 80–5.

12. Qvist J, Hill RD, Schneider RC, *et al.* Hemoglobin concentrations and blood gas tensions of free-diving Weddell seals. *J Appl Physiol* 1986; **61**: 1560–9.

13. Lynch PR. Historical and basic perspectives of SCUBA diving. *Med Sci Sports Exerc* 1996; **28**: 570–2.

14. Moon RE, Vann RD, Bennett PB. The physiology of decompresion illness. *Sci Am* Aug 1995; **273**: 54–61.

*15. Foster PD, Boriek AM, Butler BD, Gernhardt ML, Bové AA. Patent foramen ovale and paradoxical systemic embolism: a bibliographic review. *Aviat Space Environ Med* 2003; **74**: B1–B40.

16. Broome CR, Jarvis LJ, Clark RJ. Pulmonary barotrauma in submarine escape training. *Thorax* 1994; **49**: 186–7.

17. Raymond LW. Pulmonary barotrauma and related events in divers. *Chest* 1995; **107**: 1648-52.

18. Bove AA. Pulmonary barotrauma in divers: can prospective pulmonary function testing identify those at risk? *Chest* 1997; **112**: 576–8.

19. Koehle M, Lloyd-Smith R, McKenzie D, Taunton J. Asthma and recreational SCUBA diving. *Sports Med* 2003; **33**: 109–16.

20. Knauth M, Ries S, Pohimann S, *et al.* Cohort study of multiple brain lesions in sport divers: role of a patent foramen ovale. *Br Med J* 1997; **314**; 701–5.

21. Wilmshurst P. Brain damage in divers. *Br Med J* 1997; **314**: 689–90.

22. Moon RE, Sheffield PJ. Guidelines for treatment of decompression illness. *Aviat Space Environ Med* 1997; **68**: 234–43.

23. Bendrick GA, Ainscough MJ, Pilmanis AA, Bisson RU. Prevalence of decompression sickness among U-2 pilots. *Aviat Space Environ Med* 1996; **67**: 199–206.

24. Ryles MT, Pilmanis AA. The initial signs and symptoms of altitude decompression sickness. *Aviat Space Environ Med* 1996; **67**: 983–9.

25. Balldin UI, Pilmanis AA, Webb JT. Pulmonary decompression sickness at altitude: early symptoms and circulating gas emboli. *Aviat Space Environ Med* 2002; **73**: 996–9.

26. Harding RM, Mills FJ. *Aviation medicine.* London: BMJ Publishing Group, 1993.

27. Freiberger JJ, Denoble PJ, Pieper CF, Uguccioni DM, Pollock NW, Vann RD. The relative risk of decompression sickness during and after air travel following diving. *Aviat Space Environ Med* 2002; **73**: 980–4.

19 Respiration in closed environments and space

KEY POINTS

- Environments in which a closed atmosphere suitable for breathing is maintained include closed-circuit anaesthesia, submarines and space vehicles.
- Problems of maintaining acceptably low carbon dioxide concentrations and low levels of inhaled contaminants are common to all these environments.
- In the microgravity of space static lung volumes are reduced, ventilation and perfusion are better matched and airway obstruction during sleep is uncommon.
- For atmospheric regeneration in long-term space missions of the future, a combination of physicochemical and biological systems is likely to be needed.

The fascination of the human race with exploration has taken man well beyond the high-altitude and underwater environments described in Chapters 17 and 18. Our ability to maintain life in space, the most hostile of environments yet explored, was developed as a result of techniques used to sustain breathing in other seemingly unrelated environments on Earth. All these environments share the problems common to maintaining respiration while separated from the Earth's atmosphere.

CLOSED-SYSTEM ANAESTHESIA

This may not represent the most dramatic example of closed-environment breathing but it is by far the most common. Careful control of the composition of respired gas is the hallmark of inhalational anaesthesia. The anaesthetist must maintain safe concentrations of oxygen and carbon dioxide in the patient's lungs, while controlling with great precision the dose of inhaled anaesthetic. It was recognised well over 100 years ago that anaesthesia could be prolonged by allowing the patient to rebreathe

some of their expired gas, including the anaesthetic vapour.[1] Provided oxygen is added and carbon dioxide removed, other gases can be circulated round a breathing system many times, providing beneficial effects such as warm and humid inspired gas. More recently, rebreathing systems have become popular as a method of reducing both the amount of anaesthetic used and the pollution of the operating theatre environment. Some anaesthetic agents, such as xenon, are so expensive to produce that their widespread use is a practical proposition only if closed systems are used.[2]

A totally closed system during anaesthesia means that all expired gases are recirculated to the patient, with oxygen added only to replace that consumed and anaesthetic agent added to replace that absorbed by the patient. In practice, low-flow anaesthesia, in which over half of the patient's expired gases are recirculated, is much more commonly used.[1] In each case, carbon dioxide is absorbed by chemical reaction with combinations of calcium, sodium, potassium or barium hydroxides, resulting in the formation of the respective carbonate and water. The reaction cannot be reversed and the absorbent must be discarded after use. Circuit volume is typically 5–8 litres.

Widespread use of closed-circuit anaesthesia is limited by perceived difficulties with maintaining adequate circuit concentrations of gases that the patient is consuming, such as oxygen and anaesthetic agent. Differences between fresh gas and circuit oxygen concentration become larger with lower fresh gas flow rate and, so, a greater proportion of gas rebreathing. The rate of change of circuit gas concentrations is affected by the same factors. However, gas-monitoring systems are now almost universally used with low-flow and closed-circuit anaesthesia, allowing accurate control of circuit gas composition.

Accumulation of other gases in closed circuits

Closed-circuit systems with a constant inflow and consumption of oxygen will allow the accumulation of other gases entering the circuit either with the fresh gas or from the patient. This affects the patient in two quite distinct ways. First, essentially inert gases such as nitrogen and argon may accumulate to such an extent that they dilute the oxygen in the system. Second, small concentrations of more toxic gases may arise within the breathing system.

Nitrogen enters the closed circuit from the patient at the start of anaesthesia. Body stores of dissolved nitrogen are small, but air present in the lungs may contain 2–3 litres of nitrogen, which will be transferred to the circuit in the first few minutes. If nitrogen is not intended to be part of the closed-circuit gas mixture, the patient must 'denitrogenate' by breathing high concentrations of oxygen before being anaesthetised or higher fresh gas flow rates must be used initially to flush the nitrogen from the closed circuit.

Argon is normally present in air at a concentration of 0.93%. Oxygen concentrators effectively remove nitrogen from air and so concentrate argon in similar proportions to oxygen, resulting in argon concentrations of around 5%. In a study of closed-circuit breathing in volunteers using oxygen from an oxygen concentrator, argon levels in the circuit reached 40% after only 80 minutes.[3] Cylinders of medical-grade oxygen and hospital supplies from liquid oxygen evaporators contain negligible argon, so the risk of significant accumulation is low. Even so, current recommendations to 'flush' the closed circuit at least every 2 hours seem prudent.

Methane is produced in the distal colon by anaerobic bacterial fermentation and is mostly excreted directly from the alimentary tract. Some methane is, however, absorbed into the blood, where it has low solubility so is rapidly excreted by the lung, following which it will accumulate in the closed circuit. There is a large variation between subjects in methane production and, therefore, the concentrations seen during closed-circuit anaesthesia. Mean levels in the circle system in healthy patients reached over 900 ppm, well below levels regarded as unacceptable in other closed environments (see below)[4] but sufficient to cause interference with standard anaesthetic gas analysers.[5]

Acetone, ethanol and carbon monoxide all have high blood solubility, so concentrations in the closed circuit gas remain low, but rebreathing causes accumulation in the blood. Levels achieved are generally low,[4,5] but acetone accumulation may be associated with postoperative nausea.[6] Closed-circuit anaesthesia is not recommended in patients with increased excretion of acetone or alcohol, such as in uncontrolled diabetes mellitus, recent alcohol ingestion, or during prolonged starvation.[1]

Inhaled anaesthetic derivatives. Currently used volatile anaesthetics are very stable compounds, mostly consisting of halogenated hydrocarbons, and metabolism in the body is low. Under certain circumstances these compounds can, however, produce toxic metabolites and closed-circuit systems make this much more likely. Carbon monoxide may be produced when desflurane, enflurane or isoflurane react with barium hydroxide used for CO_2 absorption, and significant levels have been reported.[7] The reaction seems to occur only under dry conditions; once the CO_2 absorber has been used for a short period, generating water vapour, carbon monoxide production becomes minimal.

Sevoflurane, a relatively new volatile anaesthetic agent, is degraded in closed-circuit anaesthesia to a derivative known as compound A, which has been associated with renal damage in animals.[1] Production of compound A is increased by higher temperatures in the CO_2 absorber and may be reduced by use of CO_2 absorbers that do not contain sodium or potassium hydroxides.[8] Levels of compound A achieved in low-flow anaesthesia are variable and sevoflurane is therefore not recommended for use in closed systems.

SUBMARINES

Submersible ships have been used for almost 100 years, almost exclusively for military purposes until the last few decades, when they have become more widespread for undersea exploration and industrial use. Atmospheric pressure in the submarine remains approximately the same as at surface level during a dive, the duration of which is limited by the maintenance of adequate oxygen and carbon dioxide levels for the crew in the ship.

Diesel powered

Submarines were used extensively during both world wars and were powered by diesel engines like surface-based warships. Clearly, the oxygen requirement of the engines precluded them from use during dives and battery-powered engines were used, thus limiting the duration of dives to just a few hours. A more significant limitation to dive duration was atmospheric regulation. No attempt was made to control the internal atmosphere and, after ventilation at the surface, the submarine dived with only the air contained within. After approximately 12 hours the atmosphere contained 15% oxygen, 5% carbon dioxide and a multitude of odours and contaminants. The need to return to the surface was apparent when the submariners became short of breath and were unable to light their cigarettes due to low levels of oxygen.[9]

Nuclear powered

Short dive duration severely limited the use of diesel-powered submarines. The development of nuclear power allowed submarines to generate an ample supply of heat and electricity completely independent of oxygen supply and so allowed prolonged activity underwater. Atmospheric regeneration was therefore needed. Current nuclear-powered submarines have a crew of up to 180 and routinely remain submerged for many weeks.

Atmosphere regeneration.[9,10] The plentiful supply of sea water and electricity makes hydrolysis of water the obvious method for oxygen generation. Sea water must first have all electrolytes removed by a combination of evaporation and deionisation. Physical, though not electrical, separation of the electrolysis electrodes allows the oxygen to be taken directly from the anode, so removing the necessity to separate it from the hydrogen produced at the cathode. Theoretically, 1 litre of water can yield 620 litres of oxygen so, even with less than 100% efficient electrolysis, large volumes of oxygen are easily produced. Submarine atmosphere oxygen concentration is maintained at 21±2%.

Atmospheric CO_2 in submarines is absorbed by passage through monoethanolamine, which chemically combines with CO_2 to produce carbonates. When fully saturated, the absorber can either be replaced or be regenerated by heating with steam, when the CO_2 is released and can be vented into the sea. This method maintains the CO_2 concentration in submarines at 0.5–1.5%, and although further reduction is possible, the energy cost of doing so is prohibitive.

Atmospheric contamination during prolonged submarine patrols is well recognised, many hundreds of substances entering the atmosphere, originating from both machinery and crew. These substances include volatile hydrocarbons such as benzene, oil droplets, carbon monoxide, cadmium and microbial organisms, with varying concentrations in different parts of the submarine. Continuous monitoring of many compounds is now routine and maximum allowable levels during prolonged patrols are defined.[4,11,12] Submarine air-conditioning units include catalytic burners that oxidise carbon monoxide, hydrogen and other hydrocarbons to CO_2 and water, and charcoal absorbers to absorb any remaining contaminants. The health risks from submarine occupation are therefore believed to be extremely small.[9,11,13] To maintain crew morale, smoking continues to be permitted in most nuclear submarines and passive smoking (page 291) is therefore inevitable. Carbon monoxide levels of 9 ppm have been reported, which is close to the recommended maximum level of 10 ppm for prolonged atmospheric exposure (see Table 21.1) or 15 ppm for submarine personnel exposure.[12]

Physiological effects of prolonged hypercapnia[14]

Definition of a 'safe' level of atmospheric CO_2 over long periods has concerned submariners for some years. The respiratory response to inhalation of low concentrations of CO_2 (<3%) is similar to that at higher levels (page 62), but compensatory acid–base changes seem to be quite different.

Respiratory changes.[15,16] Atmospheric CO_2 levels of 1% cause an elevation of inspired PCO_2 of 1 kPa (7.5 mmHg), which results in an average increase in minute ventilation of 2–3 l.min^{-1}.[15,16] However, the degree of hyperventilation is highly variable between subjects and presumably relates to their central chemoreceptor sensitivity to CO_2 (page 62). Measurements of arterial blood gases in submariners show that the elevated minute volume limits the increase in arterial PCO_2 to an average of only 0.14 kPa (1 mmHg). After a few days, the increase in ventilation declines and minute volume returns towards normal, allowing arterial PCO_2 to increase further to reflect the inspired PCO_2. The time course of the decline in ventilation is too short to result from blood acid–base compensation (see below) and is believed to reflect a small attenuation of the central chemoreceptor response. On return to the surface, ventilation may be temporarily reduced following withdrawal of the CO_2 stimulus.

Calcium metabolism.[14,15,17] Elevation of arterial PCO_2 causes a respiratory acidosis, which is normally, over the course of 1 or 2 days, compensated for by the retention of bicarbonate by the kidney (page 331). The changes in pH seen when breathing less than 3% CO_2 appear to be too small to stimulate measurable renal compensation and pH remains slightly lowered for some time. During this period, CO_2 is deposited in bone as calcium carbonate, and urinary and faecal calcium excretion is drastically reduced to facilitate this. Serum calcium levels also decrease, suggesting a shift of extracellular calcium to the intracellular space.[17] After about 3 weeks, when bone stores of CO_2 are saturated, renal excretion of calcium and hydrogen ions begins to increase and pH tends to return to normal. Abnormalities of calcium metabolism have been demonstrated with inspired CO_2 concentrations as low as 0.5%.

Some other effects of low levels of atmospheric CO_2 during space travel are described below (page 279).

SPACE[10,18-20]

Space represents the most hostile environment in which man has sojourned. At 80 km (50 miles) above the Earth there is insufficient air to allow aerodynamic control of a vehicle and at 200 km (125 miles) there is an almost total vacuum. True space begins above 700 km (435 miles), where particles become so scarce that the likelihood of a collision between two atoms becomes negligible. Even under these conditions, there are estimated to be 10^8 particles (mainly hydrogen) per cubic metre compared with 10^{25} on the Earth's surface. Maintenance of a respirable atmosphere in these circumstances is challenging and both American and Soviet space pioneers lost their lives during the development of suitable technology. Current experience is based on relatively short periods in close proximity to the Earth, usually involving Earth orbit or travel to the moon. This means that the raw materials for atmosphere regeneration can be repeatedly supplied from Earth.

Atmosphere composition

A summary of manned space missions and the atmospheres used is shown in Table 19.1. Spacecraft have an almost totally sealed, closed-circuit system of atmospheric control and early Soviet space vehicles aimed to be completely sealed environments. Their designers had such confidence in the structure that emergency stores of oxygen were considered unnecessary until Soyuz 11 depressurised on reentry in 1971, tragically killing all three cosmonauts. American Apollo missions leaked approximately 1 kg of gas per day in space, even with a lower atmospheric pressure (see Table 19.1).

The use of a total pressure of 34.5 kPa (259 mmHg) in early US space vehicles required a high atmospheric

oxygen concentration to provide an adequate inspired PO_2 (see Table 19.1). Because of the fatal fire on the launch pad in 1967, the composition of the atmosphere during launch was changed from 100% oxygen to 64% oxygen in 36% nitrogen at the same pressure, which still gave an inspired PO_2 in excess of the normal sea-level value. Previous Soviet designs were all based on maintaining normal atmospheric pressure and space vehicles in current use continue to do so with inspired oxygen concentrations of near 21%. Extravehicular activity in space presents a particular problem. In order to maintain a functionally acceptable flexibility of the space suit in the vacuum of space, the internal pressure is only 28 kPa (212 mmHg). This entails the use of 100% oxygen after careful decompression and denitrogenation of the astronaut.

Oxygen supply

Storage of oxygen and other gases in space presents significant problems. The weight of the containers used is critical during launch, and storage of significant quantities of oxygen requires high pressures and therefore strong, heavy tanks. Liquid oxygen presents a greatly improved storage density, but the behaviour of stored liquids in weightless conditions is complex.

Chemical generation of oxygen has been used mainly by Soviet space missions. Potassium superoxide releases oxygen on exposure to moisture, a reaction that generates potassium hydroxide as an intermediate and so also absorbs carbon dioxide:

Table 19.1 Summary of manned space missions and their respiratory environments

Missions	Period of use	Number of crew	Habitable volume (m^3)	Cabin pressure kPa	Cabin pressure mmHg	Oxygen conc. (%)	Atmosphere regeneration methods O_2 supply	Atmosphere regeneration methods CO_2 removal
Vostok	1961–65	1	2.5	100	760	100	KO_2	KO_2
Mercury	1961–63	1	1.6	34	258	100	Pressurised O_2	LiOH
Gemini	1965–66	2	2.3	34	258	100	Liquid O_2	LiOH
Soyuz	1967–	2–3	–	100	760	22	KO_2	KO_2/LiOH
Apollo	1968–72	3	5.9	34	258	100*	Liquid O_2	LiOH
Salyut	1971–86	5	100	100	760	21	KO_2	KO_2/LiOH
Skylab	1973–74	3	361	34	258	72	Liquid O_2	Molecular sieve
Shuttle	1981–	7	74	100	760	21	Liquid O_2	LiOH
Mir	1986–01	6	150	100	760	23	Electrolysis/chemical	Molecular sieve
ISS	2001–	Variable	401/1217[†]	100	760	21	Electrolysis/chemical	Molecular sieve

* Oxygen concentration reduced to 60% during launch to reduce fire risk. [†], current/projected habitable volumes. All missions, except early Soyuz launches, carry emergency oxygen supplies as pressurised or liquid oxygen. (Data from references 10, 18 and 19.)

$$4KO_2 + 3H_2O + 2CO_2 \rightarrow 2K_2CO_3 + 3H_2O + 3O_2$$

One kilogram of KO_2 can release over 200 litres of oxygen, but the reaction is irreversible and the used canisters must be discarded. Sodium chlorate candles release oxygen when simply ignited and were used for emergency oxygen generation on older submarines and in most Soviet space missions.

Electrolysis of water, as used in submarines, is an efficient way to produce oxygen in space where solar panels provide the electricity supply. In contrast to submarines, water is scarce in space vehicles, again because of weight considerations at launch. In the International Space Station oxygen is generated by electrolysis using waste water from the occupants, though this alone does not produce sufficient oxygen for a reasonably active astronaut.

Carbon dioxide removal

Chemical absorption by lithium hydroxide has been the mainstay of the US space programme, whereas the Soviet programme used KO_2 as described above. Reversible chemical reactions such as those used in submarines have been adapted for space use and can be regenerated by exposure to the vacuum of space. These techniques are very effective, with atmospheric CO_2 concentration being maintained at less than 0.2% on Shuttle missions,[21] significantly lower than that accepted in submarines.

Molecular sieves allow CO_2 to be adsorbed into a chemical matrix without undergoing any chemical reaction. When saturated with CO_2, exposure to the space vacuum causes release of the adsorbed gas. Use of two- or four-bed molecular sieves allows continuous CO_2 removal by half the processors while the others are regenerated.

Maintenance of CO_2 levels below 0.2% on prolonged future space missions is likely to have unacceptable costs in terms of energy and consumables.[22] This fact led to three space agencies worldwide undertaking a joint research programme to study the effects of 1.2% and 0.7% atmospheric CO_2 on a wide range of physiological systems. The study involved normal volunteers spending 22 days in a closed mock 'space station' on the ground.[22] Some of the results have already been described above (page 277).[16,17] Effects at 0.7% atmospheric CO_2 were generally concluded to be minimal.[23] At 1.2%, however, changes in respiration and calcium metabolism were significant and, more importantly, mental performance was impaired, with a loss of alertness and visuomotor performance.[24]

Atmospheric contamination

Chemical contamination within space vehicles is mainly from within the habitable area of the vehicle, with external contamination from propellants etc. being very rare.[18] The greatest contribution to atmospheric contamination is the astronauts themselves, but the compounds released, such as carbon monoxide, ammonia, methane and indole, are easily dealt with by standard methods. More complex chemicals may be released into the atmosphere by a process called off-gassing. Almost any non-metallic substance, but particularly plastic, releases small quantities of volatile chemicals for many months and years after manufacture. This is more likely to occur at low atmospheric pressure, as on the earlier space missions. In a closed environment these chemicals may accumulate to toxic levels and air-conditioning units similar to those described for submarines (page 277) are required.

Long-term space travel

Manned space travel to planets more distant than the Moon requires expeditions of years' duration with no access to supplies from Earth. For example, the journey time to Mars is around 6 months, so the minimum realistic mission duration would be 2 years. The estimated mass of provisions required to sustain six crew members for this duration would be over 45 tons, which far exceeds the capacity of current interplanetary space vehicles.[25] Regenerative life support systems have, therefore, been studied extensively in recent years and aim to reverse the effects of animal metabolism on a closed atmosphere. Biological solutions are believed by many to be the only feasible option, and biospheres are discussed below. Physicochemical methods are, however, now realistic options and are likely to act as valuable back-up systems in the future.

CO_2 reduction reactions convert carbon dioxide back into oxygen and two main methods are described.[26] The Sabatier reaction requires hydrogen to produce methane and water:

$$CO_2 + 4H_2 \rightarrow CH_4 + 2H_2O$$

Methane can then be converted to solid carbon and hydrogen gas, which reenters the Sabatier reactor. The Bosch reaction produces solid carbon in one stage:

$$CO_2 + 2H_2 \rightarrow 2H_2O + solid\ C$$

Electrolysis of water generates oxygen and hydrogen gas and the latter enters the Bosch or Sabatier reactions and the water produced is recycled. Both reactions ultimately generate solid carbon, which must be removed from the reactors periodically. Use of catalysts has

Mars atmosphere
95.3% CO_2; 2.7% N_2; 1.6% Ar;
0.13% O_2; 0.07% CO

Figure 19.1 *In situ* resource utilisation on Mars. Using a series of simple physicochemical processes, the atmosphere of Mars, supplemented by hydrogen transported from Earth, may be used to provide buffer gas and oxygen for the space vehicle atmosphere, methane as propellant for the vehicle and water for use by the crew or for generation of oxygen. (After reference 27.)

allowed the development of small, efficient reactors based on a combination of the two chemical processes. Current hardware can convert CO_2 into oxygen for 60 person-days before the carbon deposits must be emptied.[26]

***In situ resource utilisation on Mars.*[27]** The atmosphere of Mars is composed of 95.3% CO_2, 2.7% N_2, 1.6% Ar, 0.13% O_2 and 0.07% CO. For any mission to Mars, these gases could be used for atmospheric regeneration as shown in Figure 19.1. Separation of the gases in the atmosphere will produce a small amount of oxygen and larger volumes of nitrogen and argon, which may be used as buffer gas in the atmosphere. On prolonged missions, loss of buffer gas from the vehicle by leakage and from activation of airlocks is a substantial problem. The abundant CO_2 on Mars could enter a Sabatier reactor and the methane produced might then be used as a propellant for the mission, the water used either by the crew or to provide oxygen for the life support systems, and the hydrogen could reenter the Sabatier reactor.

MICROGRAVITY[28,29]

All bodies with mass exert gravitational forces on each other, so zero gravity is theoretically impossible. Once in space, away from the large mass of Earth or other planets, gravitational forces become negligible and are referred to as microgravity. Space vehicles in orbit around the Earth are still subject to its considerable gravitational forces, but these are matched almost exactly by the centrifugal force from the high tangential velocity of the space vehicle.[19] Occupants of orbiting space vehicles are normally subject to a gravitational force of approximately 10^{-6} times that on Earth's surface.

Chapter 8 contains numerous references to the effect of gravity on the topography of the lung and the distribution of perfusion and ventilation. Microgravity may therefore be predicted to have significant effects on respiratory function.[30]

The first studies of short-term microgravity used a Lear jet flying in a series of Keplerian arcs, which gave 20–25 seconds of weightlessness. Unfortunately, between each period of microgravity the subject is exposed to a similar duration of increased gravitational forces (2 G) as the jet pulls out of the free-fall portion of the flight,[31] and this may influence the results of physiological studies. Sustained microgravity has been studied in space. In 1991 an extended series of investigations on seven subjects was undertaken in Spacelab SLS-1, which was carried into orbit by the space shuttle for a 9-day mission.

Lung volumes. Chest radiography in the sitting position during short-term microgravity showed no striking changes other than a tendency for the diaphragm to be slightly higher in some of the subjects at functional residual capacity (FRC).[32] This accords with a 413 ml reduction in FRC also measured in Keplerian arc studies on seated subjects.[31] Abdominal contribution to tidal excursion was increased at microgravity in the seated position, probably because of loss of postural tone in the abdominal muscles,[31] an observation recently confirmed in space studies.[33]

During sustained microgravity, subdivisions of lung volume were again found to be intermediate between the sitting and supine volumes at 1 G, except for residual volume, which was reduced below that seen in any position at 1 G (Figure 19.2).[21] The FRC was reduced by 750 ml compared with preflight standing values. These changes in lung volume are ascribed to altered respiratory mechanics and increased thoracic blood volume.

***Topographical inequality of ventilation and perfusion.*[28,29]** Early results in the Lear jet, using single-breath nitrogen washout (page 113), indicated a substantial reduction in topographical inequality of ventilation and perfusion during weightlessness, as expected.[34] However, the more detailed studies in Spacelab showed that a surprising degree of residual inequality of blood flow[35] and ventilation[36] persisted despite the major improvement at micro-gravity. Ventilatory inequality is believed to result

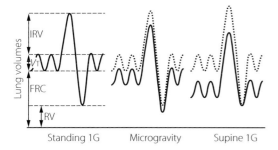

Figure 19.2 Static lung volumes during sustained microgravity after 9 days in Earth orbit. Dotted line shows the normal standing values on Earth for comparison. Volumes at microgravity are generally intermediate between standing and supine values at 1G, except residual volume, which is further reduced. FRC, functional residual capacity; IRV, inspiratory reserve volume; RV, residual volume; V_T, tidal volume.

from continued airway closure at low lung volume[24,36] and possibly from altered gas mixing in peripheral lung units.[29] Similarly, the cause of the continued small degree of perfusion inequality remains uncertain.[35] The most likely explanation is the presence of a central to peripheral 'radial' gradient within each horizontal slice of lung (page 115), which is completely overshadowed at 1 G by the large vertical perfusion gradient.[24] Early results from long-term missions in the Mir space station indicate that the changes in ventilation and perfusion may be associated with reduced arterial P_{O_2}.[28]

Diffusing capacity. SLS-1 studies have shown progressive increases in carbon monoxide diffusing capacity, the membrane component and the pulmonary capillary blood volume (page 142) all reaching 33% more than control by the ninth day in orbit.[37]

Breathing during sleep in space.[38] Snoring and airway obstruction during sleep on Earth are common and many factors are involved in their initiation (page 248). Reduced activity of pharyngeal dilator muscles and increased compliance of pharyngeal structures both encourage the normal gravitational force on Earth to initiate obstruction. This important contribution of gravity to sleep-disordered breathing has recently been confirmed by studies of astronauts sleeping in the orbiting space shuttle.[39] Compared with sleeping at 1 G before the mission, in microgravity there were dramatic reductions in their apnoea–hypopnoea index (page 248) and snoring was virtually eliminated.

BIOSPHERES[19]

A biosphere is defined as 'a closed space of two or more connected ecosystems in equilibrium with their environment'.[40] Only energy enters and leaves the biosphere.

Earth is the largest and most successful known biosphere, though the equilibrium between its ecosystems is almost certainly changing (see Chapter 1). Attempts to create smaller biospheres have mostly been driven by the prospect of long-term space travel.[41] Physicochemical methods of sustaining life, as described above, have many limitations, whereas a biological system has numerous advantages. Plants perform the complex CO_2-reduction chemistry using chlorophyll and at the same time, rather than generating carbon, they produce varying amounts of food.[42] Plants also act as efficient water purification systems via transpiration. It has been estimated that plants transpire 300 grams of water vapour for each gram of carbon dioxide used.[19]

Small-scale biological atmospheric regeneration

The first report of prolonged biological atmosphere regeneration was described in 1961 when a single mouse was maintained in a closed chamber for 66 days.[43] Air from the chamber was circulated through a second chamber containing 4 litres of *Chlorella* alga solution illuminated with artificial light. Over the course of the experiment, oxygen concentration in the chamber increased from 21% to 53% and carbon dioxide concentrations remained below 0.2%. Subsequent experiments by both American and Soviet researchers demonstrated the feasibility of human life support by *Chlorella*, culminating in a 30-day closure of a single researcher in a 4.5 m³ room, maintained by just 30 litres of alga solution. Algae alone are unsuitable for long-term life support.[19] Their excellent atmospheric regeneration properties result from a very fast rate of growth, but *Chlorella* is generally regarded as inedible and so presents a significant disposal problem in a totally closed system. In addition, if the algal solution becomes acidic for any reason, such as bacterial contamination, algae produce carbon monoxide in unacceptable quantities.

Unknown to the scientific community at large, from 1963 the Soviet Union ran a 'Bios' research centre at the Institute of Biophysics in Krasnoyarsk, Siberia.[19,44] A whole series of progressively more complex biospheres was constructed, but details of this work remain scarce. In 1983, two researchers successfully spent 5 months in a biosphere (Bios 3), which provided all their atmospheric regeneration needs and over three-quarters of their food.[44] In these studies, plants were grown hydroponically, that is, without soil with their roots bathed in carefully controlled nutrient solution. Light was provided with continuous xenon lighting to maximise growth, to such an extent that, under these conditions, wheat can be harvested six times per year. An estimated 13 m² of planted area will then produce enough oxygen for one human, though over 30 m² is probably required to produce almost enough food as well. Beds of *Chlorella* algae were also used to maximise oxygen production and, along with larger planted areas, resulted in excess oxygen. This was reduced by incineration of the non-edible portion of the plants and so enabled the researchers to exercise some control over the balance between oxygen and carbon dioxide concentration within the biosphere. In this way, levels of CO_2 in Bios 3 were maintained between 0.03% and 0.14%.[19]

American research into controlled ecological life support systems (CELSS) began in 1977 and has focused on basic plant physiology.[19] Plant species, light, humidity, nutrients and atmospheric gas concentrations all have profound effects on the design of a CELSS. Atmospheric regeneration is usually the easiest problem to overcome, and the plant species used has important implications for the dietary intake and psychological well-being of the CELSS inhabitants.[42,44]

Biosphere 2[19]

Small-scale biosphere experiments never attained a totally closed system, particularly with respect to food supplies and waste disposal. In addition, biodiversity in these systems was low, with very few species of plant, animal, insect or microbes contained within. Finally, build-up of toxic atmospheric compounds was significant, with the requirement for extensive physicochemical methods of removal similar to those used in the closed systems of submarines and space. With these problems in mind, an ambitious series of biosphere experiments was established in Arizona, USA, culminating in the Biosphere 2 project in 1991.

A totally sealed complex, covering 3.15 acres (1.3 hectares) and containing 204 000 m^3 (7.2 million ft^3) of atmosphere, was purpose built with a stainless steel underground lining and principally glass cover. Two flexible walls, or 'lungs', were included to minimise pressure changes within the complex with expansion and contraction of the atmosphere. A 2-year closure was planned, with the complex containing a wide range of flora and fauna, including eight humans, other mammals, fish and insects. The biosphere was divided into seven smaller ecosystems: rainforest, savannah, desert, ocean, saltmarsh, intensive agriculture area and a human/animal habitat. Soil was chosen as the growing medium for all plants in preference to hydroponic techniques used previously. This was to facilitate air purification by soil bed reactors, in which atmospheric air is pumped through the soil where bacterial action provides an adaptable and efficient purification system.[19] A CO_2 'scrubber' system was included in Biosphere 2 to control atmospheric CO_2 levels, particularly during winter when shorter days reduce photosynthetic activity. Also, the amount of O_2-consuming biomass relative to atmosphere volume was

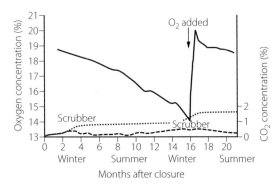

Figure 19.3 Changes in atmospheric concentrations of oxygen (solid line) and carbon dioxide (dashed line) during the 2-year closure of Biosphere 2. Less daylight during winter months reduces photosynthesis, causing increased levels of CO_2. Carbon dioxide was therefore removed using a CO_2 'scrubber' system, during the periods shown. Even when CO_2 absorption by the scrubbers is taken into account (dotted line), it can clearly be seen that the reduction in O_2 concentration exceeds the increase in CO_2 concentration; after 16 months, O_2 had to be added to the biosphere. See text for details. (Data from references 19 and 43.)

known to be high and therefore small increases in CO_2 levels were anticipated.

Biosphere 2 aimed, wherever possible, to use ecological engineering. By the inclusion of large numbers of species (3800 in total), it was hoped that there would be sufficient flexibility between systems to respond to changes in the environment. In particular, microbial diversity is believed to be extremely important in maintaining biosphere 1 (Earth) and the multiple habitats were established to facilitate this type of diversity in Biosphere 2.

Outcome from the 2-year closure. Concentrations of oxygen and carbon dioxide in Biosphere 2 were very unstable (Figure 19.3) and after 16 months, oxygen concentration had fallen to only 14%. Extensive symptoms were reported by the human inhabitants,[36] including significantly reduced work capacity, which was crucial for controlling plant growth. External oxygen therefore had to be added to the atmosphere. Carbon dioxide levels did increase slightly during winter months (see Figure 19.3) when the CO_2 was removed by the scrubber system.

It was never expected that all species introduced into Biosphere 2 would survive, and extinction of some species was seen as a natural response to stabilisation of the ecosystem. However, after 21 months, extinct species were numerous, including 19 of 25 vertebrates and most insects, including all pollinators.[46] In contrast, ants and cockroaches thrived.

The success of Biosphere 2 as a closed ecosystem was therefore limited and, in contrast to the smaller biospheres previously used, basic atmospheric regeneration was a significant problem. Any increase in CO_2 concentration should be matched by an equivalent decrease in O_2 concentration, as biological reactions between CO_2 and O_2 are generally equimolar. Even when the CO_2 removed by the recycling system is taken into account, it can clearly be seen from Figure 19.3 that oxygen losses were much greater. The explanation for this is believed to be twofold.[45] First, oxygen depletion occurred due to respiration in the biosphere proceeding faster than photosynthesis, most likely as a result of microbial activity in the soil. Second, much of the CO_2 produced by this respiration was lost from the atmosphere by chemical reaction with the concrete from which the biosphere complex was built.

Further large-scale biosphere projects are proposed,[47] but we remain some way away from being able to establish a long-term habitable atmosphere away from Earth.

REFERENCES

*1. Baum JA, Aitkenhead AR. Low-flow anaesthesia. *Anaesthesia* 1995; **50** (Supp): 37–44.
2. Nunn JF, Halsey MJ. Xenon in anaesthesia. *Lancet* 1990; **336**: 112–13.
3. Parker CJR, Snowdon SL. Predicted and measured oxygen concentrations in the circle system using low fresh gas flows with oxygen supplied by an oxygen concentrator. *Br J Anaesth* 1988; **61**: 397–402.
4. Baumgarten RK, Reynolds WJ. Much ado about nothing: trace gaseous metabolites in the closed circuit. *Anesth Analg* 1985; **64**: 1029–38.
5. Versichelen L, Rolly G, Vermeulen H. Accumulation of foreign gases during closed-system anaesthesia. *Br J Anaesth* 1996; **76**: 668–72.
6. Strauß JM, Hausdörfer J. Accumulation of acetone in blood during long-term anaesthesia with closed systems. *Br J Anaesth* 1993; **70**: 363–4.
7. Kharasch ED. Keep the blood red . . . the right way. *Anesthesiology* 1997; **87**: 202–3.
8 Filippo AD, Marini F, Pacenti M, Dugheri S, Focardi, Novelli GP. Sevoflurane low-flow anaesthesia: best strategy to reduce Compound A concentration. *Acta Anaesthesiol Scand* 2002; **46**: 1017–20.
9. Knight DR, Tappan DV, Bowman JS, O'Neill HJ, Gordon SM. Submarine atmospheres. *Toxicol Lett* 1989; **49**: 243–51.
10. Wieland PO. *Designing for human presence in space: an introduction to environmental control and life support systems.* NASA Reference Publication 1324. Houston, TX: National Aeronautics and Space Administration, 1994.
11. Dean MR. Benzene exposure in Royal Naval submarines. *J Roy Soc Med* 1996; **89**: 286P–288P.
12. Seufert KT, Kiser WR. End-expiratory carbon monoxide levels as an estimate of passive smoking exposure aboard a nuclear-powered submarine. *South Med J* 1996; **89**: 1181–3.
13. Lambert RJW. Environmental problems in nuclear submarines. *Proc Roy Soc Med* 1972; **65**: 795–6.
14. Schaefer KE. Effects of increased ambient CO_2 levels on human and animal health. *Experientia* 1982; **38**: 1163–8.
15. Pingree BJW. Acid–base and respiratory changes after prolonged exposure to 1% carbon dioxide. *Clin Sci Mol Med* 1977; **52**: 67–74.
16. Elliott AR, Prisk GK, Schöllmann C, Hoffmann U. Hypercapnic ventilatory response in humans before, during and after 23 days of low level CO_2 exposure. *Aviat Space Environ Med* 1998; **69**: 391–6.
*17. Drummer C, Friedel V, Börger A, *et al*. Effects of elevated carbon dioxide environment on calcium metabolism in humans. *Aviat Space Environ Med* 1998; **69**: 291–8.
*18. Nicogossian AE, Huntoon CL, Pool SL. *Space physiology and medicine*, 3rd edn. Philadelphia: Lea & Febiger, 1994.
19. Churchill SE. *Fundamentals of space life sciences.* Malabar, FL: Krieger Publishing, 1997.
*20. West JB. Historical aspects of the early Soviet/Russian manned space program. *J Appl Physiol* 2001; **91**: 1501–11.
21. Elliott AR, Prisk GK, Guy HJB, West JB. Lung volumes during sustained microgravity on Spacelab SLS-1. *J Appl Physiol* 1994; **77**: 2005–14.
22. Wenzel J, Luks N, Plath G, Wilke D, Gerzer R. The influence of CO_2 in a space-like environment: study design. *Aviat Space Environ Med* 1998; **69**: 285–90.
23. Frey MAB, Sulzman FM, Oser H, Ruyters G. The effects of moderately elevated ambient carbon dioxide levels on human physiology and performance: a joint NASA-ESA-DARA study – overview. *Aviat Space Environ Med* 1998; **69**: 282–4.
24. Manzey D, Lorenz B. Effects of chronically elevated CO_2 on mental performance during 26 days of confinement. *Aviat Space Environ Med* 1998; **69**: 506–14.
25. Grigoriev AI, Kozlovskaya IB, Potapov AN. Goals of biomedical support of a mission to Mars and possible approaches to achieving them. *Aviat Space Environ Med* 2002; **73**: 379–84.
26. Noyes GP. Carbon dioxide reduction processes for spacecraft ECLSS: a comprehensive review. Paper presented at the Proceedings of the 18th Intersociety Conference on Environmental Systems, July 1988, San Francisco.
27. Sridhar KR, Finn JE, Kliss MH. In-situ resource utilization technologies for Mars life support systems. *Adv Space Res* 2000; **25**: 249–55.
28. West JB, Guy HJB, Elliott AR, Prisk GK. Respiratory system in microgravity. In: Fregly MJ, Blatteis CM,

eds. *Handbook of physiology – section 4: Environmental physiology.* New York: Oxford University Press, 1996.

*29. Prisk GK. Microgravity and the lung. *J Appl Physiol* 2000; **89**: 385–96.

30. Linnarsson D. Pulmonary function and cardiopulmonary interactions at microgravity. *Med Sci Sports Exerc* 1996; **28**: S14–S17.

31. Paiva M, Estenne M, Engel LA. Lung volumes, chest wall configuration and pattern of breathing in microgravity. *J Appl Physiol* 1989; **67**: 1542–50.

32. Michels DB, Friedman PJ, West JB. Radiographic comparison of human lung shape during normal gravity and weightlessness. *J Appl Physiol* 1979; **47**: 851–7.

33. Wantier M, Estenne M, Verbanck S, Prisk GK, Paiva M. Chest wall mechanics in sustained microgravity. *J Appl Physiol* 1998; **84**: 2060–5.

34. Michels DB, West JB. Distribution of pulmonary ventilation and perfusion during short periods of weightlessness. *J Appl Physiol* 1978; **45**: 987–98.

35. Prisk GK, Guy HJB, Elliott AR, West JB. Inhomogeneity of pulmonary perfusion during sustained microgravity on SLS-1. *J Appl Physiol* 1994; **76**: 1730–8.

36. Guy HJB, Prisk GK, Elliott AR, Deutschman RA, West JB. Inhomogeneity of pulmonary ventilation during sustained microgravity as determined by single breath washouts. *J Appl Physiol* 1994; **76**: 1719–29.

37. Prisk GK, Guy HJB, Elliott AR, Deutschman RA, West JB. Pulmonary diffusing capacity, capillary blood volume and cardiac output during sustained microgravity. *J Appl Physiol* 1993; **75**: 15–26.

38. Dinges DF. Sleep in space flight. Breath easy – sleep less. *Am J Respir Crit Care Med* 2001; **164**: 337–40.

39. Elliott AR, Shea SA, Dijk D-J, *et al.* Microgravity reduces sleep-disordered breathing in humans. *Am J Respir Crit Care Med* 2001; **164**: 478–85.

40. Walford RL, Bechtel R, MacCallum T, Paglia DE, Weber LJ. 'Biospheric medicine' as viewed from the two-year first closure of biosphere 2. *Aviat Space Environ Med* 1996; **67**: 609–17.

41. Schwartzkopf SH. Human life support for advanced space exploration. *Adv Space Biol Med* 1997; **6**: 231–53.

42. Mitchell CA. Bioregenerative life-support systems. *Am J Clin Nutr* 1994; **60**: 820S–4S.

43. Bowman RO, Thomae FW. Long-term nontoxic support of animal life with algae. *Science* 1961; **134**: 55–6.

44. Ivanov B, Zubareva O. To Mars and back again on board Bios. *Soviet Life* April 1985; 22–5.

45. Severinghaus JP, Broecker WS, Dempster WF, MacCallum T, Wahlen M. Oxygen loss in biosphere 2. *EOS* 1994; **75**: 33–40.

46. Cohen JE, Tilman D. Biosphere 2 and biodiversity: the lessons so far. *Science* 1996; **274**: 1150–1.

47. Silverstone S, Nelson M, Alling A, Allen J. Development and research program for a soil-based bioregenerative agriculture system to feed a four person crew at a Mars base. *Adv Space Res* 2003; **31**: 69–75.

20 Drowning

KEY POINTS

- Immersion in thermoneutral water activates protective airway reflexes and aspiration does not occur until lung oxygen stores have been used up and hypoxia causes the airway to open.
- In cold water, the cold shock reflex causes gasping and hyperventilation under water, with inhalation of large quantities of water and rapid, severe hypoxia.
- Surface cooling of the head and 'breathing' of very cold water may cool the brain rapidly in near-drowning and so protect the victim from hypoxic brain injury.

In several countries, drowning is a major cause of accidental death, many victims being children. In the USA nearly half of the victims of drowning are under 4 years old,[1] and in most developed countries drowning is the second commonest cause of accidental death in children, exceeded only by road traffic accidents.[2,3] In adults, men are drowned more commonly than women and alcohol is a major aetiological factor.[3] For each victim of death by drowning, there are estimated to be between six and ten cases of 'near-drowning' that are severe enough to require hospital admission,[2] and probably hundreds of other less severe incidents.[3] Death from pulmonary complications ('secondary drowning') may occur a considerable time after the accident, in patients who were initially normal.

The essential feature of drowning is asphyxia, but many of the physiological responses depend on whether aspiration of water occurs and upon the substances that are dissolved or suspended in the water. The temperature of the water is crucially important and hypothermia following drowning in very cold water is a major factor influencing survival, though the mechanism underlying this observation remains controversial.

PHYSIOLOGY OF IMMERSION[3,4]

The hydrostatic pressure exerted on the body during immersion can be substantial. As a result there is a huge increase in venous return, causing increased pulmonary blood volume, cardiac output and, soon afterwards, a significant diuresis. Cephalad displacement of the diaphragm from raised abdominal pressure coupled with direct chest compression increases the work of breathing by about 65%. Three reflexes affect the respiratory system and come into play in drowning, as outlined below.

Airway irritant reflexes play a major part in drowning. Aspiration of water into the mouth initially stimulates swallowing, followed by coughing, glottic closure and laryngospasm. If water penetrates deeper into the respiratory tract, below the vocal folds, bronchospasm results.

Cold shock describes a combination of several cardiovascular and respiratory reflexes that occur in response to sudden total-body immersion in cold water.[5] Sudden immersion in water below 25°C is a potent stimulant to respiration and causes an initial large gasp followed by substantial hyperventilation. The stimulus is increased with colder temperatures, reaching a maximum at 10°C.[3] Functional residual capacity is acutely increased and individuals may find themselves breathing almost at total lung capacity, giving a sensation of dyspnoea. Breath-hold time is severely reduced, often to less than 10 seconds, which impairs the ability of victims to escape from a confined space underwater or to orientate themselves before seeking safety.

Diving reflex. In response to cold water stimulation of the face and eyes, the diving reflex produces bradycardia, peripheral vasoconstriction and apnoea in most mammals. It is particularly well developed in diving mammals, to reduce oxygen consumption and facilitate long-duration dives. The reflex is present in humans,[6] though of small magnitude compared with other species, and is believed to be more significant in infants than adults.[3]

PHYSIOLOGICAL MECHANISMS OF DROWNING

Glottic closure from inhaled water, pulmonary aspiration, cold shock and the diving response all influence the course of events following submersion in water; the relative importance of each depends, among many other factors, on the age of the victim and the temperature of the water. Conflicting influences on the heart from activation of both the parasympathetic (diving reflex) and the sympathetic (cold shock) systems are believed to contribute to death from cardiac dysrhythmia in some victims.[3]

Drowning without aspiration of water

This occurs in less than 10% of drowning victims.[7] In thermoneutral water, when cold-stimulated reflexes will be minimal, the larynx is firmly closed during submersion and some victims will lose consciousness before water is aspirated. Because of the difference in alveolar/mixed venous gas tension gradients, arterial P_{O_2} falls initially at almost ten times the rate of rise of arterial P_{CO_2}. The subsequent rate of decrease depends mainly on the lung volume and the oxygen consumption. Oxygen stored in the alveolar gas after a maximal inspiration is unlikely to exceed 1 litre and an oxygen consumption of 3 l.min^{-1} would not be unusual in a subject either swimming or struggling. Loss of consciousness from decreased alveolar P_{O_2} usually occurs very suddenly and without warning.

In cold water, hypoxia secondary to glottic closure may still occur. In addition, the cold shock and diving reflexes both leave the victim vulnerable to cardiovascular complications such as arrhythmias and sudden circulatory failure, leading to death before aspiration can occur. This is likely to be more common in elderly individuals.

Drowning with aspiration of water

Almost 90% of drowning victims have aspirated significant volumes of water. Following sudden immersion in cold water the cold shock response is believed to be more common than the diving reflex, and hyperventilation rapidly leads to aspiration. In thermoneutral water, glottic closure may either be overcome by the conscious victim or will eventually subside due to hypoxia, and in both circumstances aspiration is likely to continue. Once aspiration occurs, reflex bronchospasm quickly follows, further worsening respiratory function.

Fresh water. Aspiration of fresh water further down the bronchial tree causes rapid and profound changes to the alveolar surfactant, leading to loss of the normal elastic properties of the alveoli and a disturbed ventilation/perfusion ratio. In fresh-water drowning, alveolar water is quickly absorbed, resulting in alveolar collapse and a pulmonary shunt, this being in addition to the changes resulting from dilution of surfactant. A significant shunt is therefore quickly established, with resulting hypoxia. Some studies indicate that neurogenic pulmonary oedema due to cerebral hypoxia might coexist with alveolar flooding from aspirated water.[8] The pulmonary changes caused by immersion appear to be quickly reversible,[8] with good prospects of return to normal pulmonary function in those who survive near-drowning.[9]

A substantial volume of water may be absorbed from the lungs and profound hyponatraemia, leading to fits, has been described in infants drowned in fresh water.[10] However, most human victims absorb only small quantities of water and redistribution rapidly corrects the blood volume. Hypovolaemia is the more common problem following near-drowning.[10]

Sea water. Sea water is hypertonic, having more than three times the osmolarity of blood. Consequently, sea water in the lungs is not initially absorbed and, on the contrary, draws fluid from the circulation into the alveoli. Thus, in laboratory animals that have aspirated sea water, it is possible to recover from the lungs 50% more than the original volume that was inhaled.[11] This clearly maintains the proportion of flooded alveoli and results in a persistent shunt with reduction in arterial P_{O_2}.

Other material contaminating the lungs

It is not unusual for a drowning person to swallow large quantities of water and then to regurgitate or vomit. Material aspirated into the lungs may then be contaminated with gastric contents and the drowning syndrome complicated with features of the acid aspiration syndrome. Aspiration of solid foreign bodies is a frequent complication of near-drowning in shallow rivers and lakes.

Postmortem tests of drowning

There appears to be no conclusive test for aspiration of either fresh or sea water. Tests based on differences in specific gravity and chloride content of plasma from the right and left chambers of the heart are unreliable. The demonstration of diatoms in bone marrow tissue is also controversial. Recent work has shown the accuracy of the diatom test to be greatly improved if the species, morphology and number of diatoms found at post-mortem are compared with those in a sample of the water in which the victim allegedly drowned.[12,13]

THE ROLE OF HYPOTHERMIA[3,4]

Some degree of hypothermia is usual in near-drowned victims and body temperature is usually in the range 33–36°C.[14] Hypothermia-induced reduction in cerebral metabolism is protective during hypoxia and is believed to contribute to the numerous reports of survival after prolonged immersion in cold water, particularly in children. There have been reports of survival of near-drowned children and adults trapped for periods as long as 80 minutes beneath ice.[10] However, for the reasons outlined above, arterial hypoxia is believed to develop very quickly and there is controversy surrounding how body temperature can decrease quickly enough to provide any degree of cerebral protection. Surface cooling is not believed to allow a rapid enough fall in temperature, as normal physiological responses to cold, such as peripheral vasoconstriction and shivering, limit the decline in temperature. Even so, the greater body surface area of children relative to their body size will theoretically result in more rapid cooling by heat conduction from the body surface.[4] Absorption of cold water from either the lungs or the stomach will contribute to hypothermia during prolonged immersion, but quantitatively the volumes required are unlikely to be absorbed, particularly in sea water. Heat loss from the flushing of cold water in and out of the respiratory tract, without absorption occurring, is another possible explanation. Recent animal studies have shown that airway flushing with cold water reduces carotid artery blood temperature by several degrees within a few minutes,[15] which is sufficient to produce a useful reduction in cerebral oxygen requirement. Finally, repeated aspiration of cold water may directly cool deep areas of the brain through conductive heat loss to the nasopharynx.[4]

In spite of these potential benefits, hypothermia in most drowning victims probably does more harm than good. Consciousness is lost at around 32°C, making further aspiration almost inevitable, and ventricular fibrillation or asystole commonly occur at temperatures below 28°C. Once rescued, near-drowned patients often cool further before arrival at hospital.

PRINCIPLES OF THERAPY FOR NEAR-DROWNING

There is a high measure of agreement on general principles of treatment.[3,7,10]

Immediate treatment

Circulatory failure and loss of consciousness may occur when a patient is lifted from the water in a vertical position, as for example by a helicopter winch. This is probably due to the loss of water pressure resulting in relative redistribution of blood volume into the legs. It is now recommended that victims are removed from the water in the prone position wherever possible.

At the scene of the drowning, it can be very difficult to determine whether there has been cardiac or even respiratory arrest. However, there are many records of apparently dead victims who have recovered without evidence of brain damage after long periods of total immersion. It is therefore essential that cardiopulmonary resuscitation be undertaken in all victims until fully assessed in hospital, no matter how hopeless the outlook may appear.

Early treatment of near-drowning is crucial and this requires efficient instruction in resuscitation for those who may be available in locations where drowning is likely to occur. The normal priorities of airway clearance, artificial ventilation and cardiac massage should be observed. Out of hospital, mouth-to-mouth ventilation is the method of choice, but high inflation pressures are usually required when there has been flooding of the lungs. Attempts to drain water from the lungs by postural drainage or an abdominal thrust (the Heimlich manoeuvre) are generally unsuccessful. These manoeuvres are likely to cause regurgitation of stomach contents with possible aspiration and will delay the institution of artificial ventilation. Tracheal intubation should be performed as soon as possible to protect the airway from aspiration. Oxygen is clearly valuable if available and should be continued until hospital is reached. Most survivors will breathe spontaneously within 1–5 minutes after removal from the water. The decision to discontinue resuscitation should not be taken until assessment in hospital, particularly if the state of consciousness is confused by hypothermia.

Hospital treatment

On arrival at hospital, patients should be triaged into the following categories:

1. awake
2. impaired consciousness (but responsive)
3. comatose.

There should be better than 90% survival in the first two categories, but patients should still be admitted for observation and followed up after discharge. Late deterioration of pulmonary function may occur and is known as 'secondary drowning', which is a form of the acute lung injury (see Chapter 31). This can develop in any patient who has aspirated water and the onset is usually within 4 hours of the aspiration.[4] Patients who are comatose or hypoxic will require admission to a critical care unit. Treatment follows the general principles for hypoxic cerebral damage and aspiration lung injury. If spontaneous breathing does not result in satisfactory levels of arterial P_{O_2} and P_{CO_2}, continuous positive airway pressure (CPAP) may be tried and is frequently useful. If this is unsuccessful, or in a patient with neurological impairment, artificial ventilation is required (see Chapter 32).

REFERENCES

1. Orlowski JP. Drowning, near-drowning and ice-water submersions. *Pediatr Clin North Am* 1987; **34**: 75–92.
2. Carey VF. Childhood drownings: who is responsible? *Br Med J* 1993; **307**: 1086–7.
*3. Golden FStC, Tipton MJ, Scott RC. Immersion, near-drowning and drowning. *Br J Anaesth* 1997; **79**: 214–25.
*4. Giesbrecht GG. Cold stress, near drowning and accidental hypothermia: a review. *Aviat Space Environ Med* 2000; **71**: 733–52.
5. Tipton MJ. The initial responses to cold water immersion in man. *Clin Sci* 1989; **77**: 581–8.
6. Schagatay E, Holm B. Effects of water and ambient air temperatures on human diving bradycardia. *Eur J Appl Physiol* 1996; **73**: 1–6.
7. Modell JH. Drowning. *N Engl J Med* 1993; **328**: 253–6.
8. Rumbak MJ. The etiology of pulmonary edema in fresh water near drowning. *Am J Emerg Med* 1996; **14**: 176–9.
9. Butt MP, Jalowayski A, Modell JH, Giammona ST. Pulmonary function after resuscitation from near drowning. *Anesthesiology* 1970; **32**: 275–7.
*10. Harries M. Near drowning. *Br Med J* 2003; **327**: 1336–8.
11. Modell JH, Calderwood HW, Ruiz BC, Downs JB, Chapman R. Effects of ventilatory patterns on arterial oxygenation after near-drowning in sea water. *Anesthesiology* 1974; **40**: 376–84.
12. Pollanen MS. The diagnostic value of the diatom test for drowning. II. Validity: analysis of diatoms in bone marrow and drowning medium. *J Forensic Sci* 1997; **42**: 286–90.
13. Hurlimann J, Feer P, Elber F, Niederberger K, Dirnhofer R, Wyler D. Diatom detection in the diagnosis of death by drowning. *Int J Legal Med* 2000; **114**: 6–14.
14. Pearn J. The management of near drowning. *BMJ* 1985; **291**: 1447–52.
15. Conn AW, Miyassaka K, Katayama M, *et al*. A canine study of cold water drowning in fresh versus salt water. *Crit Care Med* 1995; **23**: 2029–36.

21 Smoking and air pollution

KEY POINTS

- Almost a third of the UK population smoke tobacco, most taking up the habit in their teenage years.
- Smoking involves the regular inhalation of a variety of toxic compounds that stimulate airway irritant receptors and activate inflammatory pathways in the lung.
- The effects of passive smoking begin *in utero* when lung development is impaired, leaving the infant susceptible to lower airway illness for the first few years of life.
- Air pollution with carbon monoxide, ozone, nitrogen dioxide and particulate matter can occur either indoors or outside and is associated with a variety of respiratory symptoms.

The air we breathe is rarely a simple mixture of oxygen, nitrogen and water vapour. For much of the world's population air also contains a highly varied collection of other, more noxious, gases and particles. In addition, a substantial proportion of people choose to further contaminate the air that they, and others, breathe with cigarette smoke.

TOBACCO SMOKE

In the Americas tobacco was used for medicinal purposes for many centuries before being introduced from the New World into Europe in the 16th century. Through his acquaintance with Queen Elizabeth I, Sir Walter Raleigh made smoking tobacco an essential fashionable activity of every gentleman. Thereafter the practice steadily increased in popularity until the explosive growth of the habit following the First World War (1914–1918).

There have always been those opposed to smoking and King James I (1603–1625) described it as 'a custom loathsome to the eye, hateful to the nose, harmful to the brain and dangerous to the lungs'. However, firm evidence to support his last conclusion was delayed by some 350 years. Only relatively recently did it become clear that smokers had a higher mortality and that the causes of the excess mortality included many respiratory diseases.[1,2] The proportion of the population who smoke has generally declined since evidence of serious health consequences emerged, though in the UK the proportion of the adult population who smoke has been static since 1992 at 27%. Unfortunately, the proportion of young smokers has also remained constant, with currently 23% of 15-year-olds regularly smoking more than one cigarette a week.

Constituents of tobacco smoke

More than 2000 potentially noxious constituents have been identified in tobacco smoke, some in the gaseous phase and others in the particulate or tar phases. The particulate phase is defined as the fraction eliminated by passing smoke through a Cambridge filter of pore size 0.1 μm. This is not to be confused with the 'filter tip', which allows the passage of considerable quantities of particulate matter.

There is great variation in the yields of the different constituents between different brands and different types of cigarette. This is achieved by using leaves of different species of plant, by varying the conditions of curing and cultivation and by using filter tips. Ventilated filters have a ring of small holes in the paper between the filter tip and the tobacco. These holes admit air during a puff and dilute all constituents of the smoke. By these means, it is possible to have wide variations in the different constituents of smoke, which do not bear a fixed relationship to one another.

The gaseous phase. Carbon monoxide is present in cigarette smoke at a yield of between 15 and 25 mg (12 and 20 ml) per cigarette.[3] The concentration issuing from the butt of the cigarette during a puff is in the range 1–5%, which is far into the toxic range. A better indication of the extent of carbon monoxide exposure is the percentage of carboxyhaemoglobin in blood. For non-smokers, the value is normally less than 1.5% but is influenced by exposure to air pollution and other people's cigarette smoke (see below). Typical values for smokers range from 2% to 12%. The value is influenced by the number of cigarettes smoked, the type of cigarette and the pattern of smoke inhalation.

Tobacco smoke also contains very high concentrations (about 400 parts per million) of the potential free radical nitric oxide (page 353) and trace concentrations of nitrogen dioxide, the former being slowly oxidised to the latter in the presence of oxygen. The toxicity of these compounds is well known. Nitrogen dioxide hydrates in alveolar lining fluid to form a mixture of nitrous and nitric acids. In addition, the nitrite ion converts haemoglobin to methaemoglobin.

Other constituents of the gaseous phase include hydrocyanic acid, cyanogen, aldehydes, ketones, nitrosamines and volatile polynuclear aromatic hydrocarbons.

The particulate phase. The material removed by a Cambridge filter is known as the 'total particulate matter', with aerosol particle size in the range 0.2–1 μm. The particulate phase comprises water, nicotine and 'tar'. Nicotine ranges from 0.05 to 2.5 mg per cigarette and 'tar' from 0.5 to 35 mg per cigarette.

Individual smoke exposure

Individual smoke exposure is a complex function of the quantity of cigarettes that are smoked and the pattern of inhalation.

The quantity of cigarettes smoked. Exposure is usually quantified in 'pack-years'. This equals the product of the number of packs (20 cigarettes) smoked per day, multiplied by the number of years that that pattern was maintained. The totals for each period are then summated for the lifetime of the subject.

The pattern of inhalation. There are very wide variations in patterns of smoking. Air is normally drawn through the cigarette in a series of 'puffs' with a volume of about 25–50 ml per puff. The puff may be simply drawn into the mouth and rapidly expelled without appreciable inhalation. However, the habituated smoker will either inhale the puff directly into the lungs or, more commonly, pass the puff from the mouth to the lungs by inhaling air either through the mouth or else through the nose while passing the smoke from the mouth into the pharynx by apposing the tongue against the palate and so obliterating the gas space in the mouth. The inspiration is often especially deep, to flush into the lung any smoke remaining in the dead space.

It will be clear that the quantity of nicotine, tar and carbon monoxide obtainable from a single cigarette is highly variable and the number and type of cigarettes smoked are not the sole determinants of effective exposure. There is good evidence that the habituated smoker adjusts his smoking pattern to maintain a particular blood level of nicotine.[4] For example, after changing to a brand with a lower nicotine yield, it is common practice to modify the pattern of inhalation to maximise nicotine absorption.

Respiratory effects of smoking

Cigarette smoking has extensive effects on respiratory function and is clearly implicated in the aetiology of a number of respiratory diseases, particularly chronic obstructive pulmonary disease and bronchial carcinoma.

Airway mucosa.[5] Airway reflexes are more sensitive in smokers when measured using either mechanical stimulation or inhalation of small concentrations of ammonia vapour.[6] This increased sensitivity almost certainly contributes to the 'smoker's cough' and is believed to contribute to anaesthetic complications in smokers. Sensitivity takes several days to resolve following smoking abstinence. The concentration of inhaled histamine required to reduce specific airway conductance by 35% is, in smokers, less than 40% of that required in non-smokers.[7]

Ciliary function is inhibited by both particulate and gas phase compounds *in vitro*, but *in vivo* studies have shown contradictory results, with some studies showing increased ciliary activity in response to cigarette smoke.

Mucus production is increased in chronic smokers, who have hyperplasia of submucosal glands and increased numbers of goblet cells even when asymptomatic. In spite of the inconsistent findings regarding ciliary activity, mucus clearance is universally found to be impaired in smokers which, coupled with increased mucus production and airway sensitivity, gives rise to the normally productive smoker's cough. Three months after smoking cessation, many of these changes are reversed except in those patients who have developed airway damage from long-term airway inflammation.

Airway diameter. Airway diameter is acutely reduced with smoking as a result of reflex bronchoconstriction in response to inhaled particles and the increased mucus production already described. Airway narrowing is greatest in those subjects with known bronchial hypersensitivity, such as asthmatics. Long-term small airway inflammation causes chronic airway narrowing that has a multitude of effects on lung function. Airway narrowing promotes premature airway closure during expiration, which results in an increase in closing volume and disturbed ventilation/perfusion relationships. Distribution of inspired gas as indicated by the single-breath nitrogen

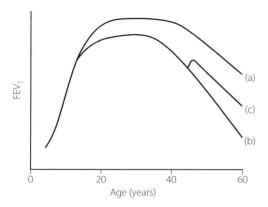

Figure 21.1 Schematic diagram showing the effects of smoking on normal lifelong changes in the forced expiratory volume in one second (FEV_1). **(a)** Normal changes. **(b)** Smoking begins at age 16 years. **(c)** Smoking stopped at 45 years of age. See text for details.

test (page 113) is therefore often abnormal in smokers. Small airway narrowing over many years gives rise to a progressive reduction in the forced expiratory volume in one second (FEV_1) described below. Many of these changes are at an advanced stage before smokers develop respiratory symptoms.

Ventilatory capacity.[8] FEV_1 normally reaches a peak in early adulthood, remains constant for some years and then declines steadily as the subject grows older (Figure 21.1). Longitudinal studies of FEV_1 in smokers reveal a very different picture, illustrated in Figure 21.1. Most smokers begin smoking in early adulthood and the rate of increase of FEV_1 immediately slows, resulting in a delayed and lower plateau. The plateau in FEV_1 is also shorter, before a more rapid decline begins. Smoking cessation is followed by a small improvement in FEV_1, followed by a return to the normal rate of decline, but rarely demonstrates a return to non-smoker values. Eventually, this decline in lung function results in lung pathology, with one in every five smokers developing chronic obstructive pulmonary disease.

Passive smoking

The non-smoker is exposed to all constituents of smoke when he is indoors in the presence of smokers. Exposure varies with many factors, including size and ventilation of the room, number of people smoking and absorption of smoke constituents on soft furnishings and clothing. Carbon monoxide concentrations of 20 ppm have been reported, which is above the recommended environmental concentration (see below). It has been estimated that non-smokers are exposed to quantities of 'tar' ranging from zero to 14 mg per day.[9] 'Sidestream' smoke from a smouldering cigarette stub produces greater quantities of potentially noxious substances than 'mainstream' smoke produced when a cigarette burns in a stream of air drawn through it during a puff. On average, 'sidestream' smoke is generated during 58 seconds in each minute of cigarette smoking and this is not included in the measured yield of a cigarette.

Evidence for adverse health effects of passive smoking is now convincing: adult passive smokers are more likely to develop lung cancer and coronary heart disease.[10,11]

Maternal smoking. Infants whose mothers smoke during pregnancy have low birthweight, are more likely to be born prematurely and are at greater risk of sudden infant death syndrome (page 235). Up to 2 years of age, infants with smoking parents are more prone to lower respiratory tract illnesses and episodes of wheezing, and when older they have reduced lung volumes, higher carboxyhaemoglobin levels and a greater likelihood of developing asthma.[8,12] It is uncertain whether this results from passive smoking *in utero* or from postnatal exposure to tobacco smoke in the home, but evidence for an *in utero* contribution is mounting.[13,14] Studies have found reduced expiratory flow rates[15] and other markers of impaired lower airway function in neonates even before they leave hospital, when their exposure to atmospheric cigarette smoke begins.[13] The same finding in neonates born on average 7 weeks before their expected date[16] indicates that maternal smoking adversely affects lung development at a crucial stage when terminal airways and alveoli are being formed (page 230). The increased risk of lower respiratory tract illness in passive-smoking infants is believed to result from smaller airway calibre at birth, causing a greater propensity to airway closure with the normal infective or allergic challenges of infancy.[13] After a few years of normal growth, airway size increases sufficiently to reduce symptoms and the child 'grows out' of their susceptibility to respiratory illness, though their lung function remains worse than in children who did not have lower airways disease in early life.[17]

Smoking and perioperative complications[18]

The increased sensitivity of the airway to inhaled irritants seen in smokers causes a greater incidence of adverse events such as cough, breath holding or laryngospasm on induction of general anaesthesia, even in passive smokers.[19,20] These complications are not necessarily associated with decreases in oxygen saturation, though episodes of desaturation in the recovery period may be more common in smokers or even in passively smoking children.[21] It is worth noting once again that commercially available pulse oximeters record carboxyhaemoglobin as if it were oxyhaemoglobin (page 195) and so will consistently overestimate oxygen saturation in recent smokers.

There is ample evidence that smokers have an increased incidence of postoperative respiratory complications, which are between two and six times more common in smokers, depending on the definitions used and the type of surgery undertaken.[22–24] This is attributable both to increased secretion and impaired clearance of mucus and to small airway narrowing. Almost all studies of the perioperative effects of smoking have been undertaken in patients having major surgery, usually coronary artery revascularisation or upper abdominal surgery. The high incidence of respiratory complications in this group makes them an ideal study population, but there remains little information regarding the respiratory effects of perioperative smoking and more minor surgery.

Preoperative smoking cessation is vital.[22,23] Nicotine, which is responsible for many untoward cardiovascular changes, has a half-life of only 30 minutes, whereas carboxyhaemoglobin has a half-life of 4 hours when breathing air. A smoking fast of just a few hours will therefore effectively remove the risks associated with carbon monoxide and nicotine. Airway reflexes take a few days to return to normal.[6] The incidence of respiratory complications after major surgery is only reduced to that of non-smokers by more than 8 weeks' abstinence. Furthermore, there is some evidence that surgery performed within this 8-week period is associated with a greater complication rate than if the patient had continued to smoke until a few hours before the operation.

MECHANISMS OF SMOKING-RELATED LUNG DAMAGE

Many of the compounds present in cigarette smoke have direct irritant and toxic effects on the lungs. There are three other mechanisms by which lung damage occurs.

Oxidative injury[25,26]

There is compelling evidence for believing that oxidative injury, including peroxidation of membrane lipids, is an important component of the pulmonary damage caused by cigarette smoke.

Direct oxidative damage. The tar phase contains quinone, the semiquinone free radical and hydroquinone in a polymeric matrix, and the gas phase contains nitric oxide. These compounds can reduce oxygen in the body, to yield the superoxide free radical and thence the highly damaging hydroxyl free radical (see Figure 26.3).

Cell-mediated oxidative damage. This results from smoking-induced activation of, or enhancement of, neutrophil and macrophage activity in the respiratory tract. Bronchoalveolar lavage in humans has shown that smokers have larger numbers of intraalveolar macrophages and also significant numbers of neutrophils that are not normally present in non-smokers.[27] It is the particulate component of smoke that is responsible for the recruitment and activation of neutrophils in the alveoli. This suggests that the interaction of particulate matter and alveolar macrophages releases a neutrophil chemattractant and that neutrophils are subsequently activated to release either proteases or oxygen-derived free radicals. This activation may be a direct response to cigarette smoke or may represent excessive free radical production in response to minor infective challenge in smokers.

Evidence of *in vivo* oxidative stress in smokers' lungs is based mainly on measures of antioxidant activity. Compared with non-smokers, human smokers have reduced levels of vitamin E in alveolar fluid, reduced plasma concentrations of vitamin C and greatly increased superoxide dismutase and catalase activity in alveolar macrophages.

Carcinogenesis[28]

Smoking contributes to the development of cancer in many organs, but the respiratory tract clearly receives substantial exposure to tobacco smoke carcinogens. There are two groups of compound with carcinogenic activity, found mostly in the tar of the particulate phase. Some hydrocarbons, in particular polynuclear aromatic hydrocarbons (PAH), are carcinogenic, whereas others such as aromatic phenols (phenol, indole and catechol) are cocarcinogens and tumour promoters, without which the carcinogenic compounds are relatively innocuous. Tobacco-related nitrosamines and nicotine derivatives are also carcinogenic and, because of their ease of absorption into the blood, are responsible for cancer formation not only in the respiratory tract and oesophagus but also in more distant organs such as the pancreas. Knowledge about these carcinogens has led to many attempts to reduce their concentration in smoke by modifying the cigarette, and tar levels in cigarettes have declined almost threefold since 1955. However, smoking cessation remains the best way of avoiding smoking-related cancers. For people who cannot achieve this goal, some early (mostly animal) research has identified several strategies that may reduce cancer risk, including ingestion of β-carotene and a reduction in dietary fat.[28]

Immunological activation[29]

Smokers have elevated serum IgE levels compared to non-smokers, the cause of which is uncertain but may be twofold. Direct toxicity and oxidative cell damage result in greater airway mucosal cell permeability, allowing better access for allergens to underlying immunologically active cells. Smoking also increases the activity of some T-lymphocyte subsets that are responsible for producing interleukin-4, a cytokine well known for stimulating IgE production.

These observations thus raise the possibility that an 'allergic' mechanism is responsible for smoking-related changes in lung function, such as small airway narrowing. An association between IgE levels and impaired lung function is well established in asthma, but has been less consistently seen in non-asthmatic smokers except in older subjects. Thus causality between smoking and an IgE-mediated mechanism is far from established. It is possible that smoking sensitises the airway to 'new' allergens and that this contributes to the development of chronic airways disease seen in some smokers.

AIR POLLUTION[30,31]

Fossil fuels have formed the major source of energy for society for many centuries and continue to do so today. Detrimental effects of air pollution were first recognised in the 13th century, though it is only in the last 50 years that effective control of pollution has been achieved. In spite of these controls, increased overall energy requirements and the internal combustion engine have ensured that air pollution remains a current problem. Production of carbon dioxide is not considered as pollution; its effects on the atmosphere are discussed in Chapter 1.

Sources of pollutants

Primary pollutants are substances that are released into the atmosphere directly from the polluting source and are mostly derived from the combustion of fossil fuels. Petrol engines that ignite the fuel in an oxygen-restricted environment produce varying quantities of carbon monoxide, nitrogen oxides and hydrocarbons such as benzene and polycyclic aromatic compounds. All of these pollutants are reduced by the use of a catalytic converter. In contrast, diesel engines burn fuel with an excess of oxygen and so produce little carbon monoxide but more nitrogen oxides and particulate matter. Burning of coal and oil is now restricted almost entirely to power generation and the pollutants produced depend on the type of fuel used and the amount of effort expended on 'cleaning' the emissions. However, particulates and nitrogen oxides are invariably produced and this remains the major source of sulphur dioxide.

Secondary pollutants are formed in the atmosphere from chemical changes to primary pollutants. Nitric oxide produced from vehicle engines is quickly converted to nitrogen dioxide and in doing so may react with ozone, reducing the atmospheric concentration of the latter.

Alternatively, when exposed to sunlight in the lower atmosphere both NO and NO_2 react with oxygen to produce ozone (O_3).[32]

Meteorological conditions have an enormous influence on air pollution. In conditions of strong wind, pollutants are quickly dispersed; in cloudy weather the development of secondary pollutants is unlikely. Ground-level pollution in urban areas is exacerbated by clear, calm weather, when 'temperature inversion' can occur. On a clear night, heat is lost from the ground to the atmosphere by radiation and the ground-level air cools dramatically (Figure 21.2a). At dawn the ground is quickly heated by the sun's radiation and warms the air, which lifts a blanket of cool air to approximately 50–100 m high. Because in still conditions mixing of air masses is slow to occur, the relatively cold air sits on top of the warm air below. In the meantime, the morning rush hour produces large amounts of pollutants that are unable to disperse and become trapped near the ground (Figure 21.2b).

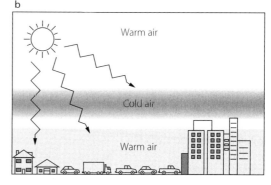

Figure 21.2 Temperature inversion producing pollution in the morning rush hour. **(a)** At night, the ground loses heat to the atmosphere by radiation and ground level air cools. **(b)** In the morning, with strong sun and still conditions, the ground heats up quickly and displaces the blanket of cold air upwards, so preventing effective air mixing and trapping vehicular pollution at ground level.

Table 21.1 Recommended air quality standards

Pollutant	Duration of exposure		
	Short ($\leq$1 hour)	Moderate (8–24 hours)	Annual
Ozone	76–110 ppb	50–60 ppb	
Particulates (PM_{10})		150 μg.m^{-3}	50 μg.m^{-3}
Sulphur dioxide	175 ppb	45 ppb	17 ppb
Nitrogen dioxide	110 ppb	80 ppb	21 ppb
Carbon monoxide	25–87 ppm	10 ppm	

Figures are derived from WHO air quality guidelines, except those for particulates which are from the National Ambient Air Quality Standards in the USA.[30,33] ppm, parts per million; ppb, parts per billion.

Respiratory effects of pollutants[30-34]

Recommended maximum levels of common pollutants are shown in Table 21.1. The extent to which these levels are achieved varies greatly between different countries and from year to year. Almost 20 million residents of the USA are believed to be regularly exposed to pollutant levels greater than the nationally agreed maxima.[33] Air pollution is now believed to be a significant public health problem.

Carbon monoxide. CO is found in the blood of patients, in trace concentrations, as a result of its production in the body, but mainly as a result of smoking and air pollution. The amount of carboxyhaemoglobin formed when breathing air polluted with CO will depend on the subject's minute volume. One study reported carboxy-haemoglobin levels of 0.4–9.7% in London taxi drivers but the highest level in a non-smoking driver was 3%.[35] Recommended levels shown in Table 21.1 are calculated to result in a carboxyhaemoglobin concentration of less than 2.5% even during moderate exercise. Carbon monoxide levels similar to those seen in smokers are only likely to occur during severe outdoor pollution episodes, though indoor pollution with CO may be more common (see below).

Nitrogen dioxide is mainly a primary pollutant, but a small amount is produced from nitric oxide. In the UK, about half of atmospheric NO_2 is derived from vehicles. Indoor levels of NO_2 commonly exceed outdoor levels and the respiratory effects of NO_2 are therefore described in the next section.

Ozone is a secondary pollutant formed by the action of sunlight on nitrogen oxides and therefore the highest levels tend to occur in rural areas downwind from cities and roads. In all areas, the dependence on sunlight means that ozone levels slowly increase throughout the day, reaching peak levels shortly after the evening rush hour.

Ozone is toxic to the respiratory tract, with effects being dependent on both concentration and duration of exposure. Exposure to concentrations of 80–100 ppb for just a few hours commonly causes throat irritation, chest discomfort and cough, resulting from both direct stimulation of irritant receptors in the airway and activation of inflammatory pathways. Bronchoconstriction may occur accompanied by a decrease in FEV_1 and exercise capacity is limited. Repeated daily exposure to ozone (200 ppb), which is common in susceptible areas, causes a gradual reduction in the response.[36] There is also large variability between individuals in their spirometric response to ozone, with approximately 10% of subjects having a severe response. This variability in response is partly a result of differing genetic susceptibilities.[31] It is interesting that laboratory studies have failed to demonstrate that asthmatic subjects are more susceptible to ozone-induced pulmonary symptoms. Even so, there is good evidence that high atmospheric ozone concentrations are associated with increased hospital attendance and admission rates for respiratory problems. Ozone therefore seems to present a respiratory challenge to some subjects, with or without asthma, even at modest atmospheric levels.[31]

Sulphur dioxide. Declining use of coal has substantially reduced the production of sulphur dioxide in recent years and two-thirds of production in the UK now originates from oil-burning power stations. Normal atmospheric levels have no short-term effect on healthy subjects, but asthmatic patients may develop broncho-constriction at between 100 and 250 ppb.

Particulate matter consists of a mixture of soot, liquid droplets, recondensed metallic vapours and organic debris. Only particles of less than 10 μm diameter are considered to be 'inhalable' into the lung (page 19), so particulate pollution is measured as the concentration of particles less than this diameter, known as PM_{10}. The disparate nature of particulate pollution reflects its very varied origins, but in the urban environment diesel engines are a major source. Acute effects of particles on lung function again include airway irritation and small reductions in lung volumes such as FVC.[37] It is, however, associations between PM_{10} levels and overall mortality that have been the focus of much research. Even when smoking habits are taken into account, particulate pollution is associated with an increased risk of death from lung cancer or other cardiopulmonary diseases.[31,38] Particulate pollution has widespread proinflammatory effects on lung epithelial cells and alveolar macrophages, causing inflammatory responses both locally in the lung, and in distant sites where activation of clotting pathways may explain PM_{10}-induced increases in death from cardiovascular disease.[31]

Indoor air pollution[10,39]

Energy-efficient homes have become the norm in recent years, with effective heating systems and extensive insulation. This has led to dramatic changes in indoor air quality, including warmer temperatures, higher humidity levels and reduced ventilation. It is estimated that most people spend in excess of 80% of their time indoors, so indoor air pollution may have a considerable impact on public health. The respiratory effects of passive smoking are described above (page 291).

Indoor air quality generally reflects that of the outdoor air except that ozone levels are invariably low indoors owing to the rapid reaction of ozone with the synthetic materials that make up much of the indoor environment. In addition to pollutants from outside, there are three specific indoor pollutants.

Allergens. Warm moist air, poor ventilation and extensive floor coverings provide ideal conditions for house dust mite infestation and the retention of numerous other allergens. This is believed to contribute to the recent upsurge in the prevalence of atopic diseases such as asthma and is discussed in Chapter 28.

Carbon monoxide.[40] Malfunctions of heating equipment in the home may release CO into the indoor environment. Acute CO poisoning from this cause is common, but the occurrence of prolonged low-level exposure to indoor CO may be underestimated. Headache, malaise and flu-like symptoms are all features of long-term CO poisoning, though these symptoms are believed to be completely reversible once the exposure to CO is stopped. Smokers, who have permanently elevated carboxyhaemoglobin levels, appear to be resistant to these symptoms.

Nitrogen dioxide. Gas-fired cookers, stoves and boilers all produce NO_2, the amount being dependent on the

arrangements for waste gas exclusion.[41] In this respect, gas cookers are the worst culprits as they are rarely associated with chimneys and flues and normally discharge their waste gases directly into the kitchen atmosphere. During cooking, NO_2 levels may reach over 400 ppb, which is well in excess of outdoor pollution targets (see Table 21.1). Mild airway irritant effects are seen at levels of around 300 ppb in asthmatic subjects or at 1000 ppb in non-asthmatic subjects,[30] so acute effects are probably uncommon. However, long-term exposure does seem to be clinically significant. Epidemiological studies have found associations between the use of gas cookers and reduced FEV_1, or indoor NO_2 concentrations and increased symptoms in subjects with asthma.[42,43]

REFERENCES

1. Doll R, Hill AB. Smoking and carcinoma of the lung. *Br Med J* 1950; **2**: 739–48.
2. Anderson DO, Ferris BG. Role of tobacco smoking in the causation of chronic respiratory disease. *N Engl J Med* 1962; **267**: 787–94.
3. Borland C, Chamberlain A, Higenbottam T, Shipley M, Rose G. Carbon monoxide yield of cigarettes and its relation to cardiorespiratory disease. *Br Med J* 1983; **287**: 1583–6.
4. Ashton H, Stepney R, Thompson PW. Self-titration by cigarette smokers. *Br Med J* 1979; **2**: 357–60.
*5. Wanner A, Salathe M, O'Riordan TG. Mucociliary clearance in the airways. *Am J Respir Crit Care Med* 1996; **154**: 1868–902.
6. Erskine RJ, Murphy PJ, Langton JA. Sensitivity of upper airway reflexes in cigarette smokers: effect of abstinence. *Br J Anaesth* 1994; **73**: 298–302.
7. Gerrard JW, Cockcroft DW, Mink JT, Cotton DJ, Poonawala R, Dosman JA. Increased nonspecific bronchial reactivity in cigarette smokers with normal lung function. *Am Rev Respir Dis* 1980; **122**: 577–81.
8. Samet JM, Lange P. Longitudinal studies of active and passive smoking. *Am J Respir Crit Care Med* 1996; **154**: S257–65.
9. Rapace JL, Lowrey AH. Tobacco smoke, ventilation and indoor air quality. *Am Soc Heating, Refrigerating and Air-conditioning Engineers, Inc Trans* 1982; **88**: 895.
*10. Samet JM, Spengler JD. Indoor environments and health: moving into the 21st century. *Am J Public Health* 2003; **93**: 1489–93.
11. Trichopoulos D, Mollo F, Tomatis L, *et al.* Active and passive smoking and pathological indicators of lung cancer risk in an autopsy study. *JAMA* 1992; **268**: 1697–701.
12. Gidding SJ, Morgan W, Perry C, Isabel-Jones J, Bricker JT. Active and passive tobacco exposure: a

serious pediatric health problem. *Circulation* 1994; **90**: 2581–90.

*13. Morgan WJ, Martinez FD. Maternal smoking and infant lung function: further evidence for an *in utero* effect. *Am J Respir Crit Care Med* 1998; **158**: 689–90.

14. Cunningham J, Dockery DW, Speizer FE. Maternal smoking during pregnancy as a predictor of lung function in children. *Am J Epidemiol* 1994; **139**: 1139–52.

15. Hanrahan JP, Tager IB, Segal MR, *et al.* The effect of maternal smoking during pregnancy on early infant lung function. *Am Rev Respir Dis* 1992; **145**: 1129–35.

16. Hoo AF, Henschen M, Dezateux C, Costeloe K, Stocks J. Respiratory function among preterm infants whose mothers smoked during pregnancy. *Am J Respir Crit Care Med* 1998; **158**: 700–5.

17. Martinez FD, Wright AL, Taussig LM, *et al.* Asthma and wheezing in the first six years of life. *N Engl J Med* 1995; **332**: 133–8.

*18. Nel MR, Morgan M. Smoking and anaesthesia revisited. *Anaesthesia* 1996; **51**: 309–11.

19. Dennis A, Curran J, Sherriff J, Kinnear W. Effects of passive and active smoking on induction of anaesthesia. *Br J Anaesth* 1994; **73**: 450–2.

20. Schwilk B, Bothner U, Schraag S, Georgieff M. Perioperative respiratory events in smokers and nonsmokers undergoing general anaesthesia. *Acta Anaesthesiol Scand* 1997; **41**: 348–55.

21. Lyons B, Frizelle H, Kirby F, Casey W. The effect of passive smoking on the incidence of airway complications in children undergoing general anaesthesia. *Anaesthesia* 1996; **51**: 324–6.

22. Egan TD, Wong KC. Perioperative smoking cessation and anesthesia: a review. *J Clin Anesth* 1992; **4**: 63–72.

23. Pearce AC, Jones RM. Smoking and anesthesia: preoperative abstinence and perioperative morbidity. *Anesthesiology* 1984; **61**: 576–84.

24. Møller AM, Maaløe R, Pedersen T. Postoperative intensive care admittance: the role of tobacco smoking. *Acta Anaesthesiol Scand* 2001; **45**: 345–8.

25. Chow CK. Cigarette smoking and oxidative damage in the lung. *Ann N Y Acad Sci* 1993; **686**: 289–98.

26. McCusker K. Mechanisms of respiratory tissue injury from cigarette smoking. *Am J Med* 1992; **93**(Supp 1A): 18S–21S.

27. Hunninghake GW, Crystal RG. Cigarette smoking and lung destruction. Accumulation of neutrophils in the lungs of cigarette smokers. *Am Rev Respir Dis* 1983; **128**: 833–8.

28. Hoffman D, Rivenson A, Chung F-L, Wynder EL. Potential inhibitors of tobacco carcinogenesis. *Ann N Y Acad Sci* 1993; **686**: 140–60.

29. Villar MTA, Holgate ST. IgE, smoking and lung function. *Clin Exp Allergy* 1995; **25**: 206–9.

30. Committee on the Medical Effects of Air Pollutants. *Handbook on air pollution and health.* London: Stationery Office, 1997.

*31. Brunekreef B, Holgate ST. Air pollution and health. *Lancet* 2002; **360**: 1233–42.

32. Tattersfield AE. Air pollution: brown skies research. *Thorax* 1996; **51**: 13–22.

33. Committee of the Environmental and Occupational Health Assembly of the American Thoracic Society. Health effects of outdoor air pollution. *Am J Respir Crit Care Med* 1996; **153**: 3–50.

34. Committee on the Medical Effects of Air Pollution. *The quantification of the effects of air pollution on health in the United Kingdom.* London: Stationery Office, 1998.

35. Jones RD, Commins BT, Cernik AA. Blood lead and carboxyhaemoglobin levels in London taxi drivers. *Lancet* 1972; **2**: 302–3.

36. Christian DL, Chen LL, Scannell CH, Ferrando RE, Welch BS, Balmes JR. Ozone-induced inflammation is attenuated with multiday exposure. *Am J Respir Crit Care Med* 1998; **158**: 532–7.

37. Scarlett JF, Abbott KJ, Peacock JL, Strachan DP, Anderson HR. Acute effects of summer air pollution on respiratory function in primary school children in southern England. *Thorax* 1996; **51**: 1109–14.

38. Dockery DW, Pope CA, Xu X, *et al.* An association between air pollution and mortality in six U.S. cities. *N Engl J Med* 1993; **329**: 1753–9.

39. Alberts WM. Indoor air pollution: NO, NO_2, CO and CO_2. *J Allergy Clin Immunol* 1994; **94**: 289–95.

40. Townsend CL, Maynard RL. Effects on health of prolonged exposure to low concentrations of carbon monoxide. *Occup Environ Med* 2002; **59**: 708–11.

41. Fuhlbrigge A, Weiss S. Domestic gas appliances and lung disease. *Thorax* 1997; **52**(Supp 3): S58–62.

42. Jarvis D, Chinn S, Luczynska C, Burney P. Association of respiratory symptoms and lung function in young adults with use of domestic gas appliances. *Lancet* 1996; **347**: 426–31.

43. Smith BJ, Nitschke M, Pilotto LS, Ruffin RE, Pisaniello DL, Willson KJ. Health effects of daily indoor nitrogen dioxide exposure in people with asthma. *Eur Respir J* 2000; **16**: 879–85.

KEY POINTS

- All anaesthetic drugs reduce resting ventilation and impair the ventilatory response to both hypercapnia and hypoxia.
- Upper airway muscle function is inhibited by anaesthesia, leading to airway obstruction, usually at the level of the soft palate.
- Functional residual capacity is reduced within a few minutes of induction of anaesthesia as a result of altered respiratory muscle activity causing changes to the shape and volume of the thoracic cavity.
- Most patients develop small areas of atelectasis during anaesthesia, reexpansion of which requires high lung inflation pressures.
- Oxygenation is impaired by these changes, with wider scatter of ventilation/perfusion ratios along with increased alveolar dead space and pulmonary shunt.

Only 12 years after the first successful public demonstration of general anaesthesia in 1846, John Snow reported the pronounced changes that occur in respiration during the inhalation of chloroform.[1] Subsequent observations have confirmed that anaesthesia has profound effects on the respiratory system. However, these effects are diverse and highly specific, some aspects of respiratory function being profoundly modified whereas others are scarcely affected at all.

CONTROL OF BREATHING[2]

Unstimulated ventilation

It has long been known that anaesthesia may diminish pulmonary ventilation and hypercapnia is commonplace if spontaneous breathing is preserved. Reduced minute volume is due partly to a reduction in metabolic demand but mainly to interference with the chemical control of breathing, in particular a reduced sensitivity to CO_2 as described below. In an uncomplicated anaesthetic, there should not be sufficient resistance to breathing to affect the minute volume. However, the minute volume may be greatly decreased if there is overt respiratory obstruction.

At lower concentrations of inhaled anaesthetics, minute volume may remain unchanged, but smaller tidal volumes with higher respiratory frequency often occur, resulting in reduced alveolar ventilation and an increase in PCO_2. With higher concentrations of anaesthetic, breathing becomes slower and spontaneous minute volume may decrease to very low levels, particularly in the absence of surgical stimulation. This will inevitably result in hypercapnia and end-expiratory PCO_2 commonly rises to 10 kPa (75 mmHg). Clearly there is no limit to the rise that may occur if the anaesthetist is prepared to tolerate gross hypoventilation.

There are anaesthetists in many parts of the world, including the UK, who do not believe that temporary hypercapnia during anaesthesia is harmful to a healthy patient. Many hundreds of millions of patients must have been subjected to this transient physiological trespass since 1846 and there seems to be no convincing evidence of harm resulting from it, except perhaps increased bleeding from the incision. In other parts of the world, particularly the USA, the departure from physiological normality is regarded with concern and it is usual either to assist spontaneous respiration by manual compression of the reservoir bag or, more commonly, to paralyse and ventilate artificially as a routine.

Quite different conditions apply during anaesthesia with artificial ventilation. The minute volume can then be set at any level that seems appropriate to the anaesthetist and in the past there was a tendency to hyperventilate patients, resulting in hypocapnia. Routine monitoring of end-expiratory PCO_2 has radically altered the control of minute volume during anaesthesia. Artificial ventilation can very easily be adjusted to maintain the target PCO_2 selected by the anaesthetist.

Effect on PCO_2/ventilation response curve

Progressive increases in the alveolar concentration of all inhalational anaesthetic agents reduce the slope of the

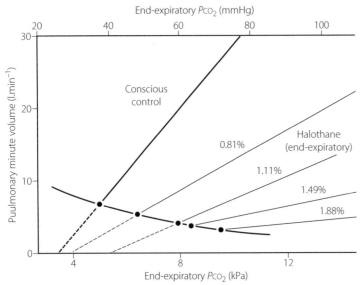

Figure 22.1 Displacement of the P_{CO_2}/ventilation response curve with different end-expiratory concentrations of halothane. The curve sloping down to the right indicates the pathway of P_{CO_2} and ventilation change resulting from depression without the challenge of exogenous carbon dioxide. The broken lines indicate extrapolation to apnoeic threshold P_{CO_2}. The curves have been constructed from the data of reference 3.

P_{CO_2}/ventilation response curve and, at deep levels of anaesthesia, there may be no response at all to P_{CO_2}. Furthermore, the anaesthetised patient, as opposed to the awake subject, always becomes apnoeic if the P_{CO_2} is reduced below this intercept, which is known as the apnoeic threshold P_{CO_2} (page 63). In Figure 22.1, the flat curve rising to the left represents the starting points for various P_{CO_2}/ventilation response curves. Without added carbon dioxide in the inspired gas, deepening anaesthesia is associated with a decreasing ventilation and a rising P_{CO_2}, points moving progressively down and to the right. At intervals along this curve are shown P_{CO_2}/ventilation response curves resulting from adding carbon dioxide to the inspired gas.

At equivalent depths of anaesthesia, currently available inhaled anaesthetics depress the ventilatory response to P_{CO_2} by a similar amount. This is conveniently shown by plotting the slope of the P_{CO_2}/ventilation response curve against equianaesthetic concentrations of different anaesthetics (Figure 22.2), shown as multiples of minimum alveolar concentration (MAC), although the validity of using MAC multiples in this way has been questioned. The currently used halogenated agents do not differ greatly from one another, but diethyl ether is exceptional in having little effect up to 1 MAC.

Surgical stimulation antagonises the effect of anaesthesia on the P_{CO_2}/ventilation response curve (Figure 22.3). It may easily be observed that in a spontaneously breathing patient a surgical incision increases the ventilation whatever the depth of anaesthesia. During prolonged anaesthesia without surgical stimulation, there is no progressive change in the response curve up to 3 hours, but some return towards the preanaesthetic position has been reported after 6 hours.[7] With the excep-

Figure 22.2 Relative depression of the ventilatory response to CO_2 by different inhalational anaesthetics as a function of minimum alveolar concentration (MAC). [●], halothane; [▲], enflurane; [■], isoflurane; [◆], sevoflurane; [○], desflurane; [□], diethylether. (Data from references 4,5 and 6.)

tion of ketamine, intravenous anaesthetics have similar effects on ventilation to the inhalational anaesthetics.

Effect on P_{O_2}/ventilation response curve[9,10]

The normal relationship between P_{O_2} and ventilation is described on pages 65 *et seq*. It was long believed that this reflex was the *ultima moriens*, or the last to go, and, unlike the P_{CO_2}/ventilation response curve, unaffected by anaesthesia. This doctrine was a source of comfort to many generations of anaesthetists in the past. Little attention was given to the observation of Gordh in 1945 that ether anaesthesia nearly abolished the ventilatory

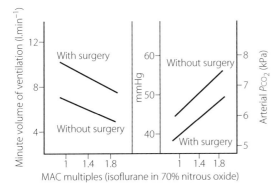

Figure 22.3 Respiratory depression by isoflurane with and without surgery at different multiples of minimum alveolar concentration (MAC) required for anaesthesia. (Data from reference 8.)

Figure 22.4 Effect of halothane anaesthesia on the ventilatory response to hypoxia. The data shown in this figure have now been challenged; see text for details. (After reference 13.)

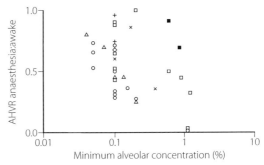

Figure 22.5 Summary of studies of the acute hypoxic ventilatory response (AHVR) and inhalational anaesthesia or sedation. The ordinate is the ratio of the increase in minute volume with hypoxia during anaesthesia or sedation and the awake (control) response. Thus a ratio of unity represents no depression of the response and zero represents a completely abolished response. All studies were performed under isocapnic conditions, except the two solid squares, which used poikilocapnia. See text for details. [O], halothane; [△], enflurane; [□], isoflurane; [◇], sevoflurane; [×], nitrous oxide; [+], desflurane. Derived from references quoted in the text and references 21–27.

response to hypoxaemia while the response to carbon dioxide was still present.[11]

Over 30 years later, halothane anaesthesia was shown to reduce the acute hypoxic ventilatory response (AHVR) in humans.[12] Shortly afterwards in 1978, Knill and Gelb[13] showed that not only was the hypoxic response affected by inhalational anaesthetics but it was also, in fact, exquisitely sensitive (Figure 22.4). Hypoxic drive was markedly attenuated at 0.1 MAC, a level of anaesthesia that would not be reached for a considerable time during recovery from anaesthesia. Similar effects were found with all the currently used inhalational agents[14–18] and with the intravenous anaesthetic propofol.[19]

These findings were widely accepted for some years, until a study by Temp et al.[20] in 1992 showed that AHVR was only diminished in hypercapnic conditions. This study initiated a great deal of further research. A summary of the findings of these and previous studies is shown in Figure 22.5. The most notable feature of these results is their diversity, with, for example, different studies of similar concentrations of isoflurane, particularly at sedative levels, resulting in completely opposite results. However, for the other agents there does seem to be a generally dose-dependent depression of the hypoxic ventilatory response, though at 0.1 MAC considerable variation remains. There are many possible explanations for these results, mostly relating to methodological differences between studies.

Anaesthetic agent. Differences between anaesthetic agents in their effects on AHVR are not obvious from Figure 22.5. However, a recent quantitative review of 37 studies did find differences, with the least depression of the response by low-dose sevoflurane, progressively increasing depression by isoflurane and enflurane, and halothane having the greatest effect.[9]

Subject stimulation. The degree of arousal of subjects is known to affect the AHVR. Studies of hypoxic response at 'sedative' levels of anaesthesia (0.2 MAC or less) have differed in the amount of stimulation provided, with some forcing the subjects to remain awake[20] and others leaving subjects undisturbed. One study comparing awake and asleep subjects with 0.1 MAC isoflurane found no depression of the hypoxic response in the awake group.[28] However, the same review described in the previous paragraph did find subject stimulation to be a significant factor in determining the degree of depression of AHVR and that this effect may be influenced by the specific anaesthetic agent used.[9]

Hypoxic challenge. The rate of onset, degree and duration of hypoxia will all affect the ventilatory response, which is normally biphasic, with hypoxic ventilatory decline (HVD) occurring a few minutes after the onset of hypoxia (see Figure 5.7). Some studies used rapid 'step' changes into hypoxic conditions,[29] whereas others used a 'ramp' onset of hypoxia over 8–10 minutes.[14] In the latter situation, the response under study will be a combination of AHVR and HVD.[20] These differences do not seem to be of practical importance. One study addressing different patterns of hypoxic onset on AHVR found no difference between the two[30] and a recent review did not find the hypoxic stimulus to be a major factor.[9] Hypoxic ventilatory decline seems to be uninfluenced by anaesthesia.[20,29,31]

Subject selection. The magnitude of the AHVR differs greatly between individuals (page 66). Some studies have been performed using only subjects found to have a 'brisk' ventilatory response to hypoxia,[29] and these results cannot therefore be extrapolated to a broader range of patients.

Carbon dioxide concentration may be maintained at normal, prehypoxic levels (isocapnia) or allowed to find its own level (poikilocapnia). This has a large effect in the awake subject, with the hypoxic response being greatly attenuated during poikilocapnia (see Figure 5.7). During anaesthesia with up to 0.85 MAC isoflurane, the hypoxic ventilatory response during poikilocapnia is essentially maintained;[32,33] that is, the increase in ventilation with hypoxic challenge is the same when asleep as when awake. This has led to the suggestion that anaesthesia has less effect on the hypoxic ventilatory response itself, but may reduce the normally additive interaction between the ventilatory responses to hypoxia and hypercapnia (see Figure 5.8).[20,33]

It is generally agreed that the effect of anaesthetics on AHVR is on the peripheral chemoreceptors,[34] possibly exclusively so at sedative levels.[35] Anaesthesia also impairs the ventilatory response to doxapram, which acts on the peripheral chemoreceptors (page 71).[13]

Implications of the depression of AHVR by anaesthetic agents

There are four important practical implications of the attenuation of AHVR by anaesthesia.

1. Patients cannot act as their own hypoxia alarm by responding with hyperventilation.
2. Patients who have already lost their sensitivity to PCO_2 (e.g. some patients with chronic respiratory failure) may stop breathing after induction of anaesthesia has abolished their hypoxic drive.
3. Anaesthesia may be dangerous at very high altitude or in other situations where survival depends on hyperventilation in response to hypoxia (see Chapter 17).
4. Because hypoxic drive is obtunded at subanaesthetic concentrations, this effect will persist into the early postoperative period after patients have regained consciousness and are apparently able to fend for themselves.

Recent uncertainty about the effect of subanaesthetic concentrations on AHVR has cast doubt on the validity of extrapolating the results of earlier studies to patients recovering from anaesthesia. The degree of stimulation of the patient is likely to affect their AHVR response, which will therefore be affected by many factors, such as pain control and the amount of activity in their surroundings. A patient should behave like a poikilocapnic subject and so depression of AHVR will be minimal.[9,32,33] Finally, patients recovering from an anaesthetic will frequently be hypercapnic secondary to opiate administration, sometimes compounded by airway obstruction. Under these circumstances the ventilatory response to the combination of hypoxia and hypercapnia is almost certainly reduced to less than that seen when awake.

There is little doubt that more research is needed to understand the complex effects of anaesthesia on ventilatory responses.[9,10,36] Though recent work may have cast some doubt on the earlier studies of Knill *et al.*[13] (see Figure 22.4), there remains plenty of evidence that a sleeping patient in the recovery room is at risk of failing to mount a suitable ventilatory response to hypoxia.

PATTERN OF CONTRACTION OF RESPIRATORY MUSCLES

One of the most remarkable examples of the specificity of anaesthetic actions is on the muscles associated with respiration. Many of these effects could hardly have been predicted but, nevertheless, have great clinical importance and underlie many of the secondary effects described later in this chapter.

The pharynx

Anaesthesia usually causes obstruction of the pharyngeal airway unless measures are taken for its protection. Figure 22.6 shows changes in the sagittal geometry of the pharynx immediately after induction of anaesthesia with

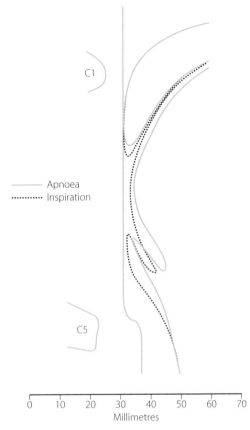

Figure 22.6 Median sagittal section of the pharynx to show changes between the conscious state (blue lines) and following induction of anaesthesia (broken lines). The most consistent change was occlusion of the nasopharynx. (Nandi PR, Charlesworth CH, Taylor SJ, Nunn JF, Doré C.J. Effect of general anaesthesia on the pharynx. *Br J Anaesth* 1991; **66**: 157–62. © The Board of Management and Trustees of the British Journal of Anaesthesia. Reproduced by permission of Oxford University Press/British Journal of Anaesthesia.)

Figure 22.7 Median sagittal section of the pharynx during anaesthesia to show changes between the apnoeic state (blue lines, corresponding to the broken lines in Figure 22.6) and following attempted inspiration (broken lines). Upstream obstruction in the nasopharynx results in downstream collapse of the oro- and hypopharynx. (Nandi PR, Charlesworth CH, Taylor SJ, Nunn JF, Doré C.J. Effect of general anaesthesia on the pharynx. *Br J Anaesth* 1991; **66**: 157–62. © The Board of Management and Trustees of the British Journal of Anaesthesia. Reproduced by permission of Oxford University Press/British Journal of Anaesthesia.)

thiopentone in the supine position.[37] The soft palate falls against the posterior pharyngeal wall, occluding the nasopharynx in almost every patient, presumably due to interference with the action of some or all of tensor palati, palatoglossus or palatopharyngeus (page 76). Similar findings are also reported using magnetic resonance imaging, when the mean anteroposterior diameter of the pharynx at the level of the soft palate decreased from 6.6 mm when awake to 2.7 mm during propofol anaesthesia.[38] Radiographic studies have shown considerable posterior movement of tongue and epiglottis, but usually not sufficient to occlude the oral or hypopharyngeal airway (see Figure 22.6). In animals, there is marked interference with genioglossus activity during anaesthesia,[39] and human observations have shown that thiopentone decreases the electromyographic (EMG)

activity of genioglossus and the strap muscles.[40] Nevertheless, Nandi *et al.*[37] showed that the posterior movement of the palate was not caused by pressure from the tongue. The changes shown in Figure 22.6 are very similar to those observed with anaesthesia and paralysis.[41]

Secondary changes occur when the patient attempts to breathe. Upstream obstruction then often causes major passive downstream collapse of the entire pharynx (Figure 22.7), a mechanism with features in common with the sleep apnoea–hyponoea syndrome (page 251). This secondary collapse of the pharynx is due to interference with the normal action of pharyngeal dilator muscles, particularly genioglossus. The epiglottis may be involved in hypopharyngeal obstruction during anaesthesia,[42] and posterior movement is clearly seen in Figures 22.6 and 22.7.

Protection of the pharyngeal airway. Extension of the neck moves the origin of genioglossus anteriorly by 1–2 cm and usually clears the hypopharyngeal airway.[41] Protrusion of the mandible, originally proposed by Heiberg in 1874,[43] moves the origin of genioglossus still further forward. The use of a pharyngeal airway, such as that of Guedel, is frequently helpful, but the tip may become lodged in the vallecula or the tongue may be pushed downwards and backwards to obstruct the tip of the airway.[44] Developed by Brain in 1983,[45] the laryngeal mask airway provides an airtight seal around the laryngeal perimeter, allowing spontaneous ventilation. Use of a laryngeal mask does not prevent regurgitated gastric contents gaining access to the larynx, and with high airway pressures, inspired gas may pass into the oesophagus or stomach during intermittent positive-pressure ventilation (IPPV). Radiographic appearances of normal and abnormal anatomical locations of the mask have been described.[46] For the most reliable maintenance of airway patency a tracheal tube is used, which requires the use of either 'deep' anaesthesia or muscle relaxants.

The inspiratory muscles[2]

John Snow's early observations of respiration during anaesthesia clearly describe that a decrease in thoracic respiratory excursion may be used as a sign of deepening anaesthesia. The effect was first quantified by Miller in 1925[47] and more precisely related to depth of anaesthesia with halothane in 1979.[48] Selective depression of some inspiratory ribcage muscles does occur. Electromyography of the parasternal intercostal muscles in humans shows their activity to be consistently abolished by 1 MAC of anaesthesia and absent in some subjects at just 0.2 MAC.[49,50] Thiopentone decreases the EMG activity of sternothyroid, sternohyoid and the scalene muscles.[40] In contrast, diaphragmatic function seems to be well preserved during anaesthesia, particularly phasic EMG activity during inspiration.

This combination of changes in muscle activity commonly gives rise to paradoxical inspiratory movements whereby diaphragmatic contraction causes expansion of the lower ribcage and abdomen, whereas the upper ribcage is drawn in due to the negative intrathoracic pressure and a lack of support from upper ribcage respiratory muscles. This pattern of breathing is seen commonly in children, who have a more compliant chest wall than adults, and in adults when respiratory resistance is increased, causing a greater decrease in intrathoracic pressure. Some studies have, however, found no reduction in ribcage movement with, for example, isoflurane

at 1 MAC[51] or ketamine.[52] It is possible that changes in spinal curvature during anaesthesia have caused earlier studies of ribcage movement to overestimate the changes.[49,53] Also, spontaneous ventilation via a tracheal tube is associated with greater airway resistance than other methods such as a laryngeal mask, which may contribute to less ribcage expansion during anaesthesia.[54] Thus earlier descriptions of selective depression of ribcage movement should not be regarded as an invariable feature of anaesthesia with spontaneous ventilation, particularly at the depth of anaesthesia used clinically and with a low-resistance, unobstructed airway. There is certainly an increased thoracic component of ventilation during IPPV of the anaesthetised paralysed patient.[55]

The resting position and dimensions of the ribcage and diaphragm during anaesthesia are described below.

The expiratory muscles[56]

General anaesthesia causes expiratory phasic activity of the abdominal muscles, which are normally silent in the conscious supine subject. Anaesthetic agents, opioids and hypercapnia are all involved in stimulating the expiratory muscle activity. This activity begins in some subjects at only 0.2 MAC of halothane[49] and is very difficult to abolish as long as spontaneous breathing continues.[57] Activation of expiratory muscles seems to serve no useful purpose and does not appear to have any significant effect on the change in functional residual capacity.[58]

Respiratory muscle coordination often becomes disturbed during anaesthesia with spontaneous ventilation.[51,54] Paradoxical movements between the upper and lower chest wall and the chest and abdominal muscles are accompanied by changes in respiratory timing between inspiratory and expiratory muscle groups. These are believed to originate in selective effects of anaesthesia on different respiratory neuronal groups in the central pattern generator[50] and are more marked when airway resistance is higher.[54] The most usual pattern seen is a phase delay between abdominal and ribcage movement, as illustrated in Figure 22.8.

CHANGE IN FUNCTIONAL RESIDUAL CAPACITY

Bergman in 1963 was the first to report a decrease of functional residual capacity (FRC) during anaesthesia.[59] This was followed by many studies, which have established the following characteristics of the change.[58,60-63]

- FRC is reduced during anaesthesia with all anaesthetic drugs that have been investigated, by a mean value of about 16–20% of the awake FRC in the supine posi-

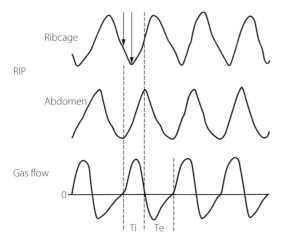

RIP

Ribcage

Abdomen

Gas flow

0

Ti Te

Figure 22.8 Respiratory inductance plethysmography (RIP) tracings of ribcage and abdominal movements during 1.5 MAC halothane anaesthesia, and the accompanying respiratory gas flows. Note the phase delay between abdominal and ribcage movements, indicated by solid arrows, which in the example shown is approximately 30% of the inspiratory time. Ti, inspiratory time; Te, expiratory time. (Reproduced with permission from Fourcade HE, Larson CP, Hickey RF et al. Effects of time on ventilation during halothane and cyclopropane anesthesia. *Anesthesiology* 1972; **36**: 83–8.)

tion. However, there is considerable individual variation and changes range from about +19% to −50%.

- FRC is reduced immediately on induction of anaesthesia, reaches its final value within the first few minutes and does not seem to fall progressively throughout anaesthesia. It does not return to normal until some hours after the end of anaesthesia.
- FRC is reduced to the same extent during anaesthesia whether the patient is paralysed or not.
- The reduction in FRC has a weak but significant correlation with the age of the patient.

The cause of the reduction in FRC

There is general agreement that there are three possible contributory factors to explain the reduced FRC, as follows.

Chest shape. Earlier studies that measured anteroposterior and lateral diameters, or the circumference, of the external chest wall gave conflicting results regarding changes in internal chest volume with anaesthesia. However, the introduction of fast computed tomography (CT) scanners led to general agreement that there is a reduction in the cross-sectional area of the ribcage corresponding to a decrease in lung volume of about 200 ml.[64,65] A dynamic spatial reconstructor (DSR) technique allows scans of half the chest to be obtained in just

0.3 s, following which a three-dimensional picture of all chest structures can be generated and analysed.[49] This has confirmed that changes in chest wall shape account for a reduction in FRC of about 200 ml. There is less agreement about why the chest wall changes shape, possible explanations including the changes in respiratory muscle activity already described, diaphragmatic position and activity, or spinal curvature.

Diaphragm position. In the conscious subject in the supine position there is evidence of residual end-expiratory tone in the diaphragm,[66] which prevents the weight of the viscera pushing the diaphragm too far into the chest in the supine position. This diaphragmatic end-expiratory tone may be lost during anaesthesia. Such a change would result in the diaphragm moving cephalad during anaesthesia, which was reported in early studies.[65,67] However, other investigators found no consistent cephalad movement of the diaphragm during anaesthesia. Studies using DSR and fast CT have provided good evidence that diaphragm *shape* alters during anaesthesia.[48,68,69] Although there is a large variation between subjects, these studies have consistently shown a cephalad movement of the dependent regions of the diaphragm, with little or no movement of the non-dependent regions.[49] One study found a significantly greater cephalad shift of the diaphragm in patients who were paralysed,[68] though this had not been observed in earlier studies. The change in FRC that can be ascribed to changes in diaphragm shape is on average less than 30 ml.[49] A summary of the changes in chest wall and diaphragm positions during anaesthesia is shown in Figure 22.9.

Thoracic blood volume. A shift of blood from the peripheral circulation into the chest during anaesthesia has been postulated as a cause of reduced FRC,[58] and one CT study seemed to demonstrate this.[77] However, this observation has not been confirmed[49,65,71] and is currently regarded as an unlikely contributory factor to the reduced FRC.

ATELECTASIS DURING ANAESTHESIA

'Miliary atelectasis' during anaesthesia was first proposed by Bendixen *et al.* in 1963 as an explanation of the increased alveolar/arterial PO_2 difference during anaesthesia.[72] Conventional radiography, however, failed to show any appreciable areas of collapse, presumably due to most atelectasis being behind the diaphragm on anteroposterior radiographs (see below). Hedenstierna's group in Sweden were the first to demonstrate pulmonary opacities on CT scans of subjects during anaesthesia. These opacities usually occurred in the dependent areas of lung just above the diaphragm and

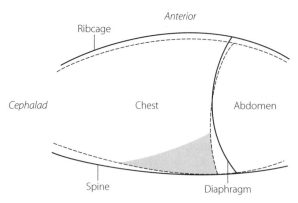

Figure 22.9 Schematic diagram showing a midsagittal section of the chest wall and diaphragm awake (solid line) and during anaesthesia (dashed line). Note the reduction in ribcage volume, increased spinal curvature and change in diaphragmatic position. The shaded area shows where atelectasis usually occurs during anaesthesia. (Reproduced with permission from Warner DO, Warner MA, Ritman EL. Atelectasis and chest wall shape during halothane anesthesia. *Anesthesiology* 1996; **85**: 49–59.)

Figure 22.10 Computed tomography of transverse sections of the thoracic cage (supine position) at the level shown in the scout view (**a**). (**b**) Control (awake) view. (**c**) Anaesthesia with zero end-expiratory pressure. Note the development of atelectasis in the dependent region of lung and some ascent of the right dome of the diaphragm. (**d**) The same patient with positive end-expiratory pressure, which reduces the amount of atelectasis. (Scans (a) and (b) are reproduced from Hedenstierna G, Tokics L, Strandberg A, Lundquist H, Brismar B. Correlation of gas exchange impairment to development of atelectasis during anaesthesia and muscle paralysis. *Acta Anaesthesiol Scand* 1986; **30**: 183–91. I am indebted to the authors for supplying the other two scans.)

were termed 'compression atelectasis' (Figure 22.10). Their extent correlated very strongly with the calculated intrapulmonary shunt.[71] Animal studies showed that the areas of opacity had a typical histological appearance of total collapse, with only moderate vascular congestion and no clear interstitial oedema.[71]

Atelectasis occurs in between 75% and 90% of healthy individuals having general anaesthesia with muscle paralysis.[61,74] It is usually quantified from a single CT scan slice, taken immediately above the dome of the right diaphragm, and expressed as the percentage of the cross-sectional area containing atelectasis. The percentage of atelectasis during anaesthesia recorded in this way seems small, usually around 3%, but the atelectatic areas contain many more alveoli per unit volume than aerated lung and this 3% of cross-sectional area equates to around 10% of lung tissue.[75]

Causes of atelectasis

There are three mechanisms involved, all closely inter-related, and it is likely that all three are involved in the formation of atelectasis *in vivo*.

Airway closure as a result of the reduced FRC may lead to atelectasis. In the supine position, the expiratory reserve volume has a mean value of approximately 1 litre in males and 600 ml in females. Therefore, the reduction in FRC following the induction of anaesthesia will bring the lung volume close to residual volume. This will tend to reduce the end-expiratory lung volume below

the closing capacity (CC), particularly in older patients (see Figure 3.10), and so result in airway closure and lung collapse. Pulmonary atelectasis can easily be demonstrated in conscious subjects who voluntarily breathe oxygen close to residual volume,[76] and Figure 22.11 shows the effect on arterial P_{O_2} of simulating the reduction in FRC that occurs during anaesthesia. Even if lung collapse does not occur, for example in younger patients, the airway narrowing caused by reduced lung volume creates areas with low ventilation/perfusion ($\dot{V}/\dot{Q}$) ratios that contribute to impaired gas exchange.[77]

An important aspect of this problem is whether CC remains constant during anaesthesia or whether it changes with FRC. Earlier studies by Hedenstierna and colleagues suggested that CC remained constant.[79] However, two other studies provided convincing evidence that FRC and CC are both reduced in parallel following the induction of anaesthesia.[80,81] It is possible that bronchodilation caused by the anaesthetic counteracts the reduction in airway calibre that would be expected to result from the reduction in FRC (see below). The results of the last two studies suggest that there should be no increased tendency towards airway closure

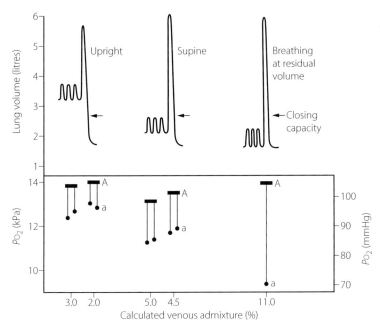

Figure 22.11 Changes in tidal excursion relative to vital capacity in Dr Nunn when aged 45; arrows indicate the closing capacity. Ideal alveolar (A) P_{O_2} is shown by the horizontal bar and arterial (a) P_{O_2} by the black circles. Venous admixture was calculated on the assumption of an arterial/mixed venous oxygen content difference of 5 ml.dl^{-1}. (Reproduced with permission from Nunn JF. Measurement of closing volume. *Acta Anaesthiol Scand Supp* 1978; **70**: 154–60.)

during anaesthesia, but this is clearly at variance with Hedenstierna's work.[77]

Compression atelectasis may occur because of changes in chest wall and diaphragm position, which lead to the transmission of high intraabdominal pressure to the chest and compression of areas of lung. As shown in Figure 22.9, the predominantly caudal distribution of atelectasis also points to a role for changes in the position of the dependent regions of the diaphragm.

Absorption atelectasis[82] develops when an airway becomes partially or totally closed and the gas contained within the pulmonary units distal to the airway is absorbed into the blood. Absorption of gas does not in itself cause atelectasis, but in effect accelerates collapse should airway closure occur from either of the preceding mechanisms. The rapid uptake of oxygen into the blood makes an important contribution to the development of absorption atelectasis (see below). The role of absorption in anaesthesia-induced atelectasis is disputed.[82]

Prevention of atelectasis[83]

Recognition of atelectasis during anaesthesia has led to great interest in ways to prevent its occurrence. Several interesting findings have emerged.

Inspired gas composition. Administration of high concentrations of oxygen during anaesthesia would be expected to promote atelectasis and there is increasing

evidence for this at a variety of stages during a general anaesthetic.

- **Preoxygenation.** An $F_{I_{O_2}}$ (fractional concentration of inspired oxygen) of 1.0 immediately prior to induction of anaesthesia leads to significantly more atelectasis than in patients with an $F_{I_{O_2}}$ of 0.3 or 0.21 during induction.[84,85] The crucial $F_{I_{O_2}}$ for worsening atelectasis seems to be above 0.6, as a recent study comparing an $F_{I_{O_2}}$ of 1.0, 0.8 or 0.6 found cross-sectional areas of atelectasis on CT scans following induction of 5.6%, 1.3% and 0.2%, respectively.[86]
- **Maintenance.** Following reexpansion of atelectasis during anaesthesia (see below), a high inspired oxygen concentration causes a more rapid recurrence of atelectasis.[87,88] However, a study comparing an $F_{I_{O_2}}$ of 0.8 or 0.3 in nitrogen throughout anaesthesia and the early postoperative period did not find any differences in oxygenation postoperatively.[89]
- **Before extubation.** Use of an $F_{I_{O_2}}$ of 1.0 before removal of the tracheal tube at the completion of surgery is associated with more CT-demonstrated atelectasis in the immediate postoperative period.[90]

Nitrous oxide. Mathematical modelling of the rate at which absorption atelectasis occurs suggests that using N_2O rather than N_2 with oxygen is unimportant.[91] Looking at diffusion of gases into and out of a closed lung unit, this model finds that the diffusion of N_2O into the lung unit from the mixed venous blood is faster than the diffusion of N_2 out of the lung unit, so its volume is maintained and collapse prevented. The *in vivo* situation is clearly more complex and clinical studies of N_2O have given conflicting results.[92,93] Partial pressures of N_2O in lung units and blood are rarely in a steady state and the time at which lung units become closed will vary, so causing unpredictable effects of N_2O on atelectasis (page 400).

Clinical implications of FI_{O_2} during anaesthesia. The use of 100% inspired oxygen before, during and at the conclusion of a general anaesthetic seems to be associated with greater severity of pulmonary atelectasis. These observations have led to the suggestion that it is time to challenge the routine use of 100% oxygen during anaesthesia.[94] Anaesthetists use 100% oxygen before induction and extubation to provide a longer period before hypoxia occurs should there be difficulty in maintaining a patent airway. However, this safety period will be shortened only slightly by preoxygenating with a FI_{O_2} of 0.8, the use of which may significantly reduce the amount of atelectasis that occurs.[86]

Positive airway pressures. Application of a tight-fitting facemask to the patient before induction allows the use of continuous positive airway pressure (CPAP) before the patient is asleep and positive end-expiratory pressure (PEEP) after induction. Using CPAP before induction may increase patient anxiety, but low levels of CPAP (6 cmH$_2$O) have been shown to abolish the formation of atelectasis[95] and also to prolong the time taken for oxygen saturation to fall to 90% during the apnoea that normally follows induction of anaesthesia.[96]

During maintenance of anaesthesia moderate levels of PEEP (10 cmH$_2$O) prevent the occurrence of atelectasis following a reexpansion manoeuvre (see below),[97] but much higher levels are needed to reexpand existing atelectasis.

Reexpansion of atelectasis

Two methods have been described to reexpand collapsed areas of lung and these are shown in Figure 22.12.

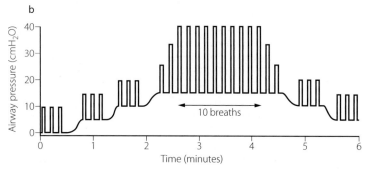

Figure 22.12 Schematic representation of manoeuvres to reexpand collapsed lung during anaesthesia. **(a)** Vital capacity manoeuvre involving three large breaths sufficient to achieve airway pressures of 30 cmH$_2$O followed by a single breath to 40 cmH$_2$O, each sustained for 15 seconds. The breaks on the abscissa represent 3–5 minutes of intermittent positive-pressure ventilation with normal tidal volume. **(b)** Positive end-expiratory pressure (PEEP) and large tidal volumes showing progressive application of PEEP up to 15 cmH$_2$O, followed by increased tidal volume until a peak airway pressure of 40 cmH$_2$O or tidal volume of 18 ml.kg^{-1} is achieved, which is then maintained for 10 breaths. (Tusman G, Böhm SH, Vazquez de Anda GF, do Campo JL, Lachmann B. 'Alveolar recruitment strategy' improves arterial oxygenation during general anaesthesia. *Br J Anaesth* 1999; **82**: 8–13 and Rothen HU, Sporre B, Engberg G, Wegenius G, Hedenstierna G. Re-expansion of atelectasis during general anaesthesia: a computed tomography study. *Br J Anaesth* 1993; **71**: 788–95. © The Board of Management and Trustees of the British Journal of Anaesthesia. Reproduced by permission of Oxford University Press/British Journal of Anaesthesia.)

Vital capacity manoeuvres. The first technique reported to reexpand atelectasis consisted of a series of hyperinflation manoeuvres using three breaths to an airway pressure of 30 cmH$_2$O followed by a final breath to 40 cmH$_2$O, each sustained for 15 seconds (Figure 22.12a).[98] Between these large breaths normal IPPV is continued for 3–5 minutes. CT assessment during this manoeuvre shows that the first hyperinflation of 30 cmH$_2$O reduces the area of atelectasis by half and the subsequent inflations to 30 cmH$_2$O have little additional effect, but the final breath to 40 cmH$_2$O completely reexpands the atelectasis. Subsequent work by the same group showed that the inflation pressure of 40 cmH$_2$O did not need to be sustained for 15 seconds, with half of the atelectasis reexpanded after only 2 seconds and all the atelactasis reexpanded after 7–8 seconds in three-quarters of patients.[100]

PEEP. High levels of PEEP are required to reexpand atelectasis. Also, resolution of atelectasis is not complete and collapse recurs within minutes when PEEP is discontinued.[101] In addition, high levels of PEEP cause significant changes to $\dot{V}/\dot{Q}$ relationships within the lung and so may not improve oxygenation of the patient. Increasing levels of PEEP are more useful if used in conjunction with large tidal volumes. One proposed technique involves increasing PEEP levels to 15 cmH$_2$O and then tidal volume is increased until peak airway pressures of 40 cmH$_2$O are achieved (Figure 22.12b).[99] This study did not use CT assessment but inferred reexpansion of atelectasis from improved arterial P_{O_2}.

In both these techniques for reexpansion of atelectasis, airway pressures reach 40 cmH$_2$O. An airway pressure this high is not without risk during anaesthesia, including the possibility of cardiovascular disturbances and pulmonary barotrauma (see Chapter 32). In a similar fashion to PEEP, these recruitment manoeuvres reduce intrapulmonary shunt, but increase $\dot{V}/\dot{Q}$ mismatch such that there is often only a small improvement in oxygenation (see below).[98,99] Obese subjects develop greater amounts of atelectasis during anaesthesia and hyperinflation is particularly effective in these patients, often leading to a sustained improvement in oxygenation.[88,98]

RESPIRATORY MECHANICS[102]

Calibre of the lower airways[103]

Effect of reduced FRC. Figures 4.5 and 22.13 both show the hyperbolic relationship between lung volume and airway resistance. Figure 22.13 clearly shows that the curve is steep in the region of FRC in the supine position, and therefore the reduction in FRC that occurs during anaesthesia might be expected to result in a marked increase in airway resistance. However, most anaesthetics are bronchodilators, as outlined in the following paragraphs, and, at least with halothane, this effect almost exactly offsets the effect of reduction in lung volume.[104] Thus total respiratory system resistance during anaesthesia is only slightly greater than in the awake supine subject, most of the change occurring in the lung/airway components rather than the chest wall

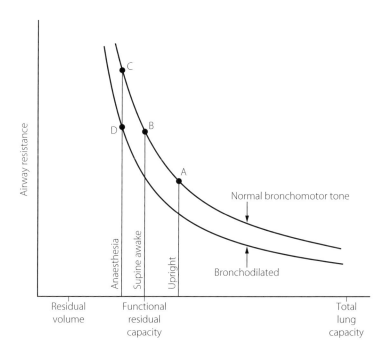

Figure 22.13 Airway resistance as a function of lung volume with normal bronchomotor tone and when bronchodilated. A = upright and awake; B = supine and awake; C = supine and anaesthetised without bronchodilation; D = supine, anaesthetised, and with the degree of bronchodilation that normally occurs during anaesthesia. Note that the airway resistance is similar at B and D, bronchodilation approximately compensating for the decrease in FRC.

Table 22.1 Respiratory mechanics during anaesthesia

Compliance (static)	Anaesthetised		Awake normal range	
	$l.kPa^{-1}$	$ml.cmH_2O^{-1}$	$l.kPa^{-1}$	$ml.cmH_2O^{-1}$
Respiratory system	0.81	81	0.5–1.9	47–190
Lungs	1.5	150	0.9–4.0	90–400
Chest wall	2.0	203	1.0–3.5	100–350
Resistance	$kPa.l^{-1}.s$	$cmH_2O.l^{-1}.s$	$kPa.l^{-1}.s$	$cmH_2O.l^{-1}.s$
Respiratory system	0.48	4.8	0.12–0.44	1.2–4.4
Lung tissue/airway	0.35	3.5	0.07–0.24	0.7–2.4
Chest wall	0.13	1.3	0.05–0.20	0.5–2.0

Data during anaesthesia are in the supine position from reference 105.

(Table 22.1).[105] As would be expected, resistance increases with increasing flow rate and decreases with increasing inflation volume during anaesthesia.[106]

Inhalational anaesthetics. All inhalational anaesthetics investigated have shown bronchodilator effects. Suppression of airway vagal reflexes, direct relaxation of airway smooth muscle[107] and inhibition of release of bronchoconstrictor mediators combine to cause an increase in airway conductance. In clinical concentrations, halothane reduces the amount of acetylcholine released from nerve terminals in response to nerve stimulation[108] and suppresses the increase in both airway and tissue resistance following vagal stimulation.[104] This appears to be more important than the direct effect of clinical concentrations of halothane on airway smooth muscle or histamine release from mast cells.[103]

Intravenous anaesthetics have similar effects to the inhalational anaesthetics. Their direct effects on smooth muscle are mostly weak in comparison with inhaled agents, and in clinical practice their ability to attenuate neural reflex bronchoconstriction predominates.

Other sites of increased airway resistance

Breathing systems. Excessive resistance or obstruction may arise in apparatus such as breathing systems, valves, connectors and tracheal tubes. The tubes may be kinked, the lumen may be blocked or the cuff may herniate and obstruct the lower end, which may also abut against the carina or the side wall of the trachea. A reduction in diameter of a tracheal tube greatly increases its resistance, the pattern of flow being intermediate between laminar and turbulent for the conditions shown in Figure 22.14. Resistance imposed by a laryngeal mask airway is less than that of a corresponding size of tracheal tube.[109]

The pharynx and larynx. The pharynx is commonly obstructed during anaesthesia by the mechanisms described earlier in this chapter, unless active steps are taken to preserve patency. Reflex laryngospasm is still possible at depths of anaesthesia that suppress other airway protective reflexes. In most cases the spasm eventually resolves spontaneously, but it may be improved by application of CPAP or terminated by neuromuscular blockade.

Compliance

Total respiratory system compliance is reduced during anaesthesia to a figure approaching the lower end of the normal range (see Table 22.1).[105] Both static and dynamic measurements (page 35) are reduced compared with the awake state.[106] Compliance seems to be reduced very early in anaesthesia and the change is not progressive.

Figure 22.15 summarises the effect of anaesthesia on the pressure/volume relationships of the lung and chest wall. The diagram shows the major differences between the conscious state and anaesthesia. There are only minor differences between anaesthesia with and without paralysis. The left-hand section shows the relationship for the whole respiratory system comprising lungs plus chest wall. The curves obtained during anaesthesia clearly show the reduction in FRC (lung volume with zero pressure gradient from alveoli to ambient). Application of a positive pressure as high as 30 cmH_2O (3 kPa) to the airways expands the lungs to barely 70% of their preoperative total capacity, which implies a reduced overall compliance. Table 22.1 and the two sections on the right of Figure 22.15 show that the major changes are in the lung rather than the chest wall.

Cause of the reduced compliance. The change seems to be due mainly to a reduction in pulmonary compliance, the cause of which has been difficult to explain. There

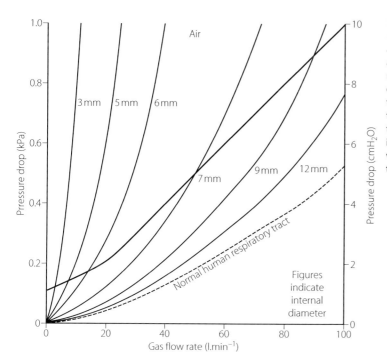

Figure 22.14 Flow rate/pressure drop plots of a range of tracheal tubes, with their connectors and catheter mounts. The heavy line is the author's suggested upper limit of acceptable resistance for an adult. Pressure drop does not quite increase according to the fourth power of the radius because the catheter mount offered the same resistance throughout the range of tubes. With 70% N_2O/30% O_2, the pressure drop is about 40% greater for the same gas flow rate when flow is turbulent, but little different when the flow is chiefly laminar.

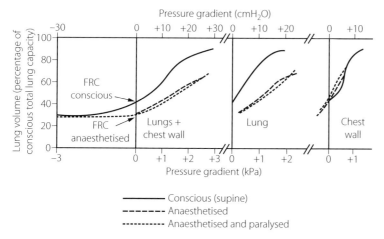

Figure 22.15 Pressure/volume relationships before and after the induction of anaesthesia and paralysis. The first section shows the relationship for the respiratory system (lungs and chest wall) The second and third sections represent the lungs and the chest wall, respectively. There are only insignificant differences between observations during anaesthesia with and without paralysis. There are, however, major differences in pressure/volume relationships of the lung and total respiratory system following the induction of anaesthesia. Arrows indicate the FRC which, during anaesthesia, is only slightly greater than the residual volume. (After reference 110.)

is no convincing evidence that anaesthesia affects pulmonary surfactant in humans at clinically used concentrations. A more likely explanation is that the reduced lung compliance is simply the consequence of breathing at reduced lung volume. Strapping the chest of volunteers, thereby decreasing their lung volume, results in a decrease in pulmonary compliance that can be restored to normal by taking a maximal inspiration.[111] This suggests that partial pulmonary atelectasis is the explanation, and the common occurrence of atelectasis during anaesthesia makes this the most likely cause of the reduced compliance.

GAS EXCHANGE

Every factor influencing gas exchange may be altered during anaesthesia and many of the changes must be considered as normal features of the anaesthetised state. These 'normal' changes usually pose no threat to the patient, since their effects can easily be overcome by such simple means as increasing the concentration of oxygen in the inspired gas and the minute volume. The 'normal' changes may be contrasted with a range of pathological alterations in gas exchange that may arise during anaesthesia from circumstances such as airway obstruction, apnoea, bronchospasm or tension pneumothorax. These may be life threatening and require urgent action for their correction.

The major changes that adversely affect gas exchange during anaesthesia are reduced minute volume of ventilation (described above), increased dead space and shunt (considered in terms of the three-compartment model described on page 116 and in Figure 8.8) and altered distribution of ventilation and perfusion in relation to ventilation/perfusion ratios.

Physiological dead space (see page 120)

The increase in physiological dead space during anaesthesia was first observed in 1958[112] and subsequently confirmed in many studies. With allowance for the apparatus dead space of the tracheal tube and its connections, the dead space/tidal volume ratio *from carina downwards* averages 32% during anaesthesia with either spontaneous or artificial ventilation.[113] This is approximately equal to the ratio for the normal conscious subject, *including trachea, pharynx and mouth* (approximately 70 ml). Physiological dead space equals the sum of its anatomical and alveolar components and the subcarinal anatomical dead space is not normally increased. There-

fore, the increase in subcarinal physiological dead space during anaesthesia must be in the alveolar component.

Anatomical dead space. In the study of Nunn and Hill[113] (Figure 22.16), subcarinal anatomical dead space was always significantly less than physiological, reaching a maximum of about 70 ml at tidal volumes above 350 ml. This roughly accords with the expected geometric dimensions of the lower respiratory tract. At smaller tidal volumes, the anatomical dead space was less than the expected geometric volume. Values of less than 30 ml were recorded in some patients with tidal volumes of less than 250 ml. This is attributed to axial streaming and the mixing effect of the heart beat, and is clearly an important and beneficial factor in patients with depressed breathing.

Alveolar dead space increases with tidal volume so that the sum of anatomical and alveolar (= physiological) dead space remains about 32% of tidal volume (see Figure 22.16). The cause of the increase in alveolar dead space during uncomplicated general anaesthesia is not immediately obvious. There is no evidence that it is due to pulmonary hypotension causing development of a zone 1 (page 97), and the reduced vertical height of the lung in the supine position would militate against this. The alternative explanation is maldistribution with overventilation of *relatively* underperfused alveoli. Studies of ventilation/perfusion relationships outlined below give some support to this view, but such patterns of maldistribution have not invariably been observed during anaesthesia.

Apparatus dead space. Use of a tracheal tube or laryngeal mask airway (LMA) will bypass much of the normal anatomical dead space arising in the mouth and pharynx.

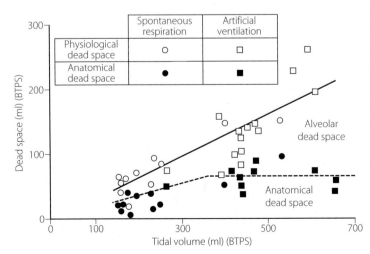

Figure 22.16 Data and regression lines for physiological and anatomical dead space (the difference indicating alveolar dead space) as a function of tidal volume. There were no significant differences between anaesthesia with and without paralysis. Note the range over which physiological dead space appeared to be a constant fraction of tidal volume. Anatomical dead space was constant above a tidal volume of 350 ml, resulting in increased alveolar dead space. (After reference 113 by permission of the Editor and publishers of the *Journal of Applied Physiology*.)

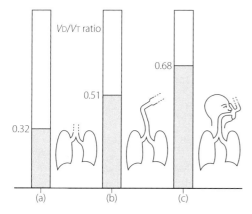

Figure 22.17 Physiological plus apparatus dead space (where applicable) as a fraction of tidal volume in anaesthetised patients: **(a)** from carina downwards; **(b)** including tracheal tube or laryngeal mask airway and connector; and **(c)** including upper airway, facemask and connector.

However, for practical purposes the apparatus dead space of the tracheal tube or LMA[114] and their connections must be included for the purpose of calculating alveolar ventilation during anaesthesia. The total dead space then increases to about 50% of tidal volume (Figure 22.17). When using a facemask, it is necessary to add the volume of the mask and its connections to the physiological dead space, which now also includes trachea, pharynx and mouth. The total dead space then amounts to about two-thirds of the tidal volume.[115] Thus, a seemingly adequate minute volume of 6 l.min^{-1} may be expected to result in an alveolar ventilation of only 2 l.min^{-1}, which would almost inevitably result in hypercapnia.

Compensation for increased dead space may be made by increasing the minute volume to maintain the alveolar ventilation. In artificially ventilated anaesthetised patients the problem hardly exists. The patient may have a large dead space, but the high minute volumes that are usually selected provide more than adequate compensation. Thus the alveolar ventilation is almost always greater than necessary for carbon dioxide homoeostasis. With monitoring of end-expiratory PCO_2, there is very seldom any difficulty in maintaining a value in the range 4–5 kPa (30–37.5 mmHg). However, the existence of an alveolar dead space means that the arterial PCO_2 during anaesthesia is usually 0.5–1 kPa (3.8–7.5 mmHg) greater than the end-expiratory PCO_2.

In the case of the hypoventilating patient who is allowed to breathe spontaneously during anaesthesia, the reduction in dead space at smaller tidal volumes shown in Figure 22.16 prevents some of the alveolar hypoventilation that would be expected if the *volume* of the dead space remained constant. This, together with the reduced metabolic rate, results in the hypercapnia being much less than the values for minute volume sometimes observed during anaesthesia might lead one to expect. No doubt, over the years, many patients have owed their lives to these factors.

Shunt

Magnitude of the change during anaesthesia. In the conscious healthy subject, the shunt or venous admixture amounts to only 1–2% of cardiac output (page 122). This results in an alveolar/arterial PO_2 gradient of less than 1 kPa (7.5 mmHg) in the young healthy subject breathing air, but the gradient increases with age. During anaesthesia, the alveolar/arterial PO_2 difference is usually increased to a value that corresponds to an average shunt of about 10%. Figure 22.18 shows the mean values for shunt, taken from a large number of different studies, plotted on the iso-shunt diagram, which is explained on page 124. Throughout the range of inspired oxygen concentrations, the means for the studies are grouped along the 10% shunt line. Formal measurements of pulmonary venous admixture, taking into account the mixed venous oxygen content, have also been made and these concur with shunts being of the order of 10%. This provides an acceptable basis for predicting arterial PO_2 during an uncomplicated anaesthetic, and it also permits calculation of the concentration of oxygen in the inspired gas that will provide an acceptable arterial PO_2. Some 30–40% inspired oxygen is usually adequate in an uncomplicated anaesthetic.

The cause of the venous admixture during anaesthesia. About half of the observed venous admixture is true shunt through the areas of atelectasis described above. There is a very strong correlation between the shunt (measured as perfusion of alveoli with a $\dot{V}/\dot{Q}$ ratio of less than 0.005) and the area or volume of atelectasis seen on CT scans.[61,64] Studies using isotope techniques have demonstrated intrapulmonary shunting in the same areas of lung where atelectasis is seen on CT scans.[124] However, the venous admixture during anaesthesia also contains components due to dispersion of the $\dot{V}/\dot{Q}$ distribution and to perfusion of alveoli with low $\dot{V}/\dot{Q}$ ratios (0.005–0.1).

Ventilation/perfusion relationships[125]

The three-compartment model of the lung (page 116) provides a definition of lung function in terms of dead space and shunt, parameters that are easily measured, reproducible, and provide a basis for corrective therapy. Nevertheless, it does not pretend to provide a true picture of what is going on in the lung. A far more

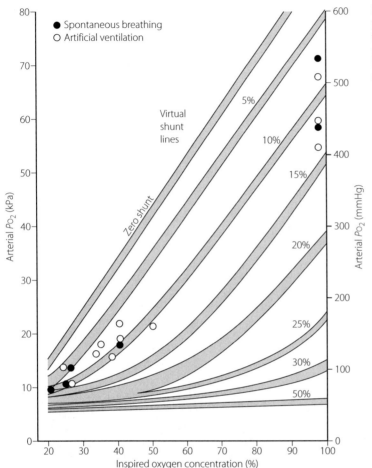

Figure 22.18 Mean values for arterial P_{O_2} are plotted against inspired oxygen concentrations for 18 published studies of anaesthetised patients, using the same coordinates as in Figure 8.11. (Data from references 63, 64,116–123.)

sophisticated approach is provided by analysis of the distribution of pulmonary ventilation and perfusion in terms of $\dot{V}/\dot{Q}$ ratios by the multiple inert gas elimination technique (page 115), and many studies during anaesthesia have been reported.[64,77,125]

During general anaesthesia and paralysis both ventilation and perfusion are found to be distributed to a wider range of $\dot{V}/\dot{Q}$ ratios than when awake (Figure 22.19).[84,126] Other studies have also found substantial $\dot{V}/\dot{Q}$ mismatch during anaesthesia and paralysis, with ventilation being distributed preferentially to ventral areas and vice versa for perfusion.[124] In the healthy young subject shown in Figure 22.19, the true intrapulmonary shunt had a mean value of less than 1% during anaesthesia, but the alveolar/arterial P_{O_2} gradient was slightly increased, and this was attributed to the increased spread of the distribution of perfusion to areas of poorer ventilation (lower $\dot{V}/\dot{Q}$ ratio). Anatomical dead space was reduced, largely because of tracheal intubation, but alveolar dead space was increased, partly due to increased spread of distribution of ventilation to areas of poorer perfusion (higher $\dot{V}/\dot{Q}$ ratio).

Effect of age on $\dot{V}/\dot{Q}$ ratios during anaesthesia. In awake subjects, increasing age causes a widening of the distribution of $\dot{V}/\dot{Q}$ ratios and the distribution widens still further with anaesthesia.[64] It would thus be expected that intrapulmonary shunt during anaesthesia would also increase with age, but studies of this effect have produced conflicting results. One study involving typical surgical patients with ages ranging from 37 to 64 found that the true intrapulmonary shunt was increased during anaesthesia.[123] However, the shunt calculated from the alveolar/arterial P_{O_2} gradient according to the three-compartment lung model would be larger still and the difference would be due to perfusion of areas of low $\dot{V}/\dot{Q}$ ratio. A second study of elderly patients (mean age 60) who all had some deterioration in pulmonary function showed wide variations in pulmonary shunt.[128] The results of this study can most easily be appreciated by considering the patients in three groups (Figure 22.20). In the first, there was only a small increase in the true shunt following the induction of anaesthesia, but there appeared a 'shelf' of perfusion of regions with very low $\dot{V}/\dot{Q}$ ratios in the range 0.01–0.1. In the second group,

Figure 22.19 Distribution of ventilation and perfusion as a function of ventilation/perfusion ratios in the awake and anaesthetised paralysed subject. (Adapted from reference 126 and reproduced from reference 127 by permission of the publishers.)

Mean values		
$\dot{Q}s/\dot{Q}t$	0%	0.9%
V_D/V_T	35%	26%
Pa_{O_2}	143 mmHg	117 mmHg

$F_{I_{O_2}}$ 30%
Age range 24–33

Figure 22.20 Changes in pulmonary perfusion as a function of ventilation/perfusion ratios following induction of anaesthesia in elderly patients. Numbers to the left of each block indicate the shunt. (Adapted from reference 128 and reproduced from reference 127 by permission of the publishers.)

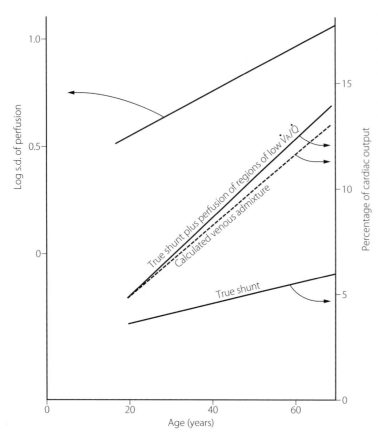

Figure 22.21 Age dependence of various factors influencing alveolar/arterial P_{O_2} difference during anaesthesia.[64] The logarithm of standard deviation of distribution of perfusion is significantly greater during anaesthesia (shown) than when awake (not shown) and has a significant regression against age under both circumstances. True shunt is significantly increased almost tenfold compared with before anaesthesia, but the correlation with age is not significant. Perfusion of areas of poorly ventilated regions ($0.005 < \dot{V}/\dot{Q} < 0.1$) was significantly increased compared with before anaesthesia and correlated with age in both circumstances. Venous admixture here refers to the value obtained from the shunt equation (page 122) and agrees well with the sum of shunt and perfusion of regions of low $\dot{V}/\dot{Q}$.

this 'shelf' was less prominent but there was a substantial increase in true shunt. Finally, in the third group, there was both a 'shelf' and an increase in true shunt. All of these changes are compatible with a decrease in FRC below closing capacity.

Finally, a study by Gunnarsson *et al.*[64] involved 45 patients of age range 23–69 years. They reached the surprising conclusion that atelectasis (as seen with CT) and true intrapulmonary shunt (determined by multiple inert gas elimination technique as alveoli with $\dot{V}/\dot{Q}$ ratio less than 0.005) did not relate to age. However, both were substantially increased during anaesthesia and correlated with each other. It is difficult to reconcile the lack of correlation between age and shunt with the striking differences seen in previous studies. Nevertheless, this study confirmed the enhanced decline in arterial P_{O_2} with increasing age during anaesthesia and venous admixture (calculated as for the three-compartment model) was increased significantly, from a mean value of 5.5% of cardiac output before anaesthesia to 9.2% during anaesthesia. Venous admixture increased steeply with age (0.17% per year), and this was attributed to an age-dependent increase in the spread of $\dot{V}/\dot{Q}$ ratios (Figure 22.21) and to greater perfusion of alveoli with low $\dot{V}/\dot{Q}$ ratios (0.005–0.1).

Effect of PEEP. It has long been known that, in contrast to the situation in intensive care, PEEP often does little to improve the arterial P_{O_2} during anaesthesia.[119] There are two reasons why PEEP is not associated with improved oxygenation. First, the decrease in cardiac output associated with PEEP reduces the saturation of the blood traversing the remaining shunt and so reduces arterial P_{O_2}.[123] Second, PEEP increases ventilation of alveoli with high $\dot{V}/\dot{Q}$ ratios, so further increasing overall $\dot{V}/\dot{Q}$ mismatch. The essential difference from the patient undergoing critical care is probably the lack of protection of intrathoracic blood vessels from raised airway pressure that is afforded by stiff lungs in most patients requiring critical care.

Other factors affecting $\dot{V}/\dot{Q}$ ratio during anaesthesia. Hypoxic pulmonary vasoconstriction (HPV) contributes to maintaining a normal $\dot{V}/\dot{Q}$ ratio by reducing perfusion to underventilated alveoli (see Chapter 7, pages 101 *et seq.*). Inhalational anaesthetics inhibit HPV (see below) and so may worsen $\dot{V}/\dot{Q}$ mismatch during anaesthesia. There is some evidence from animal studies that this is the case[125] and one human study of anaesthesia with intravenous barbiturates, which are believed to have less effect on HPV, demonstrated only a small amount of

Table 22.2 Changes in factors influencing gas exchange after induction of anaesthesia

| | Awake | Anaesthetised | | |
		Spontaneous ventilation	IPPV	IPPV + PEEP
FI_{O_2}	0.21	0.4	0.4	0.4
$\dot{Q}s/\dot{Q}t$ (%)	1.6	6.2	8.6	4.1
VD/VT (%)	30	35	38	44
Cardiac output (l.min^{-1})	6.1	5.0	4.5	3.7
Pa_{O_2} (kPa)	10.5	17.6	18.8	20.5
Pa_{O_2} (mmHg)	79	132	141	153
$\dot{V}$ – mean $\dot{V}/\dot{Q}$	0.81	1.3	2.20	3.03
$\dot{Q}$ – mean $\dot{V}/\dot{Q}$	0.47	0.51	0.83	0.55

Adapted from reference 123 and reproduced from reference 127 by permission of the publishers.

intrapulmonary shunting.[129] High concentrations of inspired oxygen will inhibit HPV by maintaining alveolar P_{O_2} at a high level even in poorly ventilated alveoli. Some work has shown that lower inspired oxygen concentrations during anaesthesia (30%) are associated with less $\dot{V}/\dot{Q}$ scatter than when breathing 100% oxygen.[84]

Summary

These studies of $\dot{V}/\dot{Q}$ relationships during anaesthesia complement one another and give us a greatly increased insight into the effect of anaesthesia on gas exchange. We are now in a position to summarise the effect of anaesthesia on gas exchange as follows.

• Uniformity of distribution of ventilation and perfusion is decreased by anaesthesia. The magnitude of the change is age related and may be affected by the inspired oxygen concentration and anaesthetic agents used.
• The increase in alveolar dead space appears to be due to increased distribution of ventilation to areas of high (but not usually infinite) $\dot{V}/\dot{Q}$ ratios.
• Venous admixture is increased in anaesthesia to a mean value of about 10%, but the change is markedly affected by age, being minimal in the young.
• The increased venous admixture during anaesthesia is due partly to an increase in true intrapulmonary shunt (due to atelectasis) and partly to increased distribution of perfusion to areas of low (but not zero) $\dot{V}/\dot{Q}$ ratios. The latter component increases with age.
• The major differences are between the awake and the anaesthetised states. Paralysis and artificial ventilation do not greatly alter the parameters of gas

exchange in spite of the different spatial distribution of ventilation.
• Both PEEP and lung hyperinflation manoeuvres reduce the shunt, but the beneficial effect on arterial P_{O_2} is offset by greater $\dot{V}/\dot{Q}$ mismatch and a decrease in cardiac output which reduces the mixed venous oxygen content.

Typical values for the various factors discussed are shown in Table 22.2.

OTHER EFFECTS OF GENERAL ANAESTHESIA ON THE RESPIRATORY SYSTEM

Response to added resistance

The preceding sections would lead one to expect that anaesthesia would cause grave impairment of patients' ability to increase their work of breathing in the face of added resistance. Surprisingly, this is not the case and anaesthetised patients preserve a remarkable ability to overcome added resistance.[130,131]

The anaesthetised patient responds to inspiratory loading in two phases. First, there is an instant augmentation of the force of contraction of the inspiratory muscles, mainly the diaphragm, during the first loaded breath.[66] This has the appearance of a typical spindle reflex (page 82). Detection of the inspiratory resistance may be mediated by either airway or lung receptors and is only slightly inhibited by anaesthesia.[132] The second response is much slower and overshoots when the loading is removed, and the time course suggests that this is mediated by an increase in P_{CO_2}.[130] In combination, these two mechanisms enable the anaesthetised

Table 22.3 Predicted values for oxygen consumption and carbon dioxide output during uncomplicated anaesthesia (ml.min^{-1}, STPD)

Age	Oxygen consumption			Carbon dioxide production		
	Small patient	Average patient	Large patient	Small patient	Average patient	Large patient
Male						
14–15		190			152	
16–17		200			160	
18–19	168	210	252	134	168	202
20–29	162	203	243	130	162	194
30–39	162	203	243	130	162	194
40–49	158	198	237	126	158	190
50–59	155	194	233	124	155	186
60–69	150	187	224	120	159	179
Female						
14–15		174			139	
16–17		188			150	
18–19	156	194	233	125	155	186
20–29	152	190	228	122	152	182
30–39	150	187	224	120	150	179
40–49	148	184	221	118	147	177
50–59	144	180	216	115	144	173
60–69	140	175	210	112	140	168

Values for CO_2 output will apply only in a steady respiratory state.
Values are probably about 6% lower during artificial ventilation.
Figures are based on 85% of basal according to the data of reference 134.

patient to achieve good compensation with inspiratory loading up to about 0.8 kPa (8 cmH$_2$O). Even more remarkable is the preservation of the elaborate response to expiratory resistance (see Figure 4.10), with a large *increase* in minute volume occurring with expiratory resistive loading during enflurane anaesthesia.[133]

Metabolic rate

During anaesthesia, the metabolic rate is reduced about 15% below basal according to the conventional standards developed over 70 years ago.[134] However, these standards do not stipulate sedation or any period of rest. In 1952, new standards were proposed for metabolic rate,[135] based on 3 hours' rest, with or without sedation. These values are about 15% below the conventional standards and so correspond fairly closely to those of the anaesthetised patient.[136] Table 22.3 lists expected values for oxygen consumption and carbon dioxide output during uncomplicated anaesthesia at normal body temperature (mean 36.5°C). In comparison with the conscious subject, there are major reductions in cerebral and cardiac oxygen consumptions during anaesthesia.

Hypoxic pulmonary vasoconstriction[137,138]

The contribution to $\dot{V}/\dot{Q}$ mismatch of disturbed HPV during anaesthesia has already been described above, but the effects of anaesthesia on HPV merit further discussion. Early animal studies using isolated lungs found that several inhalational anaesthetics inhibit HPV, but no such effect was found with intravenous anaesthetics. Although *in vitro* studies gave clear evidence that inhalational anaesthetics depressed HPV, *in vivo* studies were inconsistent. One cause of this inconsistency was found to be the concomitant depression of cardiac output by inhalational anaesthetics.[137] In Chapter 7 it was explained how hypoxia influences pulmonary vascular resistance not only by the alveolar PO_2 but also, in part, by the mixed venous PO_2. A reduction in cardiac output must decrease the mixed venous PO_2 if oxygen consumption remains unchanged and this would intensify pulmonary vasoconstriction. Thus, on the one hand, an inhalational anaesthetic will inhibit HPV by direct action while, on the other hand, it may intensify HPV by reducing mixed venous PO_2 as a result of decreasing cardiac output. Thus most investigators' results are consistent with the view that inhalational anaesthetics depress HPV provided that allowance is made for the effect of concomitant changes of cardiac output.[137] Most studies have found that intravenous anaesthesia with propofol has no effect on HPV.[139,140]

Quantitative effect of inhalational anaesthetics. Suppression of HPV by inhalational anaesthetics follows a typical sigmoid dose/response curve with an effective dose for 50% suppression (ED_{50}) of slightly less than 2 MAC and an ED_{90} of 3 MAC.[141] Thus, during a typical anaesthetic at 1.3 MAC, HPV is only attenuated by about 30%. There are no major differences between the volatile anaesthetics. Nitrous oxide (0.3 MAC) has a slight but significant effect.

SPECIAL CONDITIONS ARISING DURING ANAESTHESIA

Patient position

Lateral. In Chapter 8 it was explained that, in the lateral position, there is preferential distribution of inspired gas to the lower lung (see Table 8.1) and this accords approximately with the distribution of pulmonary blood flow. This favourable distribution of inspired gas is disturbed by anaesthesia whether respiration is spontaneous or artificial in the paralysed patient, with preferential ventilation of the non-dependent (upper) lung and continued preferential perfusion of the dependent lung. This predictably leads to a greater spread of $\dot{V}/\dot{Q}$ ratios and a further fall in PO_2 compared with the supine position.[142] Atelectasis seen on CT scanning forms only in the dependent lung, but the overall amount of atelectasis and the intrapulmonary shunt are similar to those seen when anaesthetised and paralysed when supine.[142]

Prone. A patient anaesthetised in the prone position should have the upper chest and pelvis supported, to allow free movement of the abdomen and lower chest. In subjects anaesthetised and paralysed in this position, respiratory mechanics are only minimally affected and both FRC and arterial PO_2 are greater than when supine.[105] A study using the DSR showed that with anaesthesia in the prone position, motion of non-dependent areas of the diaphragm predominates, leading the authors to suggest a difference in the anatomical structure between dorsal and ventral areas of the diaphragm.[69] Other explanations for improved oxygenation when prone include more uniform lung perfusion (page 115) and less ventilation of, or atelectasis formation in, dependent areas of lung that are reduced in volume by the presence of the mediastinum and heart.[105]

Lithotomy. In awake subjects the lithotomy position has little affect on FRC, $\dot{V}/\dot{Q}$ relationships or shunt, although some overweight subjects in lithotomy position with an epidural anaesthetic may develop atelectasis or increased shunt.[143]

One-lung ventilation (OLV)[140,144]

Surgical procedures involving the lungs, oesophagus and thoracic spine are made possible by the ability to stop the ventilation of one lung. This is normally achieved with a double-lumen tube, with the lumen connected to the non-ventilated lung being left open to atmosphere. The non-ventilated lung will then collapse, particularly when the pleura is open to the atmosphere. The physiology of OLV is complicated by the fact that most thoracic surgery is performed with the patient in the lateral position, though procedures in which OLV is required while supine are becoming more common.

Ventilation. Minute volume of ventilation during OLV is maintained at the same level as during normal ventilation, to ensure adequate CO_2 removal, but usually using a slightly smaller tidal volume (7–10 ml.kg^{-1}) and faster respiratory rate. In the lateral position, when one side of the chest is opened, the exposed lung may receive a very large proportion of the total ventilation during IPPV. Ventilation of the upper lung should therefore be stopped as soon as possible. In addition, with the non-dependent chest cavity open, the weight of the mediastinum compresses the dependent, ventilated lung, decreasing its compliance.

Perfusion. There is seldom difficulty in maintaining a satisfactory PCO_2 but oxygenation is usually compromised within a few minutes of commencing OLV. In the lateral position, gravity results in preferential perfusion of the ventilated dependent lung. Although this reduces blood flow through the collapsed lung, it is not zero and often there is a substantial shunt, usually in the range 30–50%. With OLV in the supine position this effect is absent and blood flow to the two lungs is much more even, resulting in a greater shunt and an increased alveolar/arterial PO_2 gradient in patients with lung disease.[145]

Preventing hypoxia during OLV. The surgery being performed has some bearing on the likely amount of hypoxia occurring during OLV.[144] Surgery requiring collapse of the left lung is associated with less severe hypoxia owing to the larger size of, and blood flow to, the right lung. Patients having thoracic surgery for lung resection also have less severe hypoxia, an observation believed to result from reduced blood flow through diseased lung tissue.

Strategies used to maintain oxygenation during OLV are aimed at reducing the shunt through the non-ventilated lung and maintaining good ventilation and perfusion of the ventilated lung. Suggested interventions are numerous and include the following.

- Ensuring that the double-lumen tube is positioned correctly. Current practice involves the routine use of fibreoptic bronchoscopy to confirm tube position.
- Increased FI_{O_2} will improve oxygenation in the dependent lung, particularly in areas with low $\dot{V}/\dot{Q}$ ratio, which are likely to exist in the dependent lung. However, the use of an FI_{O_2} of 1.0 may exacerbate the formation of atelectasis in the dependent lung and worsen the overall pulmonary shunt.
- PEEP may be used to prevent atelectasis formation in the dependent lung. The amount of PEEP used is crucial, with increasing levels of PEEP usually reducing arterial P_{O_2} by diverting more blood to the non-ventilated lung and reducing cardiac output. A compromise PEEP value must therefore be used, which is believed to be approximately 5 cmH$_2$O and referred to as 'best' PEEP.[146] Patients with lung disease may develop intrinsic PEEP (page 431) during OLV, and the application of further PEEP in these patients requires caution. If atelectasis has developed, then a reexpansion manoeuvre as described above may need to be performed and PEEP used to prevent recurrence of collapse.
- Ensuring adequate collapse of the non-ventilated lung. In an inflated but non-ventilated lung, pulmonary vessels are dilated by the elastic forces within the lung (see Figure 7.4) and residual oxygen in the alveoli attenuates HPV. If surgery involves resection of part or the whole of the lung then efforts should be made expedite surgical ligation of the pulmonary vessels.
- Enhancement of HPV in the non-ventilated lung. Anaesthetic techniques that avoid inhalational agents, such as a propofol infusion, may cause less severe reductions in oxygenation.[147,148] Recently, pharmacological techniques to augment HPV have been described, with one study using intravenous almitrine reporting encouraging results.[149]
- Apnoeic oxygenation of the non-ventilated lung often improves P_{O_2}, presumably by oxygenating blood flowing through the non-ventilated lung, despite the possibility of this abolishing HPV and so increasing shunt. Small amounts of CPAP applied to the non-ventilated lung are also effective at improving oxygenation, possibly by diverting blood flow away from the non-ventilated lung.

Laparoscopic surgery[150,151]

In comparison with open surgery, the benefits of laparoscopic cholecystectomy are now well established and have led to an expansion in the number of surgical procedures carried out via laparoscopy. As confidence in and

understanding of the technique improve, procedures become more complex, more prolonged, and are attempted in less fit patients.

Absorption of gas from the peritoneal cavity depends on the partial pressure of gas present and its solubility in peritoneal tissue. Gas mixtures are rarely used, so the partial pressure is normally equal to the insufflation pressure. Insoluble gases such as helium or nitrogen would be absorbed to a much smaller extent, but would also be more disastrous during the rare complication of gas embolus. Air, oxygen and nitrous oxide all support combustion and so prevent the use of diathermy, which is fundamental to laparoscopic surgery. Thus carbon dioxide remains the usual gas used for the erroneously named 'pneumoperitoneum'. Laparoscopic operations involve the insufflation of CO_2 into the peritoneum to a pressure of 10–15 mmHg, and normally also involve positioning the patient head-up (for upper abdominal surgery) or head-down (for lower abdominal and pelvic procedures). These procedures have two adverse effects on respiration.

Respiratory mechanics. In addition to the changes already described for general anaesthesia, the increased intraabdominal pressure during laparoscopy causes further restriction of the diaphragm and lower chest wall. Respiratory system compliance is significantly reduced,[150] sometimes accompanied by increased airway resistance, particularly in obese patients.[152] An increase in airway pressures invariably occurs. The head-up position may alleviate some of these changes, but patients in the head-down position during laparoscopy have a further cause for substantially reduced compliance. In healthy patients, these significant changes in respiratory system mechanics have only a small effect on $\dot{V}/\dot{Q}$ distribution. A study of nine healthy patients using MIGET to characterise $\dot{V}/\dot{Q}$ ratios found only a transient reduction in pulmonary shunt and no significant changes in alveolar dead space or in areas of abnormally high or low $\dot{V}/\dot{Q}$ ratios.[153]

Carbon dioxide absorption.[154] Transperitoneal absorption of CO_2 into the blood begins within a few minutes of commencing a laparoscopic procedure and is estimated to be 30–50 ml.min^{-1}. If ventilation remains unchanged, this will quickly increase arterial P_{CO_2} and CO_2 will begin diffusing into the medium and slow compartments of the body's huge CO_2 stores (see page 158 and Figure 10.10). After a prolonged procedure, with elevated Pa_{CO_2}, hypercapnia may be present for many hours postoperatively as the CO_2 stores empty.[150] Unfortunately, this is a period when the patient is no longer receiving artificial ventilation and is recovering from a general anaesthetic, and so may struggle to meet the increased ventilatory requirement. Increasing the minute volume during surgery should allow the maintenance of a normal Pa_{CO_2} to prevent this scenario developing. In patients who are obese or have respiratory disease, the changes in compliance described previously will further impair the excretion of CO_2 and require an even larger minute volume. End-tidal CO_2 monitoring may be used to estimate the required ventilation, but in many patients $\dot{V}/\dot{Q}$ disturbances mean that there may be a large and unpredictable end-tidal to arterial P_{CO_2} gradient,[150] and measurement of Pa_{CO_2} may be required.

REGIONAL ANAESTHESIA

Epidural or spinal anaesthesia may be expected to influence the respiratory system, either by a central effect of drugs absorbed from the spinal canal or by affecting the pattern or strength of contraction of respiratory muscle groups.[155] These effects are generally small, but of great importance in view of the tendency to use regional anaesthetic techniques in patients with respiratory disease or in obstetric practice when respiratory function is already abnormal (Chapter 14).

Control of breathing. Thoracic epidural anaesthesia may cause a small reduction in resting tidal volume as a result of reduced ribcage movement.[156,157] Predictably this does not occur following lumbar epidural anaesthesia.[158] Studies of hypercapnic and hypoxic ventilatory responses during epidural anaesthesia have produced conflicting results. Thoracic anaesthesia may reduce the ventilatory response to hypercapnia by inhibition of intercostal muscle activity. Lumbar epidurals have been reported to *increase* the response to hypercapnia,[156,159] which is believed to be stimulated by anxiety (the study was performed immediately prior to surgery)[156] or because of a direct stimulant effect of lignocaine on the respiratory centre.[159] The acute hypoxic ventilatory response is unaffected by thoracic epidural anaesthesia, but lumbar epidurals may increase ventilation in response to hypoxia by a poorly understood mechanism.[156,157]

Respiratory muscle function has been extensively studied using EMGs and the DSR during high lumbar (block up to T1 dermatome) epidural anaesthesia[160] and confirmed the reduced contribution of the ribcage to resting ventilation. Functional residual capacity was increased by 300 ml as a result of both caudad movement of the diaphragm and reduced thoracic blood volume. In spite of these changes, most respiratory function measurements remain essentially unchanged during epidural anaesthesia with only small changes in forced vital capacity and peak expiratory flow rate.[161] The situation is quite different in late pregnancy, when regional anaesthesia is

commonly employed. Significant reductions in forced vital capacity and peak expiratory flow have been reported after spinal anaesthesia,[162] with lesser changes following epidural anaesthesia.[163] Peak expiratory pressure, a measure of abdominal muscle activity, was also decreased after lumbar epidural for caesarean section, particularly when bupivacaine was used.[164]

Oxygenation during epidural anaesthesia is largely unaffected. In a study by Hedenstierna's group, lumbar epidural anaesthesia produced no changes in $\dot{V}/\dot{Q}$ relationships or pulmonary shunt and no CT evidence of atelectasis except in one subject with a higher than normal body mass index in the lithotomy position.[143]

RESPIRATORY FUNCTION IN THE POSTOPERATIVE PERIOD[165]

Early postanaesthetic recovery

In the first few minutes of recovery, alveolar P_{O_2} may be reduced by elimination of nitrous oxide, which dilutes alveolar oxygen (diffusion hypoxia) and carbon dioxide, but this effect is usually transient. Hypoxia is very common during transfer to the recovery room, when monitoring is often interrupted.[166] Airway obstruction, often associated with residual muscle paralysis, is a common potential cause of hypoxia shortly after anaesthesia. This may be compounded by the residual effects of anaesthetic agents on ventilatory control that have been described above. Both reduced FRC and the increased alveolar/arterial P_{O_2} gradient observed during anaesthesia usually return to normal during the first few hours after minor operations.

Late postoperative respiratory changes

Following major surgery, the restoration of a normal alveolar/arterial P_{O_2} gradient may take several days and episodes of hypoxia are common. There are several contributory factors.

Lung volume and atelectasis. There is a continued reduction in FRC, usually reaching its lowest value 1–2 days postoperatively, before slowly returning to normal values within a week.[167] Reduction of the FRC is greatest in patients having surgery near the diaphragm, that is, upper abdominal or thoracic incisions,[168] but is less following laparoscopic surgery in the upper abdomen.[169] Atelectasis seen on CT scans during anaesthesia persists for at least 24 hours in patients having major surgery.[170] The effects of these changes on $\dot{V}/\dot{Q}$ relationships and oxygenation will be similar to those seen during anaesthesia, but the provision of adequate inspired oxygen concentration is now far less reliable.

Effort-dependent lung function tests such as forced vital capacity, forced expiratory volume in one second and peak expiratory flow rate are all reduced significantly following surgery, particularly if pain control is inadequate. Laparoscopic surgery is again associated with lesser, but still significant, reductions in lung function and the degree of change is again related to the site of surgery.[167]

Sleep. During sleep, particularly in a patient receiving opioid analgesics, there are often episodes of obstructive apnoea. These episodes were originally described as occurring during the first postoperative night[171] but may continue for at least three nights, particularly in association with rapid eye movement (REM) sleep, which is usually absent on the first postoperative night.

Respiratory muscles.[172] Diaphragmatic dysfunction is a term that has been used to describe changes in the pattern of contraction of respiratory muscles in patients following major surgery. Impairment of diaphragmatic contraction is believed to result from reflex inhibition of phrenic nerve output in response to surgical trauma. Changes are independent of the level of pain control and are only improved by thoracic epidural, which is believed to result in neural blockade of the inhibitory reflex.[167] The existence of diaphragmatic dysfunction has been challenged, mainly on the grounds that methods used to study diaphragm function are largely indirect and greatly affected by changes in other respiratory muscle groups.[172] For example, there are well-described increases in expiratory abdominal muscle activity following surgery[173] that may be interpreted as changes in diaphragm activity.

Sputum retention occurs in many patients following surgery. General anaesthesia, particularly with a tracheal tube, causes impairment of mucociliary transport in the airways,[174] an effect that may persist into the postoperative period. This, coupled with reduced FRC, residual atelectasis and an ineffective cough, is likely to contribute to the development of chest infections, including pneumonia. Many of these factors are more pronounced in smokers, who are known to be more susceptible to chest complications following major surgery (page 291).

REFERENCES

1. Snow J. On chloroform and other anaesthetics: their action and administration. London: Churchill, 1858.
2. Nunn JF. Effects of anaesthesia on respiration. *Br J Anaesth* 1990; **65**: 54–62.
3. Munson ES, Larson CP, Babad AA, Regan MJ, Buechel DR, Eger EI. The effects of halothane, fluroxene and cyclopropane on ventilation: a comparative study in man. *Anesthesiology* 1966; **27**: 716–28.
4. Eger EI. Isoflurane: a review. *Anesthesiology* 1981; **55**: 559–76.
5. Lockhart SH, Rampil IJ, Yasuda N, Eger EI, Weiskopf RB. Depression of ventilation by desflurane in humans. *Anesthesiology* 1991; **74**: 484–8.
6. Doi M, Ikeda K. Respiratory effects of sevoflurane. *Anesth Analg* 1987; **66**: 241–4.
7. Fourcade HE, Larson CP, Hickey RF, Bahlman SH, Eger EI. Effects of time on ventilation during halothane and cyclopropane anesthesia. *Anesthesiology* 1972; **36**: 83–8.
8. Eger EI, Dolan WM, Stevens WC, Miller RD, Way WL. Surgical stimulation antagonizes the respiratory depression produced by Forane. *Anesthesiology* 1972; **36**: 544–9.
*9. Pandit JJ. The variable effect of low-dose volatile anaesthetics on the acute ventilatory response to hypoxia in humans: a quantitative review. *Anaesthesia* 2002; **57**: 632–43.
*10. Dahan A, Teppema LJ. Influence of anaesthesia and analgesia on the control of breathing. *Br J Anaesth* 2003; **91**: 40–9.
11. Gordh T. Postural circulatory and respiratory changes during ether and intravenous anesthesia. *Acta Chir Scand* 1945; **92** (Suppl 102): 26.
12. Duffin J, Triscott A, Whitwam JG. The effect of halothane and thiopentone on ventilatory responses mediated by the peripheral chemoreceptors in man. *Br J Anaesth* 1976; **48**: 975–81.
13. Knill RL, Gelb AW. Ventilatory responses to hypoxia and hypercapnia during halothane sedation and anesthesia in man. *Anesthesiology* 1978; **49**: 244–51.
14. Knill RL, Kieraszewicz HT, Dodgson BG, Clement JL. Chemical regulation of ventilation during isoflurane sedation and anaesthesia in humans. *Can Anaesth Soc J* 1983; **30**: 607–14.
15. Knill RL, Manninen PH, Clement JL. Ventilation and chemoreflexes during enflurane sedation and anaesthesia in man. *Can Anaesth Soc J* 1979; **26**: 353–60.
16. Knill RL, Clement JL. Varaible effects of anaesthetics on the ventilatory response to hypoxaemia in man. *Can Anaesth Soc J* 1982; **29**: 93–9.
17. Sarton E, Dahan A, Teppema L, et al. Acute pain and central nervous system arousal do not restore impaired hypoxic ventilatory response during sevoflurane sedation. *Anesthesiology* 1996; **85**: 295–303.
18. Dahan A, Sarton E, van den Elsen M, van Kleef J, Teppema L, Berkenbosch A. Ventilatory response to

hypoxia in humans: influences of subanesthetic desflurane. *Anesthesiology* 1996; **85**: 60–8.

19. Nagyova B, Dorrington KL, Gill EW, Robbins PA. Comparison of the effects of sub-hypnotic concentrations of propofol and halothane on the acute ventilatory response to hypoxia. *Br J Anaesth* 1995; **75**: 713–18.

*20. Temp JA, Henson LC, Ward DS. Does a subanaesthetic concentration of isoflurane blunt the ventilatory response to hypoxia? *Anesthesiology* 1992; **77**: 1116–24.

21. Knill RL. Subanaesthetic isoflurane and the ventilatory response to hypoxaemia. *Anesthesiology* 1993; **78**: 1189–91.

22. Nagyova B, Dorrington KL, Robbins PA. Effect of low-dose enflurane on the ventilatory response to hypoxia in humans. *Br J Anaesth* 1994; **72**: 509–14.

23. Gelb AW, Knill RL. Subanaesthetic halothane: its effect on regulation of ventilation and relevance to the recovery room. *Can Anaesth Soc J* 1978; **25**: 488–94.

24. Dahan A, van den Elsen MJLJ, Berkenbosch A, et al. Effects of subanesthetic halothane on the ventilatory response to hypercapnia and acute hypoxia in healthy volunteers. *Anesthesiology* 1994; **80**: 727–38.

25. Solevi A, Lindahl SGE. Hypoxic and hypercapnic ventilatory response during isoflurane sedation and anaesthesia in women. *Acta Anaesthesiol Scand* 1995; **39**: 931–8.

26. Dahan A, Ward DS. Effects of 20% nitrous oxide on the ventilatory response to hypercapnia and sustained isocapnic hypoxia in man. *Br J Anaesth* 1994; **72**: 17–20.

27. Yacoub O, Doell D, Kryger MH, Anthonisen NR. Depression of hypoxic ventilatory response by nitrous oxide. *Anesthesiology* 1976; **45**: 385–9.

28. van den Elsen MJLJ, Dahan A, Berkenbosch A, DeGoede J, van Kleef JW, Olievier ICW. Does subanesthetic isoflurane affect the ventilatory response to acute isocapnic hypoxia in healthy volunteers? *Anesthesiology* 1994; **81**: 860–7.

29. Young CH, Drummond GB, Warren PM. Effect of a sub-anaesthetic concentration of halothane on the ventilatory response to sustained hypoxia in healthy humans. *Br J Anaesth* 1993; **71**: 642–7.

30. Temp JA, Henson LC, Ward DS. Effect of a subanesthetic minimum alveolar concentration of isoflurane on two tests of the hypoxic ventilatory response. *Anesthesiology* 1994; **80**: 739–50

31. Nagyova B, Dorrington KL, Poulin MJ, Robbins PA. Influence of 0.2 minimum alveolar concentration of enflurane on the ventilatory response to sustained hypoxia in humans. *Br J Anaesth* 1997; **78**: 707–13.

32. Sjögren D, Sollevi A, Ebberyd A, Lindahl SGE. Poikilocapnic hypoxic ventilatory response in humans during 0.85 MAC isoflurane anesthesia. *Acta Anaesthesiol Scand* 1994; **38**: 149–55.

33. Sjögren D, Sollevi A, Ebberyd A, Lindahl SGE. Isoflurane anesthesia (0.6 MAC) and hypoxic ventilatory response in humans. *Acta Anaesthesiol Scand* 1995; **39**: 17–22.

34. Knill RL, Clement JL. Site of selective action of halothane on the peripheral chemoreflex pathway in humans. *Anesthesiology* 1984; **61**: 121–6.

35. van den Elsen M, Sarton E, Teppema L, Berkenbosch A, Dahan A. Influence of 0.1 minimum alveolar concentration of sevoflurane, desflurane and isoflurane on dynamic ventilatory response to hypercapnia in humans. *Br J Anaesth* 1998; **80**: 174–82.

36. Robotham JL. Do low dose inhalational anesthetic agents alter ventilatory control? *Anesthesiology* 1994; **80**: 723–6.

37. Nandi PR, Charlesworth CH, Taylor SJ, Nunn JF, Doré C.J. Effect of general anaesthesia on the pharynx. *Br J Anaesth* 1991; **66**: 157–62.

38. Mathru M, Esch O, Lang J, et al. Magnetic resonance imaging of the upper airway. Effects of propofol anesthesia and nasal continuous positive airway pressure in humans. *Anesthesiology* 1996; **84**: 273–9.

39. Ochiai R, Guthrie RD, Motoyama EK. Effects of varying concentrations of halothane on the activity of the genioglossus, intercostals and diaphragm in cats: an electromyographic study. *Anesthesiology* 1989; **70**: 812–16.

40. Drummond GB. Influence of thiopentone on upper airway muscles. *Br J Anaesth* 1989; **63**: 12–21.

41. Morikawa S, Safar P, DeCarlo J. Influence of the head-jaw position upon upper airway patency. *Anesthesiology* 1961; **22**: 265–70.

42. Boidin MP. Airway patency in the unconscious patient. *Br J Anaesth* 1985; **57**: 306–10.

43. Heiberg J. A new expedient in administering chloroform. *Medical Times and Gazette* 10 Jan 1874, p36.

44. Marsh AM, Nunn JF, Taylor SJ, Charlesworth CH. Airway obstruction associated with the use of the Guedel airway. *Br J Anaesth* 1991; **67**: 517–23.

45. Brain AIJ. The laryngeal mask: a new concept in airway management. *Br J Anaesth* 1983; **55**: 801–5.

46. Nandi PR, Nunn JF, Charlesworth CH, Taylor SJ. Radiological study of the laryngeal mask. *Eur J Anaesthesiol* Supp 1991; **4**: 33–9.

47. Miller AH. Ascending respiratory paralysis under general anaesthesia. *JAMA* 1925; **84**: 201–2.

48. Jones JG, Faithfull D, Jordan C, Minty B. Ribcage movement during halothane anaesthesia in man. *Br J Anaesth* 1979; **51**: 399–407.

*49. Warner DO, Warner MA, Ritman EL. Human chest wall function while awake and during halothane anesthesia: I Quiet breathing. *Anesthesiology* 1995; **82**: 6–19.

50. Warner DO, Warner MA, Joyner MJ, Ritman EL. The effect of nitrous oxide on chest wall function in humans and dogs. *Anesth Analg* 1998; **86**: 1058–64.

51. Lumb AB, Petros AJ, Nunn JF. Ribcage contribution to resting and carbon dioxide stimulated ventilation during 1 MAC isoflurane anaesthesia. *Br J Anaesth* 1991; **67**: 712–21.

52. Mankikian B, Cantineau JP, Sartene R, Clergue F, Viars P. Ventilatory pattern and chest wall mechanics during ketamine anesthesia in humans. *Anesthesiology* 1986; **65**: 492–9.

53. Morton CPJ, Drummond GB. Change in chest wall dimensions on induction of anaesthesia: a reappraisal. *Br J Anaesth* 1994; **73**: 135–9.

54. Reigner J, Ameur MB, Ecoffey C. Spontaneous ventilation with halothane in children: a comparative study between endotracheal tube and laryngeal mask airway. *Anesthesiology* 1995; **83**: 674–8.

55. Vellody VPS, Nassery M, Balasaraswathi K, Goldberg NG, Sharp JT. Compliances of human ribcage and diaphragm-abdomen pathways in relaxed versus paralysed states. *Am Rev Respir Dis* 1978; **118**: 479–91.

56. Drummond GB. The abdominal muscles in anaesthesia and after surgery. *Br J Anaesth* 2003; **91**: 73–80.

57. Kaul SU, Heath JR, Nunn JF. Factors influencing the development of expiratory muscle activity during anaesthesia. *Br J Anaesth* 1973; **45**: 1013–18.

58. Hewlett AM, Hulands GH, Nunn JF, Heath JR. Functional residual capacity. II: Spontaneous respiration. *Br J Anaesth* 1974; **46**: 486–94.

59. Bergman NA. Distribution of inspired gas during anesthesia and artificial ventilation. *J Appl Physiol* 1963; **18**: 1085–9.

60. Rutherford JS, Logan MR, Drummond GB. Changes in end-expiratory lung volume on induction of anaesthesia with thiopentone or propofol. *Br J Anaesth* 1994; **73**: 579–82.

*61. Warner DO, Warner MA, Ritman EL. Atelectasis and chest wall shape during halothane anesthesia. *Anesthesiology* 1996; **85**: 49–59.

62. Don HF, Wahba WM, Craig DB. Airway closure, gas trapping and the functional residual capacity during anesthesia. *Anesthesiology* 1970; **36**: 533–9.

63. Hewlett AM, Hulands GH, Nunn JF, Milledge JS. Functional residual capacity. III: Artifical ventilation. *Br J Anaesth* 1974; **46**: 495–503.

*64. Gunnarsson L, Tokics L, Gustavsson H, Hedenstierna G. Influence of age on atelectasis formation and gas exchange impairment during general anaesthesia. *Br J Anaesth* 1991; **66**: 423–32.

65. Hedenstierna G, Strandberg A, Brismar B, Lundquist H, Svensson L, Tokics L. Functional residual capacity, thoracoabdominal dimensions and central blood volume during general anesthesia with muscle paralysis and mechanical ventilation. *Anesthesiology* 1985; **62**: 247–54.

66. Muller N, Volgyesi G, Becker L, Bryan MH, Bryan AC. Diaphragmatic muscle tone. *J Appl Physiol* 1979; **47**: 279–84.

67. Froese AB, Bryan AC. Effects of anesthesia and paralysis on diaphragmatic mechanics in man. *Anesthesiology* 1974; **41**: 242–55.

*68. Reber A, Nylund U, Hedenstierna G. Position and shape of the diaphragm: implications for atelectasis formation. *Anaesthesia* 1998; **53**: 1054–61.

69. Krayer S, Rehder K, Vettermann J, Didier P, Ritman EL. Position and motion of the human diaphragm during anesthesia-paralysis. *Anesthesiology* 1989; **70**: 891–8.

70. Krayer S, Rehder K, Beck KC, Cameron PD, Didier EP, Hoffman EA. Quantification of thoracic volumes by three-dimensional imaging. *J Appl Physiol* 1987; **62**: 591–8.

71. Hedenstierna G, Lundquist H, Undh B, et al. Pulmonary densities during anaesthesia. *Eur Respir J* 1989; **2**: 528–32.

72. Bendixen HH, Hedley-Whyte J, Laver MB. Impaired oxygenation in surgical patients during general anesthesia with controlled ventilation. *N Engl J Med* 1963; **269**: 991–6.

73. Hedenstierna G, Tokics L, Strandberg A, Lundquist H, Brismar B. Correlation of gas exchange impairment to development of atelectasis during anaesthesia and muscle paralysis. *Acta Anaesthesiol Scand* 1986; **30**: 183–91.

74. Lundquist H, Hedenstierna G, Strandberg A, Tokics L, Brismar B. CT-assessment of dependent lung densities in man during general anaesthesia. *Acta Radiol* 1995; **36**: 626–32.

75. Hedenstierna G. Invited editorial on 'Kinetics of absorption atelectasis during anaesthesia: a mathematical model'. *J Appl Physiol* 1999; **86**: 1114–15.

76. Nunn JF, Williams IP, Jones JG, Hewlett AM, Hulands GH, Minty BD. Detection and reversal of pulmonary absorption collapse. *Br J Anaesth* 1978; **50**: 91–100.

77. Rothen HU, Sporre B, Engberg G, Wegenius G, Hedenstierna G. Airway closure, atelectasis and gas exchange during general anaesthesia. *Br J Anaesth* 1998; **81**: 681–6.

78. Nunn JF. Measurement of closing volume. *Acta Anaesthiol Scand Supp* 1978; **70**: 154–60.

79. Hedenstierna G, McCarthy G, Bergström M. Airway closure during mechanical ventilation. *Anesthesiology* 1976; **44**: 114–23.

80. Juno P, Marsh M, Knopp TJ, Rehder K. Closing capacity in awake and anesthetized-paralyzed man. *J Appl Physiol* 1978; **44**: 238–44.

81. Bergman NA, Tien YK. Contribution of the closure of pulmonary units to impaired oxygenation during anesthesia. *Anesthesiology* 1983; **59**: 395–401.

82. Joyce CJ, Baker AB. What is the role of absorption atelectasis in the genesis of perioperative pulmonary collapse? *Anaesth Intens Care* 1995; **23**: 691–6.

*83. Magnusson L, Spahn DR. New concepts of atelectasis during general anaesthesia. *Br J Anaesth* 2003; **91**: 61–72.

84. Rothen HU, Sporre B, Engberg G, Wegenius G, Reber A, Hedenstierna G. Prevention of atelectasis during general anaesthesia. *Lancet* 1996; **345**: 1387–91.

85. Reber A, Engberg G, Wegenius G, Hedenstierna G. Lung aeration: the effect of pre-oxygenation and hyperoxygenation during total intravenous anaesthesia. *Anaesthesia* 1996; **51**: 733–7.

86. Edmark L, Kostova-Aherdan K, Enlund M, Hedenstierna G. Optimal oxygen concentration during induction of general anesthesia. *Anesthesiology* 2003; **98**: 28–33.

87. Rothen HU, Sporre B, Engberg G, Wegenius G, Högman M, Hedenstierna G. Influence of gas composition on recurrence of atelectasis after a reexpansion maneuvre during general anesthesia. *Anesthesiology* 1995; **82**: 832–42.

88. Rothen HU, Sporre HU, Engberg G, Wegenius G, Hedenstierna G. Reexpansion of atelectasis during general anaesthesia may have a prolonged effect. *Acta Anaesthesiol Scand* 1995; **39**: 118–25.

89. Akça O, Podolsky A, Eisenhuber E, et al. Comparable postoperative pulmonary atelectasis in patients given 30% or 80% oxygen during and 2 hours after colon resection. *Anesthesiology* 1999; **91**: 991–8.

*90. Benoit Z, Wicky S, Fischer J-F, et al. The effect of increased FIO_2 before tracheal extubation on postoperative atelectasis. *Anesth Analg* 2002; **95**: 1777–81.

*91. Joyce CJ, Williams AB. Kinetics of absorption atelectasis during anaesthesia: a mathematical model. *J Appl Physiol* 1999; **86**: 1116–25.

92. Agarwal A, Singh PK, Dhiraj S, Pandey CM, Singh U. Oxygen in air (FIO_2 0.4) improves gas exchange in young healthy patients during general anesthesia. *Can J Anesth* 2002; **49**: 1040–3.

93. Gunnarson L, Strandberg Å, Brismar B, Tokics L, Lundquist H, Hedenstierna G. Atelectasis and gas exchange impairment during enflurane/nitrous oxide anaesthesia. *Acta Anaesthesiol Scand* 1989; **33**: 629–37.

94. Lindahl SGE, Mure M. Dosing oxygen: a tricky matter or a piece of cake? *Anesth Analg* 2002; **95**: 1472–3.

95. Rusca M, Proietti S, Schnyder P, et al. Prevention of atelectasis formation during induction of general anesthesia. *Anesth Analg* 2003; **97**: 1835–9.

96. Herriger A, Frascarolo P, Spahn DR, Magnusson L. The effect of positive airway pressure during pre-oxygenation and induction of anaesthesia upon duration of non-hypoxic apnoea. *Anaesthesia* 2004; **59**: 243–7.

97. Neumann P, Rothen HU, Berglund JE, Valtysson J, Magnusson A, Hedenstierna G. Positive end-expiratory pressure prevents atelectasis during general anaesthesia even in the presence of a high inspired oxygen concentration. *Acta Anaesthesiol Scand* 1999; **43**: 295–301.

*98. Rothen HU, Sporre B, Engberg G, Wegenius G, Hedenstierna G. Re-expansion of atelectasis during general anaesthesia: a computed tomography study. *Br J Anaesth* 1993; **71**: 788–95.

*99. Tusman G, Böhm SH, Vazquez de Anda GF, do Campo JL, Lachmann B. 'Alveolar recruitment strategy' improves arterial oxygenation during general anaesthesia. *Br J Anaesth* 1999; **82**: 8–13.

*100. Rothen HU, Neumann P, Berglund JE, Valtysson J, Magnusson A, Hedenstierna G. Dynamics of re-expansion of atelectasis during general anaesthesia. *Br J Anaesth* 1999; **82**: 551–6.

101. Hedenstierna G, Tokics L, Lundquist H, Andersson T, Strandberg A, Brismar B. Phrenic nerve stimulation during halothane anaesthesia. Effects on atelectasis. *Anesthesiology* 1994; **80**: 751–60.

102. Milic-Emili J, Robatto FM, Bates JHT. Respiratory mechanics in anaesthesia. *Br J Anaesth* 1990; **65**: 4–12.

103. Hirshman CA, Bergman NA. Factors influencing intrapulmonary airway calibre during anaesthesia. *Br J Anaesth* 1990; **65**: 30–42.

104. Joyner MJ, Warner DO, Rehder K. Halothane changes the relationships between lung resistances and lung volume. *Anesthesiology* 1992; **76**: 229–35.

105. Pelosi P, Croci M, Calappi E, et al. The prone position during general anesthesia minimally affects respiratory mechanics while improving functional residual capacity and increasing oxygen tension. *Anesth Analg* 1995; **80**: 955–60.

106. D'Angelo E, Robatto FM, Calderini E, et al. Pulmonary and chest wall mechanics in anesthetized paralyzed humans. *J Appl Physiol* 1991; **70**: 2602–10.

107. Yamakage M. Effects of anaesthetic agents on airway smooth muscle. *Br J Anaesth* 2002; **88**: 624–7.

108. Korenaga S, Takeda K, Ito Y. Differential effects of halothane on airway nerves and muscle. *Anesthesiology* 1984; **60**: 309–18.

109. Bhatt SB, Kendall AP, Lin ES, Oh TE. Resistance and additional inspiratory work imposed by the

laryngeal mask airway: a comparison with tracheal tubes. *Anaesthesia* 1992; **47**: 343–7.

110. Westbrook PR, Stubbs SE, Sessler AD, Rehder K, Hyatt RE. Effects of anesthesia and muscle paralysis on respiratory mechanics in normal man. *J Appl Physiol* 1973; **34**: 81–6.

111. Scheidt M, Hyatt RE, Rehder K. Effects of ribcage or abdominal restriction on lung mechanics. *J Appl Physiol* 1981; **51**: 1115–21.

112. Campbell EJM, Nunn JF, Peckett BW. A comparison of artificial ventilation and spontaneous respiration with particular reference to ventilation–blood-flow relationships. *Br J Anaesth* 1958; **30**: 166–75.

113. Nunn JF, Hill DW. Respiratory dead space and arterial to end-tidal CO_2 tension difference in anesthetized man. *J Appl Physiol* 1960; **15**: 383–9.

114. Casati A, Fanelli G, Torri G. Physiological dead space/tidal volume ratio during face mask, laryngeal mask and cuffed oropharyngeal airway spontaneous ventilation. *J Clin Anesth* 1998; **10**: 652–5.

115. Kain ML, Panday J, Nunn JF. The effect of intubation on the dead space during halothane anaesthesia. *Br J Anaesth* 1969; **41**: 94–102.

116. Michenfelder JD, Fowler WS, Theye RA. CO_2 levels and pulmonary shunting in anesthetized man. *J Appl Physiol* 1966; **21**: 1471–6.

117. Marshall BE, Cohen PJ, Klingenmaier CH, Aukberg S. Pulmonary venous admixture before, during and after halothane:oxygen anesthesia in man. *J Appl Physiol* 1969; **27**: 653–7.

118. Price HL, Cooperman LH, Warden JC, Morris JJ, Smith TC. Pulmonary hemodynamics during general anesthesia in man. *Anesthesiology* 1969; **30**: 629–36.

119. Nunn JF, Bergman NA, Coleman AJ. Factors influencing the arterial oxygen tension during anaesthesia with artificial ventilation. *Br J Anaesth* 1965; **37**: 898–914.

120. Nunn JF. Factors influencing the arterial oxygen tension during halothane anaesthesia with spontaneous respiration. *Br J Anaesth* 1964; **36**: 327–41.

121. Theye RA, Touhy GF. Oxygen uptake during light halothane anesthesia in man. *Anesthesiology* 1964; **25**: 627–33.

122. Gold MI, Helrich M. Ventilation and blood gases in anaesthetised patients. *Can Anaesth Soc J* 1967; **14**: 424–34.

123. Bindslev L, Hedenstierna G, Santesson J, Gottlieb I, Carvallhas A. Ventilation–perfusion distribution during inhalation anaesthesia. *Acta Anaesthesiol Scand* 1981; **25**: 360–71.

*124. Tokics L, Hedenstierna G, Svensson L, et al. V/Q distribution and correlation to atelectasis in anesthetized paralyzed humans. *J Appl Physiol* 1996; **81**: 1822–33.

125. Hedenstierna G. Contribution of the multiple inert gas elimination technique to pulmonary medicine. 6: Ventilation–perfusion relationships during anaesthesia. *Thorax* 1995; **50**: 85–91.

126. Rehder K, Knopp TJ, Sessler AD, Didier EP. Ventilation–perfusion relationship in young healthy awake and anesthetized-paralyzed man. *J Appl Physiol* 1979; **47**: 745–53.

127. Nunn JF. Oxygen – friend and foe. *J Roy Soc Med* 1985; **78**: 618–22.

128. Dueck R, Young I, Clausen J, Wagner PD. Altered distribution of pulmonary ventilation and blood flow following induction of inhalational anesthesia. *Anesthesiology* 1980; **52**: 113–25.

129. Anjou-Lindskog E, Broman L, Broman M, Holmgren A, Settergren G, Öhqvist G. Effects of intravenous anesthesia on VA/Q distribution: a study performed during ventilation with air and with 50% oxygen, supine and in the lateral position. *Anesthesiology* 1985; **62**: 485–92.

130. Nunn JF, Ezi-Ashi TI. The respiratory effects of resistance to breathing in anesthetized man. *Anesthesiology* 1961; **22**: 174–85.

131. Moote CA, Knill RL, Clement J. Ventilatory compensation for continuous inspiratory resistive and elastic loads during halothane anesthesia in humans. *Anesthesiology* 1986; **64**: 582–9.

132. Drummond GB, Cullen JP. Detection of inspiratory resistive loads after anaesthesia for minor surgery. *Br J Anaesth* 1997; **78**: 308–10.

133. Isono S, Nishino T, Sugimori K, Mizuguchi T. Respiratory effects of expiratory flow-resistive loading in conscious and anesthetized humans. *Anesth Analg* 1990; **70**: 594–9.

134. Boothby WM, Sandiford I. Basal metabolism. *Physiol Rev* 1924; **18**: 1085.

135. Roberston JD, Reid DD. Standards for the basal metabolism of normal people in Britain. *Lancet* 1952; **1**: 940–3.

136. Nunn JF, Matthews RL. Gaseous exchange during halothane anaesthesia: the steady respiratory state. *Br J Anaesth* 1959; **31**: 330–40.

137. Marshall BE, Marshall C. Anesthesia and the pulmonary circulation. In: Covino BG, Fozzard HA, Rehder K, Strichartz G, eds. *Effects of anesthesia*. Bethesda, MD: American Physiological Society, 1985.

138. Eisenkraft JB. Effects of anaesthetics on the pulmonary circulation. *Br J Anaesth* 1990; **65**: 63–78.

139. Abe K, Shimizu T, Takashina M, Shiozaki H, Yoshiya I. The effects of propofol, isoflurane and sevoflurane on oxygenation and shunt fraction during one-lung ventilation. *Anesth Analg* 1998; **87**: 1164–9.

140. Dunn PF. Physiology of the lateral decubitus position and one-lung ventilation. *Int Anesthesiol Clin* 2000; **38**: 25–53.

141. Marshall BE. Pulmonary blood flow and oxygenation. In: Marshall BE, Longnecker DE, Fairley HB, eds. *Anesthesia for thoracic procedures*. Oxford: Blackwell Scientific, 1988.

142. Klingstedt C, Hedenstierna G, Baehrendtz S, et al. Ventilation–perfusion relationships and atelectasis formation in the supine and lateral positions during conventional mechanical and differential ventilation. *Acta Anaesthesiol Scand* 1990; **34**: 421–9.

143. Reber A, Bein T, Högman M, Khan ZP, Nilsson S, Hedenstierna G. Lung aeration and pulmonary gas exchange during lumbar epidural anaesthesia and in the lithotomy position in elderly patients. *Anaesthesia* 1998; **53**: 854–61.

*144. Szegedi LL. Pathophysiology of one-lung ventilation. *Anesthesiol Clin North Am* 2001; **19**: 435–53.

145. Bardoczky GI, Szegedi LL, d'Hollander AA, Moures J-L, de Francquen P, Yernault J-C. Two-lung and one-lung ventilation in patients with chronic obstructive pulmonary disease: the effects of position and $F_{I_{O_2}}$. *Anesth Analg* 2000; **90**: 35–41.

146. Inomata S, Nishikawa T, Saito S, Kihara S. 'Best' PEEP during one-lung ventilation. *Br J Anaesth* 1997; **78**: 754–6.

147. Benumof JL, Augustine SD, Gibbons JA. Halothane and isoflurane only slightly impair arterial oxygenation during one-lung ventilation in patients undergoing thoracotomy. *Anesthesiology* 1987; **67**: 910–15.

148. Abe K, Shimizu T, Takashina M, Shiozaki H, Yoshiya I. The effects of propofol, isoflurane and sevoflurane on oxygenation and shunt fraction during one-lung ventilation. *Anesth Analg* 1998; **87**: 1164–9.

149. Dalibon N, Moutafis M, Liu N, Law-Koune J-D, Monsel S, Fischler M. Treatment of hypoxemia during one-lung ventilation using almitrine. *Anesth Analg* 2004; **98**: 590–4.

*150. Sharma C, Brandstetter R, Brensilver J, Jung L. Cardiopulmonary physiology and pathophysiology as a consequence of laparoscopic surgery. *Chest* 1996; **110**: 810–15.

151. O'Malley C, Cunningham AJ. Physiologic changes during laparoscopy. *Anesthesiol Clin North Am* 2001; **19**: 1–19.

152. Sprung J, Whalley DG, Falcone T, Warner DO, Hubmayr RD, Hammel J. The impact of morbid obesity, pneumoperitoneum and posture on respiratory system mechanics and oxygenation during laparoscopy. *Anesth Analg* 2002; **94**: 1345–50.

153. Andersson L, Lagerstrand L, Thörne A, Sollevi A, Brodin L-Å, Odeberg-Wernerman S. Effect of CO_2 pneumoperitoneum on ventilation-perfusion relationships during laparoscopic cholecystectomy. *Acta Anaesthesiol Scand* 2002; **46**: 552–60.

*154. Kazama T, Ikeda K, Kato T, Kikura M. Carbon dioxide output in laparoscopic cholecystectomy. *Br J Anaesth* 1996; **76**: 530–5.

155. Veering BT, Cousins MJ. Cardiovascular and pulmonary effects of epidural anaesthesia. *Anesth Intens Care* 2000; **28**: 620–35.

156. Sakura S, Saito Y, Kosaka Y. The effects of epidural anesthesia on ventilatory response to hypercapnia and hypoxia in elderly patients. *Anesth Analg* 1996; **82**: 306–11.

157. Sakura S, Saito Y, Kosaka Y. Effect of extradural anaesthesia on the ventilatory response to hypoxaemia. *Anaesthesia* 1993; **48**: 205–9.

158. Sakura S, Saito Y, Kosaka Y. Effect of lumbar epidural anesthesia on ventilatory response to hypercapnia in young and elderly patients. *J Clin Anesth* 1993; **5**: 109–13.

159. Labaille T, Clergue F, Samii K, Ecoffey C, Berdeaux A. Ventilatory response to CO_2 following intravenous and epidural lidocaine. *Anesthesiology* 1985; **63**: 179–85.

160. Warner DO, Warner MA, Ritman EL. Human chest wall function during epidural anesthesia. *Anesthesiology* 1996; **85**: 761–73.

161. Moir DD. Ventilatory function during epidural analgesia. *Br J Anaesth* 1963; **35**: 3–7.

162. Kelly MC, Fitzpatrick KTJ, Hill DA. Respiratory effects of spinal anaesthesia for Caesarean section. *Anaesthesia* 1996; **51**: 1120–2.

163. Gamil M. Serial peak expiratory flow rates in mothers during caesarean section under extradural anaesthesia. *Br J Anaesth* 1989; **62**: 415–18.

164. Yun E, Topulos GP, Body SC, Datta S, Bader AM. Pulmonary function changes during epidural anesthesia for Cesarean delivery. *Anesth Analg* 1996; **82**: 750–3.

165. Jones JG, Sapsford DJ, Wheatley RG. Postoperative hypoxaemia: mechanisms and time course. *Anaesthesia* 1990; **45**: 566–73.

166. Moller JT, Johannessen NW, Berg H, Espersen K, Larsen LE. Hypoxaemia during anaesthesia – an observer study. *Br J Anaesth* 1991; **66**: 437–44.

167. Liu S, Carpenter RL, Neal JM. Epidural anesthesia amd analgesia: their role in postoperative outcome. *Anesthesiology* 1995; **82**: 1474–506.

168. McKeague H, Cunningham AJ. Postoperative respiratory dysfunction: is the site of surgery crucial? *Br J Anaesth* 1997; **79**: 415–16.

169. Couture JD, Chartrand D, Gagner M, Bellemare F. Diaphragmatic and abdominal muscle activity after endoscopic cholecystectomy. *Anesth Analg* 1994; **78**: 733–9.

170. Strandberg A, Tokics L, Brismar B, Lundquist H, Hedenstierna G. Atelectasis during anaesthesia and in the postoperative period. *Acta Anaesthesiol Scand* 1986; **30**: 154–8.

171. Catley DM, Thornton C, Jordan C, Lehane JR, Royston D, Jones JG. Pronounced, episodic oxygen desaturation in the postoperative period: its association with ventilatory pattern and analgesic regime. *Anesthesiology* 1985; **63**: 20–8.

*172. Drummond GB. Diaphragmatic dysfunction: an outmoded concept. *Br J Anaesth* 1998; **80**: 277–80.

173. Nimmo AF, Drummond GB. Respiratory mechanics after abdominal surgery measured with continuous analysis of pressure, flow and volume signals. *Br J Anaesth* 1996; **77**: 317–26.

174. Keller C, Brimacombe J. Bronchial mucus transport velocity in paralyzed anesthetized patients: a comparison of the laryngeal mask airway and cuffed tracheal tube. *Anesth Analg* 1998; **86**: 1280–2.

Chapter

23 Changes in the carbon dioxide tension

KEY POINTS

- Hypocapnia occurs when alveolar ventilation is excessive relative to carbon dioxide production and usually results from hyperventilation due to hypoxia, acidosis or lung disease.
- Hypercapnia most commonly occurs because of inadequate alveolar ventilation from a multitude of causes or, more rarely, from increased carbon dioxide production.
- Arterial P_{CO_2} affects the cerebral circulation: hypocapnia may cause potentially harmful vasoconstriction, whereas vasodilation from hypercapnia may increase intracranial pressure.
- Hypercapnia and the resulting acidosis both have depressant effects on the cardiovascular system, but these are opposed by the stimulant effects of catecholamine release.

Routine monitoring of end-expiratory and arterial P_{CO_2} means it should now be possible to avoid both hypo- and hypercapnia under almost all clinical circumstances. However, interest in hypercapnia has continued over recent years for two reasons. First, changes in the approach to artificial ventilation in severe lung injury have led to the use of 'permissive hypercapnia' (page 414). In order to minimise pulmonary damage, minute volume of ventilation is maintained deliberately low and the arterial P_{CO_2} is allowed to increase. Second, a massive expansion of laparoscopic surgical techniques, mostly using carbon dioxide for abdominal insufflation, has led to the anaesthetist having to control arterial P_{CO_2} under conditions of significantly increased pulmonary carbon dioxide output (page 318).

Before describing the effects of carbon dioxide on various physiological systems, this chapter will briefly outline the causes of changes in arterial P_{CO_2}.

CAUSES OF HYPOCAPNIA[1]

Hypocapnia can result only from an alveolar ventilation that is excessive in relation to carbon dioxide production. Low values of arterial P_{CO_2} are commonly found, resulting from artificial ventilation with a generous minute volume or from voluntary hyperventilation due to psychological disturbance such as hysteria. A low arterial P_{CO_2} may also result simply from hyperventilation during arterial puncture. Persistently low values may be due to an excessive respiratory drive resulting from one or more of the following causes.

Hypoxaemia is a common cause of hypocapnia, occurring in congenital heart disease with right-to-left shunting, residence at high altitude, pulmonary pathology, or any other condition that reduces the arterial P_{O_2} below about 8 kPa (60 mmHg). Hypocapnia secondary to hypoxaemia opposes the ventilatory response to the hypoxaemia (page 66).

Metabolic acidosis produces a compensatory hyperventilation (air hunger), which minimises the fall in pH that would otherwise occur. This is a pronounced feature of diabetic ketoacidosis; arterial P_{CO_2} values below 3 kPa (22.5 mmHg) are not uncommon in severe metabolic acidosis. This is a vital compensatory mechanism. Failure to maintain the required hyperventilation, either from fatigue or from inadequate minute volume following tracheal intubation, leads to a rapid life-threatening decrease in arterial pH.

Mechanical abnormalities of the lung may drive respiration through the vagus, resulting in moderate reduction of the P_{CO_2}. Thus conditions such as pulmonary fibrosis, pulmonary oedema and asthma are usually associated with a low to normal P_{CO_2} until the patient passes into type 2 respiratory failure (page 365).

Neurological disorders may result in hyperventilation and hypocapnia. This is most commonly seen in those conditions that lead to the presence of blood in the cerebrospinal fluid, such as occurs following head injury or subarachnoid haemorrhage.

CAUSES OF HYPERCAPNIA

It is uncommon to encounter an arterial P_{CO_2} above the normal range in a healthy subject. Any value of more than 6.1 kPa (46 mmHg) should be considered abnormal, but values up to 6.7 kPa (50 mmHg) may be attained by breath holding. It is difficult for the healthy subject to exceed this level by any respiratory manoeuvre other than by breathing mixtures of carbon dioxide in oxygen.

When a patient is hypercapnic, there are only four possible causes. These should be considered systematically, as follows.

Increased concentration of carbon dioxide in the inspired gas. This iatrogenic cause of hypercapnia is uncommon but it is dangerous and differs fundamentally from the other causes listed below. It should therefore be excluded at the outset in any patient unexpectedly found to be hypercapnic when breathing from or being ventilated by external equipment. The carbon dioxide may be endogenous from rebreathing or exogenous from carbon dioxide added to the inhaled gases. The latter is now very rare as a supply of carbon dioxide is not provided on modern anaesthetic machines. Hypercapnia from rebreathing is more common, but fortunately its severity is limited by the rate at which the P_{CO_2} can increase. If all the carbon dioxide produced by metabolism is retained and distributed in the body stores, arterial P_{CO_2} can increase no faster than about 0.4–0.8 kPa.min^{-1} (3–6 mmHg.min^{-1}).

Increased carbon dioxide production. If the pulmonary minute volume is fixed by artificial ventilation and carbon dioxide production is increased by, for example, malignant hyperpyrexia, hypercapnia is inevitable. Like the previous category, this is a rare but dangerous cause of hypercapnia, which should be excluded when there is no other obvious explanation for an increasing P_{CO_2} during anaesthesia. A less dramatic, but very common, reason for increased carbon dioxide production is sepsis leading to pyrexia, which often results in hypercapnia in artificially ventilated patients.

Though not strictly an increase in production, absorption of carbon dioxide from the peritoneum during laparoscopic surgery has the same respiratory effects and is described on page 318.

Hypoventilation. An inadequate pulmonary minute volume is by far the commonest cause of hypercapnia. Pathological causes of hypoventilation are considered in Chapter 27. In respiratory medicine, the commonest

cause of long-standing hypercapnia is chronic obstructive pulmonary disease. There are many other possible causes (see Figure 27.2), including medullary depression by drugs, neuromuscular blockade, respiratory obstruction and restriction of the lungs or chest wall.

Increased dead space. This rare cause of hypercapnia is usually diagnosed by a process of exclusion when a patient has a high P_{CO_2}, with a normal minute volume and no evidence of a hypermetabolic state or inhaled carbon dioxide. The cause may be incorrectly configured breathing apparatus or an excessively large alveolar dead space (page 120). This might be due to pulmonary embolism or a cyst communicating with the tracheobronchial tree and receiving preferential ventilation.

EFFECTS OF CARBON DIOXIDE ON THE NERVOUS SYSTEM

A number of special difficulties hinder an understanding of the effects of changes in P_{CO_2} on any physiological system. First, there is the problem of species difference, which is a formidable obstacle to the interpretation of animal studies in this as in other fields. The second difficulty arises from the fact that carbon dioxide can exert its effect either directly or in consequence of (respiratory) acidosis. The third difficulty arises from the fact that carbon dioxide acts at many different sites in the body, sometimes producing opposite effects on a particular function, such as blood pressure (see below).

Carbon dioxide has at least five major effects on the brain.

- It is a major factor governing cerebral blood flow.
- It influences the CSF pressure through changes in cerebral blood flow.
- It is the main factor influencing the intracellular pH, which is known to have important effects on the metabolism, and hence the function, of the cell.
- It may be presumed to exert the inert gas narcotic effect in accord with its physical properties, which are similar to those of nitrous oxide.
- It influences the excitability of certain neurones, particularly relevant in the case of the reticuloactivating system.

The interplay of these effects is difficult to understand, although the gross changes produced are well established.

Effects on consciousness

Carbon dioxide has long been known to cause unconsciousness in dogs entering the Grotto del Cane in Italy, where carbon dioxide issuing from a fumarole forms a layer near the ground. It has been widely used as a routine anaesthetic agent for short procedures in small laboratory animals. Inhalation of 30% carbon dioxide is sufficient for the production of anaesthesia in humans, but is complicated by the frequent occurrence of convulsions.[2] In patients with ventilatory failure, carbon dioxide narcosis occurs when the P_{CO_2} rises above 12–16 kPa (90–120 mmHg).[3]

Narcosis by carbon dioxide is probably not due primarily to its inert gas narcotic effects, because its oil solubility predicts a very much weaker narcotic than it seems to be. It is likely that the major effect on the central nervous system is by alteration of the intracellular pH, with consequent derangements of metabolic processes. In animals the narcotic effect correlates better with cerebrospinal fluid pH than with arterial P_{CO_2}.[4]

The effects of inhaling low concentrations of carbon dioxide for a prolonged period of time are described on page 279.

Cerebral blood flow[5]

Cerebral blood flow (CBF) increases with arterial P_{CO_2} at a rate of about 7–15 ml.100 g^{-1}.min^{-1} for each kPa increase in P_{CO_2} (1–2 ml.100 g^{-1}.min^{-1} per mmHg) within the approximate range 3–10 kPa (20–80 mmHg). The full response curve is S-shaped (Figure 23.1). The response at very low P_{CO_2} is probably limited by the vasodilator effect of tissue hypoxia and the response above 16 kPa (120 mmHg) seems to represent maximal vasodilation. The changes shown in Figure 23.1 represent the brain as a whole and it is not possible to generalise about regional changes. There is some evidence that considerable regional variations in carbon dioxide responsiveness exist within the human central nervous system.[6]

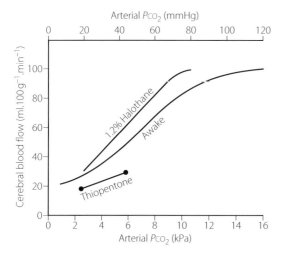

Figure 23.1 Relationship of cerebral blood flow to arterial P_{CO_2} in awake and anaesthetised patients.

Mechanisms. In the intact animal, cerebral blood flow (CBF) is increased in response to P_{CO_2} by a combination of vasodilation of cerebral blood vessels and an increase in blood pressure (see below). Changes in P_{CO_2} lead to a complex series of events that brings about vasodilation of cerebral blood vessels.[5] In adults, the effect is initiated by changes in the extracellular pH in the region of the arterioles, which alters intracellular calcium levels both directly and indirectly via nitric oxide production and the formation of cyclic GMP. With prolonged hypocapnia, and to a lesser extent hypercapnia, changes in cerebral blood flow return towards baseline after a few hours,[5,7] an effect thought to result from changes in cerebrospinal fluid pH correcting the extracellular acidosis. Hypercapnic cerebral vasodilation in neonates is believed to operate by a quite different mechanism involving the production of prostaglandins and cyclic AMP.

Pathological effects. Sensitivity of the cerebral circulation to carbon dioxide may be lost in a variety of pathological circumstances such as cerebral tumour, infarction or trauma. There is commonly a fixed vasodilation in these areas, giving rise to so-called luxury perfusion;[8] far from being luxurious, though, if widespread it may cause dangerous increases in intracranial pressure. Areas of brain with luxury perfusion may respond to altered P_{CO_2} in the opposite direction to normal. For example, a high P_{CO_2} may increase blood flow through normal brain tissue and actually decrease perfusion through ischaemic areas that have lost their response to carbon dioxide, an effect referred to as intracerebral steal. The reverse phenomenon may occur when P_{CO_2} is lowered in patients with an area of luxury perfusion. Vasoconstriction in the surrounding normal tissue may divert blood flow towards the abnormal area of luxury perfusion, which has no ability to respond to lowered P_{CO_2}, an effect known as the inverse steal.

Anaesthesia. All inhalational anaesthetics have a direct cerebral vasodilator effect and increase normocapnic CBF considerably.[9-12] They also accentuate the response to both hypocapnia and hypercapnia; that is, they increase the slope of the relationship between P_{CO_2} and CBF (see Figure 23.1). In spite of the increased slope during hypocapnia, global CBF during anaesthesia with hyperventilation is normally still greater than when awake.[5] Intravenous anaesthetics such as thiopentone[13] and propofol[14] reduce CBF at normal P_{CO_2} in accordance with the reduced cerebral oxygen consumption. Vasoconstriction in response to hyperventilation continues to occur (see Figure 23.1), but at deeper levels of anaesthesia the response is reduced compared with when awake.[5] Even so, hyperventilation during deep thiopentone anaesthesia has been shown to reduce jugular venous oxygen PO_2, indicating a significant reduction in CBF.

Intracranial pressure (ICP) tends to rise with increasing PCO_2, probably as a result of cerebral vasodilation. Hyperventilation was used for many years as a standard method of acutely reducing ICP after head injury,[15] but the reduction in ICP may only be short-lived and the effects on CBF are variable. The possibility of *increased* CBF as a result of lowered ICP must be offset against *reduced* CBF from hypocapnic vasoconstriction. It is therefore preferable to monitor ICP, an invasive technique only available in specialised units dealing with head-injured patients. Recent recommendations on the management of head injury therefore advise that hyperventilation should only be used to reduce intracranial pressure when other therapeutic approaches have failed.[16]

Effects on the autonomic and endocrine systems

Survival in severe hypercapnia is, to a large extent, dependent on the autonomic response. A great many of the effects of carbon dioxide on other systems are due wholly or in part to the autonomic response to carbon dioxide.

Animal studies[17] have clearly shown an increase in plasma levels of both adrenaline and noradrenaline in response to an elevation of PCO_2 during apnoeic mass movement oxygenation (Figure 23.2). In moderate hypercapnia there is a proportionate rise of adrenaline and noradrenaline, but in gross hypercapnia (PCO_2 more than 27 kPa or 200 mmHg) there is an abrupt rise of adrenaline. Similar, though variable, changes have been obtained over a lower range of PCO_2 in human volunteers inhaling carbon dioxide mixtures.[18,19] The increase in catecholamine levels is markedly attenuated by either epidural anaesthesia or the administration of clonidine.[20]

The effect of an increased level of circulating catecholamines is, to a certain extent, offset by a decreased sensitivity of target organs when the pH is reduced. This is additional to the general depressant direct effect of carbon dioxide on target organs. There is also evidence that the anterior pituitary is stimulated by carbon dioxide, resulting in increased secretion of ACTH.[21] Acetylcholine hydrolysis is reduced at low pH and therefore certain parasympathetic effects may be enhanced during hypercapnia.

EFFECTS ON OTHER PHYSIOLOGICAL SYSTEMS

Respiratory system

Chapter 5 describes the role of carbon dioxide in the control of breathing and this is not discussed further here.

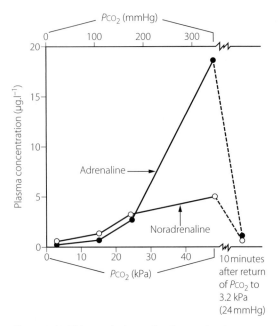

Figure 23.2 This graph shows the changes in plasma catecholamine levels in the dog during the rise of PCO_2 from 2.9 to 45 kPa (22 to 338 mmHg) in the course of 1 hour of apnoeic oxygenation. After 10 minutes of ventilation with oxygen, PCO_2 returned to 3.2 kPa (24 mmHg), following which catecholamines were almost back to control values. (Data from reference 17.)

Pulmonary circulation. An elevated PCO_2 causes vasoconstriction in the pulmonary circulation (page 102) but the effect is less marked than that of hypoxia.[22] Nevertheless, in healthy subjects an end-expiratory PCO_2 of 7 kPa (52 mmHg) increased pulmonary vascular resistance by 32% which, along with elevated cardiac output, led to a 60% increase in mean pulmonary arterial pressure.[23] Although regional variations in blood flow have not been demonstrated, this effect is believed to act in a similar fashion to hypoxic pulmonary vasoconstriction (HPV, page 101), tending to divert blood away from underventilated alveoli. Hypocapnia significantly attenuates HPV in animals, though this has not been described in humans. There is evidence from both animal[24] and human[25] studies that pH is the factor responsible for CO_2-mediated changes in the pulmonary vasculature, rather than PCO_2 *per se*.

Oxygenation of the blood. Quite apart from its effect on ventilation, carbon dioxide exerts three other important effects that influence the oxygenation of the blood. First, if the concentration of nitrogen (or other 'inert' gas) remains constant, the concentration of carbon dioxide in the alveolar gas can increase only at the expense of oxygen, which must be displaced. Second, an increase in P_{CO_2} causes a displacement of the oxygen dissociation curve to the right (page 178). Finally, in animals, changes in P_{CO_2} are known to affect the distribution of ventilation/perfusion ratios as measured by the multiple inert gas elimination technique (page 115). This results from changes in pH influencing pulmonary vessels as described in the previous paragraph, as well as causing changes in the size of small-diameter bronchi.[24]

Cardiovascular system[26]

The effects of carbon dioxide on the circulation are complicated by the alternative modes of action on different components of the system. In general, both hypercapnia and acidosis have direct depressant effects on cardiac myocytes and vascular smooth muscle cells, effects that are normally opposed by the increase in catecholamines caused by elevated P_{CO_2}. Under different circumstances these opposing effects make the overall effect of carbon dioxide on the cardiovascular system unpredictable.

Myocardial contractility and heart rate. Both contractility and heart rate are diminished by elevated P_{CO_2} in isolated preparations, probably as a result of change in pH. However, in the intact subject the direct depressant effect of carbon dioxide is overshadowed by the stimulant effect mediated through the sympathetic system. In artificially ventilated humans, increased P_{CO_2} raises cardiac output and slightly reduces total peripheral resistance,[19] and blood pressure therefore tends to be increased. Awake healthy subjects studied with non-invasive Doppler echocardiography show similar changes.[23] With an end-expiratory P_{CO_2} of 7 kPa (52 mmHg) cardiac output was increased by about 1 l.min^{-1} as a result of increases in both heart rate and stroke volume and accompanied by a small rise in blood pressure. Measurements of left ventricular systolic and diastolic function were unchanged, confirming the dominance of catecholamine stimulation compared with direct depressant effects on the heart. The response of cardiac output to hypercapnia is diminished by most anaesthetics.[19]

Arrhythmias have been reported in awake humans during acute hypercapnia, but seldom seem to be of serious import. One study of normal subjects with modest degrees of hypercapnia did, however, demonstrate an increase in QT dispersion of the electrocardiogram during hypercapnia.[23] This finding reflects regional repolarisation abnormalities of the ventricles and under other circumstances, such as ischaemic heart disease, indicates a propensity to develop life-threatening arrhythmias.

Blood pressure. As described above, an elevated P_{CO_2} usually causes a small increase in blood pressure, an effect seen in both conscious and anaesthetised patients. However, the response is variable and certainly cannot be relied upon as an infallible diagnostic sign of hypercapnia. Hypotension accompanies an elevation of P_{CO_2} if there is blockade of the sympathetic system by, for example, spinal anaesthesia. There is general agreement that hypotension follows a sudden fall of an elevated P_{CO_2}.

Effect on the kidney

Renal blood flow and glomerular filtration rate are little influenced by minor changes of P_{CO_2}. However, at high levels of P_{CO_2} there is constriction of the glomerular afferent arterioles, leading to anuria. Long-term hypercapnia results in increased resorption of bicarbonate by the kidneys, further raising the plasma bicarbonate level and constituting a secondary or compensatory metabolic alkalosis. Long-term hypocapnia decreases renal bicarbonate resorption, resulting in a further fall of plasma bicarbonate and producing a secondary or compensatory metabolic acidosis. In each case the arterial pH returns towards the normal value but the bicarbonate ion concentration departs even further from normality.

Effect on blood electrolyte levels

The acidosis that accompanies hypercapnia causes leakage of potassium ions from the cells into the plasma.[27] Hepatectomy has demonstrated that much of the potassium comes from the liver, possibly in association with glucose that is mobilised in response to the rise in plasma catecholamines.[28] Because it takes an appreciable time for the potassium ions to be transported back into the intracellular compartment, repeated bouts of hypercapnia at short intervals result in a stepwise rise in plasma potassium.

A reduction in the ionised fraction of the total calcium has, in the past, been thought to be the cause of the tetany that accompanies severe hypocapnia. However, the changes that occur are too small to account for tetany, which occurs in parathyroid disease only when there has been a fairly gross reduction of ionised calcium.[29] Hyperexcitability affects all nerves and spontaneous activity ultimately occurs. The muscle spasms probably result from activity in proprioceptive fibres causing reflex muscle contraction.

The effects of long-term small elevations in inspired carbon dioxide are described on page 279.

HYPERCAPNIA IN CLINICAL PRACTICE

Clinical signs

Hyperventilation is the cardinal sign of hypercapnia due to an increased concentration of carbon dioxide in the inspired gas, whether it be endogenous or exogenous. However, this sign will be absent in the paralysed patient and also in those in whom hypercapnia is the result of hypoventilation. Such patients, including those with chronic obstructive pulmonary disease, constitute the great majority of those with hypercapnia.

Dyspnoea may or may not be present. In patients with central failure of respiratory drive, dyspnoea may be entirely absent. On the other hand, when hypoventilation results from mechanical failure in the respiratory system (airway obstruction, pneumothorax, pulmonary fibrosis etc.), dyspnoea is usually obvious.

In patients with chronic obstructive pulmonary disease, hypercapnia is usually associated with a flushed skin and a full and bounding pulse with occasional extrasystoles. The blood pressure is often raised but this is not a reliable sign. Muscle twitchings and a characteristic flap of the hands may be observed when coma is imminent. Convulsions may occur. The patient will become comatose when the $P\text{CO}_2$ is in the range 12–16 kPa (90–120 mmHg) (see above). Hypercapnia should always be considered in cases of unexplained coma.

Hypercapnia cannot be reliably diagnosed on clinical examination. This is particularly true when there is a neurological basis for hypoventilation. Now that it has become so simple to measure the arterial $P\text{CO}_2$, an arterial sample should be taken in all cases of doubt.

Gross hypercapnia

Relatively few cases of gross hypercapnia are documented, but there are sufficient to indicate that complete recovery from gross hypercapnia without hypoxia is possible and may even be the rule.[30] One report from 1990[31] detailed five instances of hypercapnia without hypoxia in children with arterial $P\text{CO}_2$ values in the range 21–36 kPa (155–269 mmHg). All were comatose or stuporose, but recovered. A single case report of massive grain aspiration reported survival following a $P\text{CO}_2$ of 66.8 kPa (501 mmHg).[32] These cases indicate that, *of the reported cases*, full recovery seems to be the usual outcome. Hypoxia seems to be much more dangerous than hypercapnia.

REFERENCES

*1. Laffey JG, Kavanagh BP. Hypocapnia. *N Engl J Med* 2002; **347**: 43–53.

2. Leake CD, Waters RM. The anesthetic properties of carbon dioxide. *J Pharmacol Exp Ther* 1928; **33**: 280–1.

3. Refsum HE. Relationship between state of consciousness and arterial hypoxaemia and hypercapnia in patients with pulmonary insufficiency, breathing air. *Clin Sci* 1963; **25**: 361–7.

4. Eisele JH, Eger EI, Muallem M. Narcotic properties of carbon dioxide in the dog. *Anesthesiology* 1967; **28**: 856–65.

*5. Brian JE. Carbon dioxide and the cerebral circulation. *Anesthesiology* 1998; **88**: 1365–86.

6. Wilkinson IMS, Browne DRG. The influence of anaesthesia and of arterial hypocapnia on regional blood flow in the normal human cerebral hemisphere. *Br J Anaesth* 1970; **42**: 472–82.

7. Raichle ME, Posner JB, Plum F. Cerebral blood flow during and after hyperventilation. *Arch Neurol* 1970; **23**: 394–403.

8. Lassen NA. The luxury-perfusion syndrome and its possible relation to acute metabolic acidosis localised within the brain. *Lancet* 1966; **2**: 1113–15.

9. Strebel S, Kaufmann M, Baggi M, Zenklusen U. Cerebrovascular carbon dioxide reactivity during exposure to equipotent isoflurane and isoflurane in nitrous oxide anaesthesia. *Br J Anaesth* 1993; **71**: 272–6.

10. Christensen MS, Hoedt-Rasmussen K, Lassen NA. Cerebral vasodilation by halothane anaesthesia in man and its potentiation by hypotension and hypercapnia. *Br J Anaesth* 1967; **39**: 927–34.

11. Ornstein E, Young WL, Fleischer LH, Ostapkovich N. Desflurane and isoflurane have similar effects on cerebral blood flow in patients with intracranial mass lesions. *Anesthesiology* 1993; **79**: 498–502.

12. Cho S, Kujigaki T, Uchiyama Y, Fukusai M, Shibata O, Somikawa K. Effects of sevoflurane with and without nitrous oxide on human cerebral circulation. *Anesthesiology* 1996; **85**: 755–60.

13. Pierce EC, Lambertson CJ, Deutsch S, *et al*. Cerebral circulation and metabolism during thiopental anesthesia and hyperventilation in man. *J Clin Invest* 1962; **41**: 1664–71.

14. Eng C, Lam AM, Mayberg TS, Lee C, Mathisen T. The influence of propofol with and without nitrous oxide on cerebral blood flow velocity and CO_2 reactivity in humans. *Anesthesiology* 1992; **77**: 872–9.

15. Shenkin HA, Bouzarth WF. Clinical methods of reducing intracranial pressure. *N Engl J Med* 1970; **282**: 1465–71.

*16. Yundt KD, Diringer MN. The use of hyperventilation and its impact on cerebral ischaemia in the treatment of traumatic brain injury. *Crit Care Clin* 1997; **13**: 163–84.

17. Millar RA. Plasma adrenaline and noradrenaline during diffusion respiration. *J Physiol* 1960; **150**: 79–90.

18. Sechzer PH, Egbert LD, Linde HW, Cooper DY, Dripps RD, Price HL. Effect of CO_2 inhalation on arterial pressure ECG and plasma catecholamines and 17-OH corticosteroids in normal man. *J Appl Physiol* 1960; **15**: 454–8.

19. Cullen DJ, Eger EI. Cardiovascular effects of carbon dioxide in man. *Anesthesiology* 1974; **41**: 345–9.

20. Nishikawa T, Naito H. Clonidine modulation of hemodynamic and catecholamine responses associated with hypoxia or hypercapnia in dogs. *Anesthesiology* 1996; **84**: 672–85.

21. Tenney SM. The effect of carbon dioxide on neurohumeral and endocrine mechanisms. *Anesthesiology* 1960; **21**: 674–85.

22. Barer GR, Howard P, McCurrie JR. The effect of carbon dioxide and changes in blood pH on pulmonary vascular resistance in cats. *Clin Sci* 1967; **32**: 361–76.

*23. Kiely DG, Cargill RI, Lipworth BJ. Effects of hypercapnia on hemodynamic, inotropic, lusitropic and electrophysiological indices in humans. *Chest* 1996; **109**: 1215–21.

24. Domino KB, Swenson ER, Hlastala MP. Hypocapnia-induced ventilation/perfusion mismatch: a direct CO_2 or pH-mediated effect. *Am J Respir Crit Care Med* 1995; **152**: 1534–9.

25. Loeppky JA, Scotto P, Riedel CE, Roach RC, Chick TW. Effects of acid–base status on acute hypoxic pulmonary vasoconstriction and gas exchange. *J Appl Physiol* 1992; **72**: 1787–97.

26. Foëx P. Effects of carbon dioxide on the systemic circulation. In: Prys-Roberts C, ed. *The circulation in anaesthesia*. Oxford: Blackwell Scientific,1980.

27. Clowes GHA, Hopkins AL, Simeone FA. A comparison of physiological effects of hypercapnia and hypoxia in the production of cardiac arrest. *Ann Surg* 1955; **142**: 446–60.

28. Fenn WO, Asano T. Effects of carbon dioxide inhalation on potassium liberation from the liver. *Am J Physiol* 1956; **185**: 567–9.

29. Tenney SM, Lamb TW. Physiological consequences of hypoventilation and hyperventilation. In: Fenn WO, Rahn H, eds. *Handbook of physiology; section 3, volume 2 – Respiration*. Washington DC: American Physiological Society, 1965.

30. Potkin RT, Swenson ER. Resuscitation from severe acute hypercapnia. Determinants of tolerance and survival. *Chest* 1992; **102**: 1742–5.

31. Goldstein B, Shannon DC, Todres ID. Supercarbia in children: clinical course and outcome. *Crit Care Med* 1990; **18**: 166–8.

32. Slinger P, Blundell PE, Metcalf IR. Management of massive grain aspiration. *Anesthesiology* 1997; **87**: 993–5.

KEY POINTS

■ Intracellular acidosis from anaerobic metabolism occurs soon after the onset of cellular hypoxia and is worse when there is a plentiful supply of glucose to the cell.

■ Lack of high-energy substrates such as ATP and direct effects of hypoxia both inhibit the activity of ion channels, decreasing the transmembrane potential of the cell, leading to increased intracellular calcium levels.

■ In nervous tissue the uncontrolled release of excitatory amino acids exacerbates the hypoxic damage.

■ Hypoxia also causes the activation of a transcription protein, HIF-1, which induces the production of several proteins with diverse biological functions.

Chapter 1 explained how all but the simplest forms of life have evolved to exploit the immense advantages of oxidative metabolism. The price they have paid is to become dependent on oxygen for their survival. The essential feature of hypoxia is the cessation of oxidative phosphorylation (page 184) when the mitochondrial PO_2 falls below a critical level. Anaerobic pathways, in particular the glycolytic pathway (see Figure 11.13), then come into play. These trigger a complex series of cellular changes leading first to reduced cellular function and ultimately to cell death.

BIOCHEMICAL CHANGES IN HYPOXIA

Depletion of high-energy compounds

Anaerobic metabolism produces only one-nineteenth of the yield of the high-energy phosphate compound adenosine triphosphate (ATP) per mole of glucose compared to aerobic metabolism (page 186). In organs with a high metabolic rate, such as the brain, it is impossible to increase glucose transport sufficiently to main-

tain the normal level of ATP production. Therefore, during hypoxia, the ATP/ADP (adenosine diphosphate) ratio falls and there is a rapid decline in the level of all high-energy compounds (Figure 24.1). Very similar changes occur in response to arterial hypotension. These changes will rapidly block cerebral function, but organs with a lower energy requirement will continue to function for a longer time and are thus more resistant to hypoxia (see below).

Under hypoxic conditions, there are two ways in which reductions in ATP levels may be minimised, both of which are effective for only a short time. First, the high-energy phosphate bond in phosphocreatine may be used to create ATP,[2] and initially this slows the rate of reduction of ATP (see Figure 24.1). Second, two molecules of ADP may combine to form one of ATP and one of adenosine monophosphate (AMP) (the adenylate kinase reaction). This reaction is driven forward by the removal of AMP, which is converted to adenosine (a potent vasodilator) and thence to inosine, hypoxanthine, xanthine and uric acid, with irreversible loss of adenine nucleotides. The implications for production of reactive oxygen species are discussed on page 353.

End-products of metabolism

The end-products of aerobic metabolism are carbon dioxide and water, both of which are easily diffusible and lost from the body. The main anaerobic pathway produces hydrogen and lactate ions which, from most of the body, escape into the circulation, where they may be conveniently quantified in terms of the base deficit, excess lactate or lactate/pyruvate ratio. However, the blood–brain barrier is relatively impermeable to charged ions and therefore hydrogen and lactate ions are retained within the neurones of the hypoxic brain. Lactacidosis can only occur when circulation is maintained to provide the large quantities of glucose required for conversion to lactic acid.

In severe cerebral hypoxia, a major part of the dysfunction and damage is due to intracellular acidosis rather than simply depletion of high-energy compounds (see below). Gross hypoperfusion is more damaging than

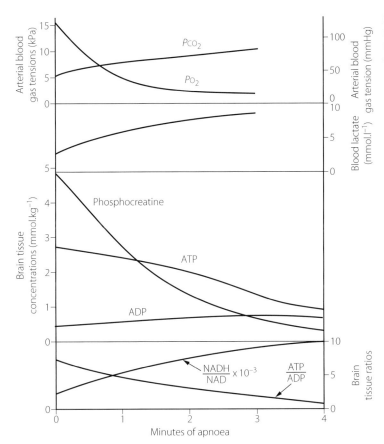

Figure 24.1 Biochemical changes during 4 minutes of respiratory arrest in rats previously breathing 30% oxygen. Recovery of all values, except blood lactate, was complete within 5 minutes of restarting pulmonary ventilation. (Data from reference 1.)

total ischaemia, because the latter limits glucose supply and therefore the formation of lactic acid. Similarly, patients who have an episode of cerebral ischaemia while hyperglycaemic (e.g. a stroke) have been found to have more severe brain injury than those with normal or low blood glucose levels at the time of the hypoxic event.[3]

Initiation of glycolysis[4]

The enzyme 6-phosphofructokinase (PFK) is the rate-limiting step of the glycolytic pathway (see Figure 11.13). Activity of PFK is enhanced by the presence of ADP, AMP and phosphate, which will rapidly accumulate during hypoxia, thus accelerating glycolysis. PFK is, however, inhibited by acidosis, which will therefore quickly limit the formation of ATP from glucose and may even result in hyperglycaemia. The intracellular production of phosphate from ATP breakdown also promotes the activity of glycogen phosphorylase, which cleaves glycogen molecules to produce fructose-1,6-diphosphate. This enters the glycolytic pathway below the rate-limiting PFK reaction and also avoids the expenditure of two molecules of ATP in its derivation from

glucose. Therefore four molecules of ATP are produced from one of fructose-1,6-diphosphate, in comparison with two from one molecule of glucose. There is no subsequent stage in the glycolytic pathway that is significantly rate limited by acidosis. Provided glycogen is available within the cell, this second pathway therefore provides a valuable reserve for the production of ATP.

MECHANISMS OF HYPOXIC CELL DAMAGE

Many mechanisms contribute to cell damage or death from hypoxia. The precise role of each is unclear, but there is general agreement that different tissues respond to hypoxia in quite varied ways. Also, the nature of the hypoxic insult has a large effect, with differing speed of onset, degree of hypoxia, blood flow, blood glucose concentration and tissue metabolic activity all influencing the resulting tissue dysfunction.

Immediate cellular responses to hypoxia[5]

Because of the dramatic clinical consequences of nervous system damage, neuronal cells are the most widely studied and therefore form the basis for the mechanisms

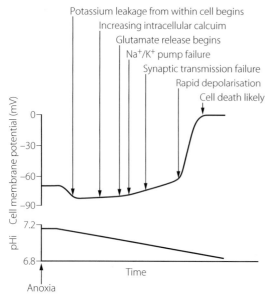

Figure 24.2 Changes in transmembrane potential and intracellular pH (pHi) in a neuronal cell following the sudden onset of anoxia. Significant physiological events in the course of the hypoxic insult are shown. Once membrane potential reaches zero, cell death is almost inevitable (see text for details). The time between anoxia and rapid depolarisation is highly variable, between about 4 minutes with complete ischaemia to almost an hour with hypoxia and preserved blood flow. (After reference 2.)

described in this section.[2] Changes in the transmembrane potential of a hypoxic neurone are shown in Figure 24.2, along with the major physiological changes that occur. At the onset of anoxia, CNS cells immediately become either slightly hyperpolarised (as shown in Figure 24.2) or depolarised, depending on the cell type. This is followed by a gradual reduction in membrane potential until a 'threshold' value is reached, when a spontaneous rapid depolarisation occurs. At this stage there are gross abnormalities in ion channel function and the normal intracellular and extracellular ionic gradients are abolished, leading to cell death.

Potassium and sodium flux. Hypoxia has a direct effect on potassium channels, increasing transmembrane K^+ conductance and causing the immediate hyperpolarisation. Potassium begins to leak out from the cell, increasing the extracellular K^+ concentration and thus tending to depolarise the cell membrane. Potassium leakage and sodium influx are accelerated when falling ATP levels cause failure of the Na^+/K^+-ATPase pump. Following rapid depolarisation, sodium and potassium channels probably simply remain open, allowing free passage of

ions across the cell membrane, leading to cellular destruction.

Calcium. Intracellular calcium concentration increases shortly after the onset of hypoxia. Voltage-gated calcium channels open in response to the falling transmembrane potential and the increasing intracellular sodium concentration causes the membrane-bound Na/Ca exchanger to reverse its activity. An altered transmembrane potential is detected within the cell by ryonidine receptors on intracellular organelles, leading to release of calcium from the endoplasmic reticulum and mitochondria.[6] This increase in intracellular calcium is generally harmful, causing the activation of ATPase enzymes just when ATP may be critically low, the activation of proteases to damage sarcolemma and the cytoskeleton, and the uncontrolled release of neurotransmitters (see below). At this stage, the cell has probably not been irretrievably damaged by spontaneous depolarisation, but derangement of calcium channel function effectively prevents normal synaptic transmission and therefore cellular function. Extracellular adenosine, formed from the degradation of AMP, is also believed to play a role in blocking calcium channels during anoxia.[2]

Excitatory amino acid release.[7] The excitatory amino acids glutamate and aspartate are released from many neurones at concentrations of 2–5 times normal early in the course of a hypoxic insult, followed by further dramatic increases after rapid depolarisation. Glutamate reuptake mechanisms also fail and extracellular concentrations quickly reach neurotoxic levels,[7,8] acting via the N-methyl-D-aspartate (NMDA) receptor. Cells with depleted energy stores are particularly susceptible,[9] but the mechanism by which glutamate and aspartate bring about cell damage is currently unknown.

Delayed cellular responses to hypoxia

Following brain injury in humans, cerebral oedema often continues to develop for some hours after the initial insult. There are several possible explanations for this delayed neuronal damage, with activation of many different cellular systems being implicated. However, it is a quite different clinical problem that has recently focused attention on cellular adaptations to hypoxia. The core of many solid malignant tumours has a poor blood supply, caused by the failure of angiogenesis to keep up with the rapid tumour growth. Tumour hypoxia is associated with highly malignant, aggressive tumours, which often respond poorly to treatment. For this reason, much recent research has focused on understanding the cellular effects of hypoxia, with a view to developing new therapeutic approaches.

Table 24.1 Genes induced by hypoxia and their effects

Function	Gene	Biological action
Oxygen transport	Erythropoietin	Stimulation of red cell production
	Transferrin	Iron transport
Increased blood flow	VEGF	Angiogenesis
	NO synthase	Vasodilation
ATP production	Glucose transporter-1	Transfer of glucose into cell
	Hexokinase	
	Aldolase	Glycolysis (see Figure 11.13)
	Pyruvate kinase	
	Lactate dehydrogenase	
pH correction	Carbonic anhydrase	Buffering of metabolic acidosis
Inflammation	Interleukin-6, -8	Activation of inflammatory cells

VEGF, Vascular endothelial growth factor; NO, nitric oxide.

Table 24.1 shows the numerous genes that may be induced by hypoxia. Most of the systems activated by hypoxia assist the cell in overcoming the hypoxic conditions, for example erythropoietin to increase haemoglobin concentration or glycolytic enzymes to increase anaerobic ATP formation. Some activated genes may accelerate cell proliferation and therefore increase tumour malignancy, whereas others are activated that encourage apoptosis and impair tumour growth.[10]

Hypoxia-inducible factor 1 (HIF-1).[11,12] Many of these cellular adaptations to hypoxia are mediated by a transcription-regulating protein called HIF-1. Under normal conditions cytoplasmic HIF-1 is ubiquitous, but a prolyl-hydroxylase protein (PHD-1) rapidly hydroxylates HIF-1, rendering it inactive. Oxygen is required as a cosubstrate for this reaction, such that when cellular hypoxia occurs hydroxylation by PHD-1 fails and HIF-1 remains stable for long enough to initiate transcription of some of the hypoxia-induced genes shown in Table 24.1. The HIF-1 system is now seen as a major potential target for therapeutic agents to treat malignancies prone to tumour hypoxia.

Ischaemic preconditioning[13,14]

Prior exposure of a tissue to a series of short periods of hypoxia, interspersed with normal oxygen levels, has been found to influence the tissue's subsequent response to a prolonged ischaemic insult, a phenomenon known as ischaemic preconditioning. Though mostly studied in heart muscle, ischaemic preconditioning has been demonstrated in many other tissues.

Early protection. Reduction in the damage occurring from an ischaemic period begins immediately after the preconditioning has occurred and lasts for 2–3 hours. Activation of sarcolemmal and mitochondrial ATP-dependent K channels (K_{ATP}) is believed to be the main mechanism by which protection from ischaemia occurs. After preconditioning, the enhanced activity of K_{ATP} channels helps to maintain the transmembrane potential nearer to normal values and so slows the rate of progression of the immediate cellular responses to hypoxia described above. During prolonged hypoxia, fluid and electrolyte imbalances also occur across the mitochondrial membrane, impairing the ability of the cell to make the best use of any oxygen remaining in the cell. Activated mitochondrial K_{ATP} channels will again reduce the rate at which these changes occur. Extracellular triggers that bring about preconditioning include adenosine, purines, bradykinin or catecholamines, all acting via G-proteins and protein kinase C to cause activation of the K_{ATP} channels.

Late protection. This describes the protection from ischaemia seen about 12 hours after the preconditioning and is less effective than early protection. It is again mediated by activation of K_{ATP} channels, this time brought about by gene transcription of proteins such as inducible nitric oxide synthase, superoxide dismutase (page 355) or cyclooxygenase (page 205).

Anaesthetic preconditioning.[13,15] Several drugs, but particularly inhalational anaesthetics, can precondition cardiac muscle in a manner similar to brief ischaemic episodes. The mechanism is also similar, with most of the effective drugs somehow enhancing K_{ATP} channel activity. Unfortunately, impressive laboratory studies of anaesthetic preconditioning have so far failed to translate into clinically useful benefits, possibly because of an inability of diseased cardiac muscle to show the same response to preconditioning as that of normal myocardium.[14]

Po_2 LEVELS AT WHICH HYPOXIA OCCURS

Cellular Po_2

'Critical Po_2' refers to the oxygen tension below which oxidative cellular metabolism fails. For isolated mitochondria, this is known to be below 0.13 kPa (1 mmHg) and possibly as low as 0.01 kPa (0.1 mmHg) in muscle cells[4] despite their large oxygen consumption. Venous Po_2 approximates to end-capillary Po_2 and, though highly variable, this is usually in excess of 3 kPa ($\approx$20 mmHg), even in maximally working skeletal muscle. Thus with the minimal Po_2 in the nearby capillary being approximately 200 times greater than that required by the mitochondria, it is difficult to envisage how cellular hypoxia can occur in all but the most extreme situations. There are reasons why this is not the case *in vivo*.

Measurement of intracellular Po_2 is difficult. The most widely used technique is applicable only to muscle cells and involves measurement of myoglobin saturation, from which Po_2 may be determined. These studies have indicated that intracellular Po_2 is in the range 0.5–2 kPa (3–15 mmHg) depending on cell activity.[4] Many studies have also indicated a minimal difference between the Po_2 in extracellular fluid and within cells.[16] This would indicate a possibly substantial barrier to oxygen diffusion between the capillary and extracellular fluid. Finally, diffusion of oxygen within cells is believed to be slow because of the proteinaceous nature of the cytoplasm and therefore large variations in intracellular Po_2 are likely to exist. Thus in intact cells, as opposed to isolated mitochondria, critical Po_2 is more likely to be of the order of 0.5–1.3 kPa (3–10 mmHg), much closer to the end-capillary value.[17]

Venous Po_2 was for many years thought to reflect the Po_2 at the cell surface but, as indicated in the previous paragraph, this is no longer believed to be so. However, the factors that alter Po_2 between capillary and cell probably remain fairly constant, so venous Po_2 remains a useful and practicable measure of the functional state of oxygenation of an organ. For example, consciousness is usually lost when the internal jugular venous Po_2 falls below about 2.7 kPa (20 mmHg) whatever the cause.

Critical arterial Po_2 for cerebral function

The minimal safe level of arterial Po_2 is that which will maintain a safe tissue Po_2. This will depend on many factors besides arterial Po_2, including haemoglobin concentration, tissue perfusion and tissue oxygen consumption. These factors accord with Barcroft's classification of 'anoxia' into anoxic, anaemic and stagnant (page 188), which has previously been shown as a Venn diagram (see Figure 11.16).

This argument may be extended to consider in which circumstances the venous Po_2 (and by implication tissue Po_2) may fall below its critical level corresponding, in normal blood, to 32% saturation and oxygen content of 6.4 ml.dl^{-1}. If the brain has a mean oxygen consumption of 46 ml.min^{-1} and a blood flow of 620 ml.min^{-1}, the arterial/venous oxygen content difference will be 7.4 ml.dl^{-1}. Therefore, *with normal cerebral perfusion, haemoglobin concentration, pH etc.*, this would correspond to a critical arterial oxygen content of 13.8 ml.dl^{-1}, saturation 68% and Po_2 4.8 kPa (36 mmHg). This calculation and others under various different conditions are set out in Table 24.2.

However, the other factors in italics (above) will probably not be normal. They may be unfavourable as a result of multiple pathologies in the patient (e.g. anaemia or a decreased cerebral blood flow). Alternatively, there may be favourable factors, such as polycythaemia in chronic arterial hypoxaemia or reduced cerebral oxygen requirements during hypothermia or anaesthesia. The possible combinations of circumstances are so great that it is not feasible to consider every possible situation. Instead, certain important examples have been selected which illustrate the fundamentals of the problem, and these are shown in Table 24.2.

A twofold increase in cerebral blood flow would allow the arterial Po_2 to decrease further from 4.8 to 3.6 kPa (36 to 27 mmHg) before the cerebral venous Po_2 reached 2.7 kPa (20 mmHg). This is important, as an increase in cerebral blood flow may be expected to follow severe hypoxia. Polycythaemia (e.g. a haemoglobin concentration of 18 g.dl^{-1}) does not confer the same degree of benefit and the critical arterial Po_2 would then be 4.3 kPa (32 mmHg). Alkalosis, which may be expected to result from the hypoxic drive to respiration, confers no advantage at all. Considerable advantage derives from hypothermia, owing to the reduction in cerebral metabolism, but not the shift of the dissociation curve.

Uncompensated ischaemia is dangerous and, with a 45% reduction in cerebral blood flow, any reduction in arterial Po_2 exposes the brain to the risk of hypoxia. Uncompensated anaemia is almost equally dangerous, although an increase in cerebral blood flow restores a satisfactory safety margin. In the example in Table 24.2, a 40% reduction of blood oxygen-carrying capacity and a 40% increase of cerebral blood flow permits the arterial Po_2 to fall to 5.3 kPa (40 mmHg) without the cerebral venous Po_2 falling below 2.7 kPa (20 mmHg). The last

Table 24.2 Lowest arterial oxygen levels compatible with a cerebral venous PO_2 of 2.7 kPa (20 mmHg) under various conditions

| | Blood O_2 capacity ml.dl⁻¹ | Brain O_2 consumption ml.min⁻¹ | Cerebral blood flow ml.min⁻¹ | Cerebral venous blood | | | | Art./ven. O_2 content difference ml.dl⁻¹ | Arterial blood | | | |
				PO_2 kPa	PO_2 mmHg	Sat. %	O_2 content ml.dl⁻¹		O_2 content ml.dl⁻¹	Sat. %	PO_2 kPa	PO_2 mmHg
Normal values	20	46	620	4.4	33	63	12.6	7.4	20.0	98	13	100
Uncompensated arterial hypoxaemia	20	46	620	2.7	20	32	6.4	7.4	13.8	68	4.8	36
Arterial hypoxaemia with increased cerebral blood flow	20	46	1240	2.7	20	32	6.4	3.7	10.1	50	3.6	27
Arterial hypoxaemia with polycythaemia	25	46	620	2.7	20	32	8.0	7.4	15.4	61	4.3	32
Arterial hypoxaemia with alkalosis*	20	46	620	2.7	20	46	9.2	7.4	16.6	82	4.9	37
Arterial hypoxaemia with hypothermia†	20	23	620	2.7	20	57	11.4	3.7	15.1	75	3.6	27
Uncompensated cerebral ischaemia	20	46	340	2.7	20	32	6.4	13.5	19.9	98	15	112
Uncompensated anaemia	12	46	620	2.7	20	32	3.8	7.4	11.2	93	8.9	67
Anaemia with increased cerebral blood flow	12	46	870	2.7	20	32	3.8	5.3	9.1	75	5.3	40
Combined anaemia and ischaemia	15	46	460	2.7	20	32	4.8	10.0	14.8	97	12	92

* pH 7.6.
† temperature 30°C; cerebral O_2 consumption reduced to half normal.

line in Table 24.2 shows the very dangerous combination of anaemia (haemoglobin concentration 11 g.dl⁻¹) and cerebral blood flow three-quarters of normal. Neither abnormality is very serious considered separately, but in combination the arterial PO_2 cannot be reduced below its normal value without the risk of cerebral hypoxia.

Table 24.2 is not to be taken too literally, because there are many minor factors that have not been considered. However, it is a general rule that maximal cerebral vasodilation may be expected to occur in any condition (other than cerebral ischaemia) that threatens cerebral oxygenation. Also, there are circumstances in which the critical organ is not the brain but the heart, liver or kidney.

The most important message of this discussion is that there is no simple answer to the question 'What is the safe lower limit of arterial PO_2?'. Acclimatised mountaineers have remained conscious during exercise at high altitude with arterial PO_2 values as low as 2.7 kPa (20 mmHg) (see Chapter 17). Patients presenting with severe respiratory disease tend to remain conscious down to the same level of arterial PO_2.[18] However, both acclimatised mountaineers and patients with chronic respiratory disease have compensatory polycythaemia and maximal cerebral vasodilation. Uncompensated subjects who are acutely exposed to hypoxia are unlikely to remain conscious with an arterial PO_2 of less than about 3.6 kPa (27 mmHg), but considerable individual variation must be expected.

Organ survival times *in vivo*

Lack of oxygen stops the machine and then wrecks the machinery. The time of circulatory arrest up to the first event (survival time) must be distinguished from the duration of anoxia that results in the second event (revival time), the latter being defined as the time beyond which no recovery of function is possible. Incomplete recovery of function may follow anoxia lasting more than the survival time but less than the revival time. Revival times tend to be about four times as long as survival times.

From the complex sequence of cellular events already described, it will be clear that tissue survival times depend on many factors. There is a very large difference between different organs, ranging from less than 1 minute for the cerebral cortex to about 2 hours for skeletal muscle. Heart is intermediate, with a survival time of about 5 minutes, liver and kidney probably being about 10 minutes. Similarly, survival time is also influenced by oxygen consumption and oxygen stores in the tissue concerned. An inactive organ (such as a heart in asystole or the brain in hypothermia) has increased resistance to hypoxia, and there is a small but definite increase in survival time when tissue PO_2 has been increased by hyperbaric oxygenation. Hypothermia both decreases oxygen demand and increases the solubility of oxygen in the tissue.

EFFECTS OF HYPOXIA

Hypoxia presents a serious threat to the body and compensatory mechanisms usually take priority over other changes. Thus, for example, in hypoxia with concomitant hypocapnia, hyperventilation and an increase in cerebral blood flow occur in spite of the decreased P_{CO_2}. Certain compensatory mechanisms will come into play whatever the reason for the hypoxia, although their effectiveness will depend to a large extent on the cause. For example, hyperventilation will be largely ineffective in stagnant or anaemic hypoxia, because hyperventilation while breathing air can do little to increase the oxygen content of arterial blood and usually nothing to increase perfusion.

Hyperventilation results from a decreased arterial P_{O_2} but the response is non-linear (see Figure 5.8). There is little effect until arterial P_{O_2} is reduced to about 7 kPa (52.5 mmHg): maximal response is at 4 kPa (30 mmHg). The interrelationship between hypoxia and other factors in the control of breathing is discussed in Chapter 5.

Pulmonary distribution of blood flow is improved by hypoxia as a result of hypoxic pulmonary vasoconstriction (page 101).

The sympathetic system is concerned in many of the responses to hypoxia, particularly the increase in organ perfusion. The immediate response is reflex and is initiated by chemoreceptor stimulation: it occurs before there is any measurable increase in circulating catecholamines, although this does occur in due course. Reduction of cerebral and probably myocardial vascular resistance is not dependent on the autonomic system but depends on local responses in the vicinity of the vessels themselves. With the exception of pulmonary vessels, hypoxia causes vasodilation of blood vessels almost everywhere in the body. This results mainly from a direct effect of adenosine and other metabolites generated by hypoxia.

Cardiac output is increased by hypoxia, together with the regional blood flow to almost every major organ, particularly the brain.

Haemoglobin concentration is not increased in acute hypoxia in humans but it is increased in chronic hypoxia due to residence at altitude or respiratory disease.

The oxyhaemoglobin dissociation curve is displaced to the right by an increase in 2,3-DPG and by acidosis which may also be present. This tends to increase tissue P_{O_2} (see Figure 11.10).

Anaerobic metabolism is increased in severe hypoxia in an attempt to maintain the level of ATP (see above).

REFERENCES

1. Kaasik AE, Nilsson L, Siesjö BK. The effect of asphyxia upon the lactate, pyruvate and bicarbonate concentrations of brain tissue and cisternal CSF and upon the tissue concentrations of phosphocreatine and adenine nucleotides in anesthetized rats. *Acta Physiol Scand* 1970; **78**: 433–47.
2. Martin RL, Lloyd HGE, Cowan AI. The early events of oxygen and glucose deprivation: setting the scene for neuronal death? *Trends Neurosci* 1994; **17**: 251–6.
3. Candelise L, Landi G, Orazio EN, Boccardi E. Prognostic significance of hyperglycaemia in acute stroke. *Arch Neurol* 1985; 42: 661–3.
4. Connett RJ, Honig CR, Gayeski TEJ, Brooks GA. Defining hypoxia: a systems view of $\dot{V}_{O_2}$, glycolysis, energetics and intracellular P_{O_2}. *J Appl Physiol* 1990; **68**: 833–42.
*5. Ransom BR, Brown AM. Intracellular Ca^{2+} release and ischemic axon injury: the Trojan horse is back. *Neuron* 2003; **40**: 2–4.
6. Katchman AN, Hershkowitz N. Early anoxia-induced vesicular glutamate release results from mobilization of calcium from intracellular stores. *J Neurophysiol* 1993; **70**: 1–7.
7. Choi DW. Cerebral hypoxia: some new approaches and unanswered questions. *J Neurosci* 1990; **10**: 2493–501.
8. Ohmori T, Hirashima Y, Kurimoto M, Endo S, Takaku A. In vitro hypoxia of cortical and hippocampal CA1 neurons: glutamate, nitric oxide and platelet activating factor participate in the mechanism of selective neural death in CA1 neurons. *Brain Res* 1996; **743**: 109–15.
9. Novelli A, Reilly JA, Lysko PG, Henneberry RC. Glutamate becomes neurotoxic via the N-methyl-D-aspartate receptor when intracellular energy levels are reduced. *Brain Res* 1988; **451**: 205–12.
*10. Harris AL. Hypoxia – a key regulatory factor in tumour growth. *Nat Rev Cancer* 2002; **2**: 38–46.
11. Höpfl G, Ogunshola O, Gassman M. HIFs and tumors – causes and consequences. *Am J Physiol Regul Integr Comp Physiol* 2004; **286**: R608–23.
*12. Semenza GL. HIF-1: mediator of physiological and pathophysiological responses to hypoxia. *J Appl Physiol* 2000; **88**: 1474–80.
13. Zaugg M, Lucchinetti E, Uecker M, Pasch T, Schaub MC. Anaesthetics and cardiac preconditioning. Part I.

Signalling and cytoprotective mechanisms. *Br J Anaesth* 2003; **91**: 551–65.

14. Zaugg M, Lucchinetti E, Garcia C, Pasch T, Spahn DR, Schaub MC. Anaesthetics and cardiac preconditioning. Part II. Clinical implications. *Br J Anaesth* 2003; **91**: 566–76.

15. Tanaka K, Ludwig LM, Kersten JR, Pagel PS, Warltier DC. Mechanisms of cardioprotection by volatile anaesthetics. *Anesthesiology* 2004; **100**: 707–21.

16. Rumsey WL, Wilson DF. Tissue capacity for mitochondrial oxidative phosphorylation and its adaptation to stress. In: Fregly MJ, Blatteis CM, eds. *Handbook of physiology, section 4: Environmental physiology*. New York: Oxford University Press, 1996.

17. Epstein FH, Agmon Y, Brezis M. Physiology of renal hypoxia. *Ann N Y Acad Sci* 1995; **718**: 72–81.

18. McNicol MW, Campbell EJM. Severity of respiratory failure. *Lancet* 1965; **1**: 336–8.

KEY POINTS

■ Anaemia has little effect on pulmonary gas exchange but decreases oxygen carriage in the arterial blood in direct proportion to the reduction in haemoglobin concentration.

■ Mechanisms that compensate for the reduced oxygen delivery include increased cardiac output, increased tissue oxygen extraction and a right shift of the oxyhaemoglobin dissociation curve.

■ Older patients or those with poor cardiac reserve compensate less well when anaemic.

Anaemia is a widespread pathophysiological disorder that interferes with oxygen transport to the tissues. In developed countries it has a varied aetiology, including iron deficiency, chronic haemorrhage, end-stage renal failure or depletion of vitamin B$_{12}$. However, in the third world it is endemic, major factors including malnutrition and infestation with various parasites such as hookworm and bilharzia. In many countries, haemoglobin concentrations within the range 6–10 g.dl^{-1} are regarded as normal.

Anaemia *per se* has no major direct effects on pulmonary function. Arterial PO$_2$ and saturation should remain within the normal range in uncomplicated anaemia and the crucial effect is on the arterial oxygen content and hence oxygen delivery. Important compensatory changes are increases in cardiac output, greater oxygen extraction from the arterial blood and, to a lesser extent, the small rightward displacement of the oxyhaemoglobin dissociation curve. However, there are limits to these adaptations, which define the minimal tolerable haemoglobin concentration and also the exercise limits attainable at various levels of severity of anaemia.

Physiological aspects of blood transfusion and blood substitutes are discussed on page 182 *et seq*.

PULMONARY FUNCTION

Gas exchange

Alveolar PO$_2$ is determined by dry barometric pressure, inspired oxygen concentration and the ratio of oxygen consumption to alveolar ventilation (page 167). Assuming that the first two factors are unchanged, and there being good evidence that the latter two are unaffected in the resting state by anaemia down to a haemoglobin concentration of at least 5 g.dl^{-1} (see below), then there is no reason why alveolar PO$_2$ or PCO$_2$ should be affected by uncomplicated anaemia down to this degree of severity.

The increased cardiac output (see below) will cause a small reduction in pulmonary capillary transit time which, together with the reduced mass of haemoglobin in the pulmonary capillaries, causes a modest decrease in diffusing capacity or transfer factor (page 141). However, such is the reserve in the capacity of pulmonary capillary blood to reach equilibrium with the alveolar gas (see Figure 9.2) that it is highly unlikely that this would have any measurable effect on the alveolar/end-pulmonary capillary PO$_2$ gradient, which in the normal subject is now believed to be of the order of only 10^{-6} mmHg. Thus pulmonary end-capillary PO$_2$ should also be normal in uncomplicated anaemia.

Continuing down the cascade of oxygen partial pressures from ambient air to the site of use in the tissues, the next step is the gradient in PO$_2$ between pulmonary end-capillary blood and mixed arterial blood. The PO$_2$ gradient at this stage is caused by shunting and the perfusion of relatively underventilated alveoli. There is no evidence that these factors are altered in anaemia and arterial PO$_2$ should therefore be normal. Because the peripheral chemoreceptors are stimulated by reduction in arterial PO$_2$ and not arterial oxygen content (page 64), there should be no stimulation of respiration unless the degree of hypoxia is sufficient to cause anaerobic metabolism and lactacidosis.

The haemoglobin dissociation curve

It is well established that red blood cell 2,3-diphospho-glycerate levels are increased in anaemia (page 178), typical changes being from a normal value of 5 mmol.l^{-1} to 7 mmol.l^{-1} at a haemoglobin concentration of 6 g.dl^{-1}.[1] This results in an increase in P_{50} from 3.6 to 4.0 kPa (27 to 30 mmHg). This rightward shift of the dissociation curve would have a negligible effect on arterial saturation, which has indeed been reported to be normal in anaemia. The rightward shift will, however, increase the P_{O_2} at which oxygen is unloaded in the tissues, mitigating to a small extent the effects of reduction in oxygen delivery so far as tissue P_{O_2} is concerned.

Arterial oxygen content

Although the arterial oxygen saturation usually remains normal in anaemia, the oxygen content of the arterial blood will be reduced in approximate proportion to the decrease in haemoglobin concentration. Arterial oxygen content can be expressed as follows:

$$
\begin{array}{llllll}
Ca_{O_2} & = ([Hb] & \times & Sa_{O_2} & \times & 1.31) & + & 0.3 \\
ml.dl^{-1} & g.dl^{-1} & & \%/100 & & ml.g^{-1} & & ml.dl^{-1} \\
19 & = (14.7 & \times & 0.97 & \times & 1.31) & + & 0.3 \quad (1)
\end{array}
$$

where Ca_{O_2} is arterial oxygen content, [Hb] is haemoglobin concentration, Sa_{O_2} is arterial oxygen saturation, 1.31 is the combining power of haemoglobin with oxygen (page 176) and 0.3 is dissolved oxygen at normal arterial P_{O_2}.

OXYGEN DELIVERY

The important concept of oxygen delivery ($\dot{D}_{O_2}$) is considered in detail on page 187. It is defined as the product of cardiac output ($\dot{Q}$) and Ca_{O_2}.

$$
\begin{array}{lll}
\dot{D}_{O_2} & = & \dot{Q} & \times & Ca_{O_2} \\
ml.min^{-1} & & l.min^{-1} & & ml.dl^{-1} \\
1000 & = & 5.25 & \times & 19 \quad (2)
\end{array}
$$

(the right-hand side is multiplied by a scaling factor of 10 to account for the differing units of volume).

Combining equations (1) and (2):

$$
\begin{array}{ll}
\dot{D}_{O_2} & = \dot{Q} \times \{([Hb] \times Sa_{O_2} \times 1.31) + 0.3\} \\
ml.min^{-1} & l.min^{-1} \quad g.dl^{-1} \quad \%/100 \quad ml.g^{-1} \quad ml.dl^{-1} \\
1000 & = 5.25 \times \{(14.7 \times 0.97 \times 1.31) + 0.3\} \quad (3)
\end{array}
$$

(the right-hand side is again multiplied by a scaling factor of 10).

Normal values give an oxygen delivery of approximately 1000 ml.min^{-1}, which is about four times the normal resting oxygen consumption of 250 ml.min^{-1}. Extraction of oxygen from the arterial blood is thus 25% and this accords with an arterial saturation of 97% and mixed venous saturation of 72%.

If the small quantity of dissolved oxygen (0.3 ml. dl^{-1}) is ignored, then oxygen delivery is seen to be proportional to the product of cardiac output, haemoglobin concentration and arterial oxygen saturation. There is, of course, negligible scope for any compensatory increase in saturation in a patient with uncomplicated anaemia at sea level.

Effect of anaemia on cardiac output

Equation (3) shows that, if other factors remain the same, a reduction in haemoglobin concentration will result in a proportionate reduction in oxygen delivery. Thus a haemoglobin concentration of 7.5 g.dl^{-1}, with unchanged cardiac output, would halve delivery to give a resting value of 500 ml.min^{-1}, which would be approaching the likely critical value. However, patients with quite severe anaemia usually show little evidence of hypoxia at rest and, furthermore, achieve surprisingly good levels of exercise. Because arterial saturation cannot be increased, full compensation can be achieved only by a reciprocal relationship between cardiac output and haemoglobin concentration. Thus, if haemoglobin concentration is halved, maintenance of normal delivery will require a doubling of cardiac output. Full compensation may not occur, but fortunately a reduction in haemoglobin concentration is usually accompanied by some increase in cardiac output.

Acute anaemia. Early studies of cardiac output and anaemia involved measurement of cardiovascular parameters in patients before and after treatment for uncomplicated anaemia.[2] Cardiac output was significantly greater before the patients' haemoglobin concentration increased from 5.9 to 10.9 g.dl^{-1}. There was, however, a negative correlation between age and cardiac index in the anaemic state, reflecting the relative inability of the older patient to compensate. More recent studies have involved deliberately reducing the haemoglobin concentration isovolaemically in volunteers and patients.[3-6] One of these studies reduced the haemoglobin concentration from 13.1 to 5.0 g.dl^{-1} and the effects of this on the cardiovascular system are shown in Figure 25.1.[4] In these healthy volunteers the predictable linear relationship between cardiac index and haemoglobin concentration can easily be seen (Figure 25.1b). The increase in cardiac output seen in response to acute anaemia is much less in anaesthetised patients.[5]

The mechanism underlying the increase in cardiac output is not clear, but is due to increases in both stroke volume and heart rate.[4] Likely explanations for these changes include reduced cardiac afterload due to lowered blood viscosity (Figure 25.1a) and increased preload due to greater venous return secondary to increased tone in capacitance vessels.[7]

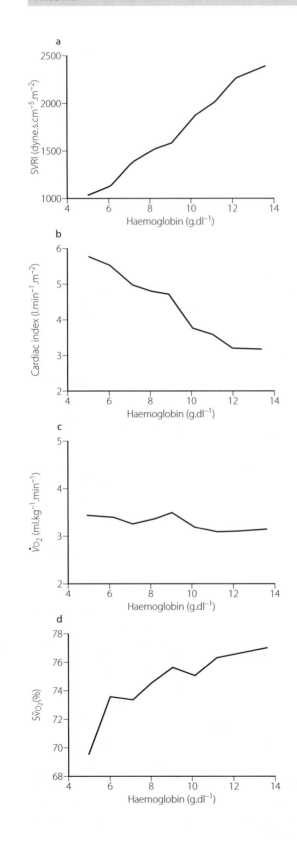

a SVRI (dyne.s.cm^{-5}.m^{-2}) vs Haemoglobin (g.dl^{-1})

b Cardiac index (l.min^{-1}.m^{-2}) vs Haemoglobin (g.dl^{-1})

c $\dot{V}_{O_2}$ (ml.kg^{-1}.min^{-1}) vs Haemoglobin (g.dl^{-1})

d $S\bar{v}_{O_2}$(%) vs Haemoglobin (g.dl^{-1})

Chronic anaemia. In one study of isovolaemic reduction of haemoglobin concentration, down to a mean value of 10 g.dl^{-1}, the anaemia was then maintained at the same level for 14 days.[3] Immediately after induction of anaemia there was a marked increase in cardiac output (55%), but this decreased to only 14% above control levels after 14 days.

The influence of cardiac output on oxygen delivery

Following the acute reduction of haemoglobin concentration in healthy subjects,[3,4] cardiac output increased sufficiently to maintain normal or near-normal oxygen delivery (Figure 25.1c). However, in sustained anaemia, the increase in cardiac output (only 14%) is insufficient to maintain oxygen delivery, which decreases to 25% below control values. Similarly, in a study of anaemic patients,[2] oxygen delivery was reduced in proportion to the degree of anaemia.

Without an increase in cardiac output, it is likely that a haemoglobin concentration of 6–8 g.dl^{-1} would be the minimum level compatible with life. It is clear that the ability of the cardiovascular system to respond to anaemia with an increase in cardiac output is an essential aspect of accommodation to anaemia, and this is less effective in anaesthetised patients, the elderly, or other subjects with reduced cardiac reserve.

Relationship between oxygen delivery and consumption

The relationship between oxygen delivery and consumption is considered on page 189 *et seq*. When oxygen delivery is reduced, for whatever reason, oxygen consumption is at first maintained at its normal value, but with increasing oxygen extraction and therefore decreasing mixed venous saturation (Figure 25.1d). Below a 'critical' value for oxygen delivery, oxygen consumption decreases as a function of delivery and is usually accompanied by evidence of hypoxia, such as increased lactate in peripheral blood. Values for critical oxygen delivery

Figure 25.1 Cardiovascular changes in response to acute isovolaemic reduction of mean haemoglobin concentration from 13.1 to 5.0 g.dl^{-1}. **(a)** Systemic vascular resistance index (SVRI) falls in direct proportion to Hb concentration as blood viscosity decreases. **(b)** Cardiac index (CI) doubles when Hb has fallen to 5.0 g.dl^{-1} in these healthy volunteers. **(c)** Oxygen delivery ($\dot{V}_{O_2}$) remains constant due to the increase in cardiac output exactly matching the decrease in arterial oxygen content. **(d)** Mixed venous oxygen saturation ($S\bar{v}_{O_2}$) falls as the tissues extract more oxygen. (After reference 4.)

depend upon the pathophysiological state of the patient and vary from one condition to another.

The critical level of oxygen delivery in uncomplicated anaemia in humans has not been clearly established. Studies of acutely induced anaemia have found no evidence of tissue hypoxia, though in one study, at a haemoglobin concentration of 5 g.dl^{-1}, oxygen consumption was reduced in spite of oxygen delivery being well maintained. In volunteers maintained at a haemoglobin concentration of 10 g.dl^{-1} for 14 days, oxygen delivery decreased from about 1200 to 900 ml.min^{-1} whereas oxygen consumption remained virtually unchanged.[3] Similarly, a study of treated anaemic patients found no increase in oxygen consumption when haemoglobin concentration was increased from a mean value of 6 to 11 g.dl^{-1}.[2] Thus these patients with long-term anaemia seemed to have all remained above the critical value for oxygen delivery down to haemoglobin values of about 6 g.dl^{-1}.

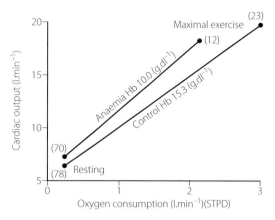

Figure 25.2 Cardiac output as a function of oxygen consumption during rest and maximal exercise under control and isovolaemic anaemic conditions. Numbers in parentheses indicate mean mixed venous oxygen saturation. (Redrawn from reference 3 on the assumption that mean weight of the subjects was 70 kg, by permission of the author and the Editors and publishers of *Journal of Applied Physiology*.)

ANAEMIA AND EXERCISE

Maintenance of constant oxygen consumption in the face of reduced delivery can only be achieved at the expense of a reduction in mixed venous saturation, as a result of increased extraction of oxygen from the arterial blood. This has been clearly demonstrated in both acute (Figure 25.1d) and sustained anaemia.[3] A reduction in the oxygen content of mixed venous blood curtails the ability of the anaemic patient to encroach on a useful reserve of oxygen, which is an important response to exercise. Reduction of haemoglobin to 10 g.dl^{-1} resulted in a curtailment of oxygen consumption attained at maximal exercise from the control values of 3.01 l.min^{-1} (normalised to 70 kg body weight) down to 2.53 l.min^{-1} in the acute stage and 2.15 l.min^{-1} after 14 days of sustained anaemia (Figure 25.2).[3] The increase in cardiac output required for the same increase in oxygen consumption was greater in the anaemic state and cardiac output at maximal oxygen consumption was slightly less than under control conditions. Maximal exercise in the anaemic state resulted in a reduction of mixed venous oxygen saturation to the exceptionally low value of 12%, compared with control values of 23% during maximal exercise with a normal haemoglobin concentration.

Brisk walking on level ground normally requires an oxygen consumption of about 1 l.min^{-1} and a cardiac output of about 10 l.min^{-1}. At a haemoglobin level of 5 g.dl^{-1}, this would require a cardiac output of about 20 l.min^{-1} to permit an oxygen consumption of 1 l.min^{-1} with a satisfactory residual level of mixed venous oxygen saturation. It will be clear that, at this degree of anaemia, cardiac function is a critical factor determining the mobility of a patient.

Exercise tolerance may be limited by either respiratory or circulatory capacity. In uncomplicated anaemia, there is no reason to implicate respiratory limitation and exercise tolerance is therefore, to a first approximation, governed by the remaining factors in the oxygen delivery equation (3) (above). On the assumption that the maximal sustainable cardiac output is only marginally affected by anaemia, it is to be expected that exercise tolerance will be reduced in direct proportion to the haemoglobin concentration. Available evidence supports this hypothesis (Figure 25.3).

Using haemoglobin to enhance athletic performance

The corollary of the preceding description is the question of improving athletic performance by increasing haemoglobin concentration above the normal range. This used to be achieved by removal of blood for replacement of red cells after a few weeks, when the subject has already partially restored his haemoglobin concentration, a procedure known as blood doping. The same effect is now much more conveniently achieved by the administration of erythropoietin. Studies of trained athletes in this area are notoriously difficult and it is easy to confuse the effects of changes in blood volume and haemoglobin concentration. Furthermore, blood doping involves the subject continuing his training after removal of blood while he is anaemic. This may well make his training more effective, as is the case when training is undertaken at altitude.

Figure 25.3 Relationship between capacity for exercise and haemoglobin concentration. (After reference 8 by permission of the authors and the Editor and publishers of *Clinics in Haematology*.)

In the pioneer study of Ekblom *et al.* in 1972,[9] it was reported that, following reinfusion of blood (resulting in an increase in haemoglobin concentration from 13.2 to 14.9 g.dl⁻¹), maximal oxygen consumption was increased from 4.40 to 4.79 l.min⁻¹ and time to exhaustion during uphill treadmill running was extended from 5.43 to 6.67 minutes. These findings were challenged in subsequent studies but confirmed in a well-controlled study of highly trained runners,[10] in which a mean haemoglobin concentration of 16.7 g.dl⁻¹ was attained with significant increases in maximal oxygen uptake from 4.85 to 5.10 l.min⁻¹. Differences of this magnitude are critically important in the arena of modern athletic competition.

WHAT IS THE OPTIMAL HAEMOGLOBIN CONCENTRATION IN THE CLINICAL SETTING?[11]

Evolution has resulted in a haemoglobin concentration of 13–16 g.dl⁻¹, presumably for sound biological reasons, and this value must represent the best compromise between oxygen carriage, cardiac output and blood viscosity. However, blood transfusion has always been, and currently remains, a hazardous procedure and a haemoglobin concentration of over 10 g.dl⁻¹ was for many years regarded as acceptable. At this level cardiac output increases are modest, and though exercise tolerance may be reduced this is unlikely to trouble the patient.

There is some evidence that lower values will be acceptable in some circumstances. Jehovah's Witnesses, whose religious beliefs prevent them from consenting to blood transfusion, frequently undergo major surgery and survival is reported following haemoglobin values of under 3 g.dl⁻¹, albeit with substantial cardiovascular and respiratory support.[12] Studies of these patients[13] indicate that perioperative death is uncommon if haemoglobin concentration remains above 5 g.dl⁻¹. There is also a suggestion that low haemoglobin values may actually be beneficial, with lowered blood viscosity improving blood flow through diseased vessels and so increasing tissue oxygenation, though evidence for a clinically relevant effect is lacking.

A target haemoglobin concentration of 10 g.dl⁻¹ may therefore be too conservative in fit healthy patients, or those with chronic anaemia,[14] and a haemoglobin level of 7 g.dl⁻¹ is probably acceptable in these groups.[11] This view was confirmed in a randomised controlled trial of intensive care patients in whom haemoglobin values of 7–9 g.dl⁻¹ were associated with improved outcome compared with those in whom haemoglobin was maintained at over 10 g.dl⁻¹.[15] The benefits were most pronounced in patients under 55 years old who were less acutely ill and did not have significant cardiac disease.

The organ that limits the acceptable degree of anaemia is the heart, where oxygen extraction is normally in excess of 50%. Increased oxygen extraction as a compensatory mechanism is therefore limited and coronary blood flow must increase to facilitate the greater oxygen requirement of a raised cardiac output. Thus any patient with ischaemic heart disease will be considerably less tolerant of anaemia than those with normal coronary arteries, as shown in the study of intensive care patients already described.[15] For these patients, particularly in the postoperative period when cardiac output is elevated, the optimal haemoglobin may be as high as 12.8 g.dl⁻¹.[16]

Chronic renal failure leads to a lack of renal erythropoietin release and chronic severe anaemia results, with patients commonly having haemoglobin levels of less than 8 g.dl⁻¹. The availability of recombinant human erythropoietin has allowed partial correction of anaemia in many patients, leading to a substantial improvement in quality of life for most. There is, however, debate about the optimal target haemoglobin concentration to aim for.[17] There is good evidence that the chronic severe anaemia associated with renal disease commonly leads to cardiac complications.[18] Unfortunately, there is also some evidence that correction of haemoglobin to normal values is associated with increased cardiac complications in these patients, and a value of 10–12 g.dl⁻¹ is therefore still recommended.[17]

REFERENCES

1. Torrance J, Jacobs P, Restrepo A, Eschbach J, Lenfant C, Finch CA. Intraerythrocytic adaptation to anemia. *N Engl J Med* 1970; **283**: 165–9.

2. Duke M, Abelmann WH. The hemodynamic response to chronic anemia. *Circulation* 1969; **39**: 503–15.

*3. Woodson RD, Wills RE, Lenfant C. Effect of acute and established anemia on O_2 transport at rest, submaximal and maximal work. *J Appl Physiol* 1978; **44**: 36–43.

*4. Weiskopf RB, Viele MK, Feiner J, *et al.* Human cardiovascular and metabolic response to acute, severe isovolemic anemia. *JAMA* 1998; **279**: 217–21.

*5. Ickx BE, Rigolet M, Van der Linden PJ. Cardiovascular and metabolic response to acute normovolemic anemia. *Anesthesiology* 2000; **93**: 1011–16.

6. Leung J, Weiskopf R, Feiner J, *et al.* Electrocardiographic ST-segment changes during acute, severe isovolemic hemodilution in humans. *Anesthesiology* 2000; **93**: 1004–10.

7. Chapler CK, Cain SM. The physiologic reserve in oxygen carrying capacity: studies in experimental haemodilution. *Can J Physiol Pharmacol* 1986; **64**: 7–12.

8. Viteri FE, Torun B. Anaemia and physical work capacity. *Clin Hematol* 1974; **3**: 609–26.

9. Ekblom B, Goldbarg AN, Gullbring B. Response to exercise after blood loss and reinfusion. *J Appl Physiol* 1972; **33**: 175–80.

10. Buick FJ, Gledhill N, Froese AB, Spriet L, Meyers EC. Effect of induced erythrocythemia on aerobic work capacity. *J Appl Physiol* 1980; **48**: 636–42.

11. Wedgwood JJ, Thomas JG. Peri-operative haemoglobin: an overview of current opinion regarding the acceptable level of haemoglobin in the peri-operative period. *Eur J Anaesthesiol* 1996; **13**: 316–24.

12. Olugbenga A, Akingbola A, Custer JR, Bunchman TE, Sedman A. Management of severe anemia without transfusion in a pediatric Jehovah's Witness patient. *Crit Care Med* 1994; **22**: 524–8.

13. Viele MK, Weiskopf RB. What can we learn about the need for transfusion from patients who refuse blood? The experience with Jehovah's Witnesses. *Transfusion* 1994; **34**: 396–401.

14. Welch HG, Meehan KR, Goodnough LT. Prudent strategies for elective red blood cell transfusion. *Ann Intern Med* 1992; **116**: 393–402.

*15. Hébert PC, Wells G, Blajchman MA, *et al.* A multicenter, randomized, controlled clinical trial of transfusion requirements in critical care. *N Engl J Med* 1999; **340**: 409–17.

16. Kettler D. 'Permissive anaemia' compared with blood transfusion in patients with cardiac disease: another point of view. *Curr Opin Anaesthesiol* 1994; **7**: 908–18.

17. Ritz E, Amann K. Optimal haemoglobin during treatment with recombinant human erythropoietin. *Nephrol Dial Transplant* 1998; **13**(Supp 2): 16–22.

18. Schunkert H, Hense H-W. A heart price to pay for anaemia. *Nephrol Dial Transplant* 2001; **16**: 445–8.

KEY POINTS

- Breathing oxygen at increased atmospheric pressure achieves very high arterial P_{O_2} values but venous P_{O_2}, and therefore minimum tissue P_{O_2}, only increases at 3 atmospheres absolute pressure.

- Hyperbaric oxygen is used to treat a variety of conditions, such as tissue infections, carbon monoxide poisoning and sports injuries, but its use remains controversial.

- Normal metabolic processes, particularly in the mitochondria, produce a range of powerful oxidising derivatives of oxygen, collectively referred to as reactive oxygen species.

- The harmful effects of reactive oxygen species are countered by a combination of ubiquitous enzymes that inactivate reactive oxygen species and endogenous antioxidant molecules.

- The lungs are susceptible to oxygen toxicity, the first measurable signs occurring in healthy subjects after breathing 100% oxygen for about 24 hours.

Chapter 24 described the disastrous consequences of lack of oxygen for life forms that depend on it, but for most organisms hypoxia is an infrequent event. However, oxygen itself also has toxic effects at the cellular level, which organisms have had to oppose by the development of complex antioxidant systems. Indeed, toxic derivatives of oxygen have now become so well controlled by animals that they are used to kill other invading organisms such as bacteria. The activity of toxic oxygen derivatives and antioxidant systems is perfectly balanced for most of the time. Nevertheless, there is a strengthening opinion that over many years oxidative mechanisms predominate and may be responsible for the generalised deterioration in function associated with ageing.[1] In a variety of diseases, or when exposed to extra oxygen, the balance is radically disturbed and oxidative tissue damage results.

Hyperoxia

Hyperventilation, while breathing air, can raise the arterial P_{O_2} to about 16 kPa (120 mmHg). Higher levels can be obtained only by oxygen enrichment of the inspired gas and/or by elevation of the ambient pressure. Although the arterial P_{O_2} can be raised to very high levels, the increase in arterial oxygen content is usually relatively small (Table 26.1). The arterial oxygen saturation is normally close to 95% and, apart from raising saturation to 100%, additional oxygen can be carried only in physical solution. Provided that the arterial/mixed venous oxygen content difference remains constant, it follows that venous oxygen content will rise by the same value as the arterial oxygen content. The consequences in terms of venous P_{O_2} (see Table 26.1) are important because minimum tissue P_{O_2} approximates more closely to venous than to arterial P_{O_2}. The rise in venous P_{O_2} is trivial when breathing 100% oxygen at normal barometric pressure, and it is necessary to breathe oxygen at 3 atmospheres absolute (ATA) pressure before there is a large increase in venous and hence tissue P_{O_2}. This is because most of the body requirement can then be met by dissolved oxygen and the saturation of capillary and venous blood remains close to 100%.

It is convenient to consider two degrees of hyperoxia. The first applies to the inhalation of oxygen-enriched gas at normal pressure; the second involves inhaling oxygen at raised pressure and is termed hyperbaric oxygenation.

HYPEROXIA AT NORMAL ATMOSPHERIC PRESSURE

The commonest indication for oxygen enrichment of the inspired gas is the prevention of arterial hypoxaemia ('anoxic anoxia') caused either by hypoventilation (page 371) or by venous admixture (page 122). Oxygen enrichment of the inspired gas may also be used to mitigate the effects of hypoperfusion ('stagnant hypoxia'). The data in Table 26.1 show that there will be only marginal improvement in oxygen flux (page 187), but it may be critical in certain situations. 'Anaemic anoxia' will be

Table 26.1 Oxygen levels attained in the normal subject by changes in the oxygen tension of the inspired gas

Inspired gas	At normal barometric pressure		At 2 ATA	At 3 ATA
	Air	Oxygen	Oxygen	Oxygen
Inspired gas P_{O_2} (humidified)				
(kPa)	20	95	190	285
(mmHg)	150	713	1425	2138
Arterial P_{O_2}*				
(kPa)	13	80	175	270
(mmHg)	98	600	1313	2025
Arterial oxygen content[†]				
(ml.dl^{-1})	19.3	21.3	23.4	25.5
Arterial/venous oxygen content difference				
(ml.dl^{-1})	5.0	5.0	5.0	5.0
Venous oxygen content				
(ml.dl^{-1})	14.3	16.3	18.4	20.5
Venous P_{O_2}				
(kPa)	5.2	6.4	9.1	48.0
(mmHg)	39	48	68	360

Oxygen-induced vasoconstriction means tissue perfusion may be reduced by elevation of P_{O_2}. This tends to increase the arterial/venous oxygen content difference, which will limit the rise in venous P_{O_2}. The increases in venous P_{O_2} shown in this table are therefore likely to be greater than *in vivo*.

* Reasonable values have been assumed for P_{CO_2} and alveolar/arterial P_{O_2} difference.

† Normal values assumed for Hb, pH etc.

only partially relieved by oxygen therapy but, because the combined oxygen is less than in a subject with normal haemoglobin concentration, the effect of additional oxygen carried in solution will be relatively more important.

Clearance of gas loculi in the body may be greatly accelerated by the inhalation of oxygen, which greatly reduces the *total* tension of the dissolved gases in the venous blood (Table 26.2). This results in the capillary blood having additional capacity to carry away gas dissolved from the loculi. Total gas tensions in venous blood are always slightly less than atmospheric and this is of critical importance in preventing the accumulation of air in potential spaces such as the pleural cavity, where the pressure is subatmospheric. Oxygen is useful in the treatment of air embolus and pneumothorax and has also been used to relieve intestinal distension.[2]

HYPERBARIC OXYGENATION

Mechanisms of benefit

Effect on P_{O_2}. Hyperbaric oxygenation is the only means by which arterial P_{O_2} values in excess of 90 kPa (675 mmHg) may be obtained. However, it is easy to be deluded into thinking that the tissues will be exposed to a similar P_{O_2} to that found in the chamber. Terms such

Table 26.2 Normal arterial and mixed venous blood gas tensions

	kPa		mmHg	
	Arterial blood	Venous blood	Arterial blood	Venous blood
Breathing air				
P_{O_2}	13.3	5.2	98	39
P_{CO_2}	5.3	6.1	40	46
P_{N_2}	76.0	76.0	570	570
Total gas tension	94.6	87.3	708	655
Breathing oxygen				
P_{O_2}	80.0	6.4	600	48
P_{CO_2}	5.3	6.1	40	46
P_{N_2}	0	0	0	0
Total gas tension	85.3	12.5	640	94

as 'drenching the tissues with oxygen' have been used but are meaningless. In fact, the simple calculations shown in Table 26.1, supported by experimental observations, show that large increases in venous and presumably therefore minimum tissue P_{O_2} do not occur until the P_{O_2} of the arterial blood is of the order of

270 kPa (2025 mmHg), when the whole of the tissue oxygen requirements can be met from the dissolved oxygen. However, the relationship between arterial and tissue PO_2 is highly variable (page 166) and hyperoxia-induced vasoconstriction in the brain and other tissues limits the rise in venous and tissue PO_2. Direct access of ambient oxygen will increase PO_2 in superficial tissues, particularly when the skin is breached.

Effect on P_{CO_2}. An increased haemoglobin saturation of venous blood reduces its buffering power and carbamino carriage of carbon dioxide, possibly resulting in carbon dioxide retention. In fact, the increase in tissue PCO_2 from this cause is unlikely to exceed 1 kPa (7.5 mmHg). However, in the brain this might result in a significant increase in cerebral blood flow, causing a secondary rise in tissue PO_2.

Vasoconstriction. An increase in PO_2 causes vasoconstriction, which may be valuable for reduction of oedema in the reperfusion of ischaemic limbs and in burns (see below).

Angiogenesis. The growth of new blood vessels is improved when oxygen is increased to more than 1 ATA pressure.[3] There seems to be no effect with 100% oxygen at 1 ATA,[4] and the mechanism by which angiogenesis is promoted is uncertain. When normoxia follows a period of hypoxia, reactive oxygen species (see below) are produced, and these are known to stimulate the production of a variety of growth factors that initiate angiogenesis.[5] The same mechanism may occur during hyperbaric oxygenation.

Antibacterial effect. Oxygen plays a major role in bacterial killing by the formation of reactive oxygen species, particularly in polymorphs and macrophages (see below). Apart from its direct effect, particularly on anaerobic bacteria, relief of hypoxia improves the performance of polymorphs.[6]

Boyle's law effect. The volume of gas spaces within the body is reduced inversely to the absolute pressure according to Boyle's law (page 456). This effect is additional to that resulting from reduction of the total tension of gases in venous blood (see above).

Clinical applications of hyperbaric oxygenation[7]

In practice, hyperbaric oxygen therapy means placing a patient into a chamber at 2–3 ATA and providing apparatus to allow them to breathe 100% oxygen, normally a tight-fitting facemask. Treatment is usually for about 1–2 hours and repeated daily for up to 30 days. Since its first use in 1960 enthusiasm for hyperbaric oxygenation

has waxed and waned, but its use is still confined to relatively few centres. Clear indications of its therapeutic value have been slow to emerge from controlled trials, which are admittedly very difficult to conduct in the conditions for which benefit is claimed. In particular, a proper 'control' group of patients must undergo a sham treatment in a hyperbaric chamber, which has been used in very few trials. The most commonly accepted indications are as follows.

Infection is the most enduring field of application for hyperbaric oxygenation, particularly anaerobic bacterial infections. High partial pressures of oxygen increase the production of reactive oxygen species, which are cidal not only to anaerobes but also to aerobes. The strongest indications are for clostridial myonecrosis (gas gangrene), refractory osteomyelitis and necrotising soft-tissue infections, including cutaneous ulcers.

Gas embolus and decompression sickness are unequivocal indications for hyperbaric therapy and the rationale of treatment is considered above and in Chapter 18.

Carbon monoxide poisoning. In spite of the exploitation of natural gas, there remains a high incidence of carbon monoxide poisoning from automobile exhausts, fires and defective domestic heating appliances. Carbon monoxide poisoning associated with loss of consciousness is generally regarded as an indication for hyperbaric oxygenation, but demonstration of clinical benefit remains controversial in this area.[7-10] The rationale of therapy – increased rate of dissociation of carboxyhaemoglobin (COHb) – seems simple when the half-life of COHb is approximately 4–5 hours while breathing air and only 20 minutes with hyperbaric oxygen. However, breathing 100% oxygen at normal pressure reduces the half-life of COHb to just 40 minutes and therefore in many cases, by the time transport to a hyperbaric chamber is achieved, COHb levels will already be considerably reduced. Other potential benefits of hyperbaric oxygen are believed to derive from minimising the effects of carbon monoxide on cytochrome-c oxidase[11] and neutrophil function.[12]

Burns. There is experimental evidence that in thermal burns hyperbaric oxygen causes vasoconstriction, reduces oedema, improves phagocytic killing of bacteria, improves angiogenesis and encourages collagen formation. Early studies reported many clinical benefits from these theoretical advantages. Subsequent advances in the general treatment of burns, however, led to the publication of studies that failed to find any outcome benefits with the use of hyperbaric oxygen.

Wound healing is improved by hyperbaric oxygenation, even when used intermittently. It is particularly useful when ischaemia contributes to the ineffective healing, for example in diabetes mellitus or peripheral vascular disease. The mechanisms are similar to those for burns and, in both cases, improved tissue oxygen levels probably result from direct diffusion of oxygen into the affected superficial tissues.

Sports injuries. Hyperbaric oxygen is believed to expedite recovery from soft tissue injuries and fractures incurred during competitive sports.[13] Early treatment (within 8 hours) is most effective, indicating a probable effect on neutrophil activity at the site of injury.[14]

Multiple sclerosis. In the early 1980s there was great interest in the therapeutic value of hyperbaric oxygenation in multiple sclerosis. A study in 1983 reported a favourable response after 12 months in a double-blind controlled trial of 40 patients, in which the treated group received 2 ATA oxygen while the placebo group inhaled 10% oxygen in nitrogen, also at 2 atmospheres.[15] Unfortunately, these findings were not confirmed in subsequent studies and a review of 14 controlled trials concluded that hyperbaric oxygen cannot be recommended for the treatment of multiple sclerosis.[16]

OXYGEN TOXICITY

The oxygen molecule and reactive oxygen species (ROS)[17,18]

Although ground state oxygen (dioxygen) is a powerful oxidising agent, the molecule is stable and has an indefinite half-life. However, the oxygen molecule can be transformed into a range of ROS and other highly toxic substances, most of which are far more reactive than oxygen itself.

The dioxygen molecule (Figure 26.1) is unusual in having two unpaired electrons in the outer (2P) shell.

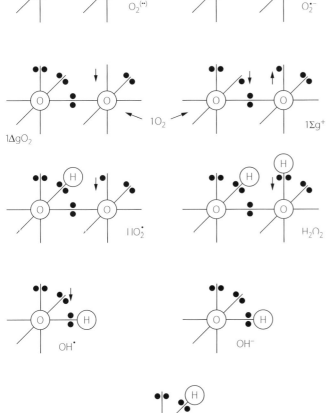

Figure 26.1 Outer orbital ring of electrons in (from the top left): ground state oxygen or dioxygen (O_2); superoxide anion ($O_2^{\bullet-}$); two forms of singlet oxygen ($^1O_2$); hydroperoxyl radical ($HO_2^{\bullet}$); hydrogen peroxide (H_2O_2); hydroxyl radical ($OH^{\bullet}$); hydroxyl ion (OH^-); and water. The arrows indicate the direction of rotation of unpaired electrons. See text for properties and interrelationships.

Thus dioxygen itself qualifies as a 'double' free radical, but stability is conferred by the fact that the orbits of the two unpaired electrons are parallel. The two unpaired electrons also confer the property of paramagnetism, which has been exploited as a method of gas analysis that is almost specific for oxygen (page 193).

Singlet oxygen. Internal rearrangements of the unpaired electrons of dioxygen result in the formation of two highly reactive species, both known as singlet oxygen ($1O_2$). In $1\Delta gO_2$ one unpaired electron is transferred to the orbit of the other (see Figure 26.1), imparting an energy level 22.4 kcal.mol^{-1} above the ground state. There being no remaining unpaired electron, $1\Delta gO_2$ is not a ROS. In $1\Sigma g^+$, the rotation of one unpaired electron is reversed, which imparts an energy level 37.5 kcal.mol^{-1} above the ground state and this molecule is a ROS. $1\Sigma g^+$ is extremely reactive and rapidly decays to the $1\Delta gO_2$ form, which is particularly relevant in biological systems and especially to lipid peroxidation.

Superoxide anion. Under a wide range of circumstances, considered below, the oxygen molecule may be partially reduced by receiving a single electron which pairs with one of the unpaired electrons, forming the superoxide anion ($O_2^{\bullet-}$ in Figure 26.1), which is both an anion and a ROS. It is the first and crucial stage in the production of a series of toxic oxygen-derived ROS and other compounds. The superoxide anion is relatively stable in aqueous solution at body pH, but has a rapid biological decay owing to the ubiquitous presence of superoxide dismutase (see below). Being charged, the superoxide anion does not readily cross cell membranes.

Hydroperoxyl radical. The superoxide anion may acquire a hydrogen ion to form the hydroperoxyl radical thus:

$$O_2^{\bullet-} + H^+ = HO_2^{\bullet}$$

The reaction is pH dependent with a pK of 4.8, so the equilibrium is far to the left in biological systems.

Hydrogen peroxide. Superoxide dismutase (SOD) catalyses the transfer of an electron from one molecule of the superoxide anion to another. The donor molecule becomes dioxygen, whereas the recipient rapidly combines with two hydrogen ions to form hydrogen peroxide (see Figure 26.1). Although hydrogen peroxide is not a ROS, it is a powerful and toxic oxidising agent that plays an important role in oxygen toxicity. The overall reaction is as follows:

$$2O_2^{\bullet-} + 2H^+ \rightarrow H_2O_2 + O_2$$

Hydrogen peroxide is continuously generated in the body. Two enzymes ensure its rapid removal. Catalase is a highly specific enzyme active against only hydrogen,

methyl and ethyl peroxides. Hydrogen peroxide is reduced to water thus:

$$2H_2O_2 \rightarrow 2H_2O + O_2$$

Glutathione peroxidase acts against a much wider range of peroxides (R–OOH), which react with glutathione (G–SH) thus:

$$R–OOH + 2G–SH \rightarrow R–OH + G–S–S–G + H_2O$$

Catalase and glutathione peroxidase are discussed further below. Obligatory anaerobic bacteria are normally without catalase.

Three-stage reduction of oxygen. Figure 26.2 summarises the three-stage reduction of oxygen to water, which is the fully reduced and stable state. This contrasts with the more familiar single-stage reduction of oxygen to water that occurs in the terminal cytochrome (page 187). Unlike the single-stage reduction of oxygen, the three-stage reaction shown in Figure 26.2 is not inhibited by cyanide.

Secondary derivatives of the products of dioxygen reduction

The Fenton reaction. Although both the superoxide anion and hydrogen peroxide have direct toxic effects, they interact to produce even more dangerous species. To the right of Figure 26.3 is shown the Fenton or Haber-Weiss reaction, which results in the formation of the harmless hydroxyl ion together with two extremely reactive species, the hydroxyl free radical (OH$^{\bullet}$) and singlet oxygen ($1O_2$).

Figure 26.2 Three-stage reduction of oxygen to water. The first reaction is a single electron reduction to form the superoxide anion reactive oxygen species. In the second stage the first products of the dismutation reaction are dioxygen and a short-lived intermediate, which then receives two protons to form hydrogen peroxide. The final stage forms water, the fully reduced form of oxygen.

Figure 26.3 Interaction of superoxide anion and hydrogen peroxide in the Fenton or Haber-Weiss reaction to form hydroxyl free radical, hydroxyl ion and singlet oxygen. Hypochlorous acid is formed from hydrogen peroxide by the myeloperoxidase system. (After reference 19 by courtesy of the Editor of the *Journal of the Royal Society of Medicine*.)

$$O_2^{\cdot-} + H_2O_2 \rightarrow OH^- + OH^\cdot + 1O_2$$

The hydroxyl free radical is much the most dangerous ROS derived from oxygen. The Fenton reaction is more likely than the Haber-Weiss reaction to take place under biological circumstances and it is catalysed by metals, particularly ferrous iron (Fe^{2+}).

The myeloperoxidase reaction.[20] To the left of Figure 26.3 is shown the reaction of hydrogen peroxide with chloride ion to form hypochlorous acid. This occurs in the phagocytic vesicle of the neutrophil and plays a major role in bacterial killing. The reaction is accelerated by the enzyme myeloperoxidase, which comprises some 7% of the dried weight of a neutrophil. Hypochlorite has long been known as an effective antibacterial agent and was used in the First World War as Dakin's solution. The myeloperoxidase reaction also occurs immediately after fertilisation of the ovum, and hypochlorous acid so formed causes polymerisation of proteins to form the membrane that prevents the further entry of spermatozoa.

Relationship to ionising radiation. The changes described above have many features in common with those caused by ionising radiation, the hydroxyl radical ($OH^\cdot$) being the most dangerous product in both cases. It is, therefore, hardly surprising that the effect of radiation is increased by high partial pressures of oxygen. As tissue P_{O_2} is reduced below about 2 kPa (15 mmHg), there is progressively increased resistance to radiation damage until, at zero P_{O_2}, resistance is increased threefold. This unfortunate effect promotes resistance to radiotherapy of malignant cells in hypoxic areas of tumours (page 336).

Nitric oxide may behave as a free radical by reacting with the superoxide anion to produce peroxynitrite ($ONOO^-$).[17] This molecule can either rearrange itself into relatively harmless nitrite or nitrate (page 180) or give rise to derivatives with similar biological activity to the hydroxyl radical. Conversely, nitric oxide may act as an antioxidant, binding to ferrous iron molecules and preventing them from contributing to the formation of superoxide anion (see below) or the Fenton reaction. The *in vivo* role of nitric oxide as a free radical or antioxidant therefore remains unclear.

Sources of electrons for the reduction of oxygen to superoxide anion

Figure 26.3 shows the superoxide anion as the starting point for the production of many other ROS. The first-stage reduction of dioxygen to the superoxide anion is therefore critically important in oxygen toxicity.

Mitochondrial enzymes. NADH dehydrogenase and a variety of other mitochondrial enzymes may 'leak' electrons to molecular oxygen and so produce superoxide anion radicals during normal oxidative respiration.[17,21] Animal studies indicate that this may account for almost 8% of total oxygen consumption, indicating the importance of the highly efficient mitochondrial form of SOD (see below).

The NADPH oxidase system is the major electron donor in neutrophils and macrophages. The electron is donated from NADPH by the enzyme NADPH oxidase, which is located within the membrane of the phagocytic vesicle. This mechanism is activated during phagocytosis and is accompanied by a transient increase in the oxygen consumption of the cells, a process known to be cyanide resistant. This is the so-called respiratory burst and occurs in all phagocytic cells in response to a wide range of stimuli, including bacterial endotoxin, immunoglobulins and interleukins. The superoxide anion is released into the phagocytic vesicle, where it is reduced to hydrogen peroxide, which then reacts with chloride ions to form hypochlorous acid in the myeloperoxidase reaction (see Figure 26.3).

Although the NADPH oxidase system has extremely important biological advantages, there seems little doubt that its inappropriate activation in marginated neutrophils can damage the endothelium of the lung and it may well play a part in the production of acute lung injury (see Chapter 31).

Xanthine oxidoreductase (XOR) and reperfusion injury.[22] The existence of the superoxide anion was first deduced from a reaction in which the electron was donated by the conversion of xanthine to uric acid by the enzyme

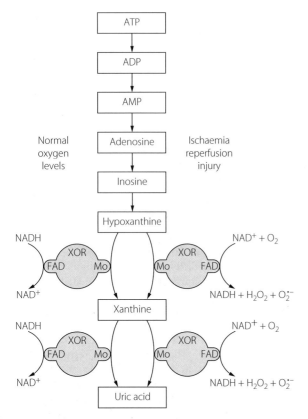

Figure 26.4 Generation of superoxide anion from oxygen by the activity of xanthine oxidoreductase (XOR). With normal cellular oxygen levels (left side) NADH is the cofactor, binding at the flavine adenine dinucleotide (FAD) site whilst the substrate reacts with the molybdenum binding site at the opposite side of the XOR molecule. Following a period of ischaemia (right side), reperfusion causes NAD^+ and oxygen rather than NADH to react at the FAD binding site of XOR, resulting in the production of hydrogen peroxide or superoxide anion.

XOR (Figure 26.4).[23] XOR is a large (300 kDa) protein involving two separate substrate-binding sites, one including flavine adenine dinucleotide cofactor and the other a molybdenum molecule. *In vivo*, XOR exists in two interchangeable forms, with about 80% existing as xanthine dehydrogenase and the remainder as xanthine oxidase. In both forms XOR catalyses the conversion of both hypoxanthine to xanthine and xanthine to uric acid, and under normal conditions uses NADH as a cofactor. In ischaemic or hypoxic tissue large quantities of hypoxanthine accumulate (page 334), the availability of NADH declines and the ratio of the oxidase and dehydrogenase forms of XOR may be reversed. As a result of these changes, when oxygen is restored to the cell, the XOR catalysis of xanthine and hypoxanthine is altered, with NAD^+ and dioxygen now being used as cofactors,

resulting in the production of hydrogen peroxide and superoxide anions (see Figure 26.4).[22] Thus during reperfusion there may be extensive production of oxygen-derived free radicals. It seems probable that, under certain circumstances, this mechanism may play a role in reperfusion tissue damage or postischaemic shock.[24]

Ferrous iron (Fe^{2+}) loses an electron during conversion to the ferric (Fe^{3+}) state. This is an important aspect of the toxicity of ferrous iron and has been proposed as a mechanism of rheumatoid arthritis.[25] A similar reaction also occurs during the spontaneous oxidation of haemoglobin to methaemoglobin (page 181). It is for this reason that large quantities of SOD, catalase and other protective agents are present in the young red blood cell. Their depletion may well determine the life of the cell. Apart from ferrous iron acting as an electron donor, it is a catalyst in the Fenton reaction (see above).

High P_{O_2}. Whatever other factors may apply, the production of ROS is increased at high levels of P_{O_2} by the law of mass action. It would seem that the normal tissue defences against ROS (discussed below) are usually effective only up to a tissue P_{O_2} of about 60 kPa (450 mmHg). This accords with the development of clinical oxygen toxicity as discussed below. There is also evidence that generation of ROS is increased when normal oxygen usage is increased, for example during exercise.[26]

Exogenous compounds. Various drugs and toxic substances can act as an analogue of NADPH oxidase and transfer an electron from NADPH to molecular oxygen. The best example of this is paraquat which can, in effect, insert itself into an electron transport chain, alternating between its singly and doubly ionised forms. This process is accelerated at high levels of P_{O_2} and so there is a synergistic effect between paraquat and oxygen. Paraquat is concentrated in the alveolar epithelial type II cell where the P_{O_2} is as high as anywhere in the body. Owing to the very short half-life of the oxygen-derived free radicals, damage is confined to the lung. Bleomycin and some antibiotics (e.g. nitrofurantoin) can act in a similar manner. Reactions usually occur at high dose levels, are again potentiated by increased oxygen levels or radiation, and eventually lead to pulmonary fibrosis.

Biological effects of ROS

Their use in phagocytosis for killing microorganisms is a clear beneficial role for ROS. Elsewhere within cells, the balance between the harmful effects of ROS and the antioxidants that counter these (see below) is described as the redox state of the cell. Cellular redox state is believed to be part of an essential cell signalling system.[27] Otherwise, most effects of ROS on biological systems are harmful and alterations in redox state are linked to a diverse range of diseases.

Biochemical targets for ROS

The three main targets are deoxyribonucleic acid (DNA), lipids and sulphydryl-containing proteins. All three are also sensitive to ionising radiation. The mechanisms of both forms of damage have much in common and synergism occurs.

DNA. Breakage of chromosomes in cultures of animal lung fibroblasts by high concentrations of oxygen was demonstrated by Sturrock and Nunn in 1978[28] (Figure 26.5). The same authors showed that 48 hours' exposure to 95% oxygen increased the rate of mutations by a factor of 25. *In vivo* studies of therapeutic hyperbaric oxygen in humans have also shown DNA damage. However, adverse clinical outcomes from hyperbaric oxygen have not been demonstrated, though susceptible subgroups, who have less effective cellular antioxidant or DNA repair systems, may exist.[29]

Lipids. There is little doubt that lipid peroxidation is a major mechanism of tissue damage by ROS. The interaction of a ROS with an unsaturated fatty acid not only disrupts that particular lipid molecule but also generates another ROS, so that a chain reaction ensues until stopped by an antioxidant.[18] Lipid peroxidation disrupts cell membranes and accounts for the loss of integrity of the alveolar/capillary barrier in pulmonary oxygen toxicity.

Proteins. Damage to sulphydryl-containing proteins results in formation of disulphide bridges, which inactivate a range of proteins.

Pathophysiological effects of ROS

Interference with these fundamental cellular processes has widespread physiological implications. Superoxide anion and the peroxynitrite formed from nitric oxide intiate a wide range of pathological processes, including the inactivation of neurotransmitters, inhibition of proteins, release of cytokines and direct cytotoxic effects (Figure 26.6).[30] Inevitably, cell dysfunction will rapidly occur, followed over the long term by the occurrence of inflammation, malignancy or cell death. Over an animal's lifetime, ROS-induced damage is now closely linked with cardiovascular[31] and neurological disease, cancer[32] and the degenerative changes of ageing.[1]

DEFENCES AGAINST REACTIVE OXYGEN SPECIES

Life in an oxidising environment is possible only because of powerful antioxidant defences, which all aerobes have developed (see Chapter 1). The defensive systems are freely duplicated and operate in depth.

Antioxidant enzymes

These enzymes are widely distributed in different organs and different species but are deficient in most obligatory anaerobic bacteria. Young animals normally have increased levels of SOD and catalase, which confers greater resistance to oxygen toxicity. The reactions catalysed by antioxidant enzymes have been described above.

Superoxide dismutase. Three types of SOD exist, each derived from a separate gene:[33–35] extracellular SOD, cytoplasmic SOD containing manganese (MnSOD), and mitochondrial SOD containing both copper and zinc (CuZnSOD). Extra production of SOD may be induced by several mechanisms, of which hyperoxia is the most notable,[36] but inflammatory cytokines such as interferon, TNF, interleukins and lipopolysaccharide are important stimulants of SOD production in the intact animal.[34,35]

Animal studies have consistently shown that induction of SOD confers some protection against the toxic effects of oxygen[17] and, by implication, enhanced SOD activity may be protective against the wide range of pathological processes described above. There are difficulties in the therapeutic use of SOD because the most important forms are intracellular or mitochondrial enzymes which

Figure 26.5 Breakage of chromosomes in a culture of Chinese hamster lung fibroblasts by oxygen at various concentrations and for varying durations of exposure. (Reproduced from reference 28 by courtesy of the Editors of *Mutation Research*.)

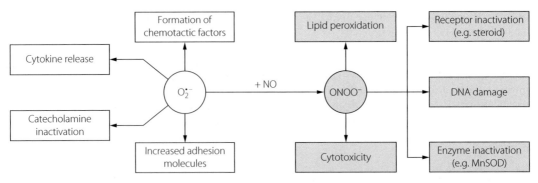

Figure 26.6 Biochemical effects of superoxide anion and peroxynitrite. These potent cellular effects initiate numerous pathological processes, including inflammation, malignancy or cell death. MnSOD, manganese superoxide dismutase. (Reproduced with permission from reference 30.)

have very short half-lives in plasma. There is therefore little scope for their use by direct intravenous injection. It is possible for SOD to enter cells if it is administered in liposomes and extracellular SOD has been used by direct instillation into the lungs.[37] Recent attempts to enhance SOD activity for therapeutic purposes have switched to the development of SOD mimetics.[30] A number of small polycyclic compounds, mostly containing a central manganese molecule, have been found to catalyse the same reactions as SOD, but because of their small size and non-peptide nature they can freely enter the intracellular environment. SOD mimetics have yet to begin clinical trials, but their therapeutic potential for the future looks promising.

Catalase has a cellular and extracellular distribution similar to SOD, with which it is closely linked in disposing of superoxide anion (see Figure 26.2). Although studied less extensively, catalase production is believed to be induced by the same factors as SOD. Similarly, trials of exogenous antioxidant enzymes have usually given better results when both SOD and catalase are administered.

Glutathione peroxidase system scavenges not only the ROS themselves but also free radicals formed during lipid peroxidation. Two molecules of the tripeptide (glycine–cysteine–glutamic acid) glutathione (GSH) are oxidised to one molecule of reduced glutathione (GSSG) by the formation of a disulphide bridge linking the cysteine residues. GSH is reformed from GSSG by the enzyme glutathione reductase, protons being supplied by NADPH.

Endogenous antioxidants

Ascorbic acid is a small molecule with significant antioxidant properties, being particularly important for removal of the hydroxyl free radical. Humans, along with guinea-pigs and bats, lack the enzyme required for the production of ascorbate and so must ingest sufficient vitamin C to compensate. In these mammals, SOD activity is markedly higher than in those able to produce endogenous ascorbate.[38]

Vitamin E (α-tocopherol) is a highly fat-soluble compound and is therefore found in high concentrations in cell membranes. Predictably, its main antioxidant role is in the prevention of lipid peroxidation chain reactions described above.

Surfactant may act as an antioxidant in the lung. Animal studies have shown that administration of exogenous surfactant prolongs the duration of oxygen exposure required to cause lung damage.[39]

Exogenous antioxidants

Allopurinol. Because XOR plays a pivotal role in the reactions shown in Figure 26.4 it seemed logical to explore the use of allopurinol, which inhibits a range of enzymes including XOR. As might have been expected, benefit was seen mainly following ischaemia/reperfusion injury, but under these conditions allopurinol has multiple effects on purine metabolism and may not be acting as an XOR inhibitor at all.[22]

Iron-chelating agents. Since ferrous iron is both a potent source of electrons for conversion of oxygen to the superoxide anion and a catalyst in the Fenton reaction, desferrioxamine has antioxidant properties *in vitro*.[40]

Steroids showed great promise as clinically useful antioxidants, including in animal studies of pulmonary oxygen toxicity.[41] These results have not translated into a clinically useful effect in humans.

These compounds, along with other *in vitro* antioxidants such as *n*-acetyl cysteine, β-carotene and dimethylsulphoxide, have generally failed to live up to their expectations in human disease.[32] There are three possible explanations. First, studies of ROS production and antioxidants in human cells are relatively rare and there is known to be considerable species variability.[17] Second, penetration of the exogenous antioxidant to the site of ROS generation (e.g. mitochondria) or damage (e.g. nuclear DNA) is likely to be poor. Finally, ROS production for bacterial killing is fundamental to mammalian defence systems, so any non-specific antioxidant activity may be detrimental. Their therapeutic role in oxygen toxicity or diseases known to involve ROS is therefore far from fully clarified.

CLINICAL OXYGEN TOXICITY

The most important clinical conditions in which oxygen has been identified as the sole precipitating cause are oxygen convulsions, pulmonary oxygen toxicity and retrolental fibroplasia.

Oxygen convulsions (the Paul Bert effect)

It is well established that exposure to oxygen at a partial pressure in excess of 2 atmospheres absolute (2 ATA) may result in convulsions, which are usually lethal to divers. This limits the depth to which closed-circuit oxygen apparatus can be used. It is interesting that the threshold for oxygen convulsions is close to that at which brain tissue P_{O_2} is likely to be sharply increased (see Table 26.1). The relationship to cerebral tissue P_{O_2} is supported by the observation that an elevation of P_{CO_2} lowers the threshold for convulsions. High P_{CO_2} increases cerebral blood flow and therefore raises the tissue P_{O_2} relative to the arterial P_{O_2}. Hyperventilation and anaesthesia each provide limited protection.

Convulsions result from poorly understood changes in cellular interactions between γ-aminobutyric acid (GABA) and nitric oxide. GABA concentrations decrease in the brain prior to convulsion and the change correlates with the severity of the convulsion.[42] As GABA is an inhibitory neurotransmitter, it is not unreasonable to suggest that a reduced level might result in convulsions. Nitric oxide is known to sensitise neurones to the toxic effects of GABA in hypoxia and is also involved in hyperoxic convulsions. Nitric oxide inhibitors delay the onset of convulsions in hyperoxia[43,44] but paradoxically, the same effect is seen with some NO donors.[44] Whatever the role of NO, the final common pathway seems to be mediated by disturbed calcium fluxes and increased cyclic-GMP concentration.[43]

Incidence. Hyperbaric oxygen used therapeutically as described above (that is, intermittent exposure to less than 3 ATA) carries little risk of oxygen convulsions. At 2 ATA, a large series reported no convulsions in over 12 000 treatments.[45] Treatment for CO poisoning is associated with a greater incidence of convulsions because of the higher pressures used (normally 2.8–3.0 ATA) and the toxic effects of CO on the brain itself. In this case, 1–2% of patients experience convulsions.[46]

Pulmonary oxygen toxicity

Pulmonary tissue P_{O_2} is the highest in the body. In addition, a whole range of other oxidising substances may be inhaled, including common air pollutants and the constituents of cigarette smoke (see Chapter 21). The lung is therefore the organ most vulnerable to oxygen toxicity and a range of defence mechanisms have developed. Overall antioxidant activity from both enzymes and other endogenous antioxidants is very high in the fluid lining the respiratory tract. Extracellular SOD is abundant in pulmonary airway tissues and abnormalities in its regulation may contribute to some lung diseases.[47] Type II alveolar epithelial cells, which produce surfactant (page 21), are believed to also incorporate vitamin E into the surfactant lipids.[48]

Pulmonary oxygen toxicity is unequivocal and lethal in laboratory animals such as the rat. Humans seem to be far less sensitive, but there are formidable obstacles to investigation of both human volunteers and patients. Study of oxygen toxicity in the clinical environment is complicated by the presence of the pulmonary pathology that necessitated the use of oxygen.

Symptoms.[49] High concentrations of oxygen cause irritation of the tracheobronchial tree, which gives rise initially to a sensation of retrosternal tightness. Continued exposure leads to chest pain, cough and an urge to take deep breaths. Reduced vital capacity is the first measurable change in lung function, occurring after about 24 hours of normobaric 100% oxygen. Oxygen exposure beyond this point leads to the widespread structural changes described below, which ultimately give rise to acute lung injury and possibly irreversible changes in lung function.

Cellular changes.[50] Electron microscopy has shown that, in rats exposed to 1 atmosphere of oxygen, the primary change is in the capillary endothelium, which becomes vacuolated and thin. Permeability is increased and fluid accumulates in the interstitial space. At a later stage, in monkeys, the epithelial lining is lost over large areas of the alveoli. This process affects the type I cell (page 21) and is accompanied by proliferation of the type II cell, which is relatively resistant to oxygen. The alveolar/

capillary membrane is greatly thickened, partly because of the substitution of type II for type I cells and partly because of interstitial accumulation of fluid.

Limits of survival. Pulmonary effects of oxygen vary greatly between species, probably because of different levels of provision of defences against free radicals. Most strains of rat will not survive for much more than 3 days in 1 atmosphere of oxygen. Monkeys generally survive oxygen breathing for about 2 weeks, and man is probably even more resistant. Oxygen tolerance for normal man has been investigated,[51] but these studies are based on reduction in vital capacity etc., which is a very early stage of oxygen toxicity. There is an approximately inverse relationship between PO_2 and duration of tolerable exposure. Thus 20 hours of 1 atmosphere had a similar effect to 10 hours of 2 atmospheres or 5 hours of 4 atmospheres.

Pulmonary oxygen toxicity seems to be related to PO_2 rather than inspired concentration. Early American astronauts breathed 100% oxygen at a pressure of about one-third of an atmosphere for many days (see Table 19.1) with no apparent ill effects. There is abundant evidence that prolonged exposure to this environment does not result in demonstrable pulmonary oxygen toxicity, thus establishing a PO_2 of 34 kPa (255 mmHg) as a safe level. It also confirms that the significant factor is partial pressure and not concentration. In contrast, the concentration of oxygen rather than its partial pressure is the important factor in absorption collapse of the lung (see below).

Clinical studies. Some limited information on human pulmonary oxygen toxicity has been obtained from patients in the course of therapeutic administration of oxygen. In 1967, a review of 70 patients who died after prolonged artificial ventilation reported a greater number of pulmonary abnormalities (fibrin membranes, oedema and fibrosis) in those who had received more than 90% oxygen.[52] However, the higher concentrations of oxygen would probably have been used in the patients with more severe defects in gas exchange and it is therefore difficult to distinguish between the effects of oxygen itself and the conditions that required its use. A similar group of patients ventilated for long periods with high concentrations of oxygen were reviewed in 1980,[53] and these authors concluded that adverse effects of oxygen on the alveolar epithelium were rarely of practical importance in hypoxaemic patients. An elegant attempt to avoid the complicating factor of preexisting pulmonary disease was made in 1970 by Singer *et al.*,[54] who ventilated a group of patients with 100% oxygen for 24 hours after cardiac surgery. Two further patients received oxygen for 5 and 7 days, respectively. Various indices of pulmonary function (VD/VT ratio, shunt and compli-

ance) were not significantly different from a control group receiving less than 42% oxygen.

In contrast to these essentially negative findings, a study in 1987 obtained positive findings in a randomised trial involving patients ventilated after cardiac surgery.[55] Venous admixture was significantly greater and arterial PO_2 less in patients receiving 50% oxygen than in the group receiving less than 30%. There are many possible causes for these changes, but the authors concluded that unnecessary elevation of inspired oxygen concentration should be avoided, a view from which few would dissent in the current state of knowledge.

Pulmonary absorption collapse. Whatever the uncertainties about the susceptibility of humans to pulmonary oxygen toxicity, there is no doubt that high concentrations of oxygen in zones of the lung with low ventilation/perfusion ratios will result in collapse. This occurs routinely during anaesthesia (page 303) and may be demonstrated in the healthy but middle-aged awake volunteer. A few minutes of breathing oxygen at residual lung volume results in radiological evidence of collapse, a reduced arterial PO_2 and substernal pain on attempting a maximal inspiration.[56]

Balancing the risks. Prevention of dangerous hypoxia is always the first priority and must be treated in spite of the various hazards associated with the use of oxygen. A reasonably safe arterial PO_2 is 10 kPa (75 mmHg), normally giving a saturation of 95% but, if this cannot be maintained without resorting to dangerous levels of inspired oxygen concentrations (in excess of 65%, see page 416), it may be necessary to settle for a lower arterial PO_2. The safe lower level of arterial PO_2 for an individual patient depends on many factors and no general rule can be formulated.

The key to avoiding the potentially harmful effects of oxygen in the clinical environment is prevention. Although brief periods of exposure to 100% oxygen appear safe, inspired oxygen concentrations should be titrated against arterial PO_2. This is particularly important in patients exposed to paraquat or bleomycin.

Retrolental fibroplasia (RLF)[57]

Shortly after RLF was first described in 1942, it became established that hyperoxia was the major aetiological factor that led to the use of oxygen being strictly curtailed in the management of neonates. This resulted in an increase in morbidity and mortality attributable to hypoxia, and thereafter oxygen was carefully monitored and titrated in the hope of steering the narrow course between the Scylla of hypoxia and the Charybdis of RLF. This policy has not eradicated the condition and there is some evidence that RLF may occur in infants who have never received additional oxygen. Vitamin E has been used in the attempt to prevent RLF, but it is currently believed that hyperoxia is but one of a variety of factors that may cause RLF by changes in the retinal oxygen supply. RLF is increasingly likely to occur with greater degrees of prematurity and there is a well-established inverse relationship between birth weight and its incidence.

REFERENCES

1. Sohal RS, Mockett RJ, Orr WC. Mechanisms of aging: an appraisal of the oxidative stress hypothesis. *Free Radic Biol Med* 2002; **33**: 575–86.
2. Down RHL, Castleden WM. Oxygen therapy for pneumatosis coli. *Br Med J* 1975; **1**: 493–4.
3. Thom SR. Hyperbaric oxygen therapy. *Intens Care Med* 1989; **4**: 58–63.
4. Marx RE, Ehler WJ, Tayapongsak P, Pierce LW. Relationship of oxygen dose to angiogenesis induction in irradiated tissue. *Am J Surg* 1990; **160**: 519–24.
5. Maulik N, Das DK. Redox signalling in vascular angiogenesis. *Free Radic Biol Med* 2002; **33**: 1047–60.
6. Mandell G. Bactericidal activity of aerobic and anaerobic polymorphonuclear neutrophils. *Infect Immun* 1974; **9**: 337–41.
7. Tibbles PM, Edelsberg JS. Hyperbaric-oxygen therapy. *N Engl J Med* 1996; **334**: 1642–8.
8. Seger D, Welch L. Carbon monoxide controversies: neuropsychologic testing, mechanism of toxicity and hyperbaric oxygen. *Ann Emerg Med* 1994; **24**: 242–8.
9. Juurlink DN, Stanbrook MB, McGuigan MA. Hyperbaric oxygen for carbon monoxide poisoning. *Cochrane Database Syst Rev* 2000; **2**: CD002041.
*10. Thom SR. Hyperbaric-oxygen therapy for acute carbon monoxide poisoning. *N Engl J Med* 2002; **347**: 1105–6.
11. Brown SD, Piantadosi CA. *In vivo* binding of carbon monoxide to cytochrome *c* oxidase in rat brain. *J Appl Physiol* 1990; **68**: 604–10.
12. Thom SR. Dehydrogenase conversion to oxidase and lipid peroxidation in brain after carbon monoxide poisoning. *J Appl Physiol* 1992; **73**: 1584–9.
13. Babul S, Rhodes EC. The role of hyperbaric oxygen therapy in sports medicine. *Sports Med* 2000; **30**: 395–403.
14. Staples J, Clement D. Hyperbaric oxygen chambers and the treatment of sports injuries. *Sports Med* 1996; **22**: 219–27.
15. Fischer BH, Marks M, Reich T. Hyperbaric-oxygen treatment of multiple sclerosis. A randomized, placebo controlled, double blind study. *N Engl J Med* 1983; **308**: 181–4.
16. Kleijnen J, Knipschild P. Hyperbaric oxygen for multiple sclerosis. Review of controlled trials. *Acta Neurol Scand* 1995; **91**: 330–4.
17. Kinnula VL, Crapo JD, Raivio KO. Generation and disposal of reactive oxygen metabolites in the lung. *Lab Invest* 1995; **73**: 3–19.
18. Webster NR, Nunn JF. Molecular structure of free radicals and their importance in biological reactions. *Br J Anaesth* 1988; **60**: 98–108.
19. Nunn JF. Oxygen – friend or foe? *J Roy Soc Med* 1985; **78**: 618–22.
20. Fantone JC, Ward PA. Role of oxygen-derived free radicals and metabolites in leukocyte-dependent inflammatory reactions. *Am J Pathol* 1982; **107**: 397–418.
*21. Turrens JF. Mitochondrial formation of reactive oxygen species. *J Physiol* 2003; **552**: 335–44.
*22. Harrison R. Structure and function of xanthine oxidoreductase: where are we now? *Free Radic Biol Med* 2002; **33**: 774–97.
23. McCord JM, Fridovich I. The reduction of cytochrome c by milk xanthine oxidase. *J Biol Chem* 1968; **243**: 5753–60.
24. Traystman RJ, Kirsch JR, Koehler RC. Oxygen radical mechanisms of brain injury following ischaemia and reperfusion. *J Appl Physiol* 1991; **71**: 1185–95.
25. Larrick JW, Wright SC. Cytotoxic mechanism of tumor necrosis factor-α. *FASEB J* 1990; **4**: 3215–23.
26. Kantner M. Free radicals, exercise and antioxidant supplementation. *Proc Nutrit Soc* 1998; **57**: 9–13.
27. Forman HJ, Torres M. Reactive oxygen species and cell signalling. Respiratory burst in macrophage signaling. *Am J Respir Crit Care Med* 2002; **166**: S4–S8.
28. Sturrock JE, Nunn JF. Chromosomal damage and mutations after exposure of Chinese hamster cells to high concentrations of oxygen. *Mutat Res* 1978; **57**: 27–31.
*29. Speit G, Dennog C, Radermacher P, Rothfuss A. Genotoxicity of hyperbaric oxygen. *Mutat Res* 2002; **512**: 111–19.
*30. Salvemini D, Riley DP, Cuzzocrea S. SOD mimetics are coming of age. *Nat Rev Drug Discov* 2002; **1**: 367–74.
31. Rapola JM. Should we prescribe antioxidants to patients with coronary heart disease? *Eur Heart J* 1998; **19**: 530–2.
32. Hennekens CH, Buring JE, Manson JE, *et al*. Lack of effect of long-term supplementation with beta carotene on the incidence of malignant neoplasms and cardiovascular disease. *N Engl J Med* 1996; **334**: 1145–9.
33. Tsan MF. Superoxide dismutase and pulmonary oxygen toxicity. *Proc Soc Exp Biol Med* 1997; **214**: 107–13.

34. Zelko IN, Mariani TJ, Folz RJ. Superoxide dismutase multigene family: a comparison of the CuZn-SOD (SOD1), Mn-SOD (SOD2) and EC-SOD (SOD3) gene structures, evolution and expression. *Free Radic Biol Med* 2002; **33**: 337–49.

*35. Kinnula VL, Crapo JD. Superoxide dismutases in the lung and human lung diseases. *Am J Respir Crit Care Med* 2003; **167**: 1600–19.

36. Crapo JD, Tierney DF. Superoxide dismutase and pulmonary oxygen toxicity. *Am J Physiol* 1974; **226**: 1401–7.

37. Barnard ML, Baker RR, Matalon S. Mitigation of oxidant injury to lung microvasculature by intratracheal instillation of antioxidant enzymes. *Am J Physiol* 1995; **265**: L340–67.

38. Nandi A, Mukhopadhyay CK, Ghosh MK, Chattopadhyay DJ, Chatterjee IB. Evolutionary significance of vitamin C biosynthesis in terrestrial vertebrates. *Free Radic Biol Med* 1997; **22**: 1047–54.

39. Ghio AJ, Fracica PJ, Young SL, Piantadosi CA. Synthetic surfactant scavenges oxidants and protects against hyperoxic lung injury. *J Appl Physiol* 1994; **77**: 1217–23.

40. Gutteridge JMC, Rowley DA, Griffiths E, Halliwell B. Low-molecular-weight iron complexes and oxygen radical reactions in idiopathic haemochromatosis. *Clin Sci* 1985; **68**: 463–7.

41. Koizumi M, Frank L, Massaro D. Oxygen toxicity in rats: varied effect of dexamethasone treatment depending on duration of hyperoxia. *Am Rev Respir Dis* 1985; **131**: 907–11.

42. Wood JD, Watson WJ. Gamma-aminobutyric acid levels in the brain of rats exposed to oxygen at high pressures. *Can J Biochem Physiol* 1963; **41**: 1907–13.

43. Wang WJ, Ho XP, Yan YL, Yan TH, Li CL. Intrasynaptosomal free calcium and nitric oxide metabolism in central nervous system toxicity. *Aviat Space Environ Med* 1998; **69**: 551–5.

44. Bitterman N, Bitterman H. L-arginine-NO pathway and CNS oxygen toxicity. *J Appl Physiol* 1998; **84**: 1633–8.

45. Hill RK. Is more better? A comparison of different clinical hyperbaric treatment pressures – a preliminary report. *Undersea Hyperb Med* 1993; **20**(Supp): 12.

46. Hampson NB, Simonson SG, Kramer CC, Piantadosi CA. Central nervous system oxygen toxicity during hyperbaric treatment of patients with carbon monoxide poisoning. *Undersea Hyperb Med* 1996; **23**: 215–19.

47. Bowler RP, Crapo JD. Oxidative stress in airways. Is there a role for extracellular superoxide dismutase? *Am J Respir Crit Care Med* 2002; **166**: S38–S43.

48. Kolleck I, Sinha P, Rüstow B. Vitamin E as an antioxidant of the lung. Mechanisms of vitamin E delivery to alveolar Type II cells. *Am J Respir Crit Care Med* 2002; **166**: S62–S66.

49. Montgomery AB, Luce JM, Murray JF. Retrosternal pain is an early indicator of oxygen toxicity. *Am Rev Respir Dis* 1989; **139**: 1548–50.

50. Weibel ER. Oxygen effect on lung cells. *Arch Intern Med* 1971; **128**: 54–6.

51. Clark JM, Lambertsen CJ, Gelfand R, *et al.* Effects of prolonged oxygen exposure at 1.5, 2.0, or 2.5 ATA on pulmonary function in men (Predictive studies V). *J Appl Physiol* 1999; **86**: 243–59.

52. Nash G, Blennerhassett JB, Pontoppidan H. Pulmonary lesions associated with oxygen therapy and artificial ventilation. *N Engl J Med* 1967; **276**: 368–74.

53. Gilbe CE, Salt JC, Branthwaite MA. Pulmonary function after prolonged mechanical ventilation with high concentrations of oxygen. *Thorax* 1980; **35**: 907–11.

54. Singer MM, Wright F, Stanley LK, Roe BB, Hamilton WK. Oxygen toxicity in man. A prospective study in patients after open-heart surgery. *N Engl J Med* 1970; **283**: 1473–8.

55. Register SD, Downs JB, Stock MC, Kirby RR. Is 50% oxygen harmful? *Crit Care Med* 1987; **15**: 598–601.

56. Nunn JF, Williams IP, Jones JG, Hewlett AM, Hulands GH, Minty BD. Detection and reversal of pulmonary absorption collapse. *Br J Anaesth* 1978; **50**: 91–100.

57. Lucey JF, Dangman B. A reexamination of the role of oxygen in retrolental fibroplasia. *Pediatrics* 1984; **73**: 82–96.

Part: Three

Physiology of pulmonary disease

KEY POINTS

- Ventilatory failure occurs when alveolar ventilation becomes too low to maintain normal arterial blood gas partial pressures.
- There are many causes, involving the respiratory centre, the respiratory muscles or their nerve supply, and abnormalities of the chest wall, lung or airways.
- Modest increases in the inspired oxygen concentration will correct hypoxia due to ventilatory failure, but may worsen hypercapnia.
- Correction of hypercapnia requires an improvement in alveolar ventilation, which often requires artificial ventilation.

Definitions

Respiratory failure is defined as a failure of maintenance of normal arterial blood gas partial pressures. Hypoxia as a result of cardiac and other extrapulmonary forms of shunting is excluded from this definition. Respiratory failure may be subdivided according to whether the arterial P_{CO_2} is normal or low (type 1) or elevated (type 2). Mean of the normal arterial P_{CO_2} is 5.1 kPa (38.3 mmHg) with 95% limits (2 s.d.) of ±1.0 kPa (7.5 mmHg). The normal arterial P_{O_2} is more difficult to define because it decreases with age (page 180) and is strongly influenced by the concentration of oxygen in the inspired gas. Mechanisms that contribute to respiratory failure include ventilatory failure (reduced alveolar ventilation) and venous admixture as a result of either pure intrapulmonary shunt or ventilation/perfusion mismatch (see Chapter 8).

Ventilatory failure is defined as a pathological reduction of the alveolar ventilation below the level required for the maintenance of normal alveolar gas partial pressures. Because arterial P_{O_2} (unlike arterial P_{CO_2}) is so strongly influenced by shunting, the adequacy of ventilation is conveniently defined by the arterial P_{CO_2}, although it is also reflected in end-expiratory P_{CO_2} and P_{O_2}. This chapter is concerned mainly with pure ventilatory failure; other causes of respiratory failure are described in the next four chapters.

PATTERN OF CHANGES IN ARTERIAL BLOOD GAS TENSIONS

Figure 27.1 shows, on a P_{O_2}/P_{CO_2} diagram, the typical patterns of deterioration of arterial blood gases in respiratory failure. The shaded area indicates the normal range of values with increasing age, corresponding to a leftward shift. Pure ventilatory failure in a young person with otherwise normal lungs would result in changes along the broken line. Chronic obstructive pulmonary disease (COPD), the most common cause of predominantly ventilatory failure, occurs in older people and the observed pattern of change is shown within the upper arrow in Figure 27.1. The limit of survival, while breathing air, is reached at a P_{O_2} of about 2.7 kPa (20 mmHg) and P_{CO_2} of 11 kPa (83 mmHg). The limiting factor is not P_{CO_2} but P_{O_2}. This prevents the rise of P_{CO_2} to higher levels except when the patient's inspired oxygen concentration is increased. It may also be raised above 11 kPa by the inhalation of carbon dioxide. In either event, a P_{CO_2} in excess of 11 kPa may be considered an iatrogenic disorder. Figure 27.1 also shows the pattern of blood gas changes caused by shunting or pulmonary venous admixture (see Chapter 8).

In general, the arterial P_{O_2} indicates the severity of respiratory failure (assuming that the patient is breathing air), whereas the P_{CO_2} indicates the differential diagnosis between ventilatory failure and shunting, as shown in Figure 27.1. In respiratory disease it is, of course, common for ventilatory failure and shunting to coexist in the same patient.

Time course of changes in blood gas tensions in acute ventilatory failure

Although the upper arrow in Figure 27.1 shows the effect of established ventilatory failure on arterial blood

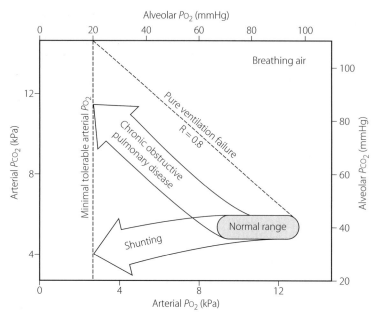

Alveolar P_{O_2} (mmHg)

Figure 27.1 Pattern of deterioration of arterial blood gases in chronic obstructive pulmonary disease and pulmonary shunting. The shaded area indicates the normal range of arterial blood gas partial pressures from 20 to 80 years of age. The oblique broken line shows the theoretical changes in alveolar P_{O_2} and P_{CO_2} resulting from pure ventilatory failure. In chronic obstructive pulmonary disease, the arterial P_{O_2} is always less than the value that would be expected in pure ventilatory failure at the same P_{CO_2} value. Discussion of shunting is to be found in Chapter 8 and further discussion of chronic obstructive pulmonary disease in Chapter 28.

gas tensions, short-term deviations from this pattern occur in acute ventilatory failure. This is because the time courses of changes of P_{O_2} and P_{CO_2} in response to acute changes in ventilation are quite different.

Body stores of oxygen are small, amounting to about 1550 ml while breathing air. Therefore, following a step change in the level of alveolar ventilation, the alveolar and arterial P_{O_2} rapidly reach the new value and the half-time for the change is only 30 seconds (see page 191 and Figure 11.19). In contrast, the body stores of carbon dioxide are very large, of the order of 120 litres. Therefore, following a step change in the level of alveolar ventilation, the alveolar and arterial P_{CO_2} only slowly attain the value determined by the new alveolar ventilation. Furthermore, the time course is slower following a reduction of ventilation than an increase (see Figure 10.11) and the half-time of rise of P_{CO_2} following a step reduction of ventilation is of the order of 16 minutes.

The practical point is that, during the early phase of acute hypoventilation, there may be a low P_{O_2} while the P_{CO_2} is increasing but is still within the normal range. Thus the pulse oximeter may, under certain circumstances, such as when breathing air, give an earlier warning of hypoventilation than the capnograph. This breaks the rule that the P_{CO_2} is the essential index of alveolar ventilation, and it may be erroneously believed that the diagnosis is shunting rather than hypoventilation.

CAUSES OF VENTILATORY FAILURE[1,2]

The causes of ventilatory failure may be conveniently considered under the headings of the anatomical sites where they arise. These sites are indicated in Figure

27.2. Lesions or malfunctions at sites a–e result in a reduction of input to the respiratory muscles. Dyspnoea may not be apparent and the diagnosis of ventilatory failure may be overlooked on superficial inspection of the patient. Lesions or malfunctions at sites g–j result in evident dyspnoea and no one is likely to miss the diagnosis of hypoventilation. The various sites will now be considered individually.

a. The respiratory neurones of the medulla are depressed by hypoxia and also by very high levels of P_{CO_2}, probably of the order of 40 kPa (300 mmHg) in the healthy unanaesthetised subject, but at a lower P_{CO_2} in the presence of some drugs (see below). Reduction of P_{CO_2} below the apnoeic threshold results in apnoea in the unconscious subject but usually not in the conscious subject. Loss of respiratory sensitivity to carbon dioxide occurs in various types of long-term ventilatory failure, particularly COPD, and this is discussed further on page 381.

A wide variety of drugs may cause central apnoea or respiratory depression and these include opioids, barbiturates and most anaesthetic agents, whether intravenous or inhalational. The respiratory neurones may also be affected by a variety of neurological conditions, such as raised intracranial pressure, stroke, trauma or neoplasm.

b. The upper motor neurones serving the respiratory muscles are most likely to be interrupted by trauma. Only complete lesions above the third or fourth cervical vertebrae will affect the phrenic nerve and result in total apnoea. However, fracture–dislocations of the lower

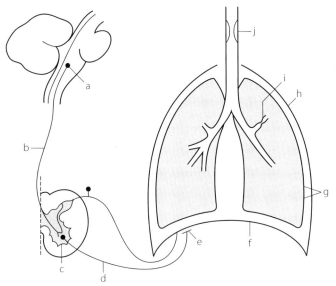

Figure 27.2 Summary of sites at which lesions, drug action or malfunction may result in ventilatory failure. a, Respiratory centre. b, Upper motor neurone. c, Anterior horn cell. d, Lower motor neurone. e, Neuromuscular junction. f, Respiratory muscles. g, Altered elasticity of lungs or chest wall. h, Loss of structural integrity of chest wall and pleural cavity. i, Increased resistance of small airways. j, Upper airway obstruction.

cervical vertebrae are relatively common and result in loss of action of the intercostal and expiratory muscles while sparing the diaphragm. Upper motor neurones may be involved in various disease processes, including tumours, demyelination and, occasionally, syringomyelia.

c. The anterior horn cell may be affected by various disease processes, of which the most important is poliomyelitis. Fortunately, this condition is now rare in the developed world but it can produce any degree of respiratory involvement, up to total paralysis of all respiratory muscles.

d. Lower motor neurones supplying the respiratory muscles are prone to normal traumatic risks, and in former times the phrenic nerves were surgically interrupted for the treatment of pulmonary tuberculosis. The later stages of motor neurone disease may cause ventilatory failure at this level. Idiopathic polyneuritis (Guillain–Barré syndrome) remains a relatively common neurological cause of ventilatory failure. The syndrome results from an immune-mediated aetiology and is characterised by a rapidly ascending motor nerve paralysis, which in one-third of patients progresses to quadriplegia and total respiratory muscle paralysis.[3] With modern ventilatory support death is fortunately rare, and 85% of sufferers make a complete neurological recovery.

e. The neuromuscular junction is affected by several causes, including botulism, neuromuscular blocking drugs used in anaesthesia, organophosphorus compounds and nerve gases. However, myasthenia gravis is by far the most common cause of ventilatory failure at this site, marked respiratory muscle weakness occurring in seemingly mild cases.[4] Myasthenia gravis is an autoimmune disease in which the acetylcholine receptors on the neuromuscular junction are destroyed, leading to progressive weakness. Administration of an anticholinesterase drug such as edrophonium increases acetylcholine concentration at the neuromuscular junction and causes an immediate improvement in symptoms. Immunosuppression or thymectomy are effective current therapies, but almost 90% of patients with generalised myasthenia still require long-term treatment.[5]

f. The respiratory muscles themselves are rarely entirely responsible for ventilatory failure, but they often contribute to reduced alveolar ventilation in a variety of respiratory diseases. For example, the efficiency of contraction of the respiratory muscles is severely impaired by the hyperinflation that normally accompanies COPD. In these patients, although the curvature of the diaphragm may remain normal, the zone of apposition is reduced (see Figures 6.1 and 6.2) and the resultant shortening of diaphragmatic muscle fibres significantly impairs their function.[2] The respiratory muscles may also become fatigued as a result of working against excessive impedance, but this is not thought to occur until very late in the course of most acute respiratory problems.[6] Patients who require critical care commonly develop a polyneuropathy and myopathy of the respiratory muscles, particularly if sepsis is the underlying cause of their multiorgan failure. Activation of cytokines and malnutrition are believed to be contributing mechanisms.[2] Furthermore, following a long period of artificial ventilation, respiratory muscles develop 'disuse atrophy'. These factors all make weaning from ventilation difficult (page 430).

Cardiac failure may result in respiratory muscle weakness owing to reduced blood supply,[7] often coupled with low compliance lungs due to pulmonary oedema (see Chapter 29).

Assessment of respiratory muscle strength is described on page 89.

g. Loss of elasticity of the lungs or chest wall is a potent cause of ventilatory failure. It may arise within the lungs (e.g. pulmonary fibrosis or acute lung injury), in the pleura (e.g. chronic empyema with fibrinous covering of the pleura), in the chest wall (e.g. kyphoscoliosis) or in the skin (e.g. contracted burn scars in children). It is frequently forgotten that seemingly mild pressures applied to the outside of the chest may seriously embarrass the breathing and even result in total apnoea. A sustained pressure of only 6 kPa (45 mmHg or a depth of 2 feet of water) is sufficient to prevent breathing. This can occur when crowds get out of control and people fall on top of one another, or when either children or adults become accidentally buried under sand or other heavy materials.

h. Loss of structural integrity of the chest wall may result in ventilatory failure, for example from multiple fractured ribs. A condition known as flail chest arises when multiple ribs are broken in two places, allowing the middle, 'flail', rib section to move independently of the anterior and posterior 'fixed' sections. Movement of the flail segment is then determined by changes in intrathoracic pressure; with spontaneous breathing, a paradoxical respiratory movement of the flail segment develops, which if large enough will compromise tidal volume. This condition, resulting from blunt trauma such as impact on the steering wheel, has become less common in the UK since the use of seat belts became compulsory. Flail chest may need to be treated by artificial ventilation with intermittent positive pressure, although conservative treatment with good analgesia, sometimes assisted by rib fixation, is becoming more common.

Closed pneumothorax causes interference with ventilation in proportion to the quantity of air in the chest. With a tension pneumothorax, the pressure rises above atmospheric, collapsing the ipsilateral lung, displacing the mediastinum and partially collapsing the contralateral lung. The function of the respiratory muscles is impaired and ventilation may become critically low. The diagnosis and correction of the condition is a matter of great urgency. In the case of open pneumothorax the reduction in overall minute volume is further complicated by pendulum breathing between the two lungs.

i. Small airway resistance remains the commonest and most important cause of ventilatory failure. The physiology of diseases affecting airway resistance is described in Chapter 28 and will not be discussed further here.

However, the relationship between airway resistance and ventilatory failure is a complex subject, which is considered below. In the clinical field, airway resistance is seldom measured but is most often inferred from measurement of ventilatory capacity.

j. Upper airway obstruction occurs in a wide range of conditions, such as airway and pharyngeal tumours, upper respiratory tract infections, inhaled foreign bodies, and tumour or bleeding in the neck causing external compression of the airway. Stridor is common and should quickly alert the clinician to the cause of respiratory distress. A smaller airway diameter in babies and children makes them more susceptible than adults to upper airway obstruction, as airway oedema from infections such as croup or epiglottitis quickly causes dramatic stridor. The excellent ability of the respiratory system to overcome increased airway resistance (page 49) is such that ventilatory failure is normally a late development.

Increased dead space

Very rarely, a large increase in the respiratory dead space may cause ventilatory failure. Minute volume may be increased but the alveolar ventilation is reduced, and the patient presents with a high $P\text{CO}_2$ accompanied by a high minute volume. An increase in the arterial/end-expiratory $P\text{CO}_2$ gradient (more than 2 kPa or 15 mmHg) indicates an increase in the alveolar dead space. This condition may be caused by ventilation of large unperfused areas of lung (e.g. an air cyst communicating with the bronchus), pulmonary emboli or pulmonary hypotension. External or apparatus dead space also tends to reduce alveolar ventilation and may be added either intentionally or accidentally.

RELATIONSHIP BETWEEN VENTILATORY CAPACITY AND VENTILATORY FAILURE

Tests for the measurement of ventilatory capacity are described on pages 88 et seq. However, a severe reduction in ventilatory capacity does not necessarily mean that a patient will be in ventilatory failure. Figure 27.3 shows the lack of correlation between FEV_1 and arterial $P\text{CO}_2$ in the grossly abnormal range of FEV_1 0.3–1 litre from a series of patients with COPD.[8]

It should again be stressed that the usual tests of ventilatory capacity depend on the expiratory muscles, whereas the work of breathing is normally achieved by the action of inspiratory muscles.

Metabolic demand and ventilatory failure

In renal failure, protein intake is a major factor in the onset of uraemia. Similarly, in ventilatory failure, the

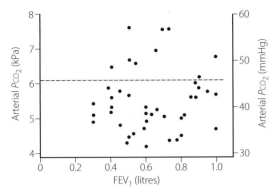

Figure 27.3 Lack of correlation between arterial $P\text{CO}_2$ and forced expiratory volume in one second (FEV_1) in 44 patients with chronic obstructive pulmonary disease. The broken line indicates the upper limit of normal for $P\text{CO}_2$. (Data from reference 8.)

onset of hypoxia and hypercapnia is directly related to the metabolic demand. Just as patients with renal failure benefit from a low-protein diet, so patients with a severe reduction of ventilatory capacity protect themselves by limiting the exercise they take.

As COPD progresses, the ventilatory capacity decreases and the minute volume of breathing required for a particular level of activity increases. The increased ventilatory requirement is because both the dead space and the oxygen cost of breathing increase. The patient is thus trapped in a pincer movement of decreasing ventilatory capacity and increasing ventilatory requirement. As the jaws of the pincer close, there is first a limitation on heavy exercise, then on moderate exercise and so on until the patient is dyspnoeic at rest. At any time his work capacity is limited by the fraction of his ventilatory capacity that he is able to maintain for a given level of oxygen uptake.

The complex interaction between these factors is demonstrated in Figure 27.4, where the upper part shows the normal state. Assuming that an untrained subject can comfortably maintain a minute volume equal to about 30% of his maximal breathing capacity (MBC) without dyspnoea, he has a reserve of ventilatory capacity that is adequate for rest and a power output of 100 watts. However, a power output of 200 watts requires a minute volume that exceeds a third of his MBC, and at this level of exercise he becomes aware of his breathing.

Figure 27.4b shows moderately severe COPD with the following changes.

1. MBC reduced from 150 to 60 l.min^{-1}.
2. Dead space/tidal volume ratio increased from 30% to 40%.
3. Oxygen cost of breathing increased by 10% for each level of activity.

Factors 2 and 3 together result in an increased minute volume for each level of activity.

Again, on the assumption that dyspnoea will not be apparent until the minute volume is 30% of MBC, the reserve of ventilation is now sufficient for rest, but 100 watts of power output will result in dyspnoea.

Finally, in Figure 27.4c, the changes have progressed to the point where resting minute volume exceeds 30% of MBC and the patient is dyspnoeic at rest.

BREATHLESSNESS[9]

Breathlessness or dyspnoea has been defined as 'undue awareness of breathing or awareness of difficulty in breathing'.[10] This definition applies to both the awareness of breathing during severe exercise in the healthy subject and the dyspnoea of a patient with respiratory failure or heart failure. In the first case the sensation is normal and to be expected. However, in the latter, it is pathological and should be considered as a symptom.

The origin of the sensation

Hypoxia and hypercapnia may force the patient to breathe more deeply but *per se* they are not responsible for the sensation of dyspnoea, which arises from the ventilatory response rather than the stimulus itself. Patients with respiratory paralysis caused by poliomyelitis did not usually complain of dyspnoea in spite of abnormal blood gas tensions. Campbell and Guz[10] advanced their reasons for believing that dyspnoea is not akin to pain, though a sensation of 'air hunger' can be induced with hypercapnia and there is evidence of sensory activation of higher cerebral centres under these conditions.[11] Neither is dyspnoea strictly related to the work of breathing. Some patients have dyspnoea at relatively low levels of work of breathing, whereas others show no dyspnoea at high levels of work. Fatigue of the respiratory muscles may be a factor in some cases but is clearly not the only cause of dyspnoea.

In 1963 it was suggested that a major factor in the origin of dyspnoea was an 'inappropriateness' between the tension generated in the respiratory muscles and the resultant shortening of the muscle fibres.[12] This sensory input from muscle spindles would indicate to the brain that breathing was in some way hindered. The theory has since been widened to include other sensory receptors in the respiratory system, again suggesting that dyspnoea results from a mismatch between motor output and sensory input in the respiratory centre.[2] These theories seem to fit observations made during breath holding (pages 69 *et seq.*), which provide some insight into the origin of the sensation of breathlessness. Blood gas tensions are by no means the only factor limiting breath-holding time, although $P\text{O}_2$ is more important than

a

b

c

Figure 27.4 Relationship between maximal breathing capacity (MBC) and ventilatory requirements at rest and work at 100 and 200 watts. The tips of the arrows indicate 30% of MBC, which can usually be maintained without dyspnoea. Ventilatory reserve is between this level and the various ventilatory requirements. **(a)** Normal. **(b)** Moderate loss of ventilatory capacity with some increase in oxygen cost of breathing. **(c)** Severe loss of ventilatory capacity with considerable increase in the oxygen cost of breathing.

P_{CO_2}. The sensation that terminates breath holding can be relieved by ventilation without change of blood gas tensions, by bilateral vagal block and by curarisation. Diaphragmatic afferents appear to be more important than those from the intercostals.

Mismatch of motor and sensory activity in respiratory neurones is unlikely to be the full explanation of breathlessness.[2,13] There is now little doubt that breathlessness involves a psychological component.[14] Dyspnoea arising from respiratory disease, particularly acutely, is often associated with anxiety and panic, which exacerbate the symptom. Conversely, many patients with primary psychological complaints, such as panic disorder, present with dyspnoea in the absence of any respiratory disease.

It cannot be said that the problem of breathlessness is completely understood at the present time.[2] The origin seems to be multifactorial and the mechanisms of its generation are clearly complex.

Treatment of breathlessness. Optimal treatment of the underlying disease process that is causing the dyspnoea is clearly the first approach to managing the symptom. However, in the later stages of many respiratory diseases, and in almost all patients with malignancy, breathlessness becomes an intractable and distressing problem. Palliation of breathlessness is now recognised as a valuable form of therapy and offers further insight into the multifactorial nature of the symptom.[9,15] Simple measures such as a fan blowing on the face are effective, and breathing oxygen relieves dyspnoea in many patients, even some who are not hypoxic.[15] Systemic opioids are effective, though whether this benefit is mediated by reducing the respiratory drive or by simply altering the patient's perception of their breathlessness is unknown.[16,17]

PRINCIPLES OF THERAPY FOR VENTILATORY FAILURE

Many patients go about their business with arterial P_{CO_2} levels as high as 8 kPa (60 mmHg). Higher levels are associated with increasing disability, largely due to the accompanying hypoxaemia when the patient is breathing air (see Figure 27.1). Treatment may be divided into symptomatic relief of hypoxaemia and attempts to improve the alveolar ventilation.

Treatment of hypoxaemia due to hypoventilation by administration of oxygen

Hypoxia must be treated as the first priority and administration of oxygen is the fastest and most effective method.

The relationship between alveolar P_{O_2} and alveolar ventilation is explained on pages 167 *et seq.* and illustrated in Figure 11.2. If other factors remain constant, an increase in inspired gas P_{O_2} will result in an equal increase in alveolar gas P_{O_2}. Therefore only small increases in inspired oxygen concentration are required for the relief of hypoxia *due to hypoventilation*. Figure 27.5 shows the rectangular hyperbola relating P_{CO_2} and alveolar ventilation (as in Figure 10.9), but superimposed are the concentrations of inspired oxygen required to restore a normal alveolar P_{O_2} for different degrees of alveolar hypoventilation. It will be seen that 30% is sufficient for the degree of alveolar hypoventilation that will result in an alveolar P_{CO_2} of 13 kPa (almost 100 mmHg). Clearly this is an unacceptable P_{CO_2}, and therefore 30% can be regarded as the upper limit of inspired oxygen concentration to be used in the palliative relief of hypoxia due to ventilatory failure, without attempting to improve the alveolar ventilation.

The use of very high concentrations of inspired oxygen will prevent hypoxia even in gross alveolar hypoventila-

Figure 27.5 Alveolar P_{CO_2} as a function of alveolar ventilation at rest. The percentages indicate the inspired oxygen concentration that is then required to restore normal alveolar P_{O_2}.

tion, which carries the risk of dangerous hypercapnia. Although this is itself a strong contraindication to the use of high concentrations of oxygen under these circumstances, the effect may be even worse in patients who have lost their ventilatory sensitivity to carbon dioxide and rely upon their hypoxic drive to maintain ventilation (page 381). Recognition of this potential problem unfortunately resulted in a tendency to withhold oxygen for fear of causing hypercapnia. The rule is that hypoxia must be treated first, because hypoxia kills quickly whereas hypercapnia kills slowly. However, it must always be remembered that administration of oxygen to a patient with ventilatory failure will do nothing to improve the P_{CO_2} and may make it worse. The arterial P_{CO_2} must be measured if there is any doubt.

Improvement of alveolar ventilation

The only way to reduce the arterial P_{CO_2} is to improve the alveolar ventilation. The first line of therapy is to improve ventilatory capacity by treatment of the underlying cause while simultaneously providing carefully controlled oxygen therapy and avoiding the use of drugs that depress breathing.

The second line is chemical stimulation of breathing. Doxapram stimulates breathing via an action on the peripheral chemoreceptors (page 71) and is effective in treating exacerbations of COPD, but only for the first few hours after admission to hospital.[18]

The third line of treatment is by tracheal intubation or tracheostomy, which may improve alveolar ventilation by reducing dead space and facilitating the control of secretions.

The fourth line of therapy is the institution of artificial ventilation (considered in detail in Chapter 32). It is difficult to give firm guidelines for the institution of artificial ventilation and the arterial P_{CO_2} should not be considered in isolation. Nevertheless, a $P\text{CO}_2$ in excess of 10 kPa (75 mmHg) that cannot be reduced by other means in a patient who is deemed recoverable is generally considered a firm indication. However, artificial ventilation may be required at much lower levels of $P\text{CO}_2$ if there is actual or impending respiratory fatigue as a result of increased work of breathing. This may be difficult to diagnose or predict. Although it is now recognised that intense activity by the respiratory muscles results in fatigue, as in the case of other skeletal muscles under similar conditions, it is also thought that ventilatory failure from this cause occurs only very late in the course of most respiratory diseases. For example, it has been mentioned above that the $P\text{CO}_2$ rises late in acute asthma, and artificial ventilation may be required before the arterial $P\text{CO}_2$ has risen much above the normal range.

REFERENCES

*1. Roussos C, Koutsoukou A. Respiratory failure. *Eur Respir J* 2003; **22** (Supp 47): 3S–14S.

*2. Laghi F, Tobin MJ. Disorders of the respiratory muscles. *Am J Respir Crit Care Med* 2003; **168**: 10–48.

3. Sharsar T, Chevret S, Bourdain F, Raphael JC. Early predictors of mechanical ventilation in Guillain–Barré syndrome. *Crit Care Med* 2003; **31**: 278–83.

4. Mier A, Brophy C, Green M. Respiratory muscle function in myasthenia gravis. *Am Rev Respir Dis* 1988; **138**: 867–74.

5. Grob D, Arsura EL, Brunner NG, Namba T. The course of myasthenia gravis and therapies affecting outcome. *Ann N Y Acad Sci* 1987; **505**: 472–99.

6. Roussos C, Zakynthinos S. Fatigue of the respiratory muscles. *Intens Care Med* 1996; **22**: 134–55.

7. Hammond MD, Bauer KA, Sharp JT, Rocha RD. Respiratory muscle strength in congestive heart failure. *Chest* 1990; **98**: 1091–4.

8. Nunn JF, Milledge JS, Chen D, Doré C. Respiratory criteria of fitness for surgery and anaesthesia. *Anaesthesia* 1988; **43**: 543–51.

*9. Meek PM, Schwartzstein RM, Adams L, *et al.* Dyspnea: mechanisms, assessment and management. A consensus statement. *Am J Respir Crit Care Med* 1999; **159**: 321–40.

10. Campbell EJM, Guz A. Breathlessness. In: Hornbein TF, ed. *Regulation of breathing*, Part II. New York: Marcel Dekker, 1981.

11. Guz A. Brain, breathing and breathlessness. *Respir Physiol* 1997; **109**: 197–204.

12. Campbell EJM, Howell JBL. The sensation of breathlessness. *Br Med Bull* 1963; **19**: 36–40.

13. Howell JBL. Breathlessness. In: Brewis RAL, Corrin B, Gedded DM, Gibson GJ, eds. *Respiratory medicine*. London: WB Saunders, 1995.

14. Smoller JW, Pollack MH, Otto MW, Rosenbaum JF, Kradin RL. Panic anxiety, dyspnea and respiratory disease – theoretical and clinical considerations. *Am J Respir Crit Care Med* 1996; **154**: 6–17.

15. Booth S, Wade R. Oxygen or air for palliation of breathlessness in advanced cancer. *J Roy Soc Med* 2002; **96**: 215–18.

16. Muers MF. Opioids for dyspnoea. *Thorax* 2002; **57**: 922–3.

17. Jennings A-L, Davies AN, Higgins JPT, Gibbs JSR, Broadley KE. A systematic review of the use of opioids in the management of dyspnoea. *Thorax* 2002; **57**: 939–44.

18. Greenstone M, Lasserson TJ. Doxapram for ventilatory failure due to exacerbations of chronic obstructive pulmonary disease. *Cochrane Database Syst Rev* 2003; **1**: CD000223.

KEY POINTS

- Whatever the cause, airway narrowing leads to expiratory flow limitation, gas trapping and hyperinflation of the lung, which manifests itself as breathlessness.
- Asthma involves intermittent, reversible airway obstruction caused by airway inflammation and bronchial smooth muscle contraction, both as a result of mediators released from mast cells and eosinophils.
- Chronic obstructive pulmonary disease is progressive and poorly reversible airway narrowing caused by airway inflammation and loss of lung tissue elasticity, mostly as a result of smoking-induced activation of airway neutrophils.
- Cystic fibrosis is an inherited disease in which abnormal chloride transport in the airway impairs the normal pulmonary defence mechanisms, leading to chronic and destructive pulmonary infections.

This chapter considers the physiological changes seen in the three most common diseases of the pulmonary airways: asthma, chronic obstructive pulmonary disease (COPD) and cystic fibrosis. The first two of these have many clinical and physiological features in common and together constitute the vast majority of respiratory disease seen in clinical practice.

ASTHMA

Lung diseases resulting from air pollution and infection have decreased dramatically in recent decades, but have been almost entirely replaced by asthma. The prevalence of asthma has now reached dramatic proportions in many areas of the world, though the causes of this differ between the 'developed' and the 'developing' world (see below).[1] In contrast to many respiratory diseases, the onset of asthma is usually in early childhood or young adulthood. The prevalence of asthma among children is now between 15% and 30% in developed countries and has approximately doubled in the last 20 years,[1-3] although there are now some signs that the epidemic may have reached its peak.[4] For many years, mortality from asthma increased in parallel with the prevalence of the disease, but deaths from asthma also now seem to have peaked in most countries.[5]

Clinical features

Asthma causes recurrent episodes of chest 'tightness', wheezing, breathlessness and coughing as a result of airway narrowing from a combination of inflammation of the small airways and contraction of bronchial smooth muscle in the lower airway. The term 'asthma' includes a wide spectrum of illnesses, varying from a wheezy 6-month-old baby with a viral infection to a young adult with multiple allergies manifested as wheeze or an older patient with chronic lung disease. In the last case, clinical features of asthma merge with those of COPD and differentiation between the two is difficult. Changing diagnostic criteria[2] have almost certainly contributed to the apparent increase in asthma prevalence, which is nevertheless still a real increase.[1] Whatever the clinical presentation, there are three closely related phases of an episode of asthma, as follows.

Bronchospasm occurs early in an asthma 'attack'. This is particularly prominent in allergic asthma when, within minutes of exposure to an allergen, wheezing develops. Narrowing of small airways occurs due to contraction of airway smooth muscle in response to the cellular mechanisms described below. Airway closure begins to occur during expiration, gas trapping follows and the lungs become hyperinflated.[6] Eventually, the patient is attempting to breathe in when the lungs are almost at total lung capacity and a sensation of inspiratory dyspnoea results, even though the defect is with expiration. Physiological effects of hyperinflation are described on page 380.

Bronchospasm may quickly subside, either spontaneously or with treatment, but more commonly progresses to a late-phase reaction.

Late-phase reactions are characterised by inflammation of the airway and develop a few hours after the acute bronchospasm. Airway obstruction continues and cough with sputum production develops. Asthma precipitated by respiratory tract infection may 'bypass' the acute bronchospasm phase and the onset of symptoms is then more gradual.

Airway hyperresponsiveness (AHR) describes the observation that asthmatic subjects become wheezy in response to a whole range of stimuli that have little effect on normal individuals. Stimuli include such things as cold air, exercise, pollution (page 294) or inhaled drugs and occur via the neural pathways present in normal lungs (page 46). Methacholine or histamine can be used to measure AHR accurately by determining the inhaled concentration that gives rise to a 20% reduction in forced expiratory volume in one second (FEV_1).[7] Inhaled adenosine also causes airway narrowing but, unlike histamine and methacholine, it does not act directly on bronchial smooth muscle.[8] Bronchoconstriction in response to adenosine involves release of mediators from inflammatory cells, so the response is sensitive to the inflammatory state of the airway. For this reason, it is

hoped that adenosine provocation may prove useful for monitoring the effectiveness of antiinflammatory treatment of asthma patients or even for differentiating between asthma and COPD.[8]

The degree of AHR seen in patients with asthma is highly variable. Severe asthma is associated with continuous AHR, whereas in mild asthma the patient's response will be normal between wheezy episodes.

Cellular mechanisms of asthma[1,9-12]

Many cell types are involved in the pathophysiology of asthma. A summary of the interactions between these cells is shown in Figure 28.1, which also shows the principal cytokines that facilitate communication between the cells.

Mast cells are plentiful in the walls of airways and alveoli and also lie free in the lumen of the airways, where they may be recovered by bronchial lavage. Mast cell activation is the main cause of the immediate bronchospasm seen in allergen-provoked asthma. The surface of the mast cell contains a large number of binding sites for the immunoglobulin IgE. Activation of the cell results from

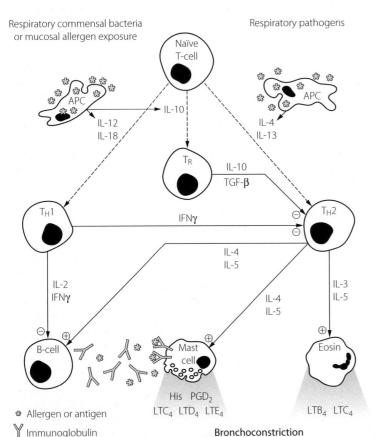

Figure 28.1 Inflammatory cells involved in the pathogenesis of asthma and the cytokines by which they communicate with each other. For details see text. The immunological pathways shown are based on a combination of animal and human studies.[3,11-14] Eosin, eosinophil; T_H2 and T_H1, subtypes of T-lymphocyte 'helper' cells; T_R, regulatory lymphocyte; B-cell, B-lymphoctye; APC, antigen-presenting cell; IL, interleukin; IFN, interferon; TGF, transforming growth factor.

Table 28.1 Mediators released from mast cells when activated by IgE

Preformed mediators	Newly generated mediators	Cytokines
Histamine	Prostaglandin D_2	Interleukins 3,4,5,6 and 13
Heparin	Thromboxane A_2	Granulocyte/macrophage
Serotonin	Leukotrienes C_4, D_4 and E_4	colony-stimulating factor
Lysosomal enzymes:		Tumour necrosis factor
Tryptase		Platelet-activating factor
Chymase		
β-Galactosidase		
β-Glucuronidase		
Hexosaminidase		

antigen bridging of only a small number of these receptors and may also be initiated by complement fractions C3a, C4a and C5a, substance P, physical stimulation, and many drugs and other organic molecules.

The triggering mechanism of the mast cell is thus extremely sensitive and is mediated by an increase in inositol triphosphate and intracellular calcium ions. Within 30 seconds of activation, there is degranulation with discharge of a range of preformed mediators listed in Table 28.1. Histamine acts directly on H_1 receptors in the bronchial smooth muscle fibres to cause contraction, on other H_1 receptors to increase vascular permeability and on H_2 receptors to increase mucus secretion. The granules also contain proteases, mainly tryptase, which can detach epithelial cells from the basement membrane, resulting in desquamation and possibly activating neuronal reflexes, causing further bronchospasm.

The second major event after mast cell activation is the initiation of synthesis of arachidonic acid derivatives (see Figure 12.2). The most important derivative of the cyclooxygenase pathway is prostaglandin PGD_2, which is a bronchoconstrictor, although its clinical significance is still not clear. The lipoxygenase pathway results in the formation of leukotriene (LT) C_4, from which two further peptide leukotrienes, LTD_4 and LTE_4, are formed (see Figure 4.9).

Finally, mast cells also release a variety of cytokines, some of which are contained within the granules whereas others are generated *de novo* on activation of the cell. Interleukin-5 (IL-5) and granulocyte/macrophage colony-stimulating factor (GM-CSF) are chemotactic for eosinophils, whereas IL-4 stimulates IgE production by B-lymphocytes and so amplifies the activation of mast cells.

Eosinophils are freely distributed alongside mast cells in the submucosa and are now believed to be the principal cell involved in the late-phase reaction of asthma. In particular, they release LTB_4 and LTC_4, which are potent bronchoconstrictors with a prolonged action. They are attracted to the area by GM-CSF, which is released by many inflammatory cells, before being activated by IL-5 and IL-3 originating from mast cells and lymphocytes.

Lymphocytes have an important role in the control of mast cell and eosinophil activation.[1,11,13] Activated B-lymphocytes are responsible for production of the antigen-specific IgE needed to cause mast cell degranulation. B-cells are in turn controlled by two subsets of T 'helper' lymphocytes, known as T_H1 and T_H2 cells.

T_H2 cells are important proinflammatory cells in asthma, promoting both bronchospasm and inflammation by stimulation of mast cells, eosinophils and B-lymphocytes with IL-3, IL-4 and IL-5. The T_H2 cell is non-specific in its response and relies on stimulation by IL-4 and IL-13 from antigen-presenting cells (APC) both for its generation from naïve T-cells and for its subsequent activation to produce its own proinflammatory cytokines. It is not clear where APCs originate, but they are probably located in the airway mucosa. Once activated by their specific antigen, the APCs migrate to lymphoid tissue in the lungs to control the division of naïve lymphocytes into their various subtypes. In the case of T_H2 stimulation the APC is responding to a range of lung pathogens, and this is the immunological pathway involved in normal pulmonary defences against infection.

T_H1 cells are also generated from naïve T-cells in lymphoid tissue in response to cytokines released by activated APC, but for T_H1 generation the cytokines concerned are IL-12 and IL-18. T_H1 cells normally act as antiinflammatory cells by producing interferon and IL-2, which inhibit the activity of T_H2 and B-cells.

The relative activity of the opposing effects of T_H1 and T_H2 lymphocytes was, until recently, believed to play an important role in the development and severity of asthma. However, this convenient explanation, based mainly on studies in animals, is now thought to be an oversimplification of the situation in humans, particularly with respect to the generation of T_H1 cells.[14]

A third subtype of T-lymphocyte is now thought to be involved in immune regulation of the lung.[11] Regulatory T-cells (T_R) are again generated from naïve T-cells, this time in response to IL-10 released by activated APCs. Activation of the APC to produce the antiinflammatory cytokines IL-10, IL-12 and IL-18 is believed to occur in response to antigens from respiratory tract commensal bacteria or from exposure to high levels of allergens.[11] T_R cells exert an anti-inflammatory effect by secretion of IL-10 and transforming growth factor β (TGF-β), which modify the activities of both T_H1 and T_H2 cells.[3]

Nitric oxide (NO) is detectable in small concentrations in the expired air of normal subjects.[15] It is produced from the mucosa of the whole respiratory tract, including the nose and nasal sinuses. Nitric oxide acts as the neurotransmitter for the non-adrenergic non-cholinergic (NANC) bronchodilator pathway in normal lungs (page 46), is involved in control of vascular tone in all tissues and is present in blood. In asthmatic patients with active disease, NO concentration in expired air is 2–10 times greater than in non-asthmatics.[16] In this situation, the extra NO is derived from inducible NO-synthase (iNOS, page 100) in the airway mucosa. Cytokines produced by the inflammatory cells already described are believed to result in increased production of iNOS.[17] This is likely to represent another means by which the inflammatory response is amplified, as NO may have an inhibitory effect on T_H1 cells.[18] Although NO seems unlikely to have a major role in the development of asthma, its presence in expired air may in future provide a useful means of quantifying the inflammatory component of asthma.[19] In addition, the discovery of another mechanism involved in bronchospasm has opened further potential therapeutic avenues.[18]

Causes of airway obstruction in asthma[2]

Bronchial smooth muscle. Stimulation of bronchial smooth muscle by the substances shown in Figure 28.1 and Table 28.1 explains some of the airway narrowing seen in asthma, particularly during the acute and early stages.

Inflammation. Airway narrowing during the late-phase response, or in severe asthma, results from inflammation of the airway. Many cytokines released during asthma have effects on blood vessel permeability and therefore cause oedema of the epithelium and basement membrane.[20] Protease enzymes (see Table 28.1) break down normal epithelial architecture, generating defects in the epithelial barrier, leading to further inflammation and

eventually detachment of the epithelium from the basement membrane. Finally, hypersecretion of mucus and impaired mucociliary clearance are both recognised features of asthma and this correlates with the flow limitation seen in individual patients. These changes in the thickness of the airway lining translate into a significant reduction in airway cross-sectional area and thus a large increase in resistance (page 40). Mucus, inflammatory cells and epithelial debris cause obstruction of small airways, compounded by flow limitation preventing an effective cough. In severe asthma, obstruction of small airways gives rise to ventilation/perfusion mismatch, shunt and hypoxaemia, and has long been recognised as a significant pathological finding in fatal asthma.

Airway remodelling.[10,21,22] Repeated activation of inflammatory pathways inevitably leads to attempts by the body to repair the tissue concerned. In the lung, this results in morphological changes to both the airway smooth muscle and the respiratory epithelium. Hyperplasia of smooth muscle cells causes thickening of the airway wall even when the muscle is relaxed and exacerbates the airway narrowing that occurs with muscle contraction because a lesser degree of muscle shortening now causes a greater reduction in the airway lumen. Goblet cell hyperplasia occurs, worsening the hypersecretion of mucus seen with airway inflammation. Finally, in asthmatic patients, there is thickening of the lamina reticularis of the epithelial basement membrane. The clinical significance of airway remodelling in asthma is unknown, but remodelling is believed to be responsible for the long-term decline in lung function seen in some asthma patients. The changes are resistant to steroid therapy, so may progress in spite of optimal treatment, and some recent studies have found that, in children, remodelling may even be occurring some years before overt symptoms of asthma develop.[23]

Aetiology of asthma

Genetics. Asthma, along with other allergic diseases, has a substantial genetic component with several genomic regions known to be linked with developing the disease.[24] Environmental factors invariably contribute to the development of clinical disease, but genetic susceptibility to asthma is strong. Two reasons explain this observation. First, the genes for most of the cytokines involved in asthma are found close together on chromosome 5 and asthmatic patients may have increased expression of these, so encouraging formation of an allergic phenotype.[1,9] Second, human lymphocyte antigens (HLA), which are involved in sensitisation of APC to specific antigens, are part of the major histocompatibility complex allowing immunological 'self recognition' and so are inherited. It is possible that some HLA types are particularly active in the processing of common allergens and thus the stimulation of T_H2 cells or the suppression of T_R cells.

Maternal allergic disease is more likely to be passed to offspring than paternal disease, though this may relate to modification of the foetal immune system *in utero* rather than a true genetic influence. During pregnancy, lymphocyte subsets T_H1 and T_H2 are closely involved in the prevention of maternal rejection and abnormalities at this stage may influence the activity of T_H1 and T_H2 cells in the offspring's immune system, leading to allergic diseases, including asthma, in later life.[25]

A genome-wide scan of patients with asthma has recently identified a specific gene that is strongly associated with bronchial hyperresponsiveness.[24,26] The gene codes for a protein named ADAM33, part of a large family of proteins with diverse functions, including the control of cell–cell and cell–matrix interactions. In lung tissue ADAM33 protein is found in smooth muscle and fibroblasts but not epithelial cells, indicating its possible role in airway remodelling in asthma.

Allergy.[1] Changes in living conditions have undoubtedly contributed to the increase in asthma prevalence. In the developing world, population shifts from rural to urban environments have reduced exposure to parasitic infections and increased exposure to other allergens, and it seems likely that the extensive IgE and mast cell systems that formally inactivated parasites now respond to urban allergens. In the developed world, changes in living conditions have resulted in a dramatic increase in allergen exposure, in particular house dust mites (HDM, *Dermatophagoides pteronyssinus*), domestic animals and fungi. Asthma is more common in affluent families and correlates with exposure to HDM, which thrives in warm, humid houses with extensive carpeting and bedding. These conditions are ideal for the HDM and its food supply of shed skin flakes. In some circumstances, up to 15% of the contents of the vacuum cleaner bag are thought to be made up of HDM or their excretory products. Simply inhaling allergens is only part of the explanation of how allergen exposure causes asthma and once again pregnancy plays a role. Allergen taken in by the mother is believed to cross the placenta and influence immunological development before birth. Neonatal T-lymphocytes taken from children who subsequently develop asthma already show a reduced production of interferon-γ in response to allergen, indicating an existing immunological susceptibility to asthma.[27]

Infection.[28] Viral respiratory tract infections cause wheezing in many asthmatics and account for over half of acute exacerbations of asthma. In infants, respiratory syncytial or parainfluenza viruses are common, whereas in adults a 'common cold' rhinovirus is the most usual

pathogen. Viral infection gives rise to an immune response involving many cells and cytokines, but T-lymphocytes are particularly important and undergo both virus-specific and generalised activation. Inevitably, T_H2 activity is increased, giving rise to wheeze and airway inflammation by the mechanisms described above (see Figure 28.1). In addition, stimulation of allergic mechanisms in susceptible individuals continues for some time after the viral symptoms have subsided. Thus, for example, after a simple rhinovirus infection allergen-induced histamine production and eosinophil-induced late-phase reactions remain increased for 4–6 weeks.[29]

Hygiene hypothesis. This hypothesis to explain the rising incidence of asthma claims that in the clean, hygienic, developed world children are exposed to fewer infections or other environmental antigens than only a few decades ago. It is known that some infections may have a protective role in preventing the initiation of asthma in early childhood.[1,28] Children who are exposed to more infections in early life, such as those with older siblings or children living on farms, are less likely to develop allergic disease. This led to a suggestion that lower infection rates in the population at large and effective immunisation programmes may have contributed to the rising incidence of asthma. Measles virus, *Mycobacterium tuberculosis*, respiratory and gastrointestinal commensal bacteria, some respiratory viral infections and hepatitis A virus all have the potential to reduce asthma development by modification of the lymphocyte subtypes shown in Figure 28.1.[1,11,30] A recent review identified three more groups of microorganisms to which the modern human is now less commonly exposed.[13] Termed 'old friends' by the authors, these include lactobacilli from untreated dairy products, saprophytic mycobacteria found in mud, and helminths (worms). All three are known to promote activity of T_R cells and so potentially protect against the development of asthma (see Figure 28.1). For many of these microorganisms exposure to the entire microbe is not required and beneficial immune responses may be gained from exposure to antigens found in the dust and dirt of the environment.

Pollution.[31] Trends in air pollution have not generally followed trends in asthma prevalence over recent decades, the levels of many pollutants declining while asthma becomes more common. Laboratory evidence described on page 294 describes how, in comparison with normal subjects, asthmatics develop wheeze when exposed to lower inhaled concentrations of nitrogen dioxide and sulphur dioxide. The levels required to cause wheezing are still higher than commonly encountered in the atmosphere, and although there is some evidence linking air pollution episodes to respiratory problems, the effect is believed to be small.

A role for air pollution in the initiation of asthma has also remained elusive. Animal experiments indicate that common air pollutants can sensitise the airway to allergens, probably by disturbance of mucociliary clearance. Prolonged pulmonary retention of allergens in the airway allows more time for sensitisation of submucosal inflammatory cells such as APC.[31] There is currently no evidence that this contributes to asthma in humans.[31]

Gastric reflux.[32] Gastro-oesophageal reflux symptoms are common in asthmatics and are involved in the production of cough or wheeze in up to a third of patients. Acid in the distal oesophagus can, via a vagally mediated reflex, provoke either bronchoconstriction itself or airway hypersensitivity to allergen. In more severe cases, oesophageal reflux leading to aspiration of small amounts of acid into the airway can provoke severe bronchospasm. In patients with asthma who are resistant to treatment or who have mainly nocturnal symptoms, reflux should be considered as a cause.

Aspirin-induced asthma (AIA)[33]

The involvement of arachidonic acid derivatives in the normal control of bronchial smooth muscle (see Table 4.2 and page 49) predicts that drugs blocking these pathways may influence the airways of asthma patients. This is indeed the case, with aspirin and the closely related non-steroidal antiinflammatory drugs sometimes causing bronchospasm in asthma patients. Based on patient history alone, only 2.7% of asthma patients report wheezing in response to aspirin, but when provocation with oral aspirin is carried out 21% of patients develop a reduction in FEV_1.[34] Many asthmatic patients who are sensitive to aspirin have a characteristic clinical presentation. Typically, AIA develops in patients at around 30 years of age, is associated with rhinitis and nasal polyps, and occurs in more female than male patients.[33]

Mechanism of aspirin sensitivity. Inhibitors of the cyclooxygenase (COX) pathway in the airway will reduce synthesis of the bronchodilator prostaglandin PGE_2. Reduced synthesis of PGE_2 cannot alone account for AIA; patients with AIA also have increased production of LTE_4, a potent bronchoconstrictor. This effect on the lipoxygenase pathway is not mediated by aspirin itself and possibly results from loss of inhibition of lipoxygenase by PGE_2. Genetic polymorphisms for the enzymes involved in leukotriene production may explain why some patients are aspirin sensitive.[35] Multiple isoforms of COX exist (page 205) and COX-1 seems to be responsible for most cases of AIA. A recently introduced group of drugs, known as coxibs, are highly specific inhibitors of COX-2 and seem to be safe for use in AIA patients.[33] The analgesic effects of paracetamol (acetaminophen) may be

mediated by inhibition of COX-3,[36] and a small subset of patients with AIA develop bronchospasm in response to paracetamol.[34] This sensitivity to paracetamol usually involves only a mild reaction in response to high doses of the drug and occurs in less than 2% of asthmatic patients. In a cohort study of over 121 000 volunteers, frequent use of paracetamol was associated with the development of asthma, leading to paracetamol use becoming the latest hypothesis to explain the increased incidence of asthma in recent years.[37]

Principles of therapy

Detailed guidelines on the treatment of asthma are published for both the UK[38] and the USA,[39] and are beyond the scope of this book. Except in very mild asthma, treatment has now moved away from the traditional bronchodilator inhaler 'when needed' approach of the past. The emphasis is now on continuous treatment with drugs and other strategies aimed at preventing exacerbations and suppressing airway inflammation.[40] Therapeutic approaches include the following.

Bronchodilators remain a common treatment for relief of acute bronchospasm. The β_2-adrenoceptor agonists (page 47) are widely used and recent developments include the introduction of longer-acting drugs such as salmeterol. Other bronchodilator drugs include inhibitors of leukotriene receptors on bronchial smooth muscle (page 49), blocking the effects of LTC_4, LTD_4 and LTE_4. They are effective in treating asthma, including the bronchospasm seen in the late-phase reaction, and may be particularly useful in patients with exercise or aspirin-induced asthma.[41]

Steroids,[42,43] either inhaled or oral, are an invaluable method of prophylaxis and treatment in asthma. The antiinflammatory effect of steroids is complex and incompletely elucidated. Steroids act on a glucocorticoid receptor found in the cytoplasm of cells, following which, the receptor–drug complex can enter the nucleus and regulate the transcription of numerous genes.[43] By a combination of direct and indirect effects on transcription, steroids inhibit the synthesis of a wide range of inflammatory proteins including cytokines, adhesion molecules and inflammatory receptors.

Allergen avoidance is an attractive strategy for the prevention of asthma in patients with known allergies. Low humidity is very effective in reducing HDM and therefore at high altitude (above 1500 m or 5000 ft) HDM allergen is non-existent. Several studies have used this to compare asthma severity in normal and HDM-free high-altitude environments and have found improvements in both clinical and cellular measures of asthma severity.[44]

However, the rather drastic intervention of moving to high altitude is clearly not practical and reduction of allergen load in the home is considerably less effective. Measures include removing carpets, reducing temperature and humidity, application of acaricides to kill HDM and encasing mattresses in allergen-impermeable membranes. Some studies have reported clinical benefits, but a metaanalysis did not support this approach.[45]

CHRONIC OBSTRUCTIVE PULMONARY DISEASE

Unlike asthma, where airway obstruction is usually intermittent, COPD is characterised by progressive chronic air flow limitation along with intermittent exacerbations. Clinical features are similar to those of asthma, with wheeze, cough and dyspnoea, but the air flow limitation is poorly reversible with bronchodilators. Older patients are more affected by COPD than by asthma, and the progressive nature of the process leads to more serious interruption of normal activities and eventually respiratory failure (page 365). COPD is now the sixth most common cause of death worldwide and its prevalence is increasing.[46]

Aetiology of COPD[47,48]

Smoking is the major aetiological factor in COPD. The accelerated decline in FEV_1 seen with smoking is shown in Figure 21.1 and the 15–20% of smokers who develop COPD probably represent an extreme response to this effect of tobacco smoke.[48] Attempts to identify the genes responsible for this susceptibility to COPD in smokers are at an early stage.[49]

Both asthma and COPD are characterised pathologically by airway narrowing and inflammation, but the causes and clinical course of the two diseases are quite different. Improved understanding of the pathology of COPD and asthma has uncovered a variety of major differences between the two and these are shown in Figure 28.2. It is believed that around 10% of patients have a mixture of the two disease processes, usually referred to as 'wheezy bronchitis'.[50]

The cellular mechanisms underlying airway inflammation in COPD relate to the disease's strong association with smoking, and with activation of neutrophils and macrophages (page 292) rather than the eosinophils and mast cells seen in asthma. Neutrophil activation causes the release of several protease enzymes, including neutrophil elastase which degrades pulmonary elastin, leading to the loss of lung tissue elasticity that is a characteristic feature of COPD. Smoking also induces oxidative stress in the airways, again potentially leading to irreversible tissue damage (page 292).

Three pathophysiological changes give rise to COPD: emphysema, mucous hypersecretion of larger airways and small airway obstruction. The last two of these are often collectively referred to as chronic bronchitis.

Emphysema may be defined as permanent enlargement of airspaces distal to the terminal bronchiole accompanied by destruction of alveolar walls.[51] The process begins by enlargement of normal interalveolar holes, followed by

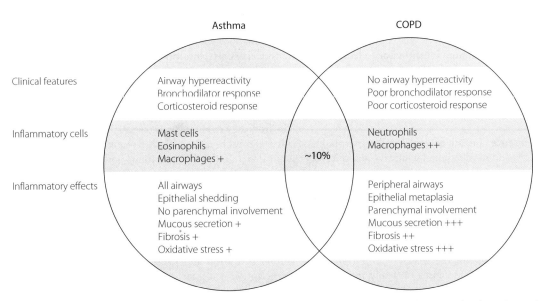

	Asthma	COPD
Clinical features	Airway hyperreactivity Bronchodilator response Corticosteroid response	No airway hyperreactivity Poor bronchodilator response Poor corticosteroid response
Inflammatory cells	Mast cells Eosinophils Macrophages +	Neutrophils Macrophages ++
Inflammatory effects	All airways Epithelial shedding No parenchymal involvement Mucous secretion + Fibrosis + Oxidative stress +	Peripheral airways Epithelial metaplasia Parenchymal involvement Mucous secretion +++ Fibrosis ++ Oxidative stress +++

~10%

Figure 28.2 Clinical and pathological differences between chronic obstructive pulmonary disease and asthma. Approximately 10% of patients have features characteristic of both diseases and may be described as having 'wheezy bronchitis'. (Reproduced with permission from Barnes PJ. Mechanisms in COPD. Differences from asthma. *Chest* 2000; **117**: 10S–14S.)

destruction of the entire alveolar septum. Both ventilation and perfusion of the emphysematous area are therefore reduced and, though some mismatch of ventilation and perfusion may occur in widespread emphysema, localised areas, as usually seen in COPD, have little effect. The loss of elastic tissue contained within the alveolar septa is, however, important and reduces the elastic recoil of the pulmonary tissue, so contributing to closure of small airways, particularly during expiration.

Current views on the cellular defect responsible for emphysema involve the relationship between protease and antiprotease activity in the lung.[51] These enzymes are normally released following activation of neutrophils (e.g. neutrophil elastase) or macrophages in response to tobacco smoke or infection. A deficiency of the most well-known antiprotease, α_1-antitrypsin, is a significant risk factor for early development of emphysema (page 202). Disturbances of less well-understood protease–antiprotease systems, such as the matrix metalloproteases group of enzymes, are now also believed to be involved in the generation of emphysema, as these proteases are normally involved in remodelling of the extracellular lung matrix.[51] Proteases with activity against elastin are likely to be responsible for generating emphysema. Elastin deposition in the lung occurs early in life and is minimal beyond late adolescence. Later, any pulmonary elastin lost through disease is likely to be replaced with collagen, so reducing lung elasticity and probably explaining the general decline in lung recoil throughout life.[52]

Small airway obstruction plays a major role in COPD, but its aetiology is controversial.[47,53,54] Part of the expiratory air flow limitation results from emphysema, as described above. It is also likely that changes in the airway wall itself contribute. Inflammatory changes in small airways are common in COPD,[54] and may lead to mucosal thickening, hypertrophy of bronchial smooth muscle, and ultimately to deposition of collagen in the outer airway wall.[47]

Large airway disease consists of goblet cell hyperplasia, mucosal oedema and production of excessive amounts of mucus. Recurrent respiratory tract infections and smoking undoubtedly contribute and a chronic productive cough is the result. This feature of COPD is not always present and its contribution to overall airway obstruction is variable. In some patients, extensive and long-standing inflammation of the large airways gives rise to permanent thickening of the airway wall within the cartilaginous airways and so causes clinically important degrees of obstruction.[54]

Hyperinflation.[55] Air flow limitation in small airways results from a combination of airway narrowing and loss of elastic recoil of lung tissue. The latter is of major importance in maintaining the patency of airways less than 1 mm in diameter (page 15), which lack supporting cartilage in their walls. Expiratory flow limitation leads to prolonged expiratory time constants in affected lung units and incomplete expiration (gas trapping).[56] Lung volume is therefore forced to increase and the patient becomes dyspnoeic, particularly during any situation that requires a greater minute volume, such as exercise or when a chest infection develops. Hyperinflation of the lung will, in theory, tend to oppose expiratory airway closure (see Figure 4.5), but it also causes a significant reduction in the efficiency of the respiratory muscles. In particular, the diaphragm becomes displaced caudally and, in severe disease, flattened, reducing the zone of apposition (see Figure 6.1) and causing much of the muscle activity to either oppose the opposite side of the diaphragm or pull the lower ribcage inwards rather outwards (see Figure 6.2). In time, lung hyperinflation becomes permanent, with expansion of the chest wall (barrel chest) and irreversible flattening of the diaphragm.

Principles of therapy[56,57]

As for asthma, detailed guidelines for the treatment of COPD have been published.[58]

Smoking cessation is central to all forms of treatment for COPD.[59] The rate of the progressive decline in lung function returns to that of a non-smoker (see Figure 21.1) and symptoms improve. Patients with COPD have often been heavy smokers for a considerable number of years and smoking cessation may therefore need great determination. Patients usually only become permanent non-smokers after multiple attempts at quitting, though nicotine replacement and other drug therapies may improve this poor success rate.

Medical treatment. Inhaled bronchodilators may be used. Their efficacy depends on the reversibility of the airways disease in each patient. Both β_2-agonists and anticholinergic drugs (page 47) are used, and long-acting drugs from both these groups now exist and are effective at improving lung function.[60] Corticosteroids are not as effective for treating COPD as they are for asthma. The inflammatory cells involved are different (see Figure 28.2) and may be less susceptible to steroid suppression Oxidative stress present in COPD airways from neutrophil activation and smoking may inhibit one of the transcription enzymes normally stimulated by steroid drugs.[61]

Medical treatment also involves active management of exacerbations, which may result from bacterial or viral infections or changes in air quality.[62] Management of the underlying disease with antibiotics and oxygen is required. Artificial ventilation is commonly required and non-invasive ventilation (page 420) is now accepted as the best initial option for these patients.[63,64]

Supplemental oxygen at low inspired concentrations for several hours a day is beneficial in the treatment of advanced COPD. Indications for its use are a Pa_{O_2} of less than 7.3 kPa (55 mmHg) with evidence of long-term hypoxia such as cor pulmonale or polycythaemia.[56] Oxygen flow is titrated to achieve an arterial PO_2 of 9–12 kPa (65–90 mmHg) and under these conditions the long-term mortality from COPD is reduced.[65]

Surgical treatment is reserved for severe COPD.[53,66] When the airspaces created in emphysema become larger than 1 cm in diameter they are referred to as a 'bulla'. Adjacent bullae can merge and result in extremely large airspaces, occupying up to one-third of the lung volume. Like emphysema, bullae have little effect on gas exchange as both tidal ventilation and blood flow to the bullae are negligible. However, with giant bullae, the airspace acts in a similar fashion to a pneumothorax and compresses surrounding normal lung tissue, causing further worsening of airways collapse and subsequently disturbing gas exchange. In these cases surgical treatment involves 'bullectomy' and, with careful patient selection, this can be a useful operation. Advances in surgical techniques have led to a resurgence of interest in surgery for COPD and extended the indications to include patients who do not have bullae. Lung volume reduction surgery involves removing 20–30% of lung volume, to include the most emphysematous areas. This procedure has yielded impressive results in some patient groups,[66] improving both symptoms and lung function tests, and is currently being evaluated in a clinical trial.[67] The physiological mechanisms of the improvement following surgery remain poorly understood, but probably include reduced pulmonary collapse adjacent to emphysematous areas, improved elastic recoil of the remaining lung tissue and better respiratory muscle function secondary to reduced hyperinflation.

Oxygen therapy in COPD

Patients with advanced COPD may be broadly classified into 'pink puffers' and 'blue bloaters', which correspond to type 1 and type 2 respiratory failure, respectively (page 365). 'Pink puffers', with predominantly emphysematous changes, maintain a considerable degree of respiratory sensitivity to carbon dioxide and struggle to keep a normal arterial PCO_2 for as long as possible, although with evident dyspnoea. On the other hand 'blue bloaters', mostly with airways disease (chronic bronchitis), have lost their sensitivity to carbon dioxide

and allow their PCO_2 to increase above the normal reference range, usually without dyspnoea. Determinants of which pattern individual patients develop are uncertain. The underlying disease process (emphysema versus airway inflammation) may determine the pattern, as may the patient's respiratory sensitivity to carbon dioxide before developing COPD.

Administration of oxygen to COPD patients commonly leads to hypercapnia. Two main mechanisms are believed to be responsible.

Ventilatory depression by oxygen. 'Blue bloaters' may be relying on their hypoxic drive to maintain ventilation. If this is abolished, as, for example, by the administration of 100% oxygen, hypoventilation or even apnoea may result. However, studies investigating oxygen-induced hypercapnia in COPD have failed to find consistent changes in minute ventilation during periods of either stable respiratory symptoms[68] or acute exacerbations.[69] Reduction in minute ventilation in response to oxygen was either too small to explain adequately the changes in PCO_2 or only transient, returning towards baseline ventilation after a few minutes. Nevertheless, in one of these reports,[69] of 22 subjects studied, two developed severe respiratory depression leading to dangerous hypercapnia after just 15 minutes of breathing 100% oxygen. A small proportion of patients with COPD are therefore clearly susceptible to oxygen-induced respiratory depression.

Altered ventilation/perfusion relationships with oxygen have been proposed to explain hypercapnia seen in COPD patients in whom minute ventilation remains essentially unchanged.[68–70] Alveolar PO_2 is known to contribute to hypoxic pulmonary vasoconstriction (page 101) and so help to minimise $\dot{V}/\dot{Q}$ mismatch. Administration of oxygen may therefore abolish hypoxic pulmonary vasoconstriction in poorly ventilated areas, increasing blood flow to these areas and so reducing blood flow to other lung regions with normal or high ventilation/perfusion ratios.[68] These areas will then contribute further to alveolar dead space and so cause an increase in arterial PCO_2 (page 118).

Which of these mechanisms predominates in an individual patient is currently difficult to predict. Administration of oxygen to patients with COPD must therefore be undertaken with great care and accompanied by suitable monitoring of both oxygenation and arterial PCO_2.

CYSTIC FIBROSIS

Cystic fibrosis (CF) is an autosomal recessive genetic disorder affecting Caucasian individuals, of whom 1 in 25 carries the gene. The disease affects approximately 1 in 2500 births[71] and abnormal CF genes can be identified prenatally, but there is a wide spectrum of clinical disease such that prediction of phenotype from genetic screening is complex.[72,73] Cystic fibrosis affects epithelial cell function in many body systems but gastrointestinal and respiratory function are the most important; this chapter discusses only the latter.

Abnormalities of pulmonary airway defence mechanisms lead to lifelong colonisation of the cystic fibrosis lung with bacteria. Recurrent airway infection produces hypersecretion of mucus, cough and, over many years, destruction of normal lung architecture, including bronchiectasis. Initial infection normally occurs early in life and progressive lung disease is the usual cause of death. Mortality from CF remains high, with a current median life expectancy of only 32 years.[74] This has improved considerably in recent years, though there continues to be a significant number of deaths in early infancy.[71] Thus, although the number of CF births is constant, improved survival means that the prevalence of CF is steadily increasing.

Aetiology of CF

Biochemical abnormality

The molecular mechanisms of CF have been the focus of extensive research for many years, which has led to CF being one of the most completely understood of inherited diseases. As long ago as 1989 the gene responsible for CF was identified.[75] It is located on chromosome 7 and codes for a protein named cystic fibrosis transmembrane conductance regulator (CFTR) found in epithelial cells. The CFTR protein functions as a membrane-bound active chloride channel and plays a major role in controlling salt concentration in epithelial secretions. Sweat production is influenced by CFTR function, allowing measurement of the sodium concentration in sweat to remain a relatively simple investigation for diagnosis, being over twice normal in CF patients.[76]

The CFTR comprises three types of protein subunit.[77,78] A ring of membrane-spanning domains forms a channel through the lipid bilayer of the cell wall (Figure 28.3). Attached to the intracellular aspect of these are two nucleotide-binding domains (NBDs) that use ATP when the channel is activated. Finally, a single regulatory domain (R) protein is loosely attached to the NBDs and can move away from them to 'open' the channel and allow chloride to pass into or out of the cell (see Figure 28.3). Intracellular protein kinase A activates the channel by binding to the regulatory domain of CFTR, whereas ATP provides the energy and is dephosphorylated by the NBDs. Over 1000 different mutations of the CF gene have been identified and can result in no CFTR being formed, failure of the different protein

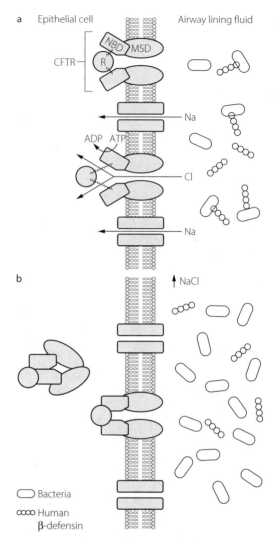

Figure 28.3 Sodium and chloride transport across the pulmonary epithelial cell wall in cystic fibrosis. **(a)** Normal lung. Cystic fibrosis transmembrane regulator (CFTR) chloride channel in the closed (upper) and open (lower) positions showing movement of the regulator domain (R). Sodium transport follows chloride via passive Na channels due to altered transmembrane potentials. Bacteria in the airway lining fluid may be inactivated by human β-defensin. **(b)** Cystic fibrosis. The CFTR proteins are defective and so do not locate in the membrane, or are non-functional when they do. Sodium and chloride concentration is therefore abnormally high in the airway, which may inactivate human β-defensin or alter airway lining fluid function and so allow bacterial proliferation. MSD, membrane-spanning domain; NBD, nucleotide-binding domain.

domains to align correctly, or failure of the CFTR to become incorporated into the cell membrane.[74,77] Almost three-quarters of clinical CF cases arise from a deletion of just three base pairs from the gene, which result in the loss of a single phenylalanine from one NBD protein and failure to locate the CFTR in its transmembrane position.[72]

Causes of lung disease

The sequence of events by which abnormal CFTR function leads to pulmonary pathology remains controversial. Abnormalities of the airway lining fluid and mucus result in poor defences against inhaled pathogens. Bacterial colonisation, particularly with *Pseudomonas aeruginosa*, occurs early in the disease process and CF patients have an exaggerated inflammatory response to a variety of other airway pathogens. A cycle becomes established in which bacterial infection leads to airway inflammation, mucus production and more infection, associated with progressive lung tissue damage.[79] Abnormal CFTR function may adversely affect the ability of the airway to remove inhaled pathogens by a variety of mechanisms, as follows.[74]

Salt-defensin hypothesis. Some work suggests that the human lung produces an endogenous antibiotic named human β-defensin (HBD), which may play an important role in preventing pulmonary infection. Consisting of a 64 amino acid peptide, HBD has been shown to be inactivated by increased sodium chloride concentrations, so allowing proliferation of bacteria in CF lungs (see Figure 28.3).[80]

Inflammation first hypothesis. This proposes that airway inflammation is the primary event in CF lungs, possibly caused by abnormal cytokine production. Inflammatory changes in the airways then lead to excessive and abnormal mucus production and colonisation with pathogens.

Cell-receptor hypothesis. In normal lung, the CFTR found on epithelial cells, along with a range of cell surface glycoproteins, binds many bacterial pathogens, including *P. aeruginosa*, as part of the normal process for killing inhaled microorganisms. Abnormal pH around epithelial cells from CF lung inhibits the binding of *P. aeruginosa* by CFTR.

Depleted airway surface liquid hypothesis. Despite the altered sodium and chloride transport in the CF lung epithelial cells, the 'sol' or periciliary layer of the airway surface liquid (ASL, page 18) is believed to be isotonic.[73] However, the volume of periciliary fluid is reduced and this disturbs the physical linkage between the cilia and the periciliary and mucous layers of ASL, effectively preventing the normal clearance of the ASL. The mucous layer becomes abnormally deep and viscous, which inhibits the function of endogenous antimicrobial systems such as HBD, lactoferrin and lysozyme, and possibly also introduces a layer of hypoxic mucus in which anaerobic bacteria can thrive.

Principles of therapy

***Conventional treatment*[74,81]** involves assisting the clearance of airway secretions by physiotherapy, postural drainage and exercise. The viscous mucous layer of ASL results in part from degradation of the numerous inflammatory cells found in infected airways, and it is DNA from these cells that tends to aggregate and increase viscosity. Treatment with inhaled recombinant human DNAase reduces the viscosity of sputum and is a useful adjunct to physical methods of mucus clearance. Antibiotic therapy, for both infective exacerbations and maintenance therapy, is now used for all patients. Despite problems with the emergence of bacterial resistance and patient hypersensitivity reactions, better strategies for antibiotic use are believed to be the main reason for improved survival in CF.[74]

Lung transplantation is now a recognised treatment for CF and is described in Chapter 33.

Gene therapy has held great potential for therapy ever since the CF gene was identified, but unfortunately this potential has not been realised.[82] A normal CFTR gene can be produced, but the problem arises in incorporating the gene into the airway cells and stimulating its expression into functioning CFTR *in vivo*.[83] Gene delivery, in either liposomes or genetically modified adenovirus vectors, has been attempted but the functional effect is poor, with only transient or small changes in CFTR expression. Viral vectors, which are the most effective technique for incorporating the new gene into the epithelial cell, may be associated with significant inflammatory reactions, which may be either harmful or protective.[82,84] A more promising approach is to incorporate the normal gene into the foetus, which bypasses immunological reactions and should provide a permanent correction of the defective gene. This has been achieved in mice,[85] but studies of this type in humans are currently prohibited by international ethical convention.

REFERENCES

1. Holgate ST. Asthma and allergy – disorders of civilisation? Q *J Med* 1998; **91**: 171–84.
2. Nadel JA, Busse WW. Asthma. *Am J Respir Crit Care Med* 1998; **157**: S130–S138.
*3. Holgate ST. The epidemic of asthma and allergy. *J Roy Soc Med* 2004; **97**: 103–10.
4. Shafazand S, Colice G. Asthma – the epidemic has ended, or has it? *Chest* 2004; **125**: 1969–70.

5. Woolcock AJ. Learning from asthma deaths. *Br Med J* 1997; **314**: 1427–8.

6. Cormier Y, Lecours R, Legris C. Mechanisms of hyperinflation in asthma. *Eur Respir J* 1990; **3**: 619–24.

7. Lötvall J, Inman M, O'Byrne P. Measurement of airway hyperresponsiveness: new considerations. *Thorax* 1998; **53**: 419–24.

8. Polosa R, Rorke S, Holgate ST. Evolving concepts on the value of adenosine hyperresponsiveness in asthma and chronic obstructive pulmonary disease. *Thorax* 2002; **57**: 649–54.

9. Lee TH. Cytokine networks in the pathogenesis of bronchial asthma: implications for therapy. *J Roy Coll Phys Lond* 1998; **32**: 56–64.

*10. Bousquet J, Jeffery PK, Busse WW, Johnson M, Vignola AM. Asthma: from bronchoconstriction to airways inflammation and remodeling. *Am J Respir Crit Care Med* 2000; **161**: 1720–45.

*11. Umetsu DT, McIntyre J, Akbari O, Macaubas C, DeKruyff RH. Asthma: an epidemic of dysregulated immunity. *Nat Immunol* 2002; **3**: 715–20.

12. Busse WW, Lemanske RF. Asthma. *N Engl J Med* 2001; **344**: 350–62.

13. Rook GAW, Adams V, Hunt J, Palmer R, Martinelli R, Brunet LR. Mycobacteria and other environmental organisms as immunomodulators for immunoregulatory disorders. *Springer Semin Immunopathol* 2004; **25**: 237–55.

14. Salvi SS, Babu KS, Holgate ST. Is asthma really due to a polarized T cell response toward a helper T cell type 2 phenotype? *Am J Respir Crit Care Med* 2001 **164**: 1343–6.

15. DuBois AB, Kelley PM, Douglas JS, Mohsenin V. Nitric oxide production and absorption in trachea, bronchi, bronchioles and respiratory bronchioles of humans. *J Appl Physiol* 1999; **86**: 159–67.

16. Frank TL, Adisesh A, Pickering AC, *et al.* Relationship between exhaled nitric oxide and chidhood asthma. *Am J Respir Crit Care Med* 1998; **158**: 1032–6.

17. Hamid Q, Springall DR, Riveros-Moreno V, *et al.* Induction of nitric oxide synthase in asthma. *Lancet* 1993; **342**: 1510–13.

18. Barnes PJ. NO or no NO in asthma. *Thorax* 1996; **51**: 218–20.

19. Lundberg JON, Lundberg JM, Alving K, Weitzberg E. Nitric oxide and inflammation: the answer is blowing in the wind. *Nat Med* 1997; **3**: 30–1.

20. Jeffery PK, Godfrey RW, Ädelroth E, Nelson F, Rogers A, Johansson S-A. Effects of treatment on airway inflammation and thickening of basement membrane reticular collagen in asthma. *Am Rev Respir Dis* 1992; **145**: 890–9.

21. Davies DE, Wicks J, Powell RM, Puddicombe SM, Holgate ST. Airway remodeling in asthma: new insights. *J Allergy Clin Immunol* 2003; **111**: 215–25.

22. McParland BE, Macklem PT, Paré PD. Airway wall remodelling: friend or foe? *J Appl Physiol* 2003; **95**: 426–34.

23. Pohunek P, Roche WR, Tarzikova J, Kurdmann J, Warner JO. Eosinophilic inflammation in the bronchial mucosa in children with bronchial asthma. *Eur Respir J* 2000; **11**(Supp 25): 160S.

*24. Van Eerdewegh P, Little RD, Dupuis J, *et al.* Association of the ADAM33 gene with asthma and bronchial hyperresponsiveness. *Nature* 2002; **418**: 426–30.

25. Warner JA, Jones AC, Miles EA, Colwell BM, Warner JO. Maternofetal interaction and allergy. *Allergy* 1996; **51**: 447–51.

26. Holgate ST, Davies DE, Murphy G, Powell RM, Holloway JW. ADAM 33: just another asthma gene or a breakthrough in understanding the origins of bronchial hyperresponsiveness? *Thorax* 2003; **58**: 466–9.

27. Tang MLK, Kemp AS, Thorburn J, Hill DJ. Reduced interferon-γ secretion in neonates and subsequent atopy. *Lancet* 1994; **344**: 983–5.

28. Folkerts G, Busse WW, Nijkamp FP, Sorkness R, Gern JE. Virus-induced airway hyperresponsiveness and asthma. *Am J Respir Crit Care Med* 1998; **157**: 1708–20.

29. Calhoun WJ, Dick EC, Schwartz LB, Busse WW. A common cold virus, rhinovirus 16, potentiates airway inflammation after segmental antigen bronchoprovocation in allergic subjects. *J Clin Invest* 1994; **94**: 2200–8.

30. Scott P. IL-12: initiation cytokine for cell-mediated immunity. *Science* 1993; **260**: 496–7.

31. Committee on the Medical Effects of Air Pollutants. *Asthma and outdoor air pollution.* London: HMSO, 1995.

32. Harding SM, Richter JE. The role of gastroesophageal reflux in chronic cough and asthma. *Chest* 1997; **111**: 1389–402.

33. Szczeklik A, Stevenson DD. Aspirin-induced asthma: advances in pathogenesis, diagnosis and management. *J Allergy Clin Immunol* 2003; **111**: 913–21.

34. Jenkins C, Costello J, Hodge L. Systematic review of prevalence of aspirin induced asthma and its implications for clinical practice. *Br Med J* 2004; **328**: 434–7.

35. Szczeklik A, Sanak M. Genetic mechanisms in aspirin-induced asthma. *Am J Respir Crit Care Med* 2000; **161**: S142–6.

36. Schwab JM, Schluesener HJ, Laufer S. COX-3: just another COX or the solitary elusive target of paracetamol? *Lancet* 2003; **361**: 981–2.

37. Barr RG, Wentowski CC, Curhan GC, *et al.* Prospective study of acetaminophen use and newly diagnosed asthma among women. *Am J Respir Crit Care Med* 2004; **169**: 836–41.

38. British Thoracic Society. British guideline on the management of asthma. *Thorax* 2003; **58** (Supp 1): 1–83.

39. National Heart, Lung and Blood Institute. *Expert Panel Report 2: guidelines for the diagnosis and management of asthma*. Publication No 97–4051. Bethesda, MD.: National Institutes of Health, 1997.

40. Lipworth BJ. Modern drug treatment of chronic asthma. *Br Med J* 1999; **318**: 380–4.

41. Salvi SS, Krishna MT, Sampson AP, Holgate ST. The anti-inflammatory effects of leukotriene-modifying drugs and their use in asthma. *Chest* 2001; **119**: 1533–46.

42. McFadden ER. Inhaled glucocorticoids and acute asthma. Therapeutic breakthrough or nonspecific effect? *Am J Respir Crit Care Med* 1998; **157**: 677–8.

43. Barnes PJ. Molecular mechanisms of corticosteroids in allergic disease. *Allergy* 2001; **56**: 928–36.

44. Custovic A, Simpson A, Chapman MD, Woodcock A. Allergen avoidance in the treatment of asthma and atopic disorders. *Thorax* 1998; **53**: 63–72.

45. Gotzsche PC, Hammarquist C, Burr M. House dust mite control measures in the management of asthma: meta-analysis. *Br Med J* 1998; **317**: 1105–10.

*46. Calverley PMA, Walker P. Chronic obstructive pulmonary disease. *Lancet* 2003; **362**: 1053–61.

*47. Barnes PJ, Shapiro SD, Pauwels RA. Chronic obstructive pulmonary disease: molecular and cellular mechanisms. *Eur Respir J* 2003; **22**: 672–88.

48. Saetta M, Turato G, Maestrelli P, Mapp CE, Fabbri LM. Cellular and structural bases of chronic obstructive pulmonary disease. *Am J Respir Crit Care Med* 2001; **163**: 1304–9.

49. Sandford AJ, Silverman EK. Chronic obstructive pulmonary disease 1: susceptibility factors for COPD – the genotype–environment interaction. *Thorax* 2002; **57**: 736–41.

50. Barnes PJ. Mechanisms in COPD. Differences from asthma. *Chest* 2000; **117**: 10S–14S.

51. Hogg JC, Senior RM. Chronic obstructive pulmonary disease. 2: Pathology and biochemistry of emphysema. *Thorax* 2002; **57**: 830–4.

52. Pierce RA, Mariani TJ, Senior RM. Elastin in lung development and disease. *Ciba Found Symp* 1995; **192**: 199–214.

53. Davies L, Calverley PMA. Lung volume reduction surgery in chronic obstructive pulmonary disease. *Thorax* 1996; **51** (Supp 2); S29–S34.

54. Tiddens HAWM, Paré PD, Hogg JC, Hop WCJ, Lambert R, De Jongste JC. Cartilaginous airway dimensions and airflow obstruction in human lungs. *Am J Respir Crit Care Med* 1995; **152**: 260–6.

55. Demedts M. Mechanisms and consequences of hyperinflation. *Eur Respir J* 1990; **3**: 617–18.

*56. Man SFP, McAlister FA, Anthonisen NR, Sin DD. Contemporary management of chronic obstructive

pulmonary disease. Clinical applications. *JAMA* 2003; **290**: 2313–16.

*57. Sutherland ER, Cherniak RM. Management of chronic obstructive pulmonary disease. *N Engl J Med* 2004; **350**: 2689–97.

58. Pauwels RA, Buist AS, Calverley PMA, Jenkins CR, Hurd SS. Global strategy for the diagnosis, management and prevention of chronic obstructive pulmonary disease. NHLBI/WHO Global Initiative for Chronic Obstructive Lung Disease (GOLD) Workshop summary. *Am J Respir Crit Care Med* 2001; **163**: 1256–76.

59. MacNee W, Calverley PMA. Chronic obstructive pulmonary disease. 7: Management of COPD. *Thorax* 2003; **58**: 261–5.

60. Tashkin DP, Cooper CB. The role of long-acting bronchodilators in the management of COPD. *Chest* 2004; **125**: 249–59.

61. Barnes PJ, Ito K, Adcock IM. Corticosteroid resistance in chronic obstructive pulmonary disease: inactivation of histone deacetylase. *Lancet* 2004; **363**: 731–3.

62. White AJ, Gompertz S, Stockley RA. Chronic obstructive pulmonary disease. 6: The aetiology of exacerbations of chronic obstructive pulmonary disease. *Thorax* 2003; **58**: 73–80.

63. Babu KS, Chauhan AJ. Non-invasive ventilation in chronic obstructive pulmonary disease. *Br Med J* 2003; **326**: 177–8.

64. Plant PK, Elliott MW. Chronic obstructive pulmonary disease. 9: Management of ventilatory failure in COPD. *Thorax* 2003; **58**: 537–42.

65. Senior RM, Anthonisen NR. Chronic obstructive pulmonary disease (COPD). *Am J Respir Crit Care Med* 1998; **157**: S139–S147.

66. Meyers BF, Patterson GA. Chronic obstructive pulmonary disease. 10: Bullectomy, lung volume reduction surgery and transplantation for patients with chronic obstructive pulmonary disease. *Thorax* 2003; **58**: 634–8.

*67. Drazen JM. Surgery for emphysema – not for everyone. *N Engl J Med* 2001; **345**: 1126–8.

68. Sassoon CSH, Hassell KT, Mahutte CK. Hyperoxic-induced hypercapnia in stable chronic obstructive pulmonary disease. *Am Rev Respir Dis* 1987; **135**: 907–11.

69. Aubier M, Murciano D, Milic-Emili J, *et al*. Effects of the administration of O_2 on ventilation and blood gases in patients with chronic obstructive pulmonary disease during acute respiratory failure. *Am Rev Respir Dis* 1980; **122**: 747–54.

70. Crossley DJ, McGuire GP, Barrow PM, Houston PL. Influence of inspired oxygen concentration on deadspace, respiratory drive and Pa_{CO_2} in intubated patients with chronic obstructive pulmonary disease. *Crit Care Med* 1997; **25**: 1522–6.

71. Dodge JA, Morison S, Lewis PA, *et al.* Incidence, population and survival of cystic fibrosis in the UK, 1968–95. *Arch Dis Child* 1997; **77**: 493–6.

72. Davidson DJ, Porteus DJ. The genetics of cystic fibrosis lung disease. *Thorax* 1998; **53**: 389–97.

*73. Boucher RC. New concepts of the pathogenesis of cystic fibrosis lung disease. *Eur Respir J* 2004; **23**: 146–58.

74. Ratjen F, Döring G. Cystic fibrosis. *Lancet* 2003; **361**: 681–9.

75. Kerem B, Rommens JM, Buchanan JA, *et al.* Identification of the cystic fibrosis gene: genetic analysis. *Science* 1989; **245**: 1073–80.

76. Wallis C. Diagnosing cystic fibrosis: blood, sweat and tears. *Arch Dis Child* 1997; **76**: 85–91.

77. Welsh MJ, Ramsey BW. Research on cystic fibrosis. *Am J Respir Crit Care Med* 1998; **157**: S148–S154.

78. Stern M, Geddes D. Cystic fibrosis: basic chemical and cellular mechanisms. *Br J Hosp Med* 1996; **55**: 237–40.

79. Bilton D, Mahadeva R. New treatments in adult cystic fibrosis. *J Roy Soc Med* 1997; **90** (Supp 31): 2–5.

80. Goldman MJ, Anderson GM, Stolzenberg ED, Kari UP, Zasloff M, Wilson J. Human β-defensin-1 is a salt-sensitive antibiotic in lung that is inactivated in cystic fibrosis. *Cell* 1997; **88**: 553–60.

81. Yankaskas JR, Marshall BC, Sufian B, Simon RH, Rodman D. Cystic fibrosis adult care: consensus conference report. *Chest* 2004; **125** (1 Supp): 1S–39S.

82. Schwiebert LM. Cystic fibrosis, gene therapy and lung inflammation: for better or worse? *Am J Physiol Lung Cell Mol Physiol* 2004; **286**: L715–16.

*83. Driskell RA, Engelhardt JF. Current status of gene therapy for inherited lung diseases. *Annu Rev Physiol* 2003; **65**: 585–612.

84. McElvaney NG, Crystal RG. IL-6 release and airway administration of human CFTR cDNA adenovirus vector. *Nat Med* 1995; **1**: 182–4.

85. Larson JE, Morrow SL, Happel L, Sharp JF, Cohen JC. Reversal of cystic fibrosis phenotype in mice by gene therapy in utero. *Lancet* 1997; **349**: 619–20.

Chapter

29 Pulmonary vascular disease

KEY POINTS

- The balance between osmotic and hydrostatic pressures normally minimises fluid transfer between the pulmonary capillary and the interstitial space.
- Pulmonary oedema occurs when increases in pulmonary capillary pressure or the permeability of the alveolar/capillary membrane cause fluid to accumulate in the interstitium and alveoli.
- Pulmonary embolism, with either thrombus or air, partially occludes the pulmonary circulation, causing an increase in alveolar dead space and pulmonary arterial hypertension.
- Pulmonary hypertension most commonly results from long-term hypoxia or elevated left atrial pressure and involves reduced nitric oxide production and remodelling of the pulmonary blood vessels.

PULMONARY OEDEMA

Pulmonary oedema is defined as an increase in pulmonary extravascular water, which occurs when transudation or exudation exceeds the capacity of the lymphatic drainage. In its more severe forms there is free fluid in the alveoli.

Anatomical factors

The pulmonary capillary endothelial cells abut against one another at fairly loose junctions which are of the order of 5 nm (50 Å) wide.[1] These junctions permit the passage of quite large molecules and the pulmonary lymph contains albumin at about half the concentration in plasma. Epithelial cells are connected by tight junctions at their alveolar surface with a gap of only about 1 nm.[1] Under normal circumstances the tightness of these junctions prevents the escape of large molecules, such as albumin, from the interstitial fluid into the alveoli. However, the proteins that make up the tight

junction are not simply passive structural units and can, for example in response to nitric oxide, be modified and allow an increase in permeability across the tight junction.[2,3]

The lung has a well-developed lymphatic system draining the interstitial tissue through a network of channels around the bronchi and pulmonary vessels towards the hilum. Lymphatic vessels are seen in the juxtaseptal alveolar region (see below) and are commonly found in association with bronchioles. Down to airway generation 11 (see Table 2.1), the lymphatics lie in a potential space around the air passages and vessels, separating them from the lung parenchyma. In the hilum of the lung, the lymphatic drainage passes through several groups of tracheobronchial lymph glands, where they receive tributaries from the superficial subpleural plexus. Most of the lymph from the left lung usually enters the thoracic duct, where it can be conveniently sampled in animals. The right side drains into the right lymphatic duct.

The normal lymphatic drainage from human lungs is astonishingly small – only about 10 ml.h^{-1}. However, lymphatic flow can increase up to ten times this value when transudation into the interstitial spaces is increased.[4] This presumably occurs when pulmonary oedema is threatened but it cannot be conveniently measured in man.

Pulmonary fluid dynamics[5]

For intravascular fluid to enter the alveoli, it must traverse three barriers. First, it must move from the microcirculation into interstitial space (across the endothelium), then through the interstitium and finally from the interstitial space into the alveoli (across the epithelium) (Figure 29.1).

Fluid exchange across the endothelium. This is promoted by the hydrostatic pressure difference between capillary and interstitium but counteracted by the osmotic pressure of the plasma proteins. The balance of pressures is normally sufficient to prevent any appreciable transudation but it may be upset in a wide variety of pathological circumstances.

P = Hydrostatic pressure (kPa or cmH₂O) – relative to atmosphere
π = Protein osmotic pressure (kPa or cmH₂O)

Figure 29.1 Normal values for hydrostatic and plasma protein osmotic pressures in the pulmonary microcirculation and interstitium. (Values taken from reference 6.)

It is customary to display the relationship between fluid flow and the balance of pressures in the form of the Starling equation. For the endothelial barrier this is as follows:

$$\dot{Q} = K[(P\text{cap} - P\text{int}) - \Sigma(\Pi\text{cap} - \Pi\text{int})]$$

$\dot{Q}$ is the flow rate of transudated fluid which, in equilibrium, will be equal to the lymphatic drainage.

K is the hydraulic conductance (i.e. flow rate of fluid per unit pressure gradient across the endothelium).

$P\text{cap}$ is the hydrostatic pressure in the pulmonary capillary.

$P\text{int}$ is the hydrostatic pressure in the interstitium.

Σ is the reflection coefficient, in this case applying to albumin. It is an expression of the permeability of the endothelium to the solute (albumin). A value of unity indicates total reflection corresponding to zero concentration of the solute in the interstitial fluid. A value of zero indicates free passage of the solute across the membrane and, with equal concentrations on both sides of the membrane, the solute can exert no osmotic pressure across the membrane. This normally applies to the crystalloids in plasma.

Πcap is the osmotic pressure the solute exerts within the pulmonary capillary.

Πint is the osmotic pressure the solute exerts in the interstitium.

Under normal circumstances in humans, the pulmonary lymph flow ($\dot{Q}$) is about 10 ml per hour with a protein content about half that of plasma. The pulmonary microvascular pressure ($P\text{cap}$) is in the range 0–2 kPa (0–15 mmHg), relative to atmosphere, depending on the vertical height in the lung field. Furthermore, there is a progressive decrease in capillary pressure from its arte-

rial to its venous end, since approximately one-half the pulmonary vascular resistance is across the capillary bed (see Figures 7.2 and 29.1). In this context, it is meaningless to think of a single value for the mean pulmonary capillary pressure.

The hydrostatic pressure in the interstitial space ($P\text{int}$) of the lung is not easy to measure. Animal studies using micropuncture techniques obtained subatmospheric pressures of –0.40 to –1.25 kPa (–4 to –12.5 cmH₂O).[7,8] In the excised lung there was no vertical gradient in interstitial pressures such as might have been expected from the effect of gravity,[7] but this was observed when measurements were made with the chest and pleura intact.[8]

The reflection coefficient for albumin (Σ) in the healthy lung is about 0.5. The overall osmotic pressure gradient between blood and interstitial fluid is about 1.5 kPa (11.5 mmHg). Thus there is a fine balance between forces favouring and opposing transudation. There is a considerable safety margin in the upper part of the lung where the capillary hydrostatic pressure is lowest. However, in the dependent part of the lung, where the hydrostatic pressure is highest, the safety margin is slender.

Fluid dynamics within the interstitium. It is now accepted that the interstitium does not simply act as a passive conduit for fluid transfer to the lymphatics.[5,9,10] Proteoglycan and hyaluron molecules are present in the pulmonary interstitium of animals and function like a gel to absorb water to minimise increases in interstitial pressure and prevent hydration of other extracellular structures such as collagen.[11] Regional differences in the properties of these molecules are believed to be responsible for the establishment of a pressure gradient between the septal interstitium and the juxtaseptal region where lymphatic channels originate. This gradient may promote, and allow some control of, fluid flow from the endothelium to the lymphatics in the normal lung.[9]

With increased fluid transfer across the endothelium, the interstitial space can accommodate large volumes of water with only small increases in pressure, the interstitial compliance being high. Some 500 ml can be accommodated in the interstitium and lymphatics of the human lungs with a pressure rise of only about 0.2 kPa (2 cmH$_2$O).[6] Eventually, the capacity of the molecules to absorb water is exceeded and the proteoglycan structure breaks down, possibly leading to disturbances of nearby collagen molecules and therefore basement membrane function, producing alveolar oedema.[9] Alterations of interstitial proteoglycan structure during lung injury may contribute to the greater likelihood of pulmonary oedema under these circumstances (Chapter 31).

Fluid exchange across the alveolar epithelium. The permeability of this barrier to gases and larger molecules is considered in Chapter 9 (page 145). It is freely permeable to gases, water and hydrophobic substances but virtually impermeable to albumin.

There is now considerable evidence of active fluid clearance from the alveoli in normal human lungs.[3,12,13] For methodological reasons, most studies of this system have involved type II alveolar epithelial cells, but the same processes are believed to occur in type I cells and in Clara cells in the distal airways. On the alveolar side of these cells, the cell membrane contains epithelial sodium channels (ENaC) and cystic fibrosis transmembrane conductance regulator (CFTR) channels (page 382), which actively pump sodium and chloride ions respectively into the cell.[3] On the interstitial border of the cells, chloride moves passively out of the cell and the Na$^+$/K$^+$-ATPase channel actively removes sodium from the cell. Water from the alveolus follows these ion transfers down an osmotic gradient into the interstitium. Aquaporins are found in human alveolar epithelial cells, suggesting that water movement may be facilitated by these water channel proteins, but their role in normal adult lung remains unclear.[3]

A small amount of active clearance of fluid from the alveoli occurs under normal circumstances, but these systems become vital when pulmonary oedema develops. Active removal of alveolar fluid by alveolar epithelial cells increases within 1 hour of the onset of oedema.[14] Stimulation of β$_2$-adrenoceptors by catecholamines increases the affinity of existing Na$^+$/K$^+$-ATPase channels for sodium and causes new channels to be incorporated into the cell membrane from intracellular endosomal stores. After a few hours, a variety of hormones[14] (e.g. thyroxine, aldosterone, glucocorticoids) and cytokines[3,13] (e.g. tumour necrosis factor) induce the transcription of new Na$^+$/K$^+$-ATPase channels and increase fluid clearance. These mechanisms are important both for minimising the severity of pulmonary oedema and for clearing oedema fluid once the precipitating cause has resolved.

Stages of pulmonary oedema

There is presumably a prodromal stage in which pulmonary lymphatic drainage is increased, but there is no increase in extravascular water. This may progress to the following stages.

Stage I. Interstitial pulmonary oedema. In its mildest form, there is an increase in interstitial fluid but without passage of oedema fluid into the alveoli. With the light microscope this is first detected as cuffs of distended lymphatics, typically '8'-shaped, around the adjacent branches of the bronchi and pulmonary artery (Figure 29.2). Electron microscopy shows fluid accumulation in the alveolar septa but this is characteristically confined to the 'service' side of the pulmonary capillary which contains the stroma, leaving the geometry of the 'active' side unchanged (see page 20 and Figure 2.8). Thus, gas exchange is better preserved than might be expected from the overall increase in lung water. Interstitial swelling is, however, not without risks and swelling on the service side will eventually cause narrowing of the capillary lumen, though this does not occur until pulmonary oedema is very advanced.

Physical signs are generally minimal in stage I, except perhaps for mild dyspnoea, particularly with exercise. The alveolar/arterial PO$_2$ gradient is normal or only slightly increased. Diagnosis relies on the chest radiograph, in which Kerley B lines may be visible, and on the demonstration of causative factors such as an increased pulmonary capillary wedge pressure.

Stage II. Crescentic filling of the alveoli. With further increase in extravascular lung water, interstitial oedema of the alveolar septa is increased and fluid begins to pass into some alveolar lumina. It first appears as crescents in the angles between adjacent septa, at least in lungs which have been fixed in inflation (see Figure 29.2). The centre of the alveoli and most of the alveolar walls remain clear and gas exchange is not grossly abnormal, but dyspnoea at rest is likely and the characteristic butterfly shadow may be visible on the chest radiograph.

Stage III. Alveolar flooding. In the third stage, there is quantal alveolar flooding. Some alveoli are totally flooded, whereas others, frequently adjacent, have only the crescentic filling or else no fluid at all in their lumina. It seems that fluid accumulates up to a point at which a critical radius of curvature results in surface tension, sharply increasing the transudation pressure gradient. This produces flooding on an all-or-none basis for each individual alveolus. Owing to the effect of gravity on pulmonary vascular pressures (page 94), alveolar flooding tends to occur in the dependent parts of the lungs. Rales can be heard during inspiration and the lung

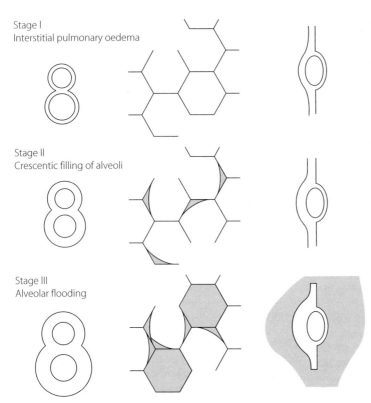

Stage I
Interstitial pulmonary oedema

Stage II
Crescentic filling of alveoli

Stage III
Alveolar flooding

Figure 29.2 Schematic diagram of the stages in the development of pulmonary oedema. On the left is shown the development of the cuff of distended lymphatics around the branches of the bronchi and pulmonary arteries. In the middle is the appearance of the alveoli by light microscopy (fixed in inflation). On the right is the appearance of the pulmonary capillaries by electron microscopy. The active side of the capillary is to the right. See text for details.

fields show an overall opacity superimposed on the butterfly shadow.

Clearly there can be no effective gas exchange in the capillaries of an alveolar septum which is flooded on both sides, and blood flow through these alveoli constitutes venous admixture or shunt.[15] This results in an increased alveolar/arterial PO_2 gradient and hypoxaemia, which may be life threatening. Blood flow to the oedematous lung regions is slightly reduced by hypoxic pulmonary vasoconstriction (page 101), possibly in conjunction with interstitial swelling causing capillary narrowing (see above), but the shunt commonly remains substantial.

Hypercapnia is not generally a problem. In less severe pulmonary oedema, there is usually an increased respiratory drive, due partly to hypoxaemia and partly to stimulation of J-receptors (page 61). As a result the PCO_2 is usually normal or somewhat decreased.

Stage IV. Froth in the air passages. When alveolar flooding is extreme, the air passages become blocked with froth, which moves to and fro with breathing. This effectively stops all gas exchange and is rapidly fatal unless treated.

Aetiology of pulmonary oedema

On the basis of the Starling equation, it is possible to make a rational approach to the aetiology of pulmonary oedema. There are three groups of aetiological factors, classified according to their effect on factors in the Starling equation.

Increased capillary pressure (haemodynamic pulmonary oedema). This group comprises the commonest causes of pulmonary oedema. There is an elevation of the hydrostatic pressure gradient across the pulmonary capillary wall, until it exceeds the osmotic pressure of the plasma proteins. Interstitial fluid accumulates until it overwhelms the ability of the interstitium to absorb fluid and transport it to the lymphatics. Fluid then begins to enter the alveoli and will initially be actively removed by the alveolar epithelial cells until this system is also overwhelmed. The oedema fluid has a protein content which is less than that of normal pulmonary lymph or plasma.[6] Apart from transudation in accord with the Starling equation, severe pulmonary capillary hypertension may result in loss of structural integrity (see below).

Causes of an increase in pulmonary capillary pressure are numerous.

- Absolute hypervolaemia may result from overtransfusion, excessive and rapid administration of other blood volume expanders or acute renal failure.
- Relative pulmonary hypervolaemia may result from redistribution of the circulating blood volume into the lungs. Examples of how this may occur include use of

the Trendelenburg position or vasopressor drugs that act on the systemic circulation to a greater extent than the pulmonary circulation and so redirect blood into the pulmonary circulation.

- Raised pulmonary capillary pressure will inevitably result from an increase in pulmonary venous pressure.[4,10] This may occur from any form of left heart failure, most commonly left ventricular failure, or mitral valve lesions.
- Increased pulmonary blood flow may raise the pulmonary capillary pressure sufficiently to precipitate pulmonary oedema. This may result from a left-to-right cardiac shunt, anaemia or, rarely, as a result of exercise.

Increased permeability of the alveolar/capillary membrane (permeability oedema). This group comprises the next commonest cause of pulmonary oedema. The mechanism is the loss of integrity of the alveolar/capillary membrane, allowing albumin and other macromolecules to enter the alveoli. The osmotic pressure gradient which opposes transudation is then lost. The oedema fluid has a protein content approaching that of plasma.

The alveolar/capillary membrane can be damaged either directly or indirectly by many agents, which are reviewed in Chapter 31. Apart from the possibility of the condition progressing to acute lung injury, permeability pulmonary oedema is always potentially very dangerous. The presence of protein in the alveoli tends to make the oedema refractory and the protein may become organised into a so-called hyaline membrane.

'Stress failure' of the pulmonary capillaries occurs when the pulmonary capillary pressure is increased in the range 3–5 kPa (30–50 cmH$_2$O). Discontinuities appear in the capillary endothelium and type I alveolar epithelial cells, but the basement membrane often remains intact.[4,16] This would seem to result in increased permeability and leakage of protein into the alveoli. The gaps tend to occur in the cell body, rather than at the junctions between the cells.

Decreased osmotic pressure of the plasma proteins. The Starling equation indicates that the osmotic pressure of the plasma proteins is a crucial factor opposing transudation. Although seldom the primary cause of pulmonary oedema, a reduced plasma albumin concentration is very common in the seriously ill patient and it must inevitably decrease the microvascular pressure threshold at which transudation commences.

Miscellaneous causes of pulmonary oedema

Pulmonary oedema occurring at high altitude is well documented although the mechanism is still open to speculation. It is considered in Chapter 17.

Neurogenic pulmonary oedema may follow head injuries or other cerebral lesions. Evidence for the existence of pulmonary venous sphincters has provided a possible mechanism for neurogenic pulmonary oedema.[17] Constriction of these sphincters, due to either circulating adrenaline or a neural response, could cause an abrupt increase in pulmonary capillary pressure. A study of neurogenic pulmonary oedema in humans supported this hypothesis by demonstrating that the oedema fluid often has a low protein content, suggesting a haemodynamic mechanism (see above).[17]

Reexpansion pulmonary oedema. Sudden expansion of a collapsed lung may result in pulmonary oedema confined to the one side and probably caused by increased permeability.[18] The problem may arise after aspiration of a pneumothorax or a pleural effusion. Large pneumothoraces, a longer duration of collapse before reexpansion and the use of suction to reexpand the lung are all associated with greater likelihood of pulmonary oedema.[19]

Principles of therapy

Immediate treatment aims to restore the arterial PO$_2$ to normal values. The inspired oxygen concentration should be increased, up to 100% if necessary. Sitting the patient up is a simple way to reduce central blood volume. Treatment of the underlying cause of pulmonary oedema follows directly from the Starling equation and an understanding of the aetiology.

Haemodynamic pulmonary oedema. Treatment aims to reduce left atrial pressure. Depending on the precise aetiology, treatment is directed towards improvement of left ventricular function and/or reduction of blood volume. The latter may be quickly and easily achieved by peripheral vasodilation. Drugs that predominantly dilate the capacitance (venous) system, such as nitrates or angiotensin-converting enzyme inhibitors, will be most effective. This mechanism is probably also responsible for the beneficial effects of furosemide and diamorphine in the acute situation. Diuretics act more slowly but are useful for long-term treatment. Essentially, the patient is titrated to the left along his Frank–Starling curve (Figure 29.3). In addition the curve is moved upwards and to the left, if this is possible, using positive inotropes as an adjunct to correction of left ventricular malfunction, for example from ischaemia. The further the curve can be moved, the greater will be that part of it lying in the safe quadrant between low cardiac output on one hand and pulmonary oedema on the other.

Permeability pulmonary oedema. Treatment should be directed towards restoration of the integrity of the alveolar/capillary membrane. Unfortunately, no particularly

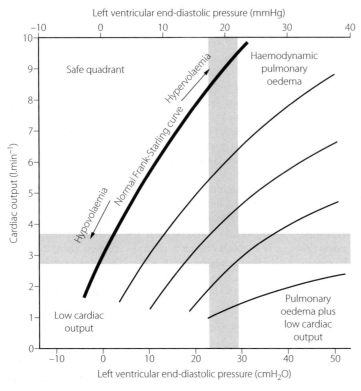

Figure 29.3 Quadrant diagram relating cardiac output to left ventricular end-diastolic pressure. The thick curve is a typical normal Frank–Starling curve. To the right are shown curves representing progressive left ventricular failure. *Top left* is the safe quadrant, which contains a substantial part of the normal curve, but much less of the curves representing ventricular failure. *Top right* is the quadrant representing normal cardiac output but raised left atrial pressure, attained at the upper end of relatively normal Frank–Starling curves (e.g. hypervolaemia). There is a danger of haemodynamic pulmonary oedema. *Bottom left* is the quadrant representing normal or low left atrial pressure but low cardiac output, attained at the lower end of all curves (e.g. hypovolaemia). The patient is in shock. *Bottom right* is the quadrant representing both low cardiac output and raised left atrial pressure. There is simultaneous danger of pulmonary oedema and shock, and the worst Frank–Starling curves hardly leave this quadrant.

successful measures are available towards this end. It is, however, important to minimise left atrial pressure even though this is not the primary cause of the oedema. Attempts may be made to increase the plasma albumin concentration if it is reduced.

Artificial ventilation and positive end-expiratory pressure (PEEP). Severe pulmonary oedema causes degrees of hypoxia that may quickly be lethal. Tracheal intubation and positive-pressure ventilation are therefore commonly required and the results are often spectacular. Froth in the airways may be aspirated and any areas of atelectasis occurring along with the oedema improved. Artificial ventilation is often combined with PEEP, resulting in further improvements in arterial PO_2. It was originally thought that the positive pressures drove the fluid back into the circulation but evidence that extravascular lung water is reduced by PEEP contradicts this, with few human studies. Animal models of pulmonary oedema indicate that by increasing the lung volume, the capacity of the interstitium to hold liquid is increased.[20] Similarly, with haemodynamic pulmonary oedema in dogs, PEEP does not alter the total amount of lung water but a greater proportion is in the extraalveolar interstitial space[21] and lymphatic drainage is increased.[22] With haemodynamic pulmonary oedema, positive-pressure ventilation has beneficial effects on the function of the

failing heart (page 436) and it is probably this effect, rather than any effect on the lungs, that causes the clinical benefit in humans.

Clinical measurement

Pulmonary vascular pressures. As an indication of impending or actual haemodynamic pulmonary oedema, the most useful clinical measurement is the pulmonary artery occlusion pressure (page 105), which equates to pulmonary venous pressure. Estimates of pulmonary capillary pressure itself may also be obtained with a Swan–Ganz catheter.[23,24] The decay curve seen on occluding a pulmonary artery branch is biphasic (Figure 29.4). The first, rapid phase reflects the fall in pressure as the arterial compartment distal to the balloon empties across the precapillary resistance. The second, slower phase represents the fall in pressure as the capillary compartment empties into the pulmonary veins across the postcapillary resistance. Thus, the inflection point of the curve should equate to mean capillary pressure.[23]

Permeability of the alveolar/capillary membrane. Laboratory methods are available for animals but the only practical approach for clinical use is measurement of the rate of loss of a γ-emitting tracer molecule from the lung into the circulation. The most sensitive tracer is ^{99m}Tc-DTPA

Figure 29.4 Estimation of pulmonary capillary pressure using the Swan–Ganz catheter. The pulmonary arterial trace has been slightly damped with air and the occlusion balloon is inflated during a prolonged expiration to prevent pressure swings with respiration. The occlusion pressure decay curve is biphasic. Pulmonary capillary pressure (PCP) is estimated as the point at which the slow component causes the decay curve to depart from its initial steep decline, and may be measured manually as shown.

(metastable technetium-99-labelled diethylene triamine pentaacetate, molecular weight 492 Da).[25] The half-time of clearance from the lung fields is usually in the range 40–100 minutes in the healthy non-smoker. The half-time is reduced below 40 minutes following a variety of lung insults. However, it is within the range 10–40 minutes in apparently healthy smokers, and this limits its scope for the early detection of a damaged alveolar/capillary membrane.

Lung water. Measurement of lung water in the intact subject has proved difficult. A great deal of effort has been devoted to the double indicator method. This uses the techniques for the measurement of pulmonary or central blood volume by dye dilution but with two indicators. One indicator is chosen to remain within the circulation while the other (usually 'coolth' or tritiated water) diffuses into the interstitial fluid. Extravascular lung water is then derived as the difference between the volumes as measured with the two indicators. These methods are limited because a high level of accuracy is required to demonstrate small changes in lung water, though clinically acceptable results may now be obtained reasonably conveniently.[26]

PULMONARY EMBOLISM

The pulmonary circulation may be occluded by embolism, which may be gas, thrombus, fat, tumour or foreign body. The architecture of the microvasculature is well adapted to minimise the effects of embolism. Large numbers of pulmonary capillaries tend to arise at right angles from metarterioles and there are abundant anastomoses throughout the microcirculation. This tends to preserve circulation distal to the impaction of a small embolus. Nevertheless, a large pulmonary embolus is a serious and potentially lethal condition.

Thromboembolism[27,28]

The commonest pulmonary embolus consists of detached venous thromboses, particularly from veins in the thigh and the pelvic venous plexuses. Smaller thrombi are filtered in the lungs without causing symptoms but larger emboli may impact in major vessels, typically at a bifurcation, thus forming a saddle embolus. There may be a catastrophic increase in pulmonary vascular resistance with acute right heart failure or cardiac arrest.

Diagnosis of pulmonary thromboembolus.[27] Massive pulmonary thromboembolus causes rapid cardiac arrest and death and over half the cases are undiagnosed except at autopsy.[29] Similarly, small pulmonary emboli may be completely asymptomatic but often precede more significant, or lethal, embolism. For patients with intermediate-sized emboli, a combination of pleuritic chest pain, dyspnoea and tachypnoea is a highly sensitive indicator of pulmonary embolus.[30] Changes in the electrocardiogram following pulmonary embolus reflect disturbed right-sided cardiac function secondary to elevated pulmonary arterial pressure and are generally non-specific. Ischaemic changes, particularly T-wave inversion in the anterior leads, do correlate with the severity of the embolism.[31] The gold standard of diagnosis is pulmonary angiography, though this is not feasible in many hospitals. More use is made of pulmonary radioisotope perfusion or ventilation/perfusion scans,[31] but several investigations have demonstrated the relatively low sensitivity of the technique.[32] Data acquisition for computed tomography (CT) scanning is now fast enough to enable imaging of thoracic vascular structures,[33] and this is now regarded as the investigation of choice for diagnosis of pulmonary thromboembolism (Figure 29.5).

Pathophysiology.[27,28,34] Three mechanisms give rise to the physiological changes seen in pulmonary embolism. First is physical occlusion of the pulmonary vascular system. Second, platelet activation within the thrombus leads to release of 5-hydroxytryptamine (5HT, serotonin) and thromboxane A_2, causing a further increase in pulmonary vascular resistance. Finally, the right ventricle commonly is unable to overcome the raised pulmonary vascular resistance and cardiac output falls, eventually culminating in right heart failure.[28]

The primary respiratory lesion is an increase in alveolar dead space with an increased arterial/end-tidal

a **b**

Figure 29.5 Spiral CT scan of pulmonary thomboemboli. Intravenous contrast injected immediately before scanning makes the blood vessels appear white. Emboli then appear as darker areas within the blood vessel lumen. **(a)** Saddle embolus (SE) situated mainly in the right pulmonary artery (RPA). **(b)** Pulmonary embolus in the basal branch of the left pulmonary artery (LPA). AA, ascending aorta; DA, descending aorta. (I am indebted to Celia Craven, Superintendent Radiographer, St James's Hospital, Leeds, for supplying the scans.)

$P\text{CO}_2$ gradient. Carbon dioxide elimination is therefore reduced and if ventilation remains unchanged, arterial $P\text{CO}_2$ slowly climbs, until elimination is restored in spite of the large dead space.[35] However, in awake patients hypercapnia is unusual because hyperventilation is almost always present and arterial $P\text{CO}_2$ is usually below the normal range.[34] The cause of respiratory stimulation is unclear but may involve stimulation of J-receptors as in air embolism (see below) or hypoxia, if present.

Arterial $P\text{O}_2$ is also decreased. This results from derangement of normal ventilation/perfusion relationships. Initially, although cardiac output remains normal, partial obstruction of the pulmonary circulation results in excessive blood flow to those lung regions that are still perfused, giving a low ventilation/perfusion ratio in these areas. When cardiac output begins to decrease as a result of a failing right ventricle, pulmonary perfusion will fall below normal levels and low mixed venous oxygen content will exacerbate the abnormal ventilation/perfusion relationships (page 124).[34,38] Elevated right atrial pressures, as a consequence of pulmonary hypertension, may cause right-to-left intracardiac shunting[28] through an unsuspected patent foramen ovale (page 201).

Bronchospasm is a well-recognised complication[36] and has been attributed to the 5HT released from platelets and also to local hypocapnia in the part of the lung without effective pulmonary circulation. Pulmonary compliance may be reduced with large pulmonary emboli, but the mechanism of this change is unknown. Pulmonary infarction, which might be expected to occur, is rarely a problem. The lung can obtain oxygen directly from air within the airways and alveoli, from backflow along pulmonary veins and from the bronchial circulation. Only when these sources are also impaired does infarction occur, for example when localised pulmonary oedema or pulmonary haemorrhage into the airways occurs in conjunction with embolism.

***Principles of therapy.*[27]** Anticoagulation with intravenous heparin is the mainstay of treatment and prevents further clot from forming, either in lung or elsewhere, and allows endogenous fibrinolysis to proceed. In more severe cases, such as patients with cardiovascular compromise, thrombolysis via a pulmonary artery catheter may be required. In the past, thrombolytic regimens were associated with high complication rates but modern treatment is much improved and believed to be underutilised in many hospitals.[37] Surgical embolectomy is now reserved for patients with significant pulmonary embolism who are unable to receive or are unresponsive to other forms of treatment.

Air embolism

An embolus may arise from pneumothorax or pulmonary barotrauma but is most commonly iatrogenic. In neurosurgery, the usual cause of air embolism is the use of the sitting position for posterior fossa surgery. A subatmospheric venous pressure at the operative site allows air to enter dural veins, which are held open by their structure. In open cardiac surgery, it is almost impossible to remove all traces of air from the cardiac chambers before closing the heart. Some small degree of air embolism is almost inevitable in all types of intravenous therapy, but catastrophic air embolism can occur when compression bags are used to accelerate the flow rate of intravenous fluids, or blood bags that accidentally already contain air.

Detection of air embolism. Early diagnosis of air embolism is essential in neurosurgery and there are three principal methods in routine use. Bubbles in circulating blood give a very characteristic sound with a precordial Doppler probe. The method is, if anything, too sensitive, because a shower of very small bubbles produces a particularly large signal. The simplest method is based on the end-expired CO_2 concentration, which is easily measured from capnography. Many factors influence the end-expiratory concentration (page 157), but a sudden decrease is likely to be either cardiac arrest or air embolism. Transoesophageal echocardiography is an efficient method of detecting air embolism[38] and, furthermore, it is the only practicable method of detecting paradoxical air embolism (see below).

Pathophysiology of air embolus. Provided there is no major intracardiac right-to-left shunt, small quantities of air are filtered out by the lungs where they are gradually excreted and no harm results. Alveolar dead space is increased according to the proportion of the pulmonary circulation that is occluded. The resultant increase in arterial/end-expiratory PCO_2 gradient is the basis of detection of air embolism by capnography as described above. Pulmonary arterial pressure is increased by a large embolus due to the right ventricle working against an increased pulmonary vascular resistance. Finally, in animal studies, airway resistance is increased following air embolism, an effect mediated by arachidonic acid metabolites, possibly in conjunction with platelet activation and stimulation of pulmonary irritant receptors.[39]

Massive air embolism (probably in excess of 100 ml) may cause cardiac arrest by accumulation in the right ventricle, where compression of the air bubble prevents ventricular ejection of blood. Treatment then requires aspiration of air through a cardiac catheter, which is difficult. In lesser degrees of embolisation during surgery, reduced cardiac output probably also contributes to the sudden reduction in end-expiratory PCO_2.

Paradoxical air embolism. Rarely, there may be passage of air emboli from the right to the left heart without there being an overt right-to-left shunt. This is important because air then enters the systemic arterial circulation where there may be embolism and infarction, particularly of the brain. It is possible to pass a probe through such a foramen ovale in over 25% of the adult population (page 201), but paradoxical embolism does not usually occur because pressure is slightly higher in the left atrium than the right. However, under many circumstances, such as following pulmonary embolism,

right atrial pressure may be elevated to the point where a right-to-left shunt occurs.

The role of paradoxical embolism in neurological damage in divers is described on page 273.

Fat embolism[40]

Fracture of long bones or major orthopaedic surgery may be associated with fat embolism.[41] This term is not strictly correct, as the features of 'fat embolism syndrome' result from release of bone marrow microemboli. Some degree of fat embolism occurs in almost all patients having hip and knee replacement surgery, but clinical sequelae occur in less than 1% of these.

Microscopic intravascular bone marrow fragments promote intravascular coagulation and platelet adherence, particularly under the conditions of venous stasis present during surgery, and so develop into larger 'mixed' emboli. There is initially an increase in physiological dead space but this is soon accompanied by an increase in shunt. Release of inflammatory mediators in the lung causes bronchospasm, increases capillary permeability leading to localised pulmonary oedema,[41] and may open anastomotic channels between pulmonary artery and vein.[42]

Lipid seems to pass through the pulmonary circulation to invade the systemic circulation. Surface forces between blood and lipid are much less than between blood and air and so would not offer the same hindrance to passage through the lungs. In the systemic circulation, fat emboli cause characteristic petechiae in the anterior axillary folds and there is often evidence of cerebral involvement.[40]

Amniotic fluid embolism[43,44]

Amniotic fluid embolism occurs rarely during delivery, but is fatal in over half of cases. Death normally results from cardiovascular disturbances and haemorrhage secondary to coagulopathy. Pulmonary vascular resistance is increased but animal studies indicate that pulmonary hypertension is only transient, returning to normal after just a few minutes. The reasons for this effect on the pulmonary circulation remain unclear. Amniotic fluid and foetal cells in the circulation may cause no cardiovascular changes, and either an immune-mediated response or the release of vasoactive mediators such as endothelin (page 99) has been suggested as the mechanism causing the clinical syndrome.

PULMONARY HYPERTENSION

There are many causes of pulmonary hypertension, which are classified as either primary or secondary (Table

Table 29.1 Causes of pulmonary hypertension

| Primary | Secondary | | |
	Respiratory	Cardiac	Other
Primary pulmonary hypertension Hepatopulmonary syndrome	COPD Emphysema Pulmonary fibrosis Cystic fibrosis Chronic embolism	Left heart failure Valvular disease Congenital disease	Sleep apnoea Lupus Scleroderma Rheumatoid arthritis HIV infection Vasculitis

29.1). The latter is much more common and is therefore considered first.

Secondary pulmonary hypertension[45]

Respiratory disease. Pulmonary vascular resistance is increased by almost any pulmonary disease that results in chronic hypoxia (see Table 29.1). Similar changes occur with intermittent hypoxia caused, for example, by sleep apnoea (see Chapter 16). The change is initially temporary and reversible but progresses to become permanent. Nitric oxide (NO) production by pulmonary endothelium contributes to the normal low resistance of the pulmonary circulation (page 101). Hypoxia has been shown to reduce this basal NO secretion,[46] and further work has identified reduced production of constitutive nitric oxide synthase as the mechanism.[47]

Cardiac disease. Valvular disease of the left heart leads to an elevation of pressure in the left atrium and pulmonary veins. Increases in pulmonary capillary pressure from this cause tend to be long term and lead to remodelling of the pulmonary circulation. Smooth muscle hypertrophy and fibrosis of the pulmonary vasculature cause pulmonary arterial hypertension and, eventually, right heart failure (cor pulmonale).[4,10] A low cardiac output, from either the original valvular heart disease or the resulting right heart failure, results in reduction of mixed venous P_{O_2}, which then causes further increases in pulmonary vascular resistance.

Treatment should first be directed towards improving the underlying condition, particularly if this is causing chronic or intermittent hypoxia. The long-term administration of oxygen to such patients, during the day and during sleep, retards the development of pulmonary hypertension, partially reverses established hypertension and improves survival.[48] Vasodilator therapy is complicated by the lack of drugs with specific action on the pulmonary circulation and is discussed below.

Primary pulmonary hypertension[49,50]

Pulmonary hypertension occurring in the absence of hypoxia is termed primary pulmonary hypertension (PPH) and has a prevalence of approximately 1300 per million. It is a progressive disease, which normally presents in early adulthood with worsening shortness of breath and eventually right heart failure. There is a familial contribution to PPH and it may rarely be associated with advanced liver disease or the use of some older appetite-suppressant drugs. Prognosis is poor, with most patients dying within a few years of diagnosis.

Pathophysiology. The disease is characterised by proliferation of endothelial cells, hypertrophy of pulmonary arterial smooth muscle, and by thrombosis within pulmonary vessels.[51] Abnormal endothelial function is believed to be where the primary defect occurs and nitric oxide-related functions are abnormal. The defect seems to arise in communication between endothelial and smooth muscle cells, though this has yet to be fully characterised.[52]

Treatment.[53–55] The only truly specific pulmonary vasodilator drugs are acetylcholine (infused into the pulmonary artery) and nitric oxide (by inhalation), but both require continuous administration. Prostacyclin is a pulmonary vasodilator (page 99) and, despite needing to be administered by continuous intravenous infusion, has been used successfully to treat PPH. Recent potential oral drug therapies for PPH have focused on endothelin receptor antagonists (page 104).[56]

PPH remains a common indication for lung transplantation (see Chapter 33).

REFERENCES

1. DeFouw DO. Ultrastructural features of alveolar epithelial transport. *Am Rev Respir Dis* 1983; **127** (Supp 5): S9–S13.

2. Bhattacharya J. The alveolar water gate. *Am J Physiol Lung Cell Mol Physiol* 2004; **286**: L257–8.

*3. Matthay MA, Folkesson HG, Clerici C. Lung epithelial fluid transport and the resolution of pulmonary edema. *Physiol Rev* 2002; **82**: 569–600.

*4. Gehlbach BK, Geppert E. The pulmonary manifestations of left heart failure. *Chest* 2004; **125**: 669–82.

5. Lai-Fook SJ. Mechanical factors in lung liquid distribution. *Annu Rev Physiol* 1993; **55**: 155–79.

6. Staub NA. Pathophysiology of pulmonary oedema. In: Staub NA, Taylor AE, eds. *Edema*. New York: Raven Press, 1984.

7. Bhattacharya J, Gropper MA, Staub NA. Interstitial fluid pressure gradient measured by micropuncture in excised dog lung. *J Appl Physiol* 1984; **56**: 271–7.

8. Miserocchi G, Negrini D, Gonano C. Direct measurement of interstitial pulmonary pressure in in situ lung with intact pleural space. *J Appl Physiol* 1990; **69**: 2168–74.

9. Bhattacharya J. The microphysiology of lung liquid clearance. *Adv Exp Med Biol* 1995; **381**: 95–108.

10. Drake RE, Doursout MF. Pulmonary edema and elevated left atrial pressure: four hours and beyond. *News Physiol Sci* 2002; **17**: 223–6.

11. Negrini D, Passi A, De Luca G, Miserocchi G. Pulmonary interstitial pressure and proteoglycans during development of pulmonary oedema. *Am J Physiol* 1996; **270**: H2000–7.

12. Matthay MA, Clerici C, Saumon G. Active fluid clearance from the distal air spaces of the lung. *J Appl Physiol* 2002; **93**: 1533–41.

13. Sznajder JI, Factor P, Ingbar DH. Lung edema clearance: role of Na^+-K^+-ATPase. *J Appl Physiol* 2002; **93**: 1860–6.

*14. Crandall ED, Matthay MA. Alveolar epithelial transport. Basic science to clinical medicine. *Am J Respir Crit Care Med* 2001; **162**: 1021–9.

15. Schumacker PT. Pulmonary edema, shunt and blood flow distribution. *Intens Care Med* 1993; **19**: 183–4.

16. Tsukimoto K, Mathieu-Costello O, Prediletto R, Elliott AR, West JB. Ultrastructural appearances of pulmonary capillaries at high transmural pressures. *J Appl Physiol* 1991; **71**: 573–82.

17. Smith WS, Matthay MA. Evidence for a hydrostatic mechanism in human neurogenic pulmonary edema. *Chest* 1997; **111**: 1326–33.

18. Pavlin DJ, Nessly ML, Cheney FW. Increased pulmonary vascular permeability as a cause of re-expansion edema in rabbits. *Am Rev Respir Dis* 1981; **124**: 422–7.

19. Sherman SC. Reexpansion pulmonary edema: a case report and review of the current literature. *J Emerg Med* 2003; **24**: 23–7.

20. Gee MH, Williams DO. Effect of lung inflation on perivascular cuff fluid volume in isolated dog lung lobes. *Microvasc Res* 1979; **17**: 192–6.

21. Paré PD, Warriner B, Baile EM, Hogg JC. Redistribution of pulmonary extravascular water with positive end-expiratory pressure in canine pulmonary edema. *Am Rev Respir Dis* 1983; **127**: 590–3.

22. Mondéjar EF, Mata GV, Càrdenas A, Mansilla A, Cantalejo F, Rivera R. Ventilation with positive end-expiratory pressure reduces extravascular lung water and increases lymphatic flow in hydrostatic pulmonary oedema. *Crit Care Med* 1996; **24**: 1562–7.

23. Cope DK, Grimbert F, Downey JM, Taylor AE. Pulmonary capillary pressure: a review. *Crit Care Med* 1992; **20**: 1043–56.

24. Baconnier PF, Eberhard A, Grimbert FA. Theoretical analysis of occlusion techniques for measuring pulmonary capillary pressure. *J Appl Physiol* 1992; **73**: 1351–9.

25. Jones JG, Royston D, Minty BD. Changes in alveolar-capillary barrier function in animals and humans. *Am Rev Respir Dis* 1983; **127**(Supp 5): S51–S59.

26. Godje O, Peyerl M, Seebauer T, Dewald O, Reichart B. Reproducibility of double indicator dilution measurements of intrathoracic blood volume compartments, extravascular lung water and liver function. *Chest* 1998; **113**: 1070–7.

27. Goldhaber SZ. Pulmonary embolism. *N Engl J Med* 1998; **339**: 93–104.

*28. Goldhaber SZ, Elliott CG. Acute pulmonary embolism. Part I. Epidemiology, pathophysiology and diagnosis. *Circulation* 2003; **108**: 2726–9.

29. Ryu JH, Olson EJ, Pellikka PA. Clinical recognition of pulmonary embolism: problem of unrecognized and asymptomatic cases. *Mayo Clin Proc* 1998; **73**: 873–9.

30. Stein PD, Terrin ML, Hales CA, *et al.* Clinical, laboratory, roentgenographic and electrocardiographic findings in patients with acute pulmonary embolism and no pre-existing cardiac or pulmonary disease. *Chest* 1991; **100**: 598–603.

31. Bone RC. Ventilation/perfusion scan in pulmonary embolism. *JAMA* 1990; **263**: 2794–5.

32. PIOPED Investigators. Value of the ventilation/perfusion scan in acute pulmonary embolism: results of the Prospective Investigation of Pulmonary Embolism Diagnosis (PIOPED). *JAMA* 1990; **263**: 2753–9.

33. Hansell DM, Flower CDR. Imaging pulmonary embolism. *Br Med J* 1998; **316**: 490–1.

34. Santolicandro A, Prediletto R, Fornai E, *et al.* Mechanisms of hypoxemia and hypocapnia in pulmonary embolism. *Am J Respir Crit Care Med* 1995; **152**: 336–47.

35. Breen PH, Mazumdar B, Skinner SC. How does experimental pulmonary embolism decrease CO_2 elimination? *Respir Physiol* 1996; **105**: 217–24.

36. Windebank WJ, Boyd G, Moran F. Pulmonary thromboembolism presenting as asthma. *Br Med J* 1973; **1**: 90–4.

37. Goldhaber SZ. Contemporary pulmonary embolism thrombolysis. *Chest* 1995; **107**: 45S–51S.

38. Furuya H, Okumura F. Detection of paradoxical air embolism by transesophageal echocardiography. *Anesthesiology* 1984; **60**: 374–7.

39. Chen HF, Lee BP, Kou YR. Mechanisms underlying stimulation of rapidly adapting receptors during pulmonary air embolism in dogs. *Respir Physiol* 1997; **109**: 1–13.

40. Mellor A, Soni N. Fat embolism. *Anaesthesia* 2001; **56**: 145–54.

41. Hofmann S, Huemer G, Salzer M. Pathophysiology and management of the fat embolism syndrome. *Anaesthesia* 1998; **53** (Supp 2): 35–7.

42. Prys-Roberts C, Greenbaum R, Nunn JF, Kelman GR. Disturbances of pulmonary function in patients with fat embolism. *J Clin Pathol* 1970; **23** (Supp 4): 143–9.

43. McDougall RJ, Duke GJ. Amniotic fluid embolism syndrome: case report and review. *Anaesth Intens Care* 1995; **23**: 735–40.

44. Davies S. Amniotic fluid embolus: a review of the literature. *Can J Anaesth* 2001; **48**: 88–98.

45. Higenbottam T, Cremona G. Acute and chronic hypoxic pulmonary hypertension. *Eur Respir J* 1993; **6**: 1207–12.

46. Adnot S, Raffestin B. Pulmonary hypertension: NO therapy? *Thorax* 1996; **51**: 762–4.

47. McQuillan L, Leung G, Marsden P, Kostyk S, Kourembanas S. Hypoxia inhibits expression of NOS via transcriptional and posttranscriptional mechanisms. *Am J Physiol* 1994; **36**: H1921–7.

48. Flenley DC. Long-term home oxygen therapy. *Chest* 1985; **87**: 99–102.

49. Rubin LJ. Primary pulmonary hypertension. *N Engl J Med* 1997; **336**: 111–17.

50. Gaine SP, Rubin LJ. Primary pulmonary hypertension. *Lancet* 1998; **352**: 719–25.

51. Rich S. Clinical insights into the pathogenesis of primary pulmonary hypertension. *Chest* 1998; **114**: 237S–241S.

*52. Budhiraja R, Tuder RM, Hassoun PM. Endothelial dysfunction in pulmonary hypertension. *Circulation* 2004; **109**: 159–65.

53. Hoeper MM, Galiè N, Simonneau G, Rubin LJ. New treatments for pulmonary arterial hypertension. *Am J Respir Crit Care Med* 2002; **165**: 1209–16.

54. Peacock AJ. Treatment of pulmonary hypertension. *Br Med J* 2003; **326** 835–6.

55. Newman JH. Treatment of primary pulmonary hypertension – the next generation. *N Engl J Med* 2002; **346**: 933–5.

56. Wilkins MR. Selective or nonselective endothelin receptor blockade in pulmonary arterial hypertension. *Am J Respir Crit Care Med* 2004; **169**: 433–6.

30 Parenchymal lung disease

KEY POINTS

- ▪ Lung collapse occurs either from compression of lung tissue or by absorption of gas from lung units with occluded, or severely narrowed, airways.
- ▪ Many forms of interstitial lung disease exist, varying from purely inflammatory conditions (alveolitis) to conditions involving progressive fibrosis with minimal lung inflammation.
- ▪ Lung fibrosis arises from an imbalance between the cellular systems responsible for inflammation and tissue repair.

PULMONARY COLLAPSE

Pulmonary collapse may be defined as an acquired state in which the lungs or part of the lungs become airless. Atelectasis is strictly defined as a state in which the lungs of a newborn have never been expanded, but the term is widely used as a synonym for pulmonary collapse.

Collapse may be caused by two different mechanisms. The first of these is loss of the forces opposing the elastic recoil of the lung, which then decreases in volume to the point at which airways are closed and gas is trapped behind the closed airways. The second is obstruction of airways at normal lung volume, which may be due to many different causes. This also results in trapping of gas behind the obstructed airway. Whatever the cause of the airway closure, there is rapid absorption of the trapped gas because the total partial pressure of gases in mixed venous blood is always less than atmospheric (see Table 26.2). This generates a subatmospheric pressure more than sufficient to overcome any force tending to hold the lung expanded.

Pulmonary collapse during anaesthesia is described in Chapter 22.

Loss of forces opposing retraction of the lung

The lungs are normally prevented from collapse by the outward elastic recoil of the ribcage and any resting tone of the diaphragm. The pleural cavity normally contains no gas but if a small bubble of gas is introduced, its pressure is subatmospheric (see Figure 3.4). Pulmonary collapse due to loss of forces opposing lung retraction may be considered under five headings as follows.

Voluntary reduction of lung volume. It seems unlikely that voluntary reduction of lung volume below closing capacity would cause overt collapse of lung in a subject breathing air. However, in older subjects, there is an increase in the alveolar/arterial PO_2 gradient, suggesting trapping of alveolar gas (see Figure 22.11). If the subject has been breathing 100% oxygen, absorption collapse may follow reduction of lung volume (see below).

Excessive external pressure. Ventilatory failure is the more prominent aspect of an external environmental pressure in excess of about 6 kPa (60 cmH₂O), which is not communicated to the airways (page 368). However, some degree of pulmonary collapse could also occur and this is a normal consequence of the great depths attained by diving mammals while breath holding. An approximately normal lung volume is maintained during conventional diving operations when respired gas is maintained at the surrounding water pressure, though this does not occur with surface diving or snorkelling (page 268).

Loss of integrity of the ribcage. Multiple rib fractures or the old operation of thoracoplasty may impair the elastic recoil of the ribcage to the point at which partial lung collapse results. This depends entirely on the extent of the injury to the ribcage, but multiple adjacent ribs fractured in two places will usually result in collapse. However, extensive trauma to the ribcage also causes interference with the mechanics of breathing, which is generally more serious than collapse (page 368).

Intrusion of abdominal contents into the chest. Extensive atelectasis results from a congenital defect of the diaphragm. Abdominal contents may completely fill one-half of the chest, with total atelectasis of that lung. In adults, similar changes may occur with a large hiatus hernia. Paralysis of one side of the diaphragm causes the diaphragm to lie higher in the chest, with a tendency to basal collapse on that side. An extensive abdominal mass (e.g. tumour or ascites) may force the diaphragm into the chest.

Space occupation of the pleural cavity. Air introduced into the pleural cavity reduces the forces opposing retraction of the lung and this is a potent cause of collapse. A closed pneumothorax is a fixed volume of air in the pleural cavity causing collapse in relation to the volume of air introduced. The intrapleural pressure rises in proportion to the volume of air in the cavity and in a tension pneumothorax is above atmospheric. The affected lung is then totally collapsed and the mediastinum is displaced towards the opposite side. This is a life-threatening condition requiring immediate relief of the pressure. An open pneumothorax communicates with the atmosphere and results in pendulum breathing in addition to collapse. The pleural cavity may also be occupied by an effusion, empyema or haemothorax, all of which may result in collapse.

Absorption of trapped gas

Absorption of alveolar gas trapped beyond obstructed airways may be the consequence of reduction in lung volume by the mechanisms described above. However, it is the primary cause of collapse when there is total or partial airway obstruction at normal lung volume. Obstruction is commonly due to secretions, pus, blood or tumour but may be due to intense local bronchospasm or mucosal oedema.

Gas trapped beyond the point of airway closure is absorbed by the pulmonary blood flow. The total of the partial pressures of the gases in mixed venous blood is always less than atmospheric (see Table 26.2), although pressure gradients for the individual component gases between alveolar gas and mixed venous blood may be quite different.

The effect of respired gases. If the patient has been breathing 100% oxygen prior to obstruction, the alveoli will contain only oxygen, carbon dioxide and water vapour. Because the last two together normally amount to less than 13.3 kPa (100 mmHg), the alveolar PO_2 will usually be in excess of 88 kPa (660 mmHg). However, the PO_2 of the mixed venous blood is unlikely to exceed about 6.7 kPa (50 mmHg), so the alveolar/mixed venous

PO_2 gradient will be of the order of 80% of an atmosphere. Absorption collapse will thus be rapid and there will be no nitrogen in the alveolar gas to maintain inflation. This has important implications during anaesthesia, when 100% oxygen is commonly administered (page 305).

The situation is much more favourable in a patient who has been breathing air, as most of the alveolar gas is then nitrogen, which is at a tension only about 0.5 kPa (4 mmHg) below that of mixed venous blood.[1] Alveolar nitrogen tension rises above that of mixed venous blood as oxygen is absorbed and eventually the nitrogen will be fully absorbed. Collapse must eventually occur but the process is much slower than in the patient who has been breathing oxygen. Figure 30.1 shows a computer simulation of the time required for collapse with various gas mixtures.[2] Nitrous oxide/oxygen mixtures may be expected to be absorbed almost as rapidly as 100% oxygen. This is partly because nitrous oxide is much more soluble in blood than nitrogen and partly because the mixed venous tension of nitrous oxide is usually much less than the alveolar tension, except after a long period of inhalation.

When the inspired gas composition is changed *after* obstruction and trapping occur, complex patterns of absorption may ensue. The inhalation of nitrous oxide, after airway occlusion has occurred while breathing air, results in temporary expansion of the trapped volume (see Figure 30.1). This is caused by large volumes of the more soluble nitrous oxide passing from blood to alveolus in exchange for smaller volumes of the less soluble nitrogen passing in the reverse direction. This phenomenon also applies to any closed airspace in the body, such as closed pneumothorax, gas emboli, bowel, and the middle ear with a blocked pharyngotympanic (Eustachian) tube. It is potentially dangerous and may contraindicate the use of nitrous oxide as an anaesthetic.

Magnitude of the pressure gradients. It needs to be stressed that the forces generated by the absorption of trapped gases are very large. The total partial pressure of gases in mixed venous blood is normally 87.3 kPa (655 mmHg). The corresponding pressure of the alveolar gases is 95.1 kPa (713 mmHg), allowing for water vapour pressure at 37°C. The difference, 7.8 kPa (58 mmHg or 78 cmH$_2$O), is sufficient to overcome any forces opposing recoil of the lung. Absorption collapse after breathing air may therefore result in drawing the diaphragm up into the chest, reducing ribcage volume or displacing the mediastinum. If the patient has been breathing oxygen, the total partial pressure of gases in the mixed venous blood is barely a tenth of an atmosphere (see Table 26.2) and absorption of trapped alveolar gas generates enormous forces.

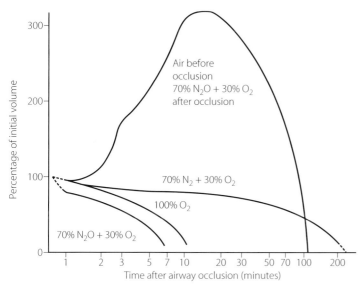

Figure 30.1 Predicted rates of absorption from alveoli of differing gas mixtures. The lower curves show the rate of absorption of the contents of sections of the lung whose air passages are obstructed, resulting in sequestration of the contents. The upper curve shows the expansion of the sequestered gas when nitrous oxide is breathed by a patient who has recently developed regional airway obstruction while breathing air. In all other cases, it is assumed that the inspired gas is not changed after obstruction has occurred. Similar considerations apply to closed gas cavities elsewhere in the body. (Reproduced from reference 2 by permission of the authors and the Editor of *Anaesthesia*.)

Effect of reduced ventilation/perfusion ratio. Absorption collapse may still occur in the absence of total airway obstruction provided that the ventilation/perfusion ($\dot{V}/\dot{Q}$) ratio is sufficiently reduced. Older subjects, as well as those with a pathological increase in scatter of $\dot{V}/\dot{Q}$ ratios, may have substantial perfusion of areas of lung with $\dot{V}/\dot{Q}$ ratios in the range 0.01–0.1. This shows as a characteristic 'shelf' in the plot of perfusion against $\dot{V}/\dot{Q}$ (Figure 30.2). These grossly hypoventilated areas are liable to collapse if the patient breathes oxygen (Figure 30.2b). If the $\dot{V}/\dot{Q}$ ratio is less than 0.05, ventilation even with 100% oxygen cannot supply the oxygen that is removed (assuming the normal arterial/mixed venous oxygen content difference of 0.05 ml.ml^{-1}). As the $\dot{V}/\dot{Q}$ ratio decreases below 0.05, so the critical inspired oxygen concentration necessary for collapse also decreases (Figure 30.2c). The flat part of the curve between $\dot{V}/\dot{Q}$ ratios of 0.001 and 0.004 means that small differences in inspired oxygen concentration in the range 20–30% may be very important in determining whether collapse occurs or not. There is no difficulty in demonstrating that pulmonary collapse may be induced in healthy middle-aged subjects breathing oxygen close to residual volume.[3,4]

Perfusion through the collapsed lung[7]

Perfusion through collapsed lung tissue is one of the most important causes of intrapulmonary shunting. At least in the short term, some perfusion continues through the collapsed area and this is regulated mainly by hypoxic pulmonary vasoconstriction. In the absence of alveolar gas, the P_{O_2} that governs pulmonary vascular resistance is the mixed venous P_{O_2} (page 101). It has

been observed that, in the presence of collapse, the shunt fraction of the pulmonary blood flow is directly proportional to the cardiac output (page 124), and this has been attributed to the effect of cardiac output on the mixed venous P_{O_2}. Thus, with a reduced cardiac output, the mixed venous P_{O_2} will be reduced and hypoxic pulmonary vasoconstriction in the area of the collapse will be increased. Therefore the shunt fraction will be decreased. However, the blood flowing through the shunt is more desaturated and these two effects counteract each other, so the arterial P_{O_2} is little changed (page 124).

Diagnosis of pulmonary collapse

The diagnosis may be made on physical signs of decreased air entry and chest dullness but reliance is usually placed on chest radiography. Pulmonary opacification is seen, along with indirect signs of thoracic volume loss such as displacement of interlobular fissures, raised diaphragms and displaced hilar or mediastinal structures.[8,9] In the upright position, collapse is commonest in the basal segments, often concealed behind the cardiac shadow unless the exposure is appropriate. Areas of atelectasis are clearly seen with CT (see Figure 22.10).

Collapse results in a reduction in pulmonary compliance, but the value of this in diagnosis is limited by the wide scatter of normal values. A sudden reduction in compliance may give an indication of collapse provided, of course, that control measurements were available before collapse.

Collapse also reduces the functional residual capacity and arterial P_{O_2}. However, in a patient with impaired

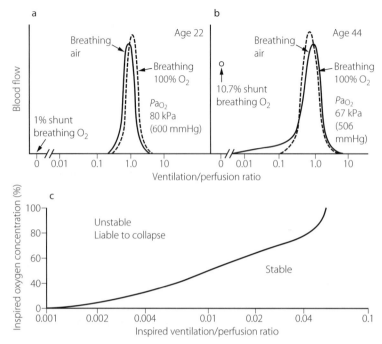

Figure 30.2 Inspiration of 100% oxygen causes collapse of alveoli with very low $\dot{V}/\dot{Q}$ ratios. **(a)** The minor change in the distribution of blood flow (in relation to $\dot{V}/\dot{Q}$ ratio) when a young subject breathes oxygen. Collapse is minimal and a shunt of 1% develops. **(b)** The changes in an older subject with a 'shelf' of blood flow distributed to alveoli with very low $\dot{V}/\dot{Q}$ ratios. Breathing oxygen causes collapse of these alveoli, and this is manifested by disappearance of the shelf and development of an intrapulmonary shunt of 10.7%. **(c)** The inspired oxygen concentration relative to the inspired $\dot{V}/\dot{Q}$ ratio that is critical for absorption collapse. (Reproduced with permission from Wagner PD, Laravuso RB, Uhl RR, West JB. Continuous distributions of ventilation–perfusion ratios in normal subjects breathing air and 100% O_2. *J Clin Invest* 1974; **54**: 54–68 and Dantzker DR, Wagner PD, West JB. Instability of lung units with low VA/Q ratios during O_2 breathing. *J Appl Physiol* 1975; **38**: 886–95.)

oxygenation a reduction in arterial P_{O_2} cannot distinguish between the three very common conditions of pulmonary collapse, consolidation and oedema.

Principles of therapy

Therapy depends on the physiological abnormality. Factors opposing the elastic recoil of the lung should be removed wherever possible. For example, pneumothorax, pleural effusion and ascites may be corrected. In other cases, particularly impaired integrity of the chest wall, it may be preferable to treat the patient with artificial ventilation. Reexpansion of collapsed lung often requires high pressures to be applied (page 306), but it is usually possible to restore normal lung volume.

When collapse is caused by regional airway obstruction, the most useful method in both treatment and prevention is chest physiotherapy, combined when necessary with tracheobronchial toilet through either a tracheal tube or a bronchoscope. Fibreoptic bronchoscopy alone will often clear an obstructed airway and permit reexpansion, particularly with lobar atelectasis.[10]

Voluntary maximal inspirations are effective in clearing areas of absorption collapse in subjects who had been breathing oxygen near residual volume.[4] This manoeuvre is the basis of the 'incentive spirometer', which is used to prevent postoperative lung collapse.

With artificial ventilation a logical approach is hyperinflation of the chest or an artificial 'sigh'. Some ventilators were designed to provide an intermittent 'sigh' but evidence of its efficacy was never found. Current strategies to prevent pulmonary collapse during artificial ventilation are described in Chapter 32.

PULMONARY CONSOLIDATION (PNEUMONIA)

Inflammation of areas of lung parenchyma, usually due to infection, can lead to the accumulation of exudate within the alveoli and small airways, causing consolidation. Areas of consolidation may be patchy, referred to as bronchopneumonia, or confined to discrete areas of the lung, forming lobar pneumonia. Pulmonary collapse frequently occurs in conjunction with pneumonia as a result of airway narrowing in surrounding lung areas.

Clinical features of pyrexia, cough, sputum production and dyspnoea occur with signs of consolidation such as bronchial breathing, chest dullness and inspiratory crackles, though physical signs may be absent in bronchopneumonia. Diagnosis again relies on chest radiography, where consolidation appears as pulmonary shadowing, sometimes accompanied by an 'air bronchogram'. With resolution of the infection, cough becomes more productive and the lung returns to normal within a few weeks.

Effects on gas exchange.[11] Patients with pneumonia are commonly hypoxic. Consolidated areas of lung behave in a similar fashion to collapse, forming an intrapulmonary shunt through which mixed venous blood flows. In addition, there is an increase in areas with low $\dot{V}/\dot{Q}$ ratios (<0.1), but the contribution of these areas to impaired oxygenation is believed to be small because of hypoxic pulmonary vasoconstriction. Administration of oxygen to patients with pneumonia causes a further widening of the scatter of $\dot{V}/\dot{Q}$ ratios, implying a reduction in hypoxic pulmonary vasoconstriction,[11] but nevertheless results in a considerable improvement in arterial P_{O_2}. In comparison with collapsed lung, consolidation is commonly associated with a worse pulmonary shunt and therefore more severe hypoxia. Many of the inflammatory mediators released as part of the response to infection act as local pulmonary vasodilators, in effect overriding hypoxic pulmonary vasoconstriction.[7]

Pathophysiology

Airway inflammation was described in detail in Chapter 28. Invasion of the lower respiratory tract with viruses and bacteria leads to further inflammatory changes characterised by migration of neutrophils from the circulation into the lung tissue. These cells, along with alveolar macrophages, provoke the production of an inflammatory exudate that leads to consolidation of the lung tissue. The exudate is a complex mixture of invading organisms, inflammatory cells (dead and alive), immunoglobulins and other immune mediators, fluid transudate from increased capillary permeability, and products resulting from destruction of lung tissue as a result of proteolytic enzyme release.

Margination of neutrophils. Before a neutrophil can contribute to the inflammatory response it must stick to the blood vessel wall (margination), migrate across the endothelium, interstitium and epithelium and become activated ready to contribute to pathogen removal (see Figure 31.3). These activities are controlled by an extensive and incompletely understood series of cytokines in a very similar fashion to airway inflammation (see Figure 28.1). Lymphocytes again play an important role, but in

parenchymal inflammation macrophages have an important control function instead of the eosinophils and mast cells involved in airway inflammation.

Neutrophil margination has been extensively studied in the systemic circulation. Selectins expressed on the surface of endothelial cells transiently bind the neutrophil, causing it to roll along the blood vessel wall. Eventually, different adhesion molecules on the endothelial cell (e.g. intercellular adhesion molecule-1, ICAM-1) bind to specific receptors on the neutrophil surface (e.g. β_2 integrins CD11/CD18), causing a more firm adhesion to the endothelium.[12] Once 'caught' by the endothelial cell, cytokines are released and neutrophil activation begins. The way in which neutrophils are marginated in the lung differs from elsewhere in the body.[13,14] Adhesion to endothelial cells occurs predominantly in the pulmonary capillary, rather than in venules as in the systemic circulation. Adhesion to the capillary wall can occur by either a CD11/CD18-dependent mechanism or by another mechanism that seems to be independent of all the adhesion molecules normally required for margination in a systemic vessel.[15] Selectin-induced rolling of neutrophils may not occur. Adhesion is facilitated by a slow transit time for neutrophils across pulmonary capillaries. Human neutrophils are of similar size to red blood cells but are much less deformable, so neutrophils take up to 120 seconds to traverse a pulmonary capillary compared to less than a second for a red blood cell.[13] Inflammatory mediators may cause changes to the biomechanical properties of neutrophils, in particular a stiffening of the cell that will further impede its movement through the pulmonary capillary.[16]

Once adhered to the pulmonary capillary wall, neutrophils may become flattened, leaving some capillary lumen available for blood flow. In this position, emigration into the pulmonary tissue begins and the neutrophil moves through small holes in the capillary basal laminae, possibly guided by fibroblasts in the interstitial space (Figure 30.3).[17]

INTERSTITIAL LUNG DISEASE AND PULMONARY FIBROSIS

Diffuse pulmonary inflammation occurs in a wide variety of conditions, which are summarised in Table 30.1. Pneumonitis may simply resolve, as in pneumonia, leaving no permanent damage, but with long-term inflammation varying degrees of pulmonary fibrosis develop.

Clinical features vary according to the aetiology. Pneumonitis alone (i.e. without fibrosis) may be asymptomatic at first, progressing to a cough and dyspnoea, and in severe cases giving rise to systemic symptoms such as

Figure 30.3 Neutrophil emigration in rabbit lung during streptococcal pneumonia. This electron micrograph shows that the neutrophils (N), which are normally the same diameter as a pulmonary capillary, are elongated, so leaving the capillary lumen (CL) partly patent. These neutrophils have already emigrated from the capillary lumen across the endothelium (En), and one is now passing into the interstitium (I) through a small hole in the capillary basement membrane (arrows). The pseudopod of the neutrophil is in close contact with fibroblasts (F), which may be guiding the neutrophil through the defect in the basement membrane. AL, alveolar lumen. (Figure kindly provided by Professor DC Walker. Reproduced with permission from Walker DC, Behzad AR, Chu F. Neutrophil migration through preexisting holes in the basal laminae of alveolar capillaries and epithelium during streptococcal pneumonia. *Microvasc Res* 1995; **50**: 397–416.)

fever. When accompanied by fibrosis, dyspnoea becomes worse and basal inspiratory crackles are present on examination. Lung function tests show a typical 'restrictive' pattern with similar reductions in both forced vital capacity and forced expiratory volume in one second (page 89). Diffuse reticular shadows develop on chest radiography and CT scanning of the lungs shows either 'ground glass' appearances, which correlate with pneumonitis, or 'honeycombing', which represents more advanced fibrosis.[12]

Causes of pulmonary fibrosis

These have been summarised in Table 30.1

Drug-induced fibrosis may follow lung injury induced by oxygen toxicity (page 354) precipitated by, for example,

bleomycin but for many drugs the mechanism is unknown.

Inorganic dusts.[20] Occupational exposure to asbestos fibres (asbestosis) or silica (silicosis) for many years leads to pulmonary fibrosis. Inhaled dust particles between 1 and 3 μm in diameter reach the alveoli and are ingested by macrophages.[21] Different dust types have variable persistence in the lung, some being rapidly cleared and others persisting within the pulmonary macrophage for many years. In addition, the total (lifetime) fibre burden probably correlates with the degree of resulting fibrosis.

Organic dusts may cause lung inflammation by an immune mechanism, a condition referred to as extrinsic allergic alveolitis. The allergen is normally derived from a fungus to which the patient has occupational exposure, giving rise to a host of disease names, such as farmer's lung, malt worker's lung etc. Bird fancier's lung differs in that it is precipitated by exposure to IgA derived from domestic birds. In extrinsic allergic alveolitis, pneumonitis results from activation of T-lymphocytes and IgG-mediated inflammation. If caught early enough and avoidance measures are taken, allergic alveolitis resolves completely, but with continued exposure fibrosis develops.

Systemic diseases that lead to fibrosis are numerous and the mechanisms obscure. Many of the diseases associated with lung fibrosis have an immunological basis. For example, sarcoidosis results from T-lymphocyte activation in response to an unknown stimulus, whereas many connective tissue diseases are known to have an autoimmune aetiology. These immune changes are therefore likely to cause activation of the pulmonary inflammatory cells described below.[21] Recurrent lung infections and some drugs used for treating systemic diseases may also contribute to the pulmonary complications seen.

Radiation lung damage[22] is seen following radiotherapy for tumours in or near the chest. Radiation pneumonitis develops over several weeks following radiotherapy, whereas fibrosis may take up to 2 years to develop. Cellular radiation damage occurs when cell division occurs, so susceptible cells in the lung are those with the greatest rate of turnover. Thus radiation injury begins with damage to type II pneumocytes and capillary endothelial cells, which results in altered surfactant and interstitial pulmonary oedema (page 391), respectively. A cascade of inflammatory cell activation will then follow.[23]

Idiopathic pulmonary fibrosis (IPF),[24] synonymous with cryptogenic fibrosing alveolitis (CFA), includes all cases of pulmonary fibrosis in which no cause can be found. It is the most common type of pulmonary fibrosis, occurs

Table 30.1 Causes of interstitial pneumonitis and pulmonary fibrosis[18,19]

Causes	Subgroups	Examples
Drug induced	Anticancer	Bleomycin, busulphan, cyclophosphamide, methotrexate
	Antibiotics	Isoniazid, nitrofurantoin, sulphonamides
	Others	Amiodarone
Dust	Inorganic	Silicosis
		Asbestosis
	Organic	Farmer's lung
Infections	Viral	Viral pneumonia
	Other	HIV
		Mycoplasma
		Opportunistic infections
Systemic disease	Connective tissue disease	Rheumatoid arthritis, scleroderma systemic lupus erythematosus, ankylosing spondylitis
	Others	Sarcoidosis, histiocytosis, uraemia
Miscellaneous	Acute inflammation	Acute lung injury
	Inhalation injury	Smoke, cadmium, sulphur dioxide
	Radiation lung damage	
	Cryptogenic fibrosing alveolitis	

more commonly in males and is of uncertain aetiology. Patients with CFA have extensive activation of pulmonary inflammatory cells and cytokines as described below. There is also accumulation of neutrophils and this indicates a role for pulmonary oxidant injury (page 353) in IPF. Whatever the cause, IPF is rapidly progressive with a median survival from diagnosis of just a few years.

Cellular mechanisms of pulmonary fibrosis[25,26]

Lung inflammation is described earlier in this chapter as well as in Chapters 28 and 31. Progression to pulmonary fibrosis is not inevitable, but predicting which patients and which underlying diseases do progress is important clinically. Male gender and smoking both indicate a worse prognosis from pulmonary fibrosis, as do increased numbers of inflammatory cells in bronchoalveolar lavage fluid.[12] These observations contributed to extensive research into the mechanisms of fibrosis, though a useful prognostic test remains a distant prospect.

Inflammation anywhere in the body is naturally succeeded by a cellular healing process that involves the laying down of new collagen. The lung is no exception and pulmonary fibrosis is a result of excessive deposition of collagen in the lung extracellular matrix.

In pulmonary fibrosis the initial disease process is diverse (see Table 30.1) and may cause changes in type I or type II alveolar epithelial cells, pulmonary macrophages, neutrophils or T-lymphocytes.[27] Interactions between these cells produce numerous cytokines, which amplify the inflammatory response and initiate cellular repair mechanisms. Once these repair mechanisms are established, apoptosis occurs in the inflammatory cells and tissue repair proceeds. Transforming growth factor-β (TGF-β) is believed to be the most important cytokine involved in stimulating tissue repair and probably acts as the final common pathway for most mechanisms leading to fibrosis.[28] Myofibroblasts are the cells responsible for repairing the extracellular matrix in lung tissue, this matrix forming the scaffolding on which new lung tissue is formed. Once myofibroblasts have completed their task, they too undergo apoptosis.

In most causes of pulmonary fibrosis this well-controlled sequence of events is abnormal. The activity of acute inflammatory cells may not subside once the stimulus has been removed and prolonged stimulation of repair mechanisms will occur. Alternatively, the normal mechanisms that terminate myofibroblast activity may be defective. A combination of inherited differences in the expression of cytokines or their receptors and the wide range of environmental stimuli described above is believed to result in pulmonary fibrosis. The intriguing possibility of abnormal apoptosis in lung cells has been suggested to explain pulmonary fibrosis.[29] Type I alveolar epithelial cells may undergo premature apoptosis and so prolong the inflammatory stimulus by continued exposure of underlying tissue. Alternatively, once tissue repair is complete, myofibroblasts may fail to respond to normal apoptotic stimuli and continue to remodel the extracellular matrix.

In a similar fashion to emphysema (page 380), excessive myofibroblast activity leads to a reduction in the amount of elastin present. Synthesis of elastin in normal lung is minimal in adults and though there is some evidence of increased production in pulmonary fibrosis, the elastic fibres formed are abnormal and probably non-functional.[30] Loss of elasticity by this mechanism causes collapse of both alveolar and small airway walls, leading to a reduction in compliance and the area available for gas exchange.

Principles of therapy[24]

Where feasible, removal of the stimulant for lung inflammation or fibrosis is vital. Although this may not halt the development of fibrosis, for example following irradiation, it may limit the degree of pulmonary damage that occurs. Very few patients with IPF gain any benefit from treatment with steroids and predicting who will respond is difficult. More specific immunosuppression of T-lymphocytes with ciclosporin provides some benefit.

Recent elucidation of the cytokines involved in pulmonary fibrosis, particularly TGF-β, has led to optimism about future therapeutic approaches.[28,31] Antibodies to TGF-β do attenuate fibrosis in experimental models, but there are considerable potential risks involved in non-specific inhibition of a fundamental inflammatory cytokine.[32]

REFERENCES

1. Klocke FJ, Rahn H. The arterial–alveolar inert gas ('N₂') difference in normal and emphysematous subjects, as indicated by the analysis of urine. *J Clin Invest* 1961; **40**: 286–94.
2. Webb SJS, Nunn JF. A comparison between the effect of nitrous oxide and nitrogen on arterial P_{O_2}. *Anaesthesia* 1967; **22**: 69–81.
3. Nunn JF, Coleman AJ, Sachithanandan T, Bergman NA, Laws JW. Hypoxaemia and atelectasis produced by forced expiration. *Br J Anaesth* 1965; **37**: 3–12.
4. Nunn JF, Williams IP, Jones JG, Hewlett AM, Hulands GH, Minty BD. Detection and reversal of pulmonary absorption collapse. *Br J Anaesth* 1978; **50**: 91–100.
5. Wagner PD, Laravuso RB, Uhl RR, West JB. Continuous distributions of ventilation-perfusion ratios in normal subjects breathing air and 100% O_2. *J Clin Invest* 1974; **54**: 54–68.
6. Dantzker DR, Wagner PD, West JB. Instability of lung units with low VA/Q ratios during O_2 breathing. *J Appl Physiol* 1975; **38**: 886–95.
7. Marshall BE, Hanson CW, Frasch F, Marshall C. Role of hypoxic pulmonary vasoconstriction in pulmonary gas exchange and blood flow distribution. 2. Pathophysiology. *Intens Care Med* 1994; **20**: 379–89.
8. Woodring JH, Reed JC. Types and mechanisms of pulmonary atelectasis. *J Thorac Imaging* 1996; **11**: 92–108.
9. Ashizawa K, Hayashi K, Aso N, Minami K. Lobar atelectasis: diagnostic pitfalls on chest radiography. *Br J Radiol* 2001; **74**: 89–97.
10. Kreider ME, Lipson DA. Bronchoscopy for atelectasis in the ICU. *Chest* 2003; **124**: 344–50.
11. Gea J, Roca J, Torres A, Agusti AGN, Wagner PD, Rodriguez-Roisin R. Mechanisms of abnormal gas exchange in patients with pneumonia. *Anesthesiology* 1991; **75**: 782–9.
12. Ward PA, Hunninghake GW. Lung inflammation and fibrosis. *Am J Respir Crit Care Med* 1998; **157**: S123–S129.
13. Hogg JC, Walker BA. Polymorphonuclear leucocyte traffic in lung inflammation. *Thorax* 1995; **50**: 819–20.
14. D'Ambrosio D, Mariani M, Panina-Bordignon P, Sinigaglia F. Chemokines and their receptors guiding T lymphocyte recruitment in lung inflammation. *Am J Respir Crit Care Med* 2001; **164**: 1266–75.
*15. Doerschuk CM, Tasaka S, Wang Q. CD11/CD18-dependent and -independent neutrophil emigration in the lungs. How do neutrophils know which route to take? *Am J Respir Cell Mol Biol* 2000; **23**: 133–6.
16. Doerschuk CM, Mizgerd JP, Kubo H, Qin L, Kumasaka T. Adhesion molecules and cellular biomechanical changes in acute lung injury. *Chest* 1999; **116**: 37S–43S.
17. Walker DC, Behzad AR, Chu F. Neutrophil migration through preexisting holes in the basal laminae of alveolar capillaries and epithelium during streptococcal pneumonia. *Microvasc Res* 1995; **50**: 397–416.
18. Egan JJ, Hasleton PS. Cryptogenic fibrosing alveolitis: diagnosis and treatment. *Hosp Med* 1998; **59**: 364–8.
19. Chan-Yeung M, Müller NL. Cryptogenic fibrosing alveolitis. *Lancet* 1997; **350**: 651–6.
20. Mossman BT, Churg A. Mechanisms in the pathogenesis of asbestosis and silicosis. *Am J Respir Crit Care Med* 1998; **157**: 1666–80.
21. Greenberger PA. Immunological aspects of lung diseases and cystic fibrosis. *JAMA* 1997; **278**: 1924–30.

22. Movsas B, Raffin TA, Epstein AH, Link CJ. Pulmonary radiation injury. *Chest* 1997; **111**: 1061–76.

23. Rubin P, Johnston CJ, Williams JP, McDonald S, Finkelstein JN. A perpetual cascade of cytokines postirradiation leads to pulmonary fibrosis. *Int J Radiat Oncol Biol Phys* 1995; **33**: 99–109.

24. Gross TJ, Hunninghake GW. Idiopathic pulmonary fibrosis. *N Engl J Med* 2001; **345**: 517–25.

*25. Thannickal VJ, Toews GB, White ES, Lynch JP, Martinez FJ. Mechanisms of pulmonary fibrosis. *Annu Rev Med* 2004; **55**: 395–417.

26. Chapman HA. Disorders of lung matrix remodelling. *J Clin Invest* 2004; **113**: 148–57.

27. Kumar RK, Lykke AWJ. Messages and handshakes: cellular interactions in pulmonary fibrosis. *Pathology* 1995; **27**: 18–26.

28. Bartram U, Speer CP. The role of transforming growth factor β in lung development and disease. *Chest* 2004; **125**: 754–65.

*29. Uhal BD. Apoptosis in lung fibrosis and repair. *Chest* 2002; **122**: 293S–298S.

30. Pierce RA, Mariani TJ, Senior RM. Elastin in lung development and disease. *Ciba Found Symp* 1995; **192**: 199–214.

31. Phan SH. New strategies for treatment of pulmonary fibrosis. *Thorax* 1995; **50**: 415–21.

32. Shull MM, Ormsby I, Kier AB, *et al*. Targeted disruption of the mouse transforming growth factor-β1 gene results in multifocal inflammatory disease. *Nature* 1992; **359**: 693–9.

31 Acute lung injury

KEY POINTS

- Acute lung injury is lung inflammation that develops in response to a variety of both pulmonary and generalised acute diseases.
- The clinical features of acute lung injury vary from mild, self-limiting dyspnoea to rapidly progressive and fatal respiratory failure.
- Widespread pulmonary inflammation causes increased permeability of the alveolar capillary membrane, leading to flooding and collapse of alveoli and severely impaired gas exchange.
- Artificial ventilation in severe acute lung injury is challenging, though a 'protective ventilation' strategy using small tidal volumes and moderate levels of positive end-expiratory pressure may be beneficial.

Acute lung injury has features in common with several of the pulmonary diseases described in the preceding four chapters, but is considered separately here. The topic has been reviewed often in recent years.[1-3]

Terminology. Acute lung injury (ALI) describes a characteristic form of parenchymal lung disease and represents a wide range of severity, from short-lived dyspnoea to a rapidly terminal failure of the respiratory system, when the term acute respiratory distress syndrome (ARDS) is normally used. The syndrome was first described in 1967 when Ashbaugh *et al.*[4] reported a condition in adults that seemed similar to the respiratory distress syndrome in infants. Later the same group introduced the term 'adult respiratory distress syndrome'.[5] One of the subjects reported in 1967 was aged only 11 years, and in recognition of the fact that respiratory distress syndrome is known to occur in children, the current recommended term is *acute* respiratory distress syndrome.[6] There are a great many other synonyms for ARDS, including acute respiratory failure, shock lung, respirator lung, pump lung and Da Nang lung.

CLINICAL ASPECTS OF ALI AND ARDS

Definition

There is no single diagnostic test and confusion has arisen in the past from differing diagnostic criteria. This has complicated comparisons of incidence, mortality, aetiology and efficacy of therapy in different centres. To address this problem, European–American consensus conferences produced the following widely accepted definitions.[6]

Acute lung injury diagnosis requires the presence of four criteria.

1. Acute onset of impaired oxygenation.
2. Severe hypoxaemia defined as a Pa_{O_2} to FI_{O_2} ratio of ≤ 40 (Pa_{O_2} in kPa) or ≤ 300 (Pa_{O_2} in mmHg).
3. Bilateral diffuse infiltration on the chest radiograph.
4. Pulmonary artery wedge pressure of ≤ 18 mmHg to exclude cardiogenic causes of pulmonary oedema.

Acute respiratory distress syndrome is defined in almost identical terms except that the impairment of gas exchange is worse, with a Pa_{O_2} to FI_{O_2} ratio of ≤ 26.7 kPa or ≤ 200 mmHg.

These definitions are now widely accepted and have been extremely helpful in researching ALI, particularly epidemiological studies. However, there are several provisos to their use in the clinical situation. For example, it is possible for patients with diseases that elevate left atrial pressure also to have ALI, but they would fall outside the strict definition. Also, many earlier definitions suggest that one or more of the known predisposing conditions should have been present and that the clinical course has followed the recognised pattern (see below). Finally, it is noted that the histology is usually diagnostic but it is seldom indicated or advisable to take a lung biopsy. There is no reliable laboratory test to confirm the diagnosis (see below).

In part, the diagnosis of ALI depends on the exclusion of other conditions. Sometimes it is not easy to separate it from other diseases such as pulmonary embolus, pulmonary oedema, fibrosing alveolitis or diffuse pneumonia, which may present with many similar features.

Table 31.1 Lung injury score[8]

Chest X-ray appearance	No alveolar consolidation		0
	Alveolar consolidation confined to 1 quadrant		1
	Alveolar consolidation confined to 2 quadrants		2
	Alveolar consolidation confined to 3 quadrants		3
	Alveolar consolidation in all 4 quadrants		4
Hypoxaemia score $Pa_{O_2} : Fi_{O_2}$	Pa_{O_2} in kPa:	Pa_{O_2} in mmHg:	
	≥40	≥300	0
	30–39.9	225–299	1
	23.3–29.9	175–224	2
	13.3–23.2	100–174	3
	<13.3	<100	4
Positive end-expiratory pressure (when ventilated)	kPa	cmH_2O	
	≤0.5	≤5	0
	0.6–0.8	6–8	1
	0.9–1.1	9–11	2
	1.2–1.4	12–14	3
	≥1.5	≥15	4
Respiratory system compliance (when available)	$l.kPa^{-1}$	$ml.cmH_2O^{-1}$	
	≥0.8	≥80	0
	0.6–0.79	60–79	1
	0.4–0.59	40–59	2
	0.2–0.39	20–39	3
	≤0.19	≤19	4

$Pa_{O_2} : Fi_{O_2}$ is the ratio of arterial Po_2 to the fractional concentration of oxygen in the inspired gas. The final lung injury score is the mean of the individual scores for each of the components which are included in the assessment.

Score

0	No lung injury
0.1–2.5	Mild to moderate ALI
>2.5	Severe ALI (ARDS)

Scoring systems

Various attempts have been made to derive a single numerical value to assess the severity of ALI. APACHE III (Acute Physiology And Chronic Health Evaluation) is widely used.[7] Murray *et al.*[8] proposed an expanded three-part definition comprising distinction between acute and chronic phases, identification of aetiological and associated conditions and a numerical lung injury score, details of which are shown in Table 31.1.

Predisposing conditions and risk factors for ALI

Although the clinical and histopathological pictures of ALI are remarkably consistent, they have been described as the sequel to a very large range of predisposing conditions (Table 31.2). There are, however, very important differences in the progression of ALI and its response to treatment, depending on the underlying cause and associated pathology.[8] Nevertheless, recognition of the predisposing conditions is crucially important for predicting which patients are at risk and the establishment of early diagnosis.

Not all the conditions listed in Table 31.2 are equally likely to proceed to ALI. Studies have consistently identified sepsis syndrome (see below) as the condition most likely to result in the development of ARDS, with about 40% of patients being affected.[9] Patients who have aspirated gastric contents, received multiple emergency

Table 31.2 Some predisposing conditions for ALI

Direct lung injury	Indirect lung injury
Common	*Common*
Pneumonia	Sepsis
Aspiration of gastric contents	Severe non-thoracic trauma
	Multiple transfusions of blood products
Less common	
Lung contusion	
Near drowning	*Less common*
Inhalation of toxic gases or vapours	Acute pancreatitis
	Cardiopulmonary bypass
Fat or amniotic fluid embolus	Severe burns
Reperfusion oedema, e.g. following lung transplantation	Drug overdose
	Disseminated intravascular coagulation

Incidence and mortality[12,13]

In the past, the lack of accepted definitions of lung injury led to widely varying estimates of the incidences of ALI and ARDS.[12] The much-quoted American Lung Program study of 1972 estimated the incidence in the USA to be 75 cases per year per 100 000 population.[14] Several studies in different regions of the world subsequently found generally lower incidences, but the range of results obtained remains wide, varying from 1.5 to 88.6 cases per year per 100 000 population.[13] The reasons for this variation in estimates of the incidence of ALI remain unknown.[3]

There is, however, considerable agreement that the overall mortality of ARDS is of the order of 50% whatever the criteria for diagnosis.[1,2] Two studies have indicated improvements in survival in comparison with historical controls, one in the USA[15] and one in the UK.[16] However, a recent review of over 20 studies of mortality from ARDS performed since 1995 does not demonstrate any consistent decline in mortality.[17]

transfusions or incurred pulmonary contusions have a 17–24% chance of developing ARDS. Overall, 25% of patients with a single risk factor develop ARDS, but this rises to 42% with two factors and 85% with three. Age and sex do not affect the likelihood of developing ARDS.

Sepsis syndrome is defined as a systemic response to proven or presumed infection, with hyper- (or hypo-) thermia, tachycardia, tachypnoea and one or more organs exhibiting signs of hypoperfusion or dysfunction. There is usually altered cerebral function, arterial hypoxaemia, lactacidosis and oliguria. Many cases of ARDS represent the pulmonary manifestation of the multiorgan dysfunction syndrome (MODS) that is a feature of this condition, and ARDS is frequently associated with circulatory failure (septic shock). Bacteraemia may or may not be present and has little effect on outcome.

Pulmonary and extrapulmonary ARDS. Gattinoni *et al.*[10] have proposed that patients with ARDS should be considered as two separate groups. Pulmonary ARDS results from clinical conditions that cause direct lung injury, whereas extrapulmonary ARDS follows indirect lung injury (see Table 31.2). These two subgroups of ARDS have been shown to differ with respect to pathological mechanisms, appearances on chest radiographs and CT scans, abnormalities of respiratory mechanics and response to ventilatory strategies.[11]

Clinical course

Four phases may be recognised in the development of severe ALI. In the first the patient is dyspnoeic and tachypnoeic but there are no other abnormalities. The chest radiograph is normal at this stage, which lasts for about 24 hours. In the next phase there is hypoxaemia but the arterial $P\text{CO}_2$ remains normal or subnormal. There are minor abnormalities of the chest radiograph. This phase may last for 24–48 hours. Diagnosis is easily missed in these prodromal stages and is very dependent on the history of one or more predisposing conditions.

It is only in phase three that the diagnostic criteria of ALI become established. There is severe arterial hypoxaemia due to an increased alveolar/arterial $P\text{O}_2$ gradient and the arterial $P\text{CO}_2$ may be slightly elevated. The lungs become stiff and the chest radiograph shows the characteristic bilateral diffuse infiltrates. Artificial ventilation is usually instituted at this stage.

The fourth phase is often terminal and comprises massive bilateral consolidation with unremitting hypoxaemia, the arterial $P\text{O}_2$ characteristically being less than 7 kPa (52.5 mmHg) when the inspired oxygen concentration is 100%. Dead space is substantially increased and the arterial $P\text{CO}_2$ is only with difficulty kept in the normal range by the use of a large minute volume.

Not every patient passes through all these phases and the condition may resolve at any stage. It is difficult to predict whether the condition will progress and there is currently no useful laboratory test, though measurement of cytokine levels has some potential in this area.[18] Serial observations of the chest radiograph, the alveolar/arterial $P\text{O}_2$ gradient and the function of other compromised organs are the best guides to progress. The more systems in failure, the worse the outlook.

Pathophysiology

Oxygen consumption by the lung. Measurement of pulmonary oxygen consumption (as the difference between spirometry and the reversed Fick method – see page 197) has repeatedly shown very high values for lungs with ARDS.[19] It is quite possible that some of this represents free radical formation (see Chapter 26), but the increase in pulmonary oxygen consumption does not seem to correlate with various markers of pulmonary inflammation at the time the measurement is made.[20]

Maldistribution of ventilation and perfusion.[21] Computed tomography (CT) of patients with ARDS shows that opacities representing collapsed areas are distributed throughout the lungs in a heterogeneous manner but predominantly in the dependent regions.[22] Following a change in posture, the opacities move to the newly dependent zones within a few minutes.[23] The most conspicuous functional disability is the shunt[21] (Figure 31.1), which is usually so large (often more than 40%)

that increasing the inspired oxygen concentration cannot produce a normal arterial PO_2 (see the iso-shunt chart, Figure 8.11). CT scans of patients with ALI also demonstrate substantial areas of lung overdistension.[24] These areas contribute to the increased dead space, which may exceed 70% of tidal volume and requires a large increase in minute volume to attempt to preserve a normal arterial PCO_2. Both shunt and dead space correlate strongly with the non-inflated lung tissue seen with CT (see Figure 31.1).

Lung mechanics. In established ARDS, lung compliance is greatly reduced and the static compliance of the respiratory system (lungs + chest wall) is of the order of 300 ml.kPa^{-1} (30 ml.cmH$_2$O^{-1}).[25,26] Patients with pulmonary and extrapulmonary forms of ARDS (see above) have different abnormalities of respiratory system mechanics.[10] Respiratory system compliance is reduced to a similar extent in both groups, but the abnormality is mostly with lung compliance when lung disease is the cause and chest wall compliance with extrapulmonary causation.

Functional residual capacity is reduced by collapse and increased elastic recoil.

Mean total resistance to air flow was found to be 1.5–2 kPa.l^{-1}.s^{-1} (15–20 cmH$_2$O.l^{-1}.s^{-1})[25,26] or about three times that of anaesthetised patients with normal lungs, measured by the same technique. Using the model shown in Figure 4.4, some two-thirds of the total resistance in patients with ARDS could be assigned to viscoelastic resistance of tissue, although the airway resistance was still about twice normal.

Alveolar/capillary permeability is increased substantially throughout the course of ALI.[27] This may be demonstrated by the enhanced transit of various tracer molecules across the alveolar/capillary membrane (page 145).[28]

MECHANISMS OF ALI

Histopathology

Although of diverse aetiologies, the histological appearances of ARDS are remarkably consistent and this lends support for ARDS being considered a discrete clinical entity. Histological changes at autopsy may be divided into two stages, as follows.[29]

Acute stage. The acute stage is characterised by damaged integrity of the blood–gas barrier. The changes are primarily in the interalveolar septa and cannot be satisfactorily seen with light microscopy. Electron microscopy shows extensive damage to the type I alveolar epithelial cells (page 21), which may be totally destroyed (Figure

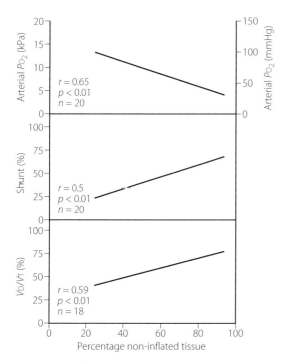

Figure 31.1 Relationship of arterial PO_2, shunt and physiological dead space (VD/VT) to the percentage of non-inflated lung tissue seen by CT in patients with acute respiratory distress syndrome, artificially ventilated with positive end-expiratory pressure of 0.5 kPa (5 cmH$_2$O). (After reference 22.)

Figure 31.2 Electron micrograph of an alveolar septum in the early stages of acute lung injury. On the right-hand side of the septum there are many examples of damage to alveolar epithelium but the endothelium tends to remain intact. The alveolar gas spaces to the left and right contain many red blood cells, leucocytes, cell debris and fibrin strands. The scale bar is 10 μm. (Reproduced from reference 29 by permission of the authors and the Editors of *Clinics in Chest Medicine*.)

31.2). Meanwhile the basement membrane is usually preserved and the endothelial cells still tend to form a continuous layer with apparently intact cell junctions. Endothelial permeability is nevertheless increased and interstitial oedema is found, predominantly on the 'service' side of the capillary, as seen in other forms of pulmonary oedema (page 389).

Protein-containing fluid leaks into the alveoli, which also contain red blood cells and leucocytes in addition to amorphous material comprising strands of fibrin (see Figure 31.2). The exudate may form into sheets that line the alveoli as the so-called hyaline membrane. Intravascular coagulation is common at this stage and, in patients with septicaemia, capillaries may be completely plugged with leucocytes and the underlying endothelium may then be damaged.

Chronic or fibroproliferative stage. Attempted repair and proliferation predominate in the chronic stage of ARDS. Within a few days of the onset of the condition, there is a thickening of endothelium, epithelium and the interstitial space. The type I epithelial cells are destroyed and replaced by type II cells, which proliferate but do not differentiate into type I cells as usual. They remain cuboidal and about ten times the thickness of the type I cells they have replaced. This appears to be a non-specific response to damaged type I cells and is similar

to that which results from exposure to high concentrations of oxygen (page 357).

The interstitial space is greatly expanded by oedema fluid, fibres and a variety of proliferating cells. In the same way as for other causes of pulmonary fibrosis, extracellular matrix remodelling begins (page 405). Fibrosis commences after the first week and ultimately fibrocytes predominate: extensive fibrosis is seen in resolving cases. These fibroproliferative changes may occur earlier in pulmonary than in extrapulmonary causes of ARDS.[30]

Cellular mechanisms[1,2,31]

The diversity of predisposing conditions suggests that there may be several possible mechanisms, at least in the early stages of development of ALI, but the end result is remarkably similar. In all cases, lung injury seems to begin with damage to the alveolar/capillary membrane. This is followed by progressive inflammation leading to alveolar epithelial cell injury, alveolar transudation, pulmonary vasoconstriction and capillary obstruction.

Cells that are capable of damaging the alveolar capillary membrane include neutrophils, basophils, macrophages and platelets. Damage may be inflicted by a large number of substances, including bacterial endotoxin, reactive oxygen species, proteases, thrombin, fibrin, fibrin degradation products, arachidonic acid metabolites and innumerable proinflammatory cytokines. It seems improbable that any one mechanism is responsible for all cases of ALI. It is more likely that different mechanisms operate in different predisposing conditions and in different animal models of ALI.

Neutrophils are now accepted as having a key role in human ALI.[32] Although ALI can still be induced in neutrophil-depleted animals, patients with ARDS have large numbers of neutrophils and associated cytokines in bronchoalveolar lavage (BAL) fluid samples.[2] Neutrophil activation may occur in response to a large number of substances, some of which are illustrated in Figure 31.3. Which of these are important in ALI is unknown, but likely to depend on the predisposing condition; for example, complement component C5a is known to be involved in sepsis-related ALI. Margination of neutrophils from the pulmonary capillary into the lung parenchyma is the first stage of neutrophil activation and is described on page 403. During margination, and once in the interstitium, the neutrophil is 'primed'; that is, stimulated to produce preformed mediators ready for release and to establish the bactericidal contents of their lysosomes. Finally, stimulation results from a whole host of cytokines, some derived from other inflammatory cells (macrophages, lymphocytes or endothelial cells) and some from other neutrophils, so amplifying the

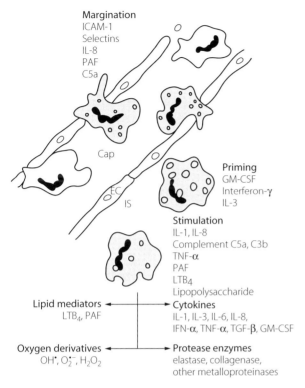

Margination
ICAM-1
Selectins
IL-8
PAF
C5a

Cap

EC
IS

Priming
GM-CSF
Interferon-γ
IL-3

Stimulation
IL-1, IL-8
Complement C5a, C3b
TNF-α
PAF
LTB₄
Lipopolysaccharide

Lipid mediators ← → Cytokines
LTB₄, PAF   IL-1, IL-3, IL-6, IL-8,
                      IFN-α, TNF-α, TGF-β, GM-CSF

Oxygen derivatives ← → Protease enzymes
OH•, O₂•⁻, H₂O₂   elastase, collagenase,
                       other metalloproteinases

Figure 31.3 Neutrophil activation and the main cytokines and mediators involved. This takes place in three stages. *Margination*, when neutrophils adhere to the capillary (Cap) wall and migrate between endothelial cells (EC) into the interstitial space (IS); *priming,* when the cells generate preformed mediators and lysozomal contents; and *stimulation*, when neutrophils release the various mediators shown. The scheme shown is based on studies of both systemic and pulmonary inflammation. Neutrophil margination may occur by different mechanisms in pulmonary capillaries (see page 403). For explanation of abbreviations, see text.

process. Stimulation causes release of a whole host of inflammatory mediators (see Figure 31.3) and is also associated with inappropriate release of lysosomal contents. Instead of being released into phagocytic vesicles containing bacteria, they come into direct contact with the endothelium, which is thereby damaged.

Four groups of substances released from neutrophils (see Figure 31.3) are considered to contribute to lung damage, as follows.

1. Cytokines.[31,33] Neutrophils are capable of producing numerous cytokines, most of which are proinflammatory. Tumour necrosis factor-α (TNF-α) and interleukin-1β (IL-1β) have widespread proinflammatory effects, including activation of endothelial cells to upregulate the adhesion molecule ICAM-1 and selectins, which facilitate margination of further inflammatory cells (page 403). Complement compo-

nent C5a, platelet-activating factor (PAF) and IL-8 accelerate margination. Granulocyte/macrophage colony-stimulating factor (GM-CSF) and IL-3 contribute to priming of further neutrophils along with interferon-γ released from other inflammatory cells. Finally, IL-1, IL-8 and TNF-α all exert positive feedback on neutrophils, causing further stimulation. Transforming growth factor-β (TGF-β) is the principal antiinflammatory cytokine produced by neutrophils and is responsible for fibroblast stimulation and the development of pulmonary fibrosis (page 405). IL-8 is involved in most stages of neutrophil activation (see Figure 31.3) and the serum concentration of IL-8 in ALI may help predict those patients with a poor prognosis.[18]

2. Protease enzymes lead to extensive tissue damage in the lung. The most damaging is elastase which, contrary to its name, is very non-specific, with proteolytic activity against collagen, fibrinogen and many other proteins as well as elastin. A group of enzymes referred to as metalloproteinases are more specific for individual substrates such as collagen.

3. Reactive oxygen species and related compounds (see Chapter 26) are powerful and important bactericidal agents, which also have the capacity to damage the endothelium by lipid peroxidation and other means. In addition, they inactivate α₁-antitrypsin, an important antiprotease enzyme (page 202).

4. Lipid-derived mediators include prostaglandins, thromboxanes and leukotrienes (LT), but LTB₄ and PAF are the most important in ALI. These two act in the same way as other cytokines to amplify neutrophil activation, and in addition, PAF damages endothelial cells directly and promotes intravascular coagulation.

Macrophages and basophils. Macrophages are already present in the normal alveolus (page 22) but their numbers increase greatly in ALI. They produce a wide range of bactericidal agents and cytokines similar to those of the neutrophil. Lung macrophages produce IL-10, which suppresses gene expression of many cytokines and so acts as one of the very few antiinflammatory cytokines so far identified in ALI.[33]

Platelets are present in the pulmonary capillaries in large numbers in ARDS. Aggregation in the capillary is associated with increased capillary hydrostatic pressure, possibly due to release of arachidonic acid metabolites.

Besides giving rise to pulmonary oedema, many of the mediators released by these inflammatory cells have other effects that contribute to the pulmonary changes seen in ALI. For example, arachidonic acid metabolites cause pulmonary venoconstriction, which will raise pulmonary capillary pressure and compound the effect of increased permeability. Accumulation of platelets and neutrophils along with intravascular coagulation will occlude pulmonary vessels, producing pulmonary hypertension and unperfused lung units. It has also been noted that many proteins, including albumin but particularly fibrin monomer, can antagonise the action of surfactant, so fundamentally altering lung mechanics.[34]

The potential contribution to ALI of lung damage secondary to artificial ventilation is described on page 437.

PRINCIPLES OF THERAPY[35,36]

Treatment of the underlying cause in conjunction with supportive therapy remains the mainstay of current management. Optimal management of the cardiovascular and renal systems is a vital component of ALI treatment as any increase in pulmonary capillary pressure (e.g. from fluid overload) may lead to catastrophic pulmonary oedema. Respiratory support requires artificial ventilation in all but the most minor degrees of ALI.

Artificial ventilation in ARDS[37–39]

General principles of artificial ventilation and the resulting physiological effects are described in detail in the next chapter. In this section, only the problems associated with ventilation of patients with ALI are described.

The lungs of patients with severe ALI may be conveniently divided into three hypothetical sections.[40] First, there will be some 'normal' areas, usually in the nondependent region. Second, there will be areas, usually in dependent regions, with such severe collapse and alveolar flooding that ventilation will be impossible. Finally, there will be an intermediate area with poorly ventilated or collapsed alveoli that are capable of being 'recruited' by appropriate artificial ventilation, with a resultant improvement in gas exchange. Although the relative amounts of each section will vary greatly according to the severity of the ALI, there will always be *some* lung in the final area and so capable of recruitment.

Tidal volume. The recognition that positive-pressure ventilation can lead to lung damage (page 437) has led to a change in ventilatory technique used in patients with ALI. Overdistension of alveoli by application of large tidal volumes is now believed to be a significant factor in lung damage. In particular, because of the extensive areas of pulmonary collapse a typical patient with ARDS may only have approximately one-third of the lung being ventilated. Thus use of a normal tidal volume (10–12 ml.kg^{-1}) will, for the few alveoli being ventilated, equate to a tidal volume of three times usual for normal healthy lungs, which in a 70 kg subject equates to over 2 litres.

Pressure-controlled ventilation (page 421) is now the preferred technique in most centres to avoid the problems outlined in the previous paragraph. However, with pressure-controlled ventilation in lungs with low compliance, such as in ALI, the delivery of an adequate minute volume may be difficult. Two techniques are advocated to deal with this problem. First, inverse inspiration/expiration ratios may be used, in which expiratory time is shorter than inspiratory time, allowing the delivery of a larger tidal volume. Second, the hypercapnia that results from the inadequate minute volume may be partially ignored. Known as 'permissive hypercapnia',[41,42] arterial $P\text{CO}_2$ is allowed to increase until such time as the respiratory acidosis is deemed detrimental, which will depend on the patient's cardiovascular function.

Positive end-expiratory pressure (PEEP).[43] At one time it seemed that the early use of PEEP might prevent the development of ARDS,[44] but it now seems unlikely that there is any such effect. PEEP does, however, reduce the amount of non-inflated lung tissue seen an CT scan,[22] particularly in dependent lung regions.[45] Shunt fraction, and therefore the arterial $P\text{O}_2$ (Figure 31.4), also improves. Reduced pulmonary compliance means that cardiac output is better maintained than might be expected (page 436), with a reduction of about 20% with PEEP of 1.5 kPa (15 cm H_2O) (see Figure 31.4). The resultant reduction in oxygen delivery is insignificant.[46]

The ideal PEEP value to use has been controversial for decades. Differing end-points (shown here in parentheses) have given rise to numerous terms such as 'optimal' PEEP (lowest physiological shunt fraction), 'best' PEEP (optimal static lung compliance), 'preferred' PEEP (best oxygen delivery) and 'least' PEEP (acceptable values for arterial $P\text{O}_2$, inspired oxygen and cardiac output). High levels of PEEP will probably result in increased alveolar recruitment and improved oxygenation, but normal alveoli can only enlarge in response to PEEP to a certain extent, above which dramatic increases in alveolar pressure and possible damage occur (page 437 *et seq.*). Identifying this point has vexed intensivists for some time. It has been suggested that PEEP be increased until the lower inflection of the patient's respiratory system static compliance curve is reached (point A in Figure 31.5), which is normally between 10 and 15 cmH$_2$O.[47] The pressure seen at the lower point of inflection is believed to represent the pressure at which most recruitable alveoli have been opened, whereas the upper inflection point (B in Figure 31.5) designates the point above which overdistension of alveoli may occur.[37] A pressure–volume curve in ARDS patients has also been compared to chest CT scans and may prove useful in ascertaining which patients have significant potentially recruitable regions of lung.[48]

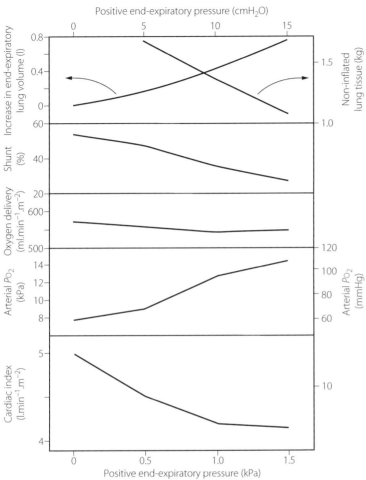

Figure 31.4 Effect of positive end-expiratory pressure on various factors influencing oxygen delivery in patients with acute respiratory distress syndrome. Although arterial Po_2 is increased, cardiac output is decreased and there is no significant change in oxygen transport. (Data on non-inflated lung tissue are from reference 22; remaining data from reference 45.)

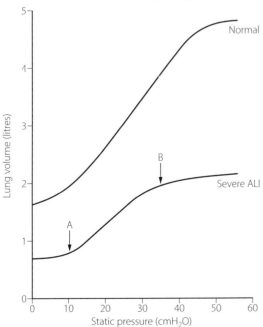

Figure 31.5 Static pressure versus lung volume curves for patients receiving positive-pressure ventilation. Note the severely reduced lung volume and compliance in ALI. Point A indicates the lower inflection of the curve, above which compliance is considerably improved. Application of positive end-expiratory pressure of approximately 12 cmH_2O in this patient will therefore improve tidal volume relative to the ventilatory pressure required. Point B indicates the upper inflection point, above which alveolar overdistension may occur. Therefore, in this patient, airway pressure should ideally be maintained below 35 cmH_2O.

Table 31.3 Summary of pharmacological interventions suggested for the treatment of ALI or ARDS

Therapy	Examples	Proposed mechanism
Pulmonary vasodilators	Prostacyclin	Non-specific pulmonary vasodilator
	Nitric oxide	Regional pulmonary vasodilator (see text)
	Almitrine	Enhancement of hypoxic pulmonary vasoconstriction
Surfactant	Artificial surfactants	Replace depleted alveolar surfactant, may also have antiinflammatory properties
Antiinflammatory	Steroids	General antiinflammatory
	Ketoconazole	Inhibits thromboxane synthesis
	Ibuprofen/Indomethacin	Inhibits prostaglandin production
	Prostaglandin E_1	Inhibits platelet aggregation, vasodilator
	Pentoxifylline	Reduces neutrophil chemotaxis and activation
	Endotoxin/TNF/IL-1 antagonists	Inhibition of specific aspects of inflammatory response
Antioxidants	N-acetylcysteine	Increased glutathione activity (page 356)
	Recombinant human manganese SOD	Replaces epithelial extracellular SOD (page 355)
Anticoagulants	Heparin	Reduces fibrin deposition in alveoli

NB All the therapies listed have been shown to have beneficial effects in *in vitro* or animal studies of ALI. There is insufficient evidence of improved outcome for any of the therapies listed to be recommended for routine use in human ALI. For further details see references 1, 36, 51, 52.
SOD, superoxide dismutase (page 355); TNF, tumour necrosis factor; IL-1, interleukin 1.

Protective ventilation strategy. In ARDS, the ventilatory strategy used must balance the conflicting requirements of maintaining adequate gas exchange in severely diseased lungs while simultaneously avoiding damaging the lungs by the use of large tidal volumes, high airway pressures or harmful levels of inspired oxygen. Protective ventilation is a widely advocated ventilatory strategy that may achieve the best compromise and involves using small tidal volumes to prevent alveolar overdistension and moderate levels of PEEP to maintain alveolar recruitment. Initial tidal volumes used for ventilation should be between 6 and 8 ml.kg^{-1} using pressure-controlled ventilation. PEEP is set using a pressure–volume curve or increased until arterial $P\text{O}_2$ is adequate or cardiovascular depression occurs. If plateau airway pressure exceeds 35 cmH$_2$O or the inspired oxygen level required to obtain acceptable arterial $P\text{O}_2$ exceeds 0.65, then an alternative ventilatory strategy should be considered.[37] There is increasing evidence of a clinically significant outcome benefit of using protective ventilation in some groups of patients with ARDS.[49]

Alternative ventilatory strategies.[37] Many other techniques have been described for ventilating patients with ARDS who continue to have unacceptably poor gas exchange despite the use of protective ventilation. None

of these has been shown to improve clinical outcome. Possible interventions include:

- inverse-ratio ventilation (page 425)
- prone position. In the prone position both ventilation and perfusion become more uniform and the areas of atelectasis in dependent lung regions change position, re-forming in the anterior (now dependent) regions.[23] About two-thirds of patients demonstrate an improvement in oxygenation on turning prone, though this is normally not sustained and repeated turning of the patient may be required
- inhaled nitric oxide (page 103)[51]
- high-frequency ventilation (page 429)
- extrapulmonary gas exchange (page 439)
- partial liquid ventilation.

Other therapeutic options

Specific therapy for ALI is the goal of much research, which is directed particularly towards the control of sepsis and the development of antagonists to the various mediators considered above.[35] In most cases it has proved difficult to demonstrate their efficacy in the clinical setting. Detailed description of these, and several other pharmacological approaches to the treatment of ALI, is beyond the scope of this book but a summary is shown in Table 31.3.

REFERENCES

1. Fulkerson WJ, MacIntyre N, Crapo JD. Pathogenesis and treatment of the adult respiratory distress syndrome. *Arch Intern Med* 1996; **156**: 29–38.
2. Luce JM. Acute lung injury and the acute respiratory distress syndrome. *Crit Care Med* 1998; **26**: 369–76.
3. Ware LB, Matthay MA. The acute respiratory distress syndrome. *N Engl J Med* 2000; **342**: 1334–49.
4. Ashbaugh DG, Bigelow DB, Petty TL, Levine BE. Acute respiratory distress in adults. *Lancet* 1967; **2**: 319–23.
5. Petty TL, Ashbaugh DG. The adult respiratory distress syndrome. *Chest* 1971; **60**: 233–8.
6. Bernard GR, Artigas A, Brigham KL, *et al.* The American-European consensus conference on ARDS: definitions, mechanisms, relevant outcomes and clinical trial coordination. *Am J Respir Crit Care Med* 1994; **149**: 818–24.
7. Knaus WA, Wagner DP, Draper EA, *et al.* The APACHE III prognostic system. Risk prediction of hospital mortality for critically ill hospitalized adults. *Chest* 1991; **100**: 1619–36.
8. Murray JF, Matthay MA, Luce JM, Flick MR. An expanded definition of the adult respiratory distress syndrome. *Am Rev Respir Dis* 1988; **138**: 720–3.
9. Hudson LD, Millberg JA, Anardi D, Maunder RJ. Clinical risks for development of the acute respiratory distress syndrome. *Am J Respir Crit Care Med* 1995; **151**: 293–301.
10. Gattinoni L, Pelosi P, Suter PM, Pedoto A, Vercesi P, Lissoni A. Acute respiratory distress syndrome caused by pulmonary and extrapulmonary disease. Different syndromes? *Am J Respir Crit Care Med* 1998; **158**: 3–11.
*11. Pelosi P, D'Onofrio D, Chiumello D, *et al.* Pulmonary and extrapulmonary acute respiratory distress syndrome are different. *Eur Respir J* 2003; **22**(Suppl 42): 48S–56S.
12. Atabai K, Matthay MA. The pulmonary physician in critical care. 5: Acute lung injury and the acute respiratory distress syndrome: definitions and epidemiology. *Thorax* 2002; **57**: 452–8.
13. Rubenfeld GD. Epidemiology of acute lung injury. *Crit Care Med* 2003; **31**(Supp): S276–84.
14. National Heart and Lung Institute. *Respiratory distress syndromes: task force on problems, research approaches, needs.* DHEW Publication No. (NIH) 73–432. Washington DC: US Government Printing Office, 1972.
15. Milberg JA, Davis DR, Steinberg KP, Hudson LD. Improved survival of patients with acute respiratory distress syndrome (ARDS): 1983–1993. *JAMA* 1995; **273**: 306–9.
16. Abel SJC, Finney SJ, Brett SJ, Keogh BF, Morgan CJ, Evans TW. Reduced mortality in association with the acute respiratory distress syndrome (ARDS). *Thorax* 1998; **53**: 292–4.
17. Vincent JL, Sakr Y, Ranieri VM. Epidemiology and outcome of acute respiratory failure in intensive care unit patients. *Crit Care Med* 2003; **31**(Supp): S296–9.
18. Pittet JF, Mackersie RC, Martin TR, Matthay MA. Biological markers of acute lung injury: prognostic and pathogenic significance. *Am J Respir Crit Care Med* 1997; **155**: 1187–205.
19. Smithies MN, Royston B, Makita K, Konieczko K, Nunn JF. Comparison of oxygen consumption measurements: indirect calorimetry versus the reversed Fick method. *Crit Care Med* 1991; **19**: 1401–6.
20. Jolliet P, Thorens JB, Nicod L, Pichard C, Kyle U, Chevrolet JC. Relationship between pulmonary oxygen consumption, lung inflammation and calculated venous admixture in patients with acute lung injury. *Intens Care Med* 1996; **22**: 277–85.
21. Sinclair SE, Albert RK. Altering ventilation-perfusion relationships in ventilated patients with acute lung injury. *Intens Care Med* 1997; **23**: 942–50.
22. Gattinoni L, Pesenti A, Bombino M, *et al.* Relationships between lung computed tomographic density, gas exchange and PEEP in acute respiratory failure. *Anesthesiology* 1988; **69**: 824–32.
23. Gattinoni L, Pelosi P, Vitale G, Pesenti A, D'Andrea L, Mascheroni D. Body position changes redistribute lung computed-tomographic density in patients with acute respiratory failure. *Anesthesiology* 1991; **74**: 15–23.
24. Vieira SRR, Puybasset L, Richecoeur J, *et al.* A lung computed tomographic assessment of positive end-expiratory pressure-induced lung overdistension. *Am J Respir Crit Care Med* 1998; **158**: 1571–7.
25. Tantucci C, Corbeil C, Chasse M, *et al.* Flow and volume dependence of respiratory system flow resistance in patients with adult respiratory distress syndrome. *Am Rev Respir Dis* 1992; **145**: 355–60.
26. Eissa NT, Ranieri VM, Corbeil C, *et al.* Analysis of behavior of the respiratory system in ARDS patients: effects of flow, volume and time. *J Appl Physiol* 1991; **70**: 2719–29.
27. Sinclair DG, Braude S, Haslam PL, Evans TW. Pulmonary endothelial permeability in patients with severe lung injury: clinical correlates and natural history. *Chest* 1994; **106**: 535–9.
28. Rocker GM. Bedside measurement of pulmonary capillary permeability in patients with acute lung injury. What have we learned? *Intens Care Med* 1996; **22**: 619–21.
29. Bachofen M, Weibel ER. Structural alterations and lung parenchyma in the adult respiratory distress syndrome. *Clin Chest Med* 1982; **3**: 35–43.

30. Negri EM, Hoelz C, Barbas CSV, Montes GS, Saldiva PHN, Capelozzi VL. Acute remodeling of parenchyma in pulmonary and extrapulmonary ARDS. An autopsy study of collagen and elastic system fibres. *Pathol Res Pract* 2002; **198**: 355–61.

*31. Bhatia M, Moochhala S. Role of inflammatory mediators in the pathophysiology of acute respiratory distress syndrome. *J Pathol* 2004; **202**: 145–56.

*32. Abraham E. Neutrophils and acute lung injury. *Crit Care Med* 2003; **31**(Supp): S195–9.

*33. Ward PA. Role of complement, chemokines and regulatory cytokines in acute lung injury. *Ann N Y Acad Sci* 1996; **796**: 104–12.

34. Seeger W, Stöhr G, Wolf HRD, Neuhof H. Alteration of surfactant function due to protein leakage. *J Appl Physiol* 1985; **58**: 326–38.

35. Artigas A, Bernard GR, Carlet J, *et al.* The American-European consensus conference on ARDS. Part 2: Ventilatory, pharmacologic, supportive therapy, study design strategies and issues related to recovery and remodelling. *Intens Care Med* 1998; **24**: 378–98.

36. Brower RG, Ware LB, Berthiaume Y, Matthay MA. Treatment of ARDS. *Chest* 2001; **120**: 1347–67.

*37. Malarkkan N, Snook NJ, Lumb AB. New aspects of ventilation in acute lung injury. *Anaesthesia* 2003; **58**: 647–67.

38. Moloney ED, Griffiths MJD. Protective ventilation of patients with acute respiratory distress syndrome. *Br J Anaesth* 2004; **92**: 261–70.

*39. Rouby J-J, Constantin J-M, Giradi CrdeA, Zhang M, Lu Q. Mechanical ventilation in patients with acute respiratory distress syndrome. *Anesthesiology* 2004; **101**: 228–34.

40. Gattinoni L, Pesenti A. ARDS: the non-homogenous lung: facts and hypotheses. *Intens Crit Care Digest* 1987; **6**: 1–4.

41. Lewandowski K. Permissive hypercapnia in ARDS: just do it? *Intens Care Med* 1996; **22**: 179–81.

42. Laffey JG, O'Croinin D, McLoughlin P, Kavanagh BP. Permissive hypercapnia – role in protective lung ventilatory strategies. *Intens Care Med* 2004; **30**: 347–56.

43. Rouby JJ, Lu Q, Goldstein I. Selecting the right level of positive end-expiratory pressure in patients with acute respiratory distress syndrome. *Am J Respir Crit Care Med* 2002; **165**: 1182–6.

44. Schmidt GB, O'Neill WW, Kotb K, Hwang KK, Bennett EJ, Bombeck CT. Continuous positive airway pressure in the prophylaxis of the adult respiratory distress syndrome. *Surg Gynecol Obstet* 1976; **143**: 613–20.

45. Gattinoni L, D'Andrea L, Pelosi P, Vitale G, Pesenti A, Fumagalli R. Regional effects and mechanism of positive end-expiratory pressure in early adult respiratory distress syndrome. *JAMA* 1993; **269**: 2122–7.

46. Ranieri VM, Eissa NT, Corbeil C, *et al.* Effects of positive end-expiratory pressure on alveolar recruitment and gas exchange in patients with the adult respiratory distress syndrome. *Am Rev Respir Dis* 1991; **144**: 544–51.

47. Rupie E, Dambrosio M, Servillo G, *et al.* Titration of tidal volume and induced hypercapnia in acute respiratory distress syndrome. *Am J Respir Crit Care Med* 1995; **152**: 121–8.

48. Rouby J-J, Lu Q, Vieira S. Pressure/volume curves and lung computed tomography in acute respiratory distress syndrome. *Eur Respir J* 2003; **22**(Suppl 42): 27S–36S.

49. Petrucci N, Iacovelli W. Ventilation with lower tidal volumes versus traditional tidal volumes in adults for acute lung injury and acute respiratory distress syndrome. *Cochrane Database Syst Rev* 2003; **3**: CD003844.

50. Adhikari N, Granton JT. Inhaled nitric oxide for acute lung injury. No place for NO? *JAMA* 2004; **291**: 1629–31.

51. Moloney ED, Evans TW. Pathophysiology and pharmacological treatment of pulmonary hypertension in acute respiratory distress syndrome. *Eur Respir J* 2003; **21**: 720–7.

52. Laterre P-F, Wittebole X, Dhainaut J-F. Anticoagulant therapy in acute lung injury. *Crit Care Med* 2003; **31**(Suppl): S329–36.

32 Respiratory support and artificial ventilation

KEY POINTS

■ Non-invasive ventilation may be used to increase airway pressure and support a failing respiratory system without the need for tracheal intubation or tracheostomy.

■ Intermittent positive-pressure ventilation can be delivered by a variety of different techniques, many of which are coordinated with the patient's own respiratory efforts.

■ Positive end-expiratory pressure increases the functional residual capacity, reduces airway resistance and may prevent or reverse lung collapse.

■ Any increase in mean intrathoracic pressure, as seen during positive-pressure ventilation, impairs venous return, increases pulmonary vascular resistance and so reduces cardiac output.

■ Artificial ventilation may damage the lung by exerting excessive pressures or volumes on lung tissue or by causing repeated opening and closure of small airways with each breath.

■ A clinically useful artificial lung remains only a distant possibility, although extracorporeal systems that partially replace pulmonary gas exchange continue to evolve and are now beneficial for some groups of patients.

The previous five chapters have outlined the numerous ways in which the respiratory system may fail to achieve its primary objective of gas exchange. This chapter describes the various techniques available to replace, either partially or totally, the gas exchange function of the respiratory system.

Respiratory support is required when there is impaired action of the patient's respiratory muscles or a severe dysfunction of the mechanics of breathing. It may also be used to improve oxygenation of arterial blood even when $P\text{CO}_2$ is within normal limits. Artificial ventilation is defined as the provision of the minute volume of res-

piration by external forces. For most clinical applications, current practice has moved more towards respiratory 'support' or 'assist', in which the patient's breathing is assisted, but not entirely replaced, by a variety of techniques described throughout this chapter.[1] Provision of the whole minute ventilation by artificial means is now only seen during anaesthesia with paralysis and in the most critically ill patients.

NON-INVASIVE VENTILATION[2,3]

Non-invasive ventilation is defined as respiratory support without establishing a tracheal airway. It may be achieved by either negative-pressure ventilation or positive-pressure ventilation via a mask or similar device.

Negative-pressure ventilation[4]

This requires the application of subatmospheric pressure to the trunk. It was first reported in 1929[5] and widely used for the following 30 years during polio epidemics. Enthusiasm for the technique has fluctuated since, but there continues to be interest in negative-pressure ventilation for a small group of patients.[6]

Cabinet ventilators, often referred to as an 'iron lung', require the whole body except the head to be encased in a cabinet with an airtight seal around the neck. An intermittent negative pressure is then applied in the tank, causing inspiration, with passive expiration as normal. A superimposed continuous negative pressure may also be applied, which provides the negative-pressure equivalent of positive end-expiratory pressure (PEEP). In terms of the airway-to-ambient pressure gradient, cabinet ventilators are identical in principle to positive-pressure ventilation, with very similar effects on cardiovascular and respiratory physiology. Collapse of the extrathoracic upper airway during inspiration may occur, particularly during sleep. Vomiting or regurgitation of gastric contents exposes the patient to the danger of aspiration during the inspiratory phase, and fatalities have occurred under particularly distressing circumstances.

Cuirass and jacket ventilators are a simplified form of cabinet ventilator in which the application of subatmospheric pressure is confined to the trunk or anterior abdominal wall. Function depends on a good airtight seal. They are less efficient than cabinet ventilators and suffer from the same disadvantages. However, they are much more convenient to use and may be useful to supplement inadequate spontaneous breathing.

The Hayek oscillator is a form of cuirass that encircles the trunk and allows high-frequency ventilation (see below) with a continuous negative pressure.[7] It facilitates a wide range of tidal volumes and some degree of control of the functional residual capacity (FRC). It may be used during surgery on the airway, so avoiding the need for any form of tracheal tube.[8]

Negative-pressure ventilation continues to have a place in the management of respiratory failure due to neuromuscular disorders[4] or central apnoeas[2] and in paediatric intensive care.[6]

Non-invasive positive-pressure ventilation[2,3]

Positive-pressure ventilation may be delivered using soft masks that fit over the mouth and nose or only the nose. With nasal ventilation, positive pressure in the nasopharynx normally displaces the soft palate anteriorly against the tongue, thus preventing escape of gas through the mouth. Most ventilator systems used are pressure generators and so are 'leak tolerant'; that is, flow automatically increases to compensate for a pressure drop due to gas leakage. Adverse effects of nasal ventilation include eye irritation, conjunctivitis and facial skin necrosis.

Techniques of ventilation are similar to invasive artificial ventilation. Ventilator modes that use patient triggering are better tolerated than controlled ventilation, particularly in awake patients, but both techniques are used. Volume-controlled ventilation is poorly tolerated and does not compensate for leaks, so is rarely used. Pressure-controlled ventilation or pressure support ventilation (PSV, see below) are commonly used, as is continuous positive airway pressure (CPAP). In bilevel positive airway pressure (bilevel PAP) the ventilator pressure steps between two preset values for inspiration and expiration and, except for the terminology used to describe the pressures, is the same as PSV with CPAP.[2]

Ventilation may be provided continually during acute respiratory problems or only at night for long-term respiratory disease.[9] The use of nasal CPAP for treating the sleep apnoea–hypopnoea syndrome has been described on page 251. In this case, benefit occurs simply by displacing the soft palate away from the posterior pharyngeal wall. Benefit in other respiratory diseases is more difficult to explain, but possible mechanisms include:[3]

- resting fatigued respiratory muscles
- delivery of a higher inspired oxygen concentration by the use of a tight-fitting facemask (page 191)
- augmentation of minute ventilation to reduce hypercapnia
- prevention or reexpansion of areas of atelectasis, as seen when using PEEP (see below)
- reduction of cardiac preload in patients with heart failure (page 436).

Clinical applications.[3,10,11] Hypoventilation and hypercapnia associated with neuromuscular disorders or central hypoventilation syndromes may be readily treated with non-invasive ventilation (NIV), with good symptom relief. The case for long-term treatment of COPD remains unproven, but there is now widespread acceptance that NIV is beneficial when treating acute exacerbations (page 380), reducing the need for tracheal intubation. Other groups in which NIV has been shown to be beneficial include immunocompromised patients with chest infections, some patients with acute lung injury and patients who prove difficult to wean from artificial ventilation.[12] Acute pulmonary oedema may be successfully treated with non-invasive positive-pressure ventilation[13] and the mechanism of this beneficial effect is explained on page 392.

INTERMITTENT POSITIVE-PRESSURE VENTILATION (IPPV)

Phases of the respiratory cycle

Inspiration. During IPPV, the mouth (or airway) pressure is intermittently raised above ambient pressure. The inspired gas then flows into the lungs in accordance with the resistance and compliance of the respiratory system. If inspiration is slow, the distribution is governed mainly by regional compliance. If inspiration is fast, there is preferential ventilation of parts of the lungs with short time constants (see Figure 3.6). Different temporal patterns of pressure may be applied, as discussed below.

Expiration. During IPPV, expiration results from allowing mouth pressure to fall to ambient. Expiration is then passive and differs from expiration during spontaneous breathing, in which diaphragm muscle tone is gradually reduced (page 56). Expiration may be impeded by the application of PEEP. In the past, expiration was sometimes accelerated by the application of a subatmospheric pressure, termed negative end-expiratory pressure (NEEP), though this technique is no longer used. Expiration to ambient pressure is termed zero end-expiratory pressure (ZEEP).

If the inflating pressure is maintained for several seconds, the resulting tidal volume will be indicated by the following relationship:

Tidal volume = sustained inflation pressure

× total static compliance

Thus, for example, a sustained inflation pressure of 10 cmH$_2$O with a static compliance of 0.5 l.kPa^{-1} (50 ml.cmH$_2$O^{-1}) would result in a lung volume 500 ml above FRC.

Time course of inflation and deflation

Equilibration according to the above equation usually takes several seconds. When the airway pressure is raised during inspiration, it is opposed by the two forms of impedance: the elastic resistance of lungs and chest wall (see Chapter 3) and resistance to air flow (see Chapter 4). At any instant, the inflation pressure equals the sum of the pressures required to overcome these two forms of impedance. The pressure required to overcome elastic resistance equals the lung volume above FRC divided by

the total (dynamic) compliance, whereas the pressure required to overcome air flow resistance equals the air flow resistance multiplied by the instantaneous flow rate.

The effect of applying a constant pressure (or square wave inflation) is shown in Figure 32.1. The two components of the inflation pressure vary during the course of inspiration but their sum remains constant. The component overcoming air flow resistance is maximal at first and declines exponentially with air flow as inflation proceeds. The component overcoming elastic resistance increases with the lung volume. With normal respiratory mechanics in the unconscious patient, the change in lung volume should be 95% complete in about 1.5 seconds, as in Figure 32.1.

The approach of the lung volume to its equilibrium value is according to an exponential function of the wash-in type (see Appendix F). The time constant, which is the time required for inflation to 63% of the equilibrium value, equals the product of resistance and

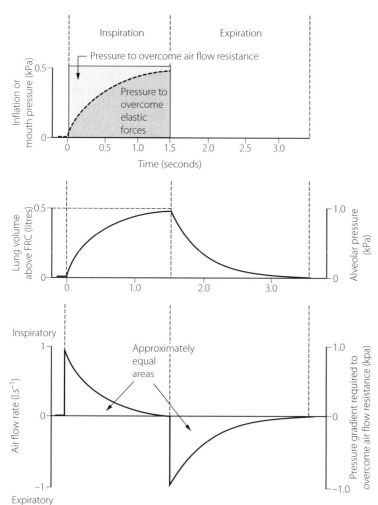

Figure 32.1 Artificial ventilation by intermittent application of a constant pressure (square wave) followed by passive expiration. Inspiratory and expiratory flow rates are both exponential. Assuming that air flow resistance is constant, it follows that the flow rate and pressure gradient required to overcome resistance may be shown on the same graph. Lung volume and alveolar pressure may be shown on the same graph if compliance is constant. Values are typical for an anaesthetised supine paralysed patient: total dynamic compliance, 0.5 l.kPa^{-1} (50 ml.cmH$_2$O^{-1}); pulmonary resistance 0.3 kPa.l^{-1}.s^{-1} (3 cmH$_2$O.l^{-1}.s^{-1}); apparatus resistance 0.7 kPa.l^{-1}.s^{-1} (7 cmH$_2$O.l^{-1}.s^{-1}); total resistance, 1 kPa.l^{-1}.s^{-1} (10 cmH$_2$O.l^{-1}.s^{-1}); time constant, 0.5 s.

compliance. Normal values for an unconscious patient are as follows:

$$\text{Time constant} = \text{resistance} \times \text{compliance}$$
$$0.5\,\text{second} = 1\,\text{kPa.l}^{-1}.\text{s}^{-1} \times 0.5\,\text{l.kPa}^{-1}$$
$$\text{or} \quad 0.5\,\text{second} = 10\,\text{cmH}_2\text{O.l}^{-1}.\text{s}^{-1} \times 0.05\,\text{l.cmH}_2\text{O}^{-1}$$

The time constant is the time that would be required to reach equilibrium if the initial inspiratory flow rate were maintained. It is sometimes more convenient to use the half-time, which is 0.69 times the time constant. The inflation curve is shown in full, with further mathematical detail in Appendix F.

It is normal practice for the inspiratory phase to be terminated after 1 or 2 seconds, at which time the lung volume will still be increasing. Inflation pressure is not then the sole arbiter of tidal volume but must be considered in relation to the duration of the inspiratory phase.

If expiration is passive and mouth pressure remains at ambient, the driving force is the elevation of alveolar pressure above ambient, caused by elastic recoil of lungs and chest wall. This pressure is dissipated in overcoming air flow resistance during expiration. In Figure 32.1, during expiration the alveolar pressure (proportional to the lung volume above FRC) is directly proportional to expiratory flow rate and all three quantities decline according to a wash-out exponential function, with a time constant which is again equal to the product of compliance and resistance.

The effect of changes in inflation pressure, resistance and compliance

The heavy line in Figure 32.2 shows the inflation curve for the normal parameters of an unconscious paralysed patient as listed in Table 32.1. These are the same values that were considered above. The basic curve is a single exponential approaching a lung volume 0.5 litre above FRC with a time constant of 0.5 seconds.

Changes in inflation pressure do not alter the time constant of inflation, but directly influence the amount of air introduced into the lungs in a given number of time constants. In Figure 32.2, each point on the curve labelled 'inflation pressure doubled' is twice the height of the corresponding point on the basic curve for the same time.

Effect of changes in compliance and resistance. If the compliance is doubled, the equilibrium tidal volume is also doubled. However, the time constant (product of compliance and resistance) is also doubled and therefore the equilibrium volume is approached more slowly (see Figure 32.2). Conversely, if the compliance is halved, the equilibrium tidal volume is also halved and so is the time constant.

Changes in resistance have a direct effect on the time constant of inflation but do not affect the equilibrium tidal volume. Thus the effect of an increased resistance on tidal volume is through the reduction in inspiratory flow rate. Within limits, this can be counteracted by prolonging inspiration or by increasing the inflation pressure and the degree of overpressure (explained below). The effects, shown in Figure 32.2, apply not only to the whole lung but also to regions that may have different compliances, resistances and time constants (page 111).

Overpressure. Increasing the inflation pressure has a major effect on the time required to achieve a particular lung volume above FRC. In Figure 32.3, the lung

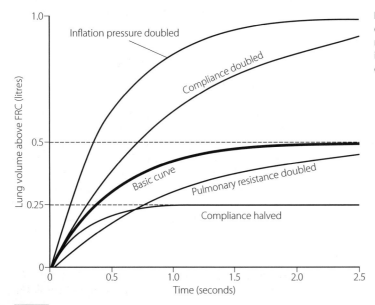

Figure 32.2 Effect of changes in various factors on the rate of inflation of the lungs. Fixed relationships: final tidal volume achieved = inflation pressure × compliance; time constant = compliance × resistance. (See also Table 32.1.)

Table 32.1 Parameters for inflation curves shown in Figure 32.2

	Basic curve	Pulmonary resistance doubled	Inflation pressure doubled	Compliance doubled	Compliance halved
Inflation pressure					
(kPa)	1	1	2	1	1
(cmH$_2$O)	10	10	20	10	10
Compliance					
(l.kPa^{-1})	0.5	0.5	0.5	1	0.25
(ml.cmH$_2$O^{-1})	50	50	50	100	25
Final tidal volume (l)	0.5	0.5	1	1	0.25
Pulmonary resistance					
(kPa.l^{-1}.s^{-1})	1	2	1	1	1
(cmH$_2$O.l^{-1}.s^{-1})	10	20	10	10	10
Time constant					
(seconds)	0.5	1	0.5	1	0.25

characteristics are the same as for the basic curve in Figure 32.2. If the required tidal volume is 475 ml, this is achieved in 1.5 seconds with an inflation pressure of 10 cmH$_2$O. However, the same lung volume is achieved in only 0.3 seconds by doubling the inflation pressure. The application of a pressure that, if sustained, would give a tidal volume higher than that which is intended is known as overpressure; it is used extensively to increase the inspiratory flow rate and so to shorten the inspiratory phase. The use of a subatmospheric pressure to increase the rate of passive expiration is similar in principle but is complicated by airway trapping (Figure 32.3b).

Deviations from true exponential character of expiration. It is helpful to assume that the patterns of air flow described above are exponential in character, as this greatly assists our understanding of the situation. However, there are many reasons why air flow should not be strictly exponential in character. Air flow is normally partly turbulent (see Chapter 4) and therefore resistance cannot be considered as a constant. Furthermore, as expiration proceeds, the calibre of the air passages decreases and there is also a transition to more laminar flow as the instantaneous flow rate decreases. Approximation to a single exponential function is nevertheless good enough for many practical purposes.

Alternative patterns of application of inflation pressure

Constant pressure or square wave inflation has been considered above because it is the easiest for mathematical analysis. There are, however, an almost infinite number of pressure profiles that may be applied for IPPV. There

is no very convincing evidence of the superiority of one over the other, except that distribution of inspired gas is improved if there is a prolongation of the period during which the applied pressure is maximal. This permits better ventilation of the 'slow' alveoli and is not very important in patients with relatively healthy lungs.

Constant flow rate ventilators are extensively used and Figure 32.4 shows pressure, volume and flow changes in a manner analogous to Figure 32.1.

Sine wave generators were popular in the days of mechanical ventilators. The pattern of inspiratory flow rate was a direct consequence of the mechanical linkage used in these ventilators, which are now only rarely used. Figure 32.5 shows the pattern of pressure, volume and flow rate changes with a sine wave generator.

Control of duration of inspiration

Three methods are in general use.

Time cycling terminates inspiration after a preset time. With mechanical ventilators delivering a sine pressure wave, the inspiratory time usually derives directly from the system itself. However, with constant pressure generators and constant flow generators, a separate and variable timing system is used. With constant flow generators, inspiratory time has a direct effect on the tidal volume. With constant pressure generators the relationship is more complex, as described above (see Figure 32.3).

Volume cycling terminates inspiration when a preset volume has been delivered. In the absence of a leak this

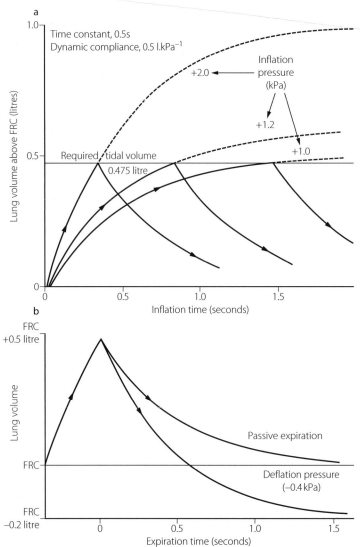

a

Time constant, 0.5 s
Dynamic compliance, 0.5 l.kPa^{-1}

Inflation
pressure
(kPa)

+2.0

+1.2

+1.0

Required tidal volume
0.475 litre

Lung volume above FRC (litres)

Inflation time (seconds)

b

FRC
+0.5 litre

Lung volume

Passive expiration

FRC

Deflation pressure
(−0.4 kPa)

FRC
−0.2 litre

Expiration time (seconds)

Figure 32.3 **(a)** How the duration of inflation may be shortened by the use of overpressure. Inflation curves are shown for +2 kPa (+20 cmH$_2$O) (equilibrium 1 litre), +1.2 kPa (+12 cmH$_2$O) (equilibrium 0.6 litre) and +1 kPa (+10 cmH$_2$O) (equilibrium 0.5 litre). With a required tidal volume of 0.475 litre, note the big reduction in duration of inflation needed when the inflation pressure is increased from 1 to 2 kPa (10 to 20 cmH$_2$O). **(b)** How expiration is influenced by the use of a subatmospheric pressure or 'negative phase'. Expiration may be terminated at the FRC after 0.6 s or may be prolonged, in which case the lung volume will fall to 0.2 litre below FRC.

should guarantee the tidal volume even if the compliance or resistance of the lungs changes within limits. Formerly, volume-cycled ventilators were usually based on a reciprocating pump of preset tidal volume. Nowadays they are more likely to be flow generators with an inspiratory flow sensor that terminates inspiration when the required volume (integral of flow rate) has entered the lungs.

Pressure cycling terminates inspiration when a particular mouth pressure is achieved. This in no way guarantees the tidal volume. Increased airway resistance, for example, would limit inspiratory flow rate and cause a more rapid increase in mouth pressure, thus terminating the inspiratory phase. Pressure-cycled ventilators are almost invariably flow generators.

Limitations on inspiratory duration. Whatever the means of cycling, it is possible to add a limitation on inspiratory duration, usually as a safety precaution. For example, a pressure limitation can be added to a time-cycled or a volume-cycled ventilator. This can either function as a pressure relief valve or it can terminate the inspiratory phase.

The inspiratory/expiratory (I/E) ratio

For a given minute volume of ventilation, it is possible to vary within wide limits the duration of inspiration and expiration and the ratio between the two. A common pattern is about 1 second for inspiration, followed by 2–4 seconds for expiration (*I/E* ratio 1/2–1/4), giving respiratory frequencies in the range 12–20 breaths per

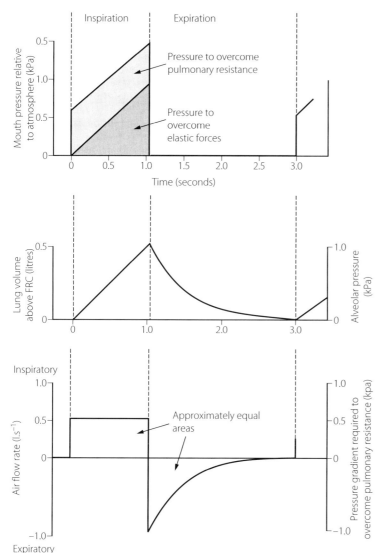

Figure 32.4 Artificial ventilation by intermittent application of a constant flow, with passive expiration. Note that inspiratory flow rate is constant. Assuming that pulmonary resistance is constant, it follows that a constant amount of the inflation pressure is required to overcome flow resistance. Lung volume and alveolar pressure may be shown on the same graph if compliance is constant. Values are typical for an anaesthetised supine paralysed patient: total dynamic compliance, 0.5 l.kPa^{-1} (50 ml.cmH$_2$O^{-1}); pulmonary resistance 0.3 kPa.l^{-1}.s^{-1} (3 cmH$_2$O.l^{-1}.s^{-1}); apparatus resistance 0.7 kPa.l^{-1}.s^{-1} (7 cmH$_2$O.l^{-1}.s^{-1}); total resistance, 1 kPa.l^{-1}.s^{-1} (10 cmH$_2$O.l^{-1}.s^{-1}); time constant, 0.5 s.

minute. The problem is whether changes from this pattern confer any appreciable benefit in terms of gas exchange. Reduction of the inspiratory time to less than 1 second may cause an increase in dead space, but there is no evidence that the duration of inspiration (in the range 0.5–3 seconds) has any appreciable effect on the alveolar/arterial $P\mathrm{O_2}$ gradient. Thus the accepted view seems to be that 1 second is a reasonable minimal time for inspiration.

Inverse I/E ratio ventilation has the effect of increasing the mean lung volume and so may be expected to achieve some of the advantages of PEEP, as considered

below. It may be achieved either by slowing the inspiratory flow rate (shallow ramp) or by holding the lung volume at the end of inspiration (inspiratory pause), the latter seeming to be more logical. I/E ratios as high as 4/1 have been used but 2/1 is generally preferable. The degree of inverse I/E ratio used is limited by the cardiovascular disturbances seen with the technique (see below) and the time available for expiration. If the latter is unduly curtailed, FRC will be increased, generating so-called 'intrinsic PEEP' (see below).

Gas redistribution during an inspiratory hold reduces the dead space (page 120) and so results in a lower $P\mathrm{CO_2}$ for the same minute volume.[14] This permits the use of a lower peak inflation pressure.

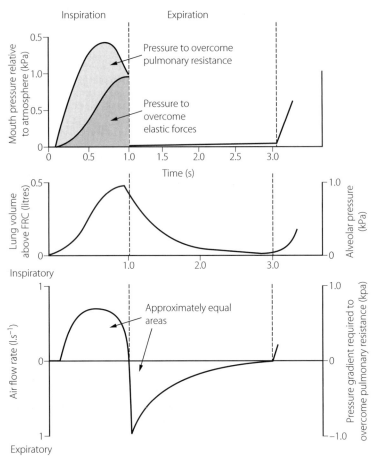

Figure 32.5 Artificial ventilation with inspiratory gas flow conforming to a sine wave, with passive expiration. Note that inspiratory gas flow rate is out of phase with the change in lung volume. (The latter conforms to a sine wave and the former to the differential of the sine, which is the cosine.) Assuming that air flow resistance is constant, it follows that flow rate and pressure gradient required to overcome resistance may be shown on the same graph. Lung volume and alveolar pressure may be shown on the same graph if compliance is constant. Peak inspiratory flow rate = π × minute volume × 1.5. (The factor 1.5 is used because in this example inspiration does not last half the respiratory cycle.) Values are typical for an anaesthetised supine paralysed patient: total dynamic compliance, 0.5 l.kPa^{-1} 50 ml.cmH$_2$O^{-1}); pulmonary resistance 0.3 kPa.l^{-1}.s^{-1} (3 cmH$_2$O.l^{-1}.s^{-1}); apparatus resistance 0.7 kPa.l^{-1}.s^{-1} (7 cmH$_2$O.l^{-1}.s^{-1}); total resistance, 1 kPa.l^{-1}.s^{-1} (10 cmH$_2$O.l^{-1}.s^{-1}); time constant, 0.5 s.

Interaction of ventilator controls

The usual controls that are provided on an artificial ventilator are drawn from the following list:

- Tidal volume
- Inspiratory flow rate
- Duration of inspiration
- Duration of expiration
- I/E ratio
- Respiratory frequency
- Minute volume.

It will be found that the maximum possible number of independent controls is three. A setting of any three on this list will determine the values for all the remaining variables. Opinion is divided on which of these controls the clinician should operate directly. With the advent of electronically controlled ventilators, many of these controls may be altered by the user while the remainder are simultaneously displayed, allowing the user to immediately see the effect of the changes being made.

CLINICAL USE OF IPPV

The previous section classifies ventilators according to the method of gas flow generation – for example, constant flow, constant pressure or sine wave generators – based on the mechanism by which the ventilator worked. Most ventilators in clinical use in the developed world are now electronically controlled. These allow accurate control of gas pressure and flow throughout the ventilator circuit and can normally perform as either flow or pressure generators, usually with a variety of inspiratory flow patterns. In addition, they have given rise to a whole host of previously impossible ventilatory techniques, a majority of which are dependent on the ventilator responding appropriately to the patient's own respiratory efforts.

Interactions between patient and ventilator

For many years there have been ventilators in which the inspiratory phase could be triggered with a spontaneous breath and mechanical ventilators could be modified to facilitate a mandatory minute volume of ventilation, as described below. Electronic ventilators continuously monitor tidal volume, whether generated by the patient (spontaneous breath) or artificially (ventilator breath). With this information available it is a simple task to achieve, by electronic means, a predetermined minute volume, number of breaths etc. by introducing extra ventilator breaths when necessary. The challenge for ventilator design in recent years has been the speed and sensitivity with which ventilators can sense and respond to the patient's own respiratory efforts in order to synchronise ventilator and spontaneous breaths. Without this synchronisation, a patient with any reasonable spontaneous respiratory effort begins to 'fight' against the ventilator,[15] leading to discomfort, poor gas exchange and cardiovascular disturbance.

There are two ways by which a ventilator may detect the onset of a spontaneous breath.[16]

Pressure sensing. At the onset of a respiratory effort, the patient will generate a reduction in pressure within the circuit, which may be detected in the ventilator. This pressure wave travels through the circuit at approximately the speed of sound and so reaches the ventilator within 12 ms, following which the pressure sensor must respond and flow into the circuit be increased to facilitate inspiration. Overall, these events take approximately 100 ms to occur, which is undetectable by the patient. The pressure drop required to trigger inspiration is now always measured relative to circuit (not atmospheric) pressure, to allow the use of CPAP during ventilation. The time taken to trigger the ventilator increases with decreased sensitivity settings, that is, when a greater pressure drop is required for triggering. Pressure triggering is also affected by the circuit compliance, which is a function of the circuit volume and the stiffness of the tubing.

Flow sensing. Detection of inspiratory flow may trigger a ventilator breath or some type of respiratory assist (see below). Many current intensive care ventilators provide a continuous base flow around the ventilator circuit of $2-20$ l.min^{-1}. Any difference between ventilator inflow and outflow represents the patient's respiration. Flow triggering occurs in approximately 80 ms, irrespective of the sensitivity setting. A high base flow provides adequate inspiratory flow for the patient at the start of inspiration and the flow rate is increased when the ventilator is triggered. Flow sensing can also detect the end of inspiration and is used in pressure support ventilation (see below).

Ventilatory modes in common use

In addition to control mode ventilation (CMV), there are now a bewildering range of ventilation patterns. Many of these are essentially the same but have different nomenclatures owing to their development by rival ventilator manufacturers. Those in common use are described below and shown graphically in Figure 32.6.

Mandatory minute volume (MMV). Introduced in the 1970s, this was a simple technique for controlling the volume of artificial ventilation so that the total of spontaneous and artificial ventilation did not fall below a preset value. If the patient was able to achieve the preset level of MMV, ventilator breaths did not occur. Electronic ventilators allow MMV to be used and can coordinate the mandatory breaths with patient respiration to a greater degree than the original mechanical technique, including provision for the spontaneous ventilation to exceed the MMV. Achievement of the preset MMV by a rapid, shallow respiratory pattern commonly seen in intensive care patients was a major disadvantage of MMV, which has now been almost entirely replaced by other techniques.

Assist-control ventilation or synchronised IPPV (Figure 32.6c). This was one of the earlier ventilatory modes that depended on patient triggering of ventilator breaths. It is essentially the same as volume preset IPPV except that breaths are triggered by the patient, normally as a result of reduced circuit pressure. A maximum time delay between breaths is incorporated, following which a breath will be generated by the ventilator if spontaneous triggering has ceased. There is no provision for spontaneous breathing between ventilator breaths.

Airway pressure release ventilation (Figure 32.6d).[17,18] This ventilation mode differs significantly from all other forms of positive-pressure ventilation and is essentially the reverse of IPPV. It consists of maintaining the breathing system at an upper airway pressure level (P_{high}), which is intermittently released to a lower airway pressure level (P_{low}), causing the patient to *exhale* to FRC. The pattern of the imposed breaths is similar to that of reversed I/E ratio. The patient is able to breathe spontaneously throughout the entire respiratory cycle, but most of the time this will be during P_{high}, when inspiration will start from a lung volume greater than FRC. Artificial breaths are thus within the conventional tidal range set by the patient's FRC, whereas spontaneous inspirations are usually within his inspiratory reserve. More frequent and longer periods at P_{low} lead to a greater minute volume, and so improved elimination of carbon dioxide and a lower mean airway pressure,[19] but are also

Figure 32.6 Airway pressure during a variety of commonly used modes of ventilation. **(a)** CPAP, continuous positive airway pressure, and sPEEP, true positive end-expiratory pressure, applied during spontaneous breathing. **(b)** CMV, control mode ventilation, showing volume and pressure-controlled inspiration. **(c)** A-CMV, assist-control mode ventilation, where breaths are triggered by a fall in circuit pressure. When apnoea occurs, ventilator breaths occur without triggering. **(d)** APRV, airway pressure release ventilation, with an upper airway pressure (P_{high}) of 8 cmH$_2$O and simultaneous spontaneous breathing. **(e)** SIMV, synchronised intermittent mandatory ventilation, as for A-CMV except that spontaneous breathing can occur between ventilator breaths. **(f)** PSV, pressure support ventilation, in which pressure-controlled breaths are triggered by the patient, who also controls the duration of each breath. In practice, many ventilators allow combinations of these modes, such as SIMV, PSV and PEEP together.

associated with greater likelihood of pulmonary collapse in injured lungs and, as a consequence, worsening of oxygenation.

Synchronised intermittent mandatory ventilation (SIMV) (Figure 32.6e). Intermittent mandatory ventilation was introduced in the 1970s, followed a few years later by the ability to synchronise ventilator breaths with the patient's own respiratory effort as described above. The essential feature of SIMV is to allow the patient to take a spontaneous breath between artificial breaths. This confers three major advantages. First, a spontaneous inspiration is not obstructed by a closed inspiratory valve and this helps to prevent the patient fighting the venti-

lator. The second advantage is the facilitation of weaning, which is considered below. Third, the patient is able to breathe spontaneously at any time during prolonged ventilation; this may prevent respiratory muscle atrophy and helps to reduce the mean intrathoracic pressure. Most ventilators now provide SIMV as a normal feature and it is used extensively in many parts of the world, often in conjunction with pressure support ventilation (see below).

Pressure support ventilation (PSV) (Figure 32.6f).[20,21] In this system a spontaneous inspiration triggers a rapid flow of gas that increases until airway pressure reaches a preselected level. Flow sensing by the ventilator is also then able to detect when the spontaneous inspiration ends, at which point the pressure support ceases and expiration occurs. The purpose is not to provide a prescribed tidal volume, but to assist the patient in making an inspiration of a pattern that lies largely within his own control. The level of support may be increased until the pressure is sufficient to provide the full tidal volume (maximal pressure support) and may be gradually reduced as the patient's ventilatory capacity improves. The amount of pressure support provided does seem to be inversely related to the work of breathing.[21]

High-frequency ventilation[22]

High-frequency ventilation may be classified into the following categories: high-frequency positive-pressure ventilation (HFPPV), high-frequency jet ventilation (HFJV) and high-frequency oscillation (HFO).

High-frequency positive-pressure ventilation (HFPPV) is applied in the frequency range 1–2 Hz (60–120 breaths.min^{-1}) and can be considered as an extension of conventional IPPV techniques. Although many conventional ventilators will operate within this frequency range, specially designed ventilators have been used.

High-frequency jet ventilation (HFJV) covers the frequency range 1–5 Hz. Inspiration is driven by a high-velocity stream of gas from a jet, which may or may not entrain gas from a secondary supply. Humidification with HFJV is technically difficult and, if done properly, requires equipment as complex as the ventilator itself. The position of the jet may be proximal to the patient, in the hope of avoiding dead space, or more distal, which is safer in terms of mucosal trauma and thermal injury from cooling due to the Joule–Kelvin effect.[22] A unique advantage is the ability to ventilate through a narrow cannula, as for example through the cricothyroid membrane.

HFJV has been extensively used both in the operating theatre and also during intensive therapy. Jet systems are extremely versatile. Jets may face towards or away from the patient and may thus power inspiration, retard expiration, assist expiration or provide PEEP.

High-frequency oscillation (HFO)[23] covers the frequency range 3–50 Hz and the flows are usually generated by an oscillating pump making a fourth connection to a T-piece. At these high frequencies, the respiratory waveform is usually sinusoidal, including active expiration. Tidal volumes are inevitably small and are difficult to measure.

The relationship between tidal volume and dead space during high-frequency ventilation is crucial to an under-

Table 32.2 Gas exchange during high-frequency ventilation

		Respiratory frequency		
		15 bpm 0.25 Hz	60 bpm 1 Hz	120 bpm 2 Hz
Arterial P_{CO_2}	kPa	4.8	4.8	4.9
	mmHg	36	36	37
$\dot{V}$	l.min^{-1}	6.8	10.2	14
V_T	ml	454	170	117
V_D (physiol.)	ml	165	96	88
V_D/V_T ratio	%	36	56	75

bpm, breaths per minute. Data from reference 24.

standing of the technique. It is useless to infer values for tidal volume and dead space from measurements made under other circumstances, and yet it is very difficult to make direct measurements of these variables under the actual conditions of high-frequency ventilation, especially in humans. Chakrabarti and colleagues[24] studied anaesthetised humans during HFPPV up to frequencies of 2 Hz, holding arterial P_{CO_2} approximately constant at about 5 kPa (37.5 mmHg). As frequency increased from conventional ventilation at 15 breaths.min^{-1} to HFPPV at 2 Hz it was necessary to double the minute volume (Table 32.2). The actual volume of the physiological dead space decreased with decreasing tidal volume to reach a minimal value of about 90 ml at 1 Hz. However, the normal proportionality between dead space and tidal volume (page 120) was not maintained. Dead space/tidal volume ratio increased from 37% at 15 breaths.min^{-1} to 75% at 2 Hz, which explains the requirement for the increased minute volume. The situation is more complex at higher frequencies. One study found that tidal volumes of at least 100 ml were still required at frequencies of 15 Hz, corresponding to an *applied* minute volume of 90 l.min^{-1}, which would indicate a dead space/tidal volume ratio of over 90%.[25] There are severe technical difficulties in the measurement of the actual delivered tidal volumes which, though undoubtedly less than the pump settings, are probably much larger than the external movements of the thorax would suggest.

End-expiratory pressure is inevitably raised at high frequencies because the duration of expiration will be inadequate for passive exhalation to FRC, the time constant of the normal respiratory system being about 0.5 second (see above). Therefore, the use of respiratory frequencies above about 2 Hz will usually result in 'intrinsic' PEEP,[26] and hence an increased end-expiratory lung volume, which is likely to be a major factor promoting favourable gas exchange.

Gas mixing and streaming is likely to be modified at high frequencies. The sudden reversals of flow direction are likely to set up eddies that blur the boundary between dead space and alveolar gas, thus improving the efficiency of ventilation. It has been suggested that such 'enhanced diffusion' or 'augmented dispersion' plays a major role in gas exchange during HFO.[25] Air passages dilated by intrinsic PEEP may contribute to this effect. Furthermore, cardiac mixing of gases becomes relatively more important at small tidal volumes.[27] It has also been suggested that high-frequency ventilation causes 'accelerated diffusion', but this is difficult to demonstrate.

The clinical indications for high-frequency ventilation remain unclear. The techniques have been used mainly for weaning from artificial ventilation in adults and for respiratory support in babies.[23] HFJV seems to have a wider acceptance than HFPPV or HFO, but randomised trials have generally failed to demonstrate any clear clinical advantage over conventional methods of ventilation.[28,29] There is no doubt that effective gas exchange is usually possible with high-frequency ventilation but the advantages over conventional artificial ventilation are less clear. Although there are enthusiasts, others believe that it is merely a technique in search of an application. There is agreement on its special role for patients with bronchopleural fistula and the technique is particularly convenient when there is no airtight junction between ventilator and the tracheobronchial tree, during surgery on the airway for example. Another attractive feature is the avoidance of high *peak* inspiratory pressures. However, *mean* airway pressure may still be high if exhalation is impeded, as it must be at very high frequencies. Whether high-frequency ventilation is less likely to produce pulmonary barotrauma than conventional techniques of ventilation will be difficult to determine in man, but animal experiments suggest this may be so. A recently developed non-invasive form of high-frequency ventilation is described above.

Weaning[30,31]

Weaning is the process by which artificial ventilation is gradually withdrawn and the patient returned to normal respiration. In practice it is useful to think of two stages: the withdrawal of respiratory support and the removal of any artificial airway, usually a tracheal tube or tracheostomy. Only the first of these stages is considered here.

Predicting successful weaning. Before weaning can be attempted, the balance between ventilatory load and capacity must be favourable. Extra demands on the respiratory system may originate from increased oxygen consumption, commonly as a result of sepsis but also

Table 32.3 Measurements of lung function used to assess suitability for weaning from artificial ventilation

Measurement	Value for successful weaning
Measured on ventilator:	
$Pa_{O_2} : Fi_{O_2}$ ratio	>20 (Pa_{O_2} in kPa) or 150 (Pa_{O_2} in mmHg)
Resting minute volume	<10 l.min^{-1}
Negative inspiratory force	−20 to −30 cmH$_2$O
PI_{max}	−15 to −30 cmH$_2$O
$P_{0.1}/PI_{max}$	>0.3
CROP score	≥13 ml.breath^{-1}.min
Measured during brief period of spontaneous breathing:	
Respiratory rate	<30 breaths.min^{-1}
Tidal volume	>4–6 ml.kg^{-1}
Respiratory rate : tidal volume ratio	>60 breaths.l^{-1}
RVR score	≤105 breaths.min^{-1}.l^{-1}

PI_{max}, maximal inspiratory pressure; $P_{0.1}$, mouth occlusion 0.1 s after the onset of inspiration; CROP and RVR scores, see text for details. (After references 31 and 32.)

occasionally from thyrotoxicosis, convulsions or shivering. Reduced respiratory system compliance or increased airway resistance also imposes additional loads on the respiratory system. The capacity of the respiratory system to wean depends on having, first, adequate ventilation perfusion matching and, second, low intrapulmonary shunt and respiratory dead space. Finally, good respiratory muscle function must be achieved (page 84), including correction of any metabolic disturbance and provision of adequate blood supply to the muscles; that is, the patient must have reasonable cardiovascular function. Over 60 different measurements of lung function have been reported to predict successful weaning from ventilatory support. Some of the more widely accepted ones are shown in Table 32.3.

No single variable is a reliable indicator of success, with most having very low predictive values. This has led to the development of more complex scoring systems, which include the Compliance, Rate, Oxygenation, Pressure (CROP) score, calculated as:

$$CROP = \text{dynamic } Crs \times PI_{max} \times (Pa_{O_2}/PA_{O_2})/\text{respiratory rate}$$

(Crs, respiratory system compliance; PI_{max} maximum inspiratory pressure).

Rate/volume ratio (RVR) score is respiratory rate (breaths.min^{-1}) divided by tidal volume (litres) measured over 1 minute without artificial ventilation.

A CROP score of ≤ 13 ml.breaths^{-1}.min^{-1} or an RVR score ≤ 105 breaths.min^{-1}.l^{-1} are both reasonable predictors of successful weaning.[32]

Techniques for weaning. Recent guidelines suggest that once these predictors indicate that discontinuation of ventilation may be possible, a trial of spontaneous breathing should be undertaken.[31] During this trial, which should last between 30 and 120 minutes, the patient breathes spontaneously with only minimal respiratory support and is closely observed to ensure that respiratory pattern, patient comfort, gas exchange and cardiovascular stability are all acceptable. If this trial of spontaneous breathing fails, appropriate degrees of ventilatory support should be recommenced and further trials of spontaneous breathing performed at 24-hour intervals if the predictors of successful weaning remain satisfactory.

Ventilation strategies to use between trials of spontaneous breathing focus on gradual withdrawal of respiratory support using the techniques described above. Control-mode ventilation is usually replaced by either SIMV or A-CMV until the patient has established adequate respiratory effort, following which the number of ventilator breaths can be gradually reduced. While breathing via an artificial airway some respiratory support is normally required, and this is most commonly provided with PSV, the level of which can again be gradually reduced.

It is important not to place excessive reliance on modern ventilator systems to wean patients from ventilatory support.[33] Close attention must also be paid to nutrition, psychological care such as establishment of normal night/day sleep patterns, and the use of non-invasive ventilation (page 420) following early extubation.

POSITIVE END-EXPIRATORY PRESSURE

A great variety of pathological conditions, as well as general anaesthesia, result in a decrease in FRC. The deleterious effect of this on gas exchange has been considered elsewhere (page 310) and it is reasonable to consider increasing the FRC by the application of PEEP, first described by Hill *et al.* in 1965.[34]

Expiratory pressure can be raised during both artificial ventilation and spontaneous breathing and the two forms are best considered together. The terminology is confusing and this chapter adheres to the definitions illustrated in Figure 32.6. Note in particular sPEEP, in which a patient inhales spontaneously from ambient pressure but exhales against PEEP. This involves him in a considerable amount of additional work of breathing because he must raise his entire minute volume to the level of PEEP that is applied. This is undesirable and CPAP is much to be preferred to sPEEP.

True CPAP is more difficult to achieve than sPEEP. Biased demand valves may be used but usually result in a pronounced dip in inspiratory pressure, increasing the total work of breathing. The simplest approach is a T-piece with a high fresh gas flow venting through a PEEP valve at the expiratory limb throughout the respiratory phase. Electronic ventilators produce CPAP in a similar fashion by circulating high flows of gas around the ventilator circuit at the required positive pressure.

PEEP may be achieved by many techniques. The simplest is to exhale through a preset depth of water, but more convenient methods are spring-loaded valves or diaphragms pressed down by gas, a column of water or a spring. It is also possible to use Venturis and fans opposing the direction of expiratory gas flow.

Intrinsic PEEP[15]

If a passive expiration is terminated before the lung volume has returned to FRC, there will be residual end-expiratory raised alveolar pressure, variously known as dynamic hyperinflation, auto-PEEP or intrinsic PEEP (PEEPi).[35] The elevated alveolar pressure will not be transmitted back to the ventilator pressure sensors, so PEEPi may go undetected,[36] but simple methods to measure it have been described.[35] Artificial ventilation with inverse I/E ratio may result in PEEPi, but it is more commonly a result of increased expiratory flow resistance due to airway disease or retention of mucus, or from the tracheal tube (Figure 32.7). Eventually, alveolar pressure and lung volume increase sufficiently to cause reductions in both lung compliance and airway resistance (pages 29 and 43); expiratory flow rate then increases and so the degree of PEEPi stabilises.

At first sight PEEPi may be perceived as beneficial – for example, leading to increased FRC and alveolar recruitment – and it is likely that improved gas exchange seen with inverse I/E ratio results, at least in part, from this mechanism. However, the first hazard of PEEPi is its variability. Small changes in airway resistance, for example with mucus retention, can lead to rapid increases in the level of PEEPi. The cardiovascular consequences of PEEPi are significant (see below) and have been described as 'applying a tourniquet to the right heart'.[36] Finally, the presence of PEEPi will impede the ability of the patient to trigger ventilators by necessitating a greater fall in alveolar pressure to initiate respiratory support.[15]

Application of external PEEP will, to some extent, attenuate the generation of PEEPi by maintaining airway patency in late expiration and so improving expiratory flow.

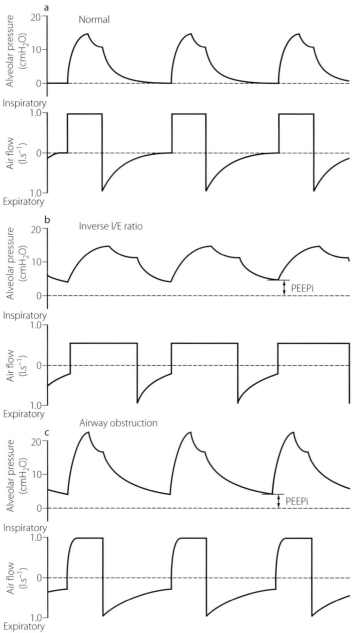

Figure 32.7 Pressure and flow curves demonstrating generation of intrinsic positive end-expiratory pressure (PEEPi). **(a)** Normal ventilation with both alveolar pressure and airway flow returning to zero before the next breath. **(b)** Inverse I/E ratio ventilation. Although the decline in pressure and flow is normal, there is insufficient time for complete expiration to occur. **(c)** Airway obstruction. Expiratory time is normal, but the decline in pressure and flow is retarded to such an extent that expiration is again incomplete.

PHYSIOLOGICAL EFFECTS OF POSITIVE-PRESSURE VENTILATION

A positive pressure in the chest cavity is a significant physiological insult that normally occurs only transiently with coughing, straining etc., although the pressure achieved in these situations may be very high. Most physiological effects of IPPV are related to the mean pressure throughout the whole respiratory cycle, which is in turn influenced by a large number of ventilatory settings, such as mode of ventilation, tidal volume, respiratory rate and I/E ratio. PEEP results in large increases in mean intrathoracic pressure. For example, IPPV in a patient with normal lungs using 10 breaths of 10 ml.kg^{-1} and an I/E ratio of 1:2 will generate mean airway pressures of approximately 5 cmH$_2$O. Addition of a modest 5 cmH$_2$O of PEEP will therefore double the mean airway pressure and thus the physiological insult associated with IPPV. For this reason, much research into the physiological effects of artificial ventilation has focused on PEEP.

Respiratory effects

Distribution of ventilation. Intermittent positive-pressure ventilation results in a spatial pattern of distribution that is determined by inflation pressure, regional compliance and time constants. Based on external measurements, the anatomical pattern of distribution of inspired gas is different from that of spontaneous breathing, there being a relatively greater expansion of the ribcage.[37] However, with spontaneous breathing regional differences in ventilation are small in the supine position (page 110) and in spite of the altered ribcage motion, changes in regional ventilation with IPPV are minimal.[38] It thus seems that, although the spatial distribution of gas appears to be altered by IPPV, the functional effect is minimal. Application of PEEP increases lung volume and, at high levels, reexpands collapsed alveoli, which changes the compliance of dependent lung regions and so improves ventilation of these areas.

Apparatus dead space. Positive-pressure ventilation, whether invasive or non-invasive, requires the provision of an airtight connection to the patient's airway. This inevitably involves the addition of some apparatus dead space. With orotracheal and tracheostomy tubes much of the normal anatomical dead space (page 119) is bypassed, such that overall anatomical dead space may be unchanged or reduced. With non-invasive ventilation using facemasks, apparatus dead space may be substantial. Ventilator tubing used to deliver IPPV is normally corrugated and expands longitudinally with each inspiration. For an average ventilator circuit, this expansion may amount to 2–3 ml per cmH_2O of positive pressure,[1] and this volume will constitute dead space ventilation.

Physiological dead space. In normal lungs during anaesthesia, IPPV alone seems to have little effect on the V_D/V_T ratio compared with the value obtained with spontaneous breathing.[39] There is a slight widening of the distribution of $\dot{V}/\dot{Q}$ ratios (page 115), mostly as a result of a reduction in pulmonary blood flow from depression of cardiac output (see below). These changes are normally not sufficient to alter gas exchange. The acute application of moderate amounts of PEEP causes only a slight increase in V_D/V_T ratio.[39]

The alveolar component of physiological dead space may be increased by ventilation in patients with lung injury or when mean intrathoracic pressure is high, such as with significant amounts of PEEP. Under the latter conditions, lung volume is increased to such an extent that not only does cardiac output fall but pulmonary vas-

cular resistance rises as well (see Figure 7.4).[40] Perfusion to overexpanded alveoli is reduced and areas of lung with high $\dot{V}/\dot{Q}$ ratios develop, which constitute alveolar dead space. In healthy lungs, this effect is not seen until PEEP levels exceed 10–15 cmH_2O.[39] However, with IPPV in lung injury there is now good evidence that overdistension occurs in the relatively small number of functional alveoli (page 414) and local perfusion to these lung units is likely to be impeded.

There is indirect evidence that long-term application of PEEP may cause a very large increase in the dead space, probably because of bronchiolar dilation (see below).

Lung volume. IPPV and ZEEP will have no effect on FRC. However, with PEEP, end-expiratory alveolar pressure will equal the level of applied PEEP and this will reset the FRC in accord with the pressure/volume curve of the respiratory system (see Figure 3.7). For example, PEEP of 10 cmH_2O will increase FRC by 500 ml in a patient with a compliance of 0.5 $l.kPa^{-1}$ (50 $ml.cmH_2O^{-1}$). In many patients this may be expected to raise the tidal range above the closing capacity (page 34) and so reduce pulmonary collapse. Prevention of alveolar collapse is probably the greatest single advantage of PEEP. It will also reduce airway resistance according to the inverse relationship between lung volume and airway resistance (see Figure 4.5). It may also change the relative compliance of the upper and lower parts of the lung (Figure 32.8), thereby improving the ventilation of the dependent overperfused parts of the lung.

Alveolar/capillary permeability. It has been found that PEEP increases the permeability of the lung to DTPA, a tracer molecule that does not readily cross the alveolar/capillary membrane. However, it appears that this effect may be related to lung volume rather than to any damage to the membrane. The effect of PEEP on extravascular lung water distribution is discussed on page 392.

Arterial Po_2. Neither IPPV nor PEEP will appreciably improve arterial oxygenation in patients with healthy lungs. During anaesthesia, it has been repeatedly observed that PEEP does little to improve arterial oxygenation in healthy patients. Pulmonary shunting is decreased, but the accompanying decrease in cardiac output reduces the mixed venous oxygen saturation, which counteracts the effect of a reduction in the shunt, resulting in minimal increase in arterial Po_2.[39] There is, however, no doubt that positive-pressure ventilation improves arterial Po_2 in a wide range of pathological situations. In most cases, the improvement in Po_2 relates to the mean airway pressure achieved and, as described above, PEEP provides an easy way of elevating airway pressures. Re-expansion of collapsed lung units, improved ventilation of alveoli with low $\dot{V}/\dot{Q}$ ratios and redistribution of extravascular lung water will all contribute to the observed improvement in oxygenation. The use of PEEP for prevention of atelectasis in anaesthesia is described on page 307, and its contributions to the treatment of pulmonary oedema and acute lung injury are described on pages 392 and 414, respectively.

The Valsalva effect

It has long been known that an increase in intrathoracic pressure has complex circulatory effects, characterised as the Valsalva effect, which is the circulatory response to a subject increasing his airway pressure to about 5 kPa (50 cmH$_2$O) against a closed glottis for about 30 seconds. The normal response is in four parts (Figure 32.9a). Initially the raised intrathoracic pressure alters the baseline for circulatory pressures and the arterial pressure (measured relative to atmosphere) is consequently increased (phase 1). At the same time, ventricular filling is decreased by the adverse pressure gradient from peripheral veins to the ventricle in diastole and cardiac output therefore decreases. The consequent decline in arterial pressure in phase 2 is normally mitigated by three factors: tachycardia, increased systemic vascular resistance (afterload) and an increase in peripheral venous pressure, which tends to restore the venous return. As a result of these compensations, the arterial pressure normally settles to a value fairly close to the level before starting the Valsalva manoeuvre. When the intrathoracic pressure is restored to normal, there is an

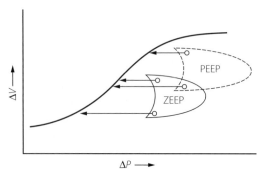

Figure 32.8 Effect of positive end-expiratory pressure (PEEP) on the relationship between regional pressure and volume in the lung (supine position). Note that compliance is greater in the upper part of the lung with zero end-expiratory pressure (ZEEP) and in the lower part of the lung with PEEP, which thus improves ventilation in the dependent zone of the lung. (Diagram kindly supplied by Professor J Gareth Jones.)

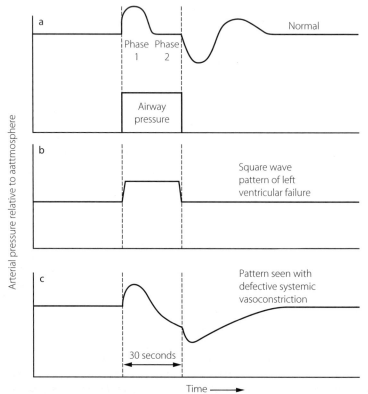

Figure 32.9 Qualitative changes in mean arterial blood pressure during a Valsalva manoeuvre as seen in the normal subject and for two abnormal responses. See text for explanation of the changes.

immediate decrease in arterial pressure due to the altered baseline. Simultaneously the venous return improves and therefore the cardiac output increases within a few seconds. However, the arteriolar bed remains temporarily constricted and there is therefore a transient overshoot of arterial pressure.

Figure 32.9b shows the abnormal 'square wave' pattern that occurs with raised end-diastolic pressure or left ventricular failure or both. The initial increase in arterial pressure (phase 1) occurs normally, but the decline in pressure in phase 2 is missing because the output of the congested heart is not usually limited by end-diastolic pressure. Because the cardiac output is unchanged, there is no increase in pulse rate or systemic vascular resistance. Therefore there is no overshoot of pressure when the intrathoracic pressure is restored to normal.

Figure 32.9c shows a different abnormal pattern, which may be seen with defective systemic vasoconstriction (e.g. autonomic neuropathy or a spinal anaesthetic). Phase 1 is normal, but in phase 2 the decreased cardiac output is not accompanied by an increase in systemic vascular resistance and the arterial pressure therefore continues to decline. The normal overshoot is replaced by a slow recovery of arterial pressure as the cardiac output returns to control values.

Cardiovascular effects of positive-pressure ventilation[41,42]

Initially there was great reluctance to use PEEP, partly because of the well-known Valsalva effect and partly because of the circulatory hazard that had been described in the classic paper of Cournand and his colleagues in 1948.[43] Not many papers in this field have two Nobel prize winners among their authors. The cardiovascular effects of IPPV and PEEP continue to cause problems in clinical practice, and after another half century of investigation the effects remain incompletely elucidated.

Cardiac output.[41] Bindslev *et al.*[39] reported a progressive decrease in cardiac output with IPPV and PEEP in anaesthetised patients without pulmonary pathology. Compared with when anaesthetised and breathing spontaneously, cardiac output was reduced by 10% with IPPV and ZEEP, 18% with 9 cmH$_2$O of PEEP and 36% with 16 cmH$_2$O of PEEP. Another study, this time in patients with severe acute lung injury, also demonstrated a progressive reduction in cardiac output for PEEP in the range 5–30 cmH$_2$O, but the effect was partially reversed by blood volume expansion (Figure 32.10).

There is general agreement that the main cause of the reduction in cardiac output is obstruction to filling of the right atrium, caused by the elevated intrathoracic pressure. With spontaneous respiration, the negative

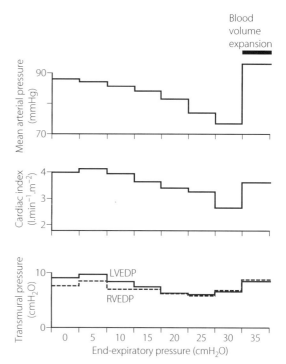

Figure 32.10 Cardiovascular responses as a function of positive end-expiratory pressure (PEEP) in patients with acute lung injury. Left and right ventricular end-diastolic pressure (LVEDP and RVEDP) were measured relative to intrapleural pressure. (Drawn from data of Jardin F, Farcot J-C, Boisante L, Curien N, Margairaz A, Bourdarias J-P. Influence of positive end-expiratory pressure on left ventricular performance. *N Engl J Med* 1981; **304**: 387–92 and reproduced with permission from Nunn JF. Positive end-expiratory pressure. *Int Anaesthesiol Clin* 1984; **22**: 149–64.)

intrathoracic pressure during inspiration draws blood into the chest from the major veins, known as the 'thoracic pump'. Positive intrathoracic pressure abolishes this effect and also imposes a further reduction in driving pressure for flow between extra- and intrathoracic vessels. Reduced right ventricle (RV) filling pressures quickly lead to reduced left ventricle (LV) filling and cardiac output falls.[46] These changes will clearly be more pronounced with hypovolaemia.

A second cause for reduced cardiac output may come into play with high airway pressures, moderate PEEP or lung hyperinflation such as occurs with PEEPi. As described above, increasing lung volume leads to elevated pulmonary vascular resistance, which will cause an increase in RV volume.[40] There is now good evidence that dilation of the RV has profound effects on LV function, preventing adequate LV filling and reducing LV compliance, both of which lead to a fall in cardiac output.[41] Contractility of the LV is not thought to change with positive intrathoracic pressure. Interactions of some

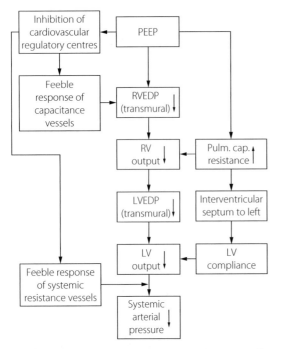

Figure 32.11 Summary of the possible cardiovascular effects of positive end-expiratory pressure (PEEP). See text for full explanation. RVEDP and LVEDP, right and left ventricular end-diastolic pressure; RV and LV, right and left ventricle.

Figure 32.12 End-expiratory alveolar and intrapleural pressures as a function of positive end-expiratory pressure (PEEP). The lower unbroken line shows intrapleural pressure in the relaxed healthy subject. The broken line shows values of intrapleural pressure in patients with acute lung injury taken from reference 44. Absolute values of pressure probably reflect experimental technique and cannot be compared between studies. (Reproduced with permission from Nunn JF. Positive end-expiratory pressure. *Int Anaesthesiol Clin* 1984; **22**: 149–64.)

of the factors by which PEEP may influence cardiac output and systemic arterial pressure are shown in Figure 32.11.

Oxygen flux. In many patients with pulmonary disease, PEEP tends to improve the arterial P_{O_2} while decreasing the cardiac output. As PEEP is increased the oxygen delivery (the product of cardiac output and arterial oxygen content; page 187) tends to rise to a maximum and then fall. Assuming that a normal or high oxygen flux is desirable, use of IPPV or PEEP therefore requires optimisation of cardiac output with fluid replacement (see Figure 32.10) or with positive inotropes and this is now standard practice in critical care units.

Arterial blood pressure. Figure 32.10 shows the decline in mean arterial pressure closely following the change in cardiac output with increasing PEEP. Although there was some increase in systemic vascular resistance, this was only about half that required for maintenance of the arterial pressure in the face of the declining cardiac output. It has been suggested that this is due to PEEP causing inhibition of the cardiovascular regulatory centres.[47]

Interpretation of vascular pressures. Atrial pressures are normally measured relative to atmospheric pressure.

With positive-pressure ventilation, atrial pressures tend to be increased relative to atmospheric. However, relative to intrathoracic pressure, they are reduced at higher levels of PEEP (see Figure 32.10). It is the transmural pressure gradient and not the level relative to atmosphere that is relevant to cardiac filling.[42]

Transmission of airway pressure to other intrathoracic structures. The intrapleural pressure is protected from the level of PEEP by the transmural pressure gradient of the lungs. Animal studies have shown that reduced pulmonary compliance is the main factor governing the transmission of airway pressure to other thoracic structures. With reduced compliance the effect of mean intrathoracic pressure on cardiac output is greatly reduced.[48] Patients with diseased lungs tend to have reduced pulmonary compliance, which limits the rise in intrapleural pressure (Figure 32.12). Therefore, their cardiovascular systems are better protected against the adverse effects of IPPV and PEEP.

Haemodynamic response in heart failure. The cardiovascular responses described thus far apply only to patients with normal cardiac function and, like the Valsalva response, are very different in patients with raised ventricular end-diastolic pressure with or without ventricular failure.[42] Reduction of venous return to an overloaded and failing right heart will return the RV to a more favourable section of its Frank–Starling curve (see Figure 29.3) and so improve its function. Reducing RV end-diastolic volume will overcome some of the adverse ventricular interactions that occur in heart failure and so also improve LV function. These factors almost certainly contribute to the success of CPAP in the treatment of cardiogenic pulmonary oedema (page 392).[3,13]

Other physiological effects

Renal effects. Patients receiving prolonged IPPV tend to become oedematous. Protein depletion and inappropriate fluid loading may be factors but there is also evidence that PEEP itself reduces glomerular filtration.[49] Arterial pressure tends to be reduced as described above, whereas central venous pressure is raised. Therefore, the pressure gradient between renal artery and vein is reduced and this has a direct effect on renal blood flow. In addition, PEEP causes elevated levels of antidiuretic hormone, possibly due to activation of left atrial receptors, although this is insufficient to fully explain the changes in urinary flow rate.

Pulmonary neutrophil retention. Neutrophils have a diameter close to that of a pulmonary capillary and this is important in slowing their transit time through the lung to facilitate margination for pulmonary defence mechanisms (page 403). Any reduction in pulmonary capillary diameter may therefore be expected to increase pulmonary neutrophil retention, which has indeed been demonstrated in humans following a Valsalva manoeuvre[50] or with the application of PEEP.[51] If the neutrophils trapped in this way have already been activated, for example following cardiopulmonary bypass, then lung injury may occur.

VENTILATOR-ASSOCIATED LUNG INJURY (VALI)[52]

The first description of the potential harm that artificial ventilation may cause to the lungs was published in 1745 by John Fothergill.[53,54] Following the successful resuscitation of a patient using expired air respiration rather than bellows, which were fashionable at the time, Fothergill wrote that *'the lungs of one man may bear, without injury, as great a force as those of another man can exert; which by the bellows cannot always be determin'd'*.

Artificial ventilation may damage *normal* lungs only after prolonged ventilation with high airway pressures or large tidal volumes and is very rarely a problem in clinical practice. However, in abnormal lungs, such as during acute lung injury (see Chapter 31), VALI may contribute not only to further lung damage but also to multisystem organ failure affecting other body systems.[55]

Barotrauma

A sustained increase in the transmural pressure gradient can damage the lung.[56] The commonest forms of barotrauma attributable to artificial ventilation with or without PEEP are subcutaneous emphysema, pneumomediastinum and pneumothorax. Tension lung cysts and hyperinflation of a lung or lobe have also been reported but the incidence of these complications is variable. Pulmonary barotrauma probably starts as disruption of the alveolar membrane, with air entering the interstitial space and tracking along the bronchovascular bundles into the mediastinum, from which it can reach the peritoneum, the pleural cavity or the subcutaneous tissues. Radiological demonstration of pulmonary interstitial gas may provide an early warning of barotrauma.

In patients who died following a prolonged period of exposure to PEEP, Slavin and his colleagues[57] demonstrated at autopsy a gross dilation of terminal and respiratory bronchioles which they termed bronchiolectasis (Figure 32.13). Another study described similar changes in 26 of 30 patients who died following artificial ventilation.[58] These studies found development of the condition to be increased by high PEEP levels, high peak airway pressures, large tidal volumes and the duration of artificial ventilation. Indirect evidence suggested that barotrauma resulted in a large increase in dead space. Follow-up of a group of patients who had survived the use of PEEP indicated a return to normal pulmonary function with normal values for dead space.[59] The condition of bronchiolectasis appears to be analogous to bronchopulmonary dysplasia described in infants ventilated for respiratory distress syndrome.[60]

Volutrauma[53,61]

Many animal studies have demonstrated pulmonary oedema following artificial ventilation with high inflation pressures. In one of these studies, lung damage with high inflation pressures was attenuated by restricting chest movement to prevent overdistension of the lungs, indicating that alveolar size rather than pressure was responsible for lung injury.[56] Termed volutrauma, this is now believed to contribute significantly to lung damage in patients with acute lung injury, in whom only a small proportion of alveoli may receive the entire tidal volume (page 414).

This form of VALI most commonly manifests itself as interstitial or alveolar pulmonary oedema. There are several possible underlying mechanisms, all of which are closely interrelated.

Alveolar distension causes permeability pulmonary oedema (page 391).[52] With extreme lung distension in animal studies this occurs quickly and probably results

Figure 32.13 Histological appearance of bronchiolectasis in a patient who died after 16 days of artificial ventilation with positive end-expiratory pressure of 5 cmH$_2$O. Terminal and respiratory bronchioles are grossly dilated and surrounding alveoli are collapsed. Diameter of normal terminal bronchiole is 0.5 mm. Scale bar is 1 mm. (Reproduced with permission from Nunn JF. Positive end-expiratory pressure. *Int Anaesthesiol Clin* 1984; **22**: 149–64.)

from direct trauma to alveolar structures. In larger animals and humans, the permeability changes occur more slowly (several hours) and are more likely to result from the alterations in surfactant and inflammatory mediators described below.

Airway trauma occurs with repeated closure and reopening of small airways with each breath and has been termed atelectrauma. Eventually, mucosal oedema will develop and the airways become progressively more difficult to open until collapse occurs. Recruitment of lung units with positive-pressure ventilation has beneficial effects on gas exchange and so encourages the use of higher pressures and volumes to recruit more airways, leading to further VALI.

Surfactant function is affected by artificial ventilation. Animal studies have demonstrated that surfactant release is *increased* by artificial ventilation, but there is also ample evidence that surfactant function is reduced.[52] Cyclical closure of airways during expiration causes surfactant to be drawn from the alveoli into the airway,[62] whereas alveolar proteins seen with permeability oedema inactivate surfactant (page 414). The resultant increase in alveolar surface tension will not only affect lung compliance but may also increase local microvascular permeability and encourage alveolar collapse.

Lung inflammation occurs with VALI as a result of neutrophil activation. Pulmonary retention of neutrophils has been described above. Once activated – for example by exposure to the alveolar basement membrane – inflammatory mediators will contribute to permeability oedema and further loss of surfactant function. Alveolar epithelial[63] and pulmonary capillary[64] cells may also contribute to lung inflammation. Results from animal studies and cultured human cells indicate that cyclical stretching of many cell types induces the production of inflammatory mediators.

Prevention of VALI

PEEP. In spite of its contribution to mean airway pressure, animal studies show that modest amounts of PEEP are helpful in reducing VALI.[61] Reduction of interstitial oedema, prevention of cyclical airway closure and preservation of surfactant function are all possible mechanisms for this effect. Determination of an acceptable level of PEEP in injured lungs is discussed on page 414.

Tidal volume and airway pressure should be minimised as far as possible. Plateau pressure is the ventilator measurement that equates most closely to the degree of alveolar distension. It is currently recommended that in patients with normal chest wall compliance, the plateau pressure should not be allowed to exceed 35 cmH$_2$O.[65]

A 'protective' ventilation strategy that combines these requirements is described on page 416 and early results of its use in the clinical setting indicate that it may be effective at reducing VALI.

ARTIFICIAL VENTILATION FOR RESUSCITATION

Until about 1960, artificial ventilation was usually attempted by applying mechanical forces directly to the trunk. Methods were based on the rescuer manipulating the trunk and arms of the victim to achieve changes in lung volume which, when performed in sequence, could produce some degree of pulmonary ventilation. These methods, which undoubtedly saved many lives in the past, are now largely obsolete.

Expired air ventilation[66]

Recognition of the inadequacy of the manual methods of artificial ventilation led directly to a radical new approach to artificial ventilation in an emergency. Around 1960 there was vigorous reexamination of the concept of the rescuer's expired air being used for inflation of the victim's lungs. Elisha has been credited with use of this technique on the son of the Shunammite woman (*2 Kings 4:32*) but the first clear and unequivocal account of the method was by Herholdt and Rafn in 1796.[67]

At first sight, it might appear that expired air would not be a suitable inspired air for the victim. However, if the rescuer doubles his ventilation he is able to breathe for two. If neither party had any respiratory dead space, the simple relationship shown in Table 32.4 would apply. In fact, the rescuer's dead space improves the situation. At the start of inflation, the rescuer's dead space is filled with fresh air and this is the first gas to enter the victim's lungs. If the rescuer's dead space is artificially increased by apparatus dead space, this will improve the freshness of the air that the victim receives and will also reduce the likelihood of hypocapnia in the rescuer.

Expired air ventilation has now displaced the manual methods in all except the most unusual circumstances and its success depends on the following factors.

1. It is normally possible to achieve adequate ventilation for long periods of time without fatigue, though symptomatic hypocapnia can occur.[68]
2. The hands of the rescuer are free to control the patency of the victim's airway.
3. The rescuer can monitor the victim's chest expansion visually and can also hear any airway obstruction and sense the tidal exchange from the proprioceptive receptors in his own chest wall.

4. The method is extremely adaptable and has been used, for example, before drowning victims have been removed from the water and on linesmen electrocuted while working on pylons. No manual method would have any hope of success in such situations.
5. The method seems to come naturally and many rescuers have achieved success with the minimum of instruction.

There have been few new developments in recent years. There is now increased fear of infection from the victim and, despite this being very rare in practice,[66] there is renewed interest in mechanical methods of ventilation[69] or even complete avoidance of expired air ventilation during resuscitation. One study of cardiac arrest victims outside hospital found that instructing bystanders to perform either chest compressions alone or chest compressions and mouth-to-mouth ventilation had no influence on survival from the cardiac arrest.[70] This study indicates that for the first few minutes after a witnessed cardiac arrest, oxygen stores in the blood and lungs may obviate the need for artificial ventilation until trained personnel and equipment arrive. The findings of this study must be interpreted with caution and are only applicable to a witnessed cardiac arrest in an urban environment where emergency services arrive an average of 4 minutes after the cardiac arrest.[66,70]

EXTRAPULMONARY GAS EXCHANGE

The development of an artificial lung remains only a distant possibility,[71,72] but techniques for short-term replacement of lung function or more prolonged partial respiratory support have existed for many years. Extracorporeal gas exchangers were first developed for cardiac surgery to facilitate cardiopulmonary bypass and so allow surgery on a motionless heart. Subsequently the use of extracorporeal and, more recently, intracorporeal gas exchange was extended into the treatment of respiratory failure.

Factors in design[73]

The lungs of an adult have an interface between blood and gas of the order of $126 \, m^2$. It is not possible to achieve this in an artificial substitute, and artificial lungs can be considered to have a very low 'diffusing capacity'. Nevertheless, they function satisfactorily within limits for many reasons.

Factors favouring performance

- The real lung is adapted for maximal exercise, whereas patients requiring extrapulmonary gas exchange are usually close to basal metabolic rate or

Table 32.4 Alveolar gas concentrations during expired air resuscitation

	Normal spontaneous respiration	Expired air resuscitation with doubled ventilation	
		Donor	Recipient
Alveolar CO_2	6%	3%	6%
Alveolar O_2	15%	18%	15%

Doubling the rescuer's ventilation increases his alveolar O_2 concentration to a value midway between the normal alveolar oxygen concentration and that of room air.

less if hypothermia is used, for example during cardiac surgery.

- Under resting conditions at sea level, there is an enormous reserve in the capacity of the lung to achieve equilibrium between pulmonary capillary blood and alveolar gas (see Figure 9.2). Therefore, a subnormal diffusing capacity does not necessarily result in arterial hypoxaemia.
- It is possible to operate an artificial lung with an 'alveolar' oxygen concentration in excess of 90%, compared with 14% for real alveolar gas under normal circumstances. This greatly increases the oxygen transfer for a given 'diffusing capacity' of the artificial lung.
- There is no great difficulty in increasing the 'ventilation/perfusion ratio' of an artificial lung above the value of about 0.8 in the normal lung at rest.
- The 'capillary transit time' of an artificial lung can be increased beyond the 0.75 second in the real lung. This facilitates the approach of blood P_{O_2} to 'alveolar' P_{O_2} (see Figure 9.2).
- It is possible to use countercurrent flow between gas and blood. This does not occur in the lungs of mammals, although it is used in the gills of fish.

Carbon dioxide exchanges much more readily than oxygen because of its greater blood and lipid solubility. Therefore, in general, elimination of carbon dioxide does not present a major problem and the limiting factor of an artificial lung is oxygenation.

Unfavourable factors

Against these favourable design considerations, there are certain advantages of the real lung – apart from its very large surface area – that are difficult to emulate in an artificial lung.

- The pulmonary capillaries have a diameter close to that of a red blood cell (RBC). Therefore, each RBC is brought into very close contact with the alveolar gas (see Figure 2.8). The diffusion distance for artificial lungs is considerably greater, and this problem is considered further below.
- The vascular endothelium is specially adapted to prevent undesirable changes in the formed elements of blood, particularly neutrophils and platelets. Most artificial surfaces cause clotting of blood, and artificial lungs therefore require the use of anticoagulants.
- No artificial lung has the extensive non-respiratory functions of the real lung, which include uptake, synthesis and biotransformation of many constituents of the blood (see Chapter 12). This function is lost when the lungs are bypassed.
- The lung is an extremely efficient filter with an effective pore size of about 10 μm for flow rates of blood

up to about 25 l.min^{-1}. This is difficult to achieve with any man-made filter.

Bubble oxygenators

By breaking up the gas stream into small bubbles, it is possible to achieve very large surface areas of interface. However, the smaller the bubbles, the greater the tendency for them to remain in suspension when the blood is returned to the patient. This is dangerous during cardiopulmonary bypass because of the direct access of the blood to the cerebral circulation. A compromise is to break the gas stream into bubbles ranging from 2 to 7 mm in diameter, giving an effective area of interface of the order of 15 m^2. With a mean RBC transit time of 1–2 seconds and an oxygen concentration of more than 90%, this gives an acceptable outflow blood P_{O_2} with blood flow rates up to about 6 l.min^{-1}. The P_{CO_2} of the outflowing blood must be controlled by admixture of carbon dioxide with the inflowing oxygen in the gas phase. Gas is passed through the blood in a reservoir of about 1 litre capacity in which foaming takes place. Blood is then passed to a second reservoir for 'debubbling' with the help of an antifoaming compound.

Cellular and protein damage (see below) at the blood–gas interface occurs in bubble oxygenators. This is not considered to have significant clinical effects during short-term use, as for example with cardiac surgery, but may become significant when used for prolonged periods in the treatment of respiratory failure.[73]

Membrane oxygenators

Diffusion properties. Unlike their predecessors, currently available membranes offer little resistance to the diffusion of oxygen and carbon dioxide. At 25–50 μm thick, artificial membranes are several times thicker than the active side of the alveolar/capillary membrane (see Figure 2.8) but they contain small (<1 μm) pores, which increase gas transfer substantially. The hydrophobic nature of the membrane material prevents water entering the pores, and in normal use membranes can withstand a hydrostatic pressure gradient of the order of normal arterial blood pressure. However, over time the pores tend to fill with protein which slowly reduces the membrane's efficiency.

Gas diffusion within the blood presents a considerable barrier to efficiency of membrane oxygenators. Slow diffusion of gases through plasma is now thought to limit gas transfer in normal lung, in which the RBC is almost in contact with the capillary wall (page 137). Streamlined flow through much wider channels in a membrane oxygenator tends to result in a stream of RBC remaining at a distance from the interface. It has been estimated that in membrane oxygenators the diffusion path for oxygen is about 25 times further than in lung. Much thought has been devoted to the creation of turbulent flow to counteract this effect by 'mixing' the blood. Unfortunately, this inevitably leads to a greater degree of cell damage (see below) and increased resistance to flow through the oxygenator.

Biocompatibility. Adsorption of proteins, particularly albumin, onto the membrane reduces platelet, neutrophil and complement activation (see below) and this technique may be used to 'prime' oxygenators before use. Attempts to mimic endothelial cell properties have led to the production of membranes with heparin bonded to the surface, which also reduces activation of most of the processes described below.

Damage to blood

Damage due to non-occlusive roller pumps and centrifugal pumps is almost negligible. Damage due to oxygenators is probably far less than that which results from surgical suction in removing blood from the operative site and, during cardiac surgery, this factor outweighs any differences attributable to the type of oxygenator. However, during prolonged extracorporeal oxygenation for respiratory failure, the influence of the type of oxygenator becomes important and membrane oxygenators are then clearly superior to bubble oxygenators.

Protein denaturation. Contact between blood and either gas bubbles or synthetic surfaces results in protein denaturation and synthetic surfaces become coated with a layer of protein. With membrane oxygenators this tends to be self-limiting and the protein products remain bound to the membrane. Bubble oxygenators cause a continuous and progressive loss of protein, including the release of denatured proteins into the circulation where they may have biological effects.

Complement activation. Complement activation occurs when blood comes into contact with any artificial surface and complement C5a is known to be formed after cardiopulmonary bypass surgery. Heparin-bonded systems cause less complement activation.[74]

RBC. Shear forces, resulting from turbulence or foaming, may cause shortened survival or actual destruction of RBC. However, without surgical suction, damage to RBC with membrane oxygenators remains within reasonable limits for many days.

Leucocytes and platelets. Counts of these elements are usually reduced by an amount in excess of the changes attributable to haemodilution. Platelets are lost by adhesion and aggregation, and following cardiac surgery, postoperative counts are commonly about half the preoperative value. Neutrophil activation may occur within the extracorporeal circuit, leading to pathological effects in distant organs.

Coagulation. No oxygenator can function without causing coagulation of the blood. Anticoagulation is therefore a *sine qua non* of the technique and heparin is usually employed for this purpose. Heparin-bonded components have significantly reduced the systemic anticoagulant requirement and allowed more prolonged use of circuits, but coagulopathy remains the most common complication of extracorporeal circulation.[75]

Systems for extrapulmonary gas exchange[76]

Cardiopulmonary bypass for cardiac surgery remains the most common situation in which patients are exposed to extrapulmonary gas exchange. The duration of such exposure is normally very short and causes few physiological disturbances postoperatively. Providing longer term respiratory support is much less common, and also considerably more difficult, but three techniques exist.

Extracorporeal membrane oxygenation (ECMO).[77-79] Provision of ECMO requires continuous blood flow from the patient to a reservoir system, from which a pump propels blood through an oxygenator and a heat exchanger back to the patient. Venovenous ECMO is acceptable for treatment of respiratory failure and may be instituted via percutaneous venous catheters. If circulatory support is also required, then venoarterial ECMO is used, which normally requires surgical access to the vessels. A typical adult ECMO circuit provides $7 m^2$ of membrane for oxygenation using 100% oxygen, with blood flows of approximately $2-4 l.min^{-1}$. The technique is only available in specialised centres, so in recent years ECMO systems have been developed for use while transporting the patient to the ECMO facilities.[80]

Extracorporeal carbon dioxide removal (ECCO₂R). A different approach to artificial gas exchange was developed by Gattinoni *et al.* in Milan.[81] They restricted an ECMO system to removal of carbon dioxide only and maintained oxygenation by a modification of apnoeic mass movement oxygenation (page 160). The lungs were either kept motionless or were ventilated two to three times per minute (low-frequency positive-pressure ventilation with extracorporeal CO_2 removal: LFPPV-ECCO₂R).[82]

The technique depends on two important differences between the exchange of carbon dioxide and oxygen.

First, membrane oxygenators remove carbon dioxide some 10–20 times more effectively than they take up oxygen. Second, the normal arterial oxygen content (20 ml.dl^{-1}) is very close to the maximum oxygen capacity, even with 100% oxygen in the gas phase (22 ml.dl^{-1}). Therefore, there is little scope for superoxygenation of a fraction of the cardiac output to compensate for a larger fraction of the cardiac output in which oxygenation does not take place. In contrast, the normal mixed venous carbon dioxide content is 52 ml.dl^{-1} compared with an arterial carbon dioxide content of 48 ml.dl^{-1}. There is therefore ample scope for removing a larger than normal fraction of carbon dioxide from a part of the cardiac output to compensate for the remaining fraction that does not undergo any removal of carbon dioxide.

It is therefore possible to maintain carbon dioxide homoeostasis by diversion of only a small fraction of the cardiac output through an extracorporeal membrane oxygenator.[81]

With $P\text{CO}_2$ held constant by extracorporeal removal of carbon dioxide, there is no obstacle to the continued uptake of oxygen by mass movement apnoeic oxygenation, a process that is otherwise terminated by a progressive increase in $P\text{CO}_2$. All that is necessary is to replace the alveolar gas with oxygen and connect the trachea to a supply of oxygen, which is then drawn into the lungs at a rate equal to the metabolic consumption of oxygen, and this should continue indefinitely.

Intravascular oxygenators (IVOX).[83] Siting the gas exchange membrane within the patient's own circulation obviates the need for any extracorporeal circulation. In return, the size of the gas exchange surface is severely limited and the blood flow around the membrane no longer controlled. However, the development of a heparin-bonded hollow-fibre oxygenator suitable for use in humans has promoted great interest in the technique. The device is inserted via surgical exposure of the femoral vein until it lies throughout the length of both inferior and superior vena cavae, through the right atrium. An IVOX device comes in different sizes between 40 and 50 cm long with 600–1100 fibres through which oxygen flows, providing a surface area of 0.21–0.52 m^2 for gas exchange.[84] Blood flow in the venae cavae is thought to be mostly laminar, even with the IVOX in place, and gas exchange is again therefore limited by diffusion within the blood.[83]

The available membrane surface area with IVOX is such that total extrapulmonary gas exchange is currently impossible and the technique is suitable only for partial respiratory support. Even so, the modest improvement in blood gases seen with IVOX allows significant reductions in several ventilator settings, such as inspiratory airway pressure and minute volume.[85]

Table 32.5 Aetiology of respiratory failure in infants treated with extracorporeal membrane oxygenation

Neonates 0–1 month old	Other infants >1 month old
Meconium aspiration syndrome	Viral pneumonitis
Congenital diaphragmatic hernia	Bacterial pneumonia
Overwhelming neonatal sepsis	Acute respiratory distress syndrome
Severe surfactant deficiency	Myocarditis and cardiomyopathy
Persistent pulmonary hypertension	

(After references 76, 77 and 79.)

Clinical applications

Neonates and infants[76,79,86]

It is estimated that worldwide in excess of 22 000 babies have received treatment involving ECMO. The indication for treatment is acute respiratory failure of such severity that predicted survival is less than 20%, and the causes are shown in Table 32.5. Although survival varies with the aetiology, there is general agreement that ECMO improves outcome substantially in infants, with some centres achieving survival figures of almost 80%.[77,79]

This benefit is not without costs. Vascular access in infants is difficult and venoarterial ECMO using the carotid and jugular vessels is often required, though venovenous ECMO with a double-lumen cannula is now widely used. In either case, there are believed to be significant disturbances to cerebral blood flow during ECMO, possibly exacerbated by altered cerebral autoregulation. As a result, a significant number of ECMO-treated infants develop clinical evidence of cerebral damage, which in some infants causes long-term disability.[79,87,88]

Adults[78]

Extrapulmonary gas exchange is occasionally used as a therapeutic 'bridge' in patients waiting for lung transplantation, but its main indication is for management of severe acute lung injury (ALI, see Chapter 30).[78] Ventilator-associated lung injury as a result of artificial ventilation (page 437) contributes to respiratory failure in severe ALI and the prospect of using extrapulmonary gas exchange to facilitate 'lung rest' is attractive. Unfortunately, the significant benefits of ECMO use in infants have not been found in adults and its place in treatment remains controversial. The invasive nature of extrapulmonary gas exchange and the serious potential complications mean that ECMO is used only in the most severely ill patients. Even in specialist centres, recruitment of enough patients for randomised trials is difficult and units have tended to simply publish results of uncontrolled case series.

IVOX as described above does allow some improvement in ventilator settings, which should alleviate the risk of lung trauma. Outcome studies are awaited, but it is unlikely that the modest improvement in gas exchange seen with current systems will have significant effects.[89]

ECMO. A multicentre randomised prospective trial of ECMO for patients with severe ALI was published in 1979.[90] Severely hypoxic patients were randomly allocated to conventional artificial ventilation or ECMO. The study was terminated after recruitment of only 90 patients when it was found that mortality was more than 90% in both groups, with no statistically significant difference between the two forms of treatment. This trial effectively stopped ECMO use in adults for several years; in the meantime, significant advances were made in the causes and treatment of ALI by other means, such as ventilator strategies to limit VALI (see Chapter 31). In addition, since 1979 there have been major advances in the technology available for ECMO, in particular the advent of heparin-bonded and intravascular devices. Current ECMO techniques do seem to offer some patients substantial benefits,[91] particularly if instituted early in the course of severe ALI,[89] but comparative trials are still awaited.[78]

ECCO₂R has been compared with currently accepted techniques of artificial ventilation and found to provide no improvement in mortality (67% with ECCO₂R versus 58% for control group).[92] This study has been criticised by the proponents of ECMO because of a high complication rate, mostly related to bleeding as a result of anticoagulation used for the non-heparin bonded circuit.[80]

REFERENCES

1. Shneerson JM. Techniques in mechanical ventilation: principles and practice. *Thorax* 1996; **51**: 756–61.
*2. Hillberg RE, Johnson DC. Noninvasive ventilation. *N Engl J Med* 1997; **337**: 1746–52.
*3. Mehta S, Hill NS. Noninvasive ventilation. *Am J Respir Crit Care Med* 2001; **163**: 540–77.
4. Hill NS. Clinical applications of body ventilators. *Chest* 1986; **90**: 897–905.
5. Drinker P, Shore LA. An apparatus for the prolonged administration of artificial respiration. *J Clin Invest* 1929; **7**: 229–47.
6. Thomson A. The role of negative pressure ventilation. *Arch Dis Child* 1997; **77**: 454–8.
7. Petros AJ, Fernando SSD, Shenoy VS, Al-Saady NM. The Hayek oscillator. Nomograms for tidal volume and minute ventilation using external high frequency oscillation. *Anaesthesia* 1995; **50**: 601–6.
8. Dilkes MG, McNeill JM, Hill AC, Monks PS, McKelvie P, Hollamby RG. The Hayek oscillator: a new method of ventilation in microlaryngeal surgery. *Ann Otol Rhinol Laryngol* 1993; **102**: 455–8.
9. Claman DM, Pipier A, Sanders MH, Stiller RA, Votteri BA. Nocturnal noninvasive positive pressure ventilatory assistance. *Chest* 1996; **110**: 1581–8.
10. Brochard L. Noninvasive ventilation for acute respiratory failure. *JAMA* 2002; **288**: 932–5.
11. Liesching T, Kwok H, Hill NS. Acute applications of non-invasive positive pressure ventilation. *Chest* 2003; **124**: 699–713.
12. Navalesi P. Weaning and non-invasive ventilation. The odd couple. *Am J Respir Crit Care Med* 2003; **168**: 5–6.
13. Bersten AD, Holt AW, Vedig AE, Skowronski GA, Baggoley CJ. Treatment of severe cardiogenic pulmonary edema with continuous positive airway pressure delivered by facemask. *N Engl J Med* 1991; **325**: 1825–30.
14. Fuleihan S, Wilson RS, Pontoppidan H. Effect of mechanical ventilation with end-expiratory pause on blood-gas exchange. *Anesth Analg* 1976; **55**: 122–30.
15. Rossi A, Appendini L. Wasted efforts and dyssynchrony: is the patient–ventilator battle back? *Intens Care Med* 1995; **21**: 867–70.
16. Sassoon CSH, Gruer SE. Characteristics of the ventilator pressure- and flow-trigger variables. *Intens Care Med* 1995; **21**: 159–68.
17. Downs J, Stock MC. Airway pressure release ventilation: a new concept in ventilatory support. *Crit Care Med* 1987; **15**: 459–61.
18. Frawley PM, Habashi N. Airway pressure release ventilation: theory and practice. *AACN Clin Issues* 2001; **12**: 234–46.
19. Neumann P, Golisch W, Strohmeyer A, Buscher H, Burchardi H, Sydow M. Influence of different release times on spontaneous breathing pattern during airway pressure release ventilation. *Intens Care Med* 2002; **28**: 1742–9.
20. Wahba RW. Pressure support ventilation. *J Cardiothorac Anesth* 1990; **4**: 624–30.
21. Dekel B, Segal E, Perel A. Pressure support ventilation. *Arch Intern Med* 1996; **156**: 369–73.
22. Smith BE. High frequency ventilation: past, present and future? *Br J Anaesth* 1990; **65**: 130–8.
23. Bouchut J-C, Godard J, Claris O. High-frequency oscillatory ventilation. *Anesthesiology* 2004; **100**: 1007–12.
24. Chakrabarti MK, Gordon G, Whitwam JG. Relationship between tidal volume and deadspace

during high frequency ventilation. *Br J Anaesth* 1986; **58**: 11–17.

25. Butler WJ, Bohn DJ, Bryan AC, Froese AB. Ventilation by high-frequency oscillation in humans. *Anesth Analg* 1980; **59**: 577–84.

26. Beamer WC, Prough DS, Royster RL, Johnston WE, Johnson JC. High frequency jet ventilation produces auto-PEEP. *Crit Care Med* 1984; **12**: 734–7.

27. Nunn JF, Hill DW. Respiratory dead space and arterial to end-tidal CO_2 tension difference in anesthetized man. *J Appl Physiol* 1960; **15**: 383–9.

28. Carlon GC, Howland WS, Ray C, Miodownik S, Griffin JP, Groeger JJ. High frequency jet ventilation. A prospective randomized evaluation. *Chest* 1983; **84**: 551–9.

29. Hurst JM, Branson RD, Davis K, Barrette RR, Adams KS. Comparison of conventional mechanical ventilation and high-frequency ventilation. A prospective randomized trial in patients with respiratory failure. *Ann Surg* 1990; **211**: 486–91.

*30. Manthous CA, Schmidt GA, Hall JB. Liberation from mechanical ventilation: a decade of progress. *Chest* 1998; **114**: 886–901.

*31. MacIntyre NR, Cook DJ, Ely EW, *et al.* Evidence-based guidelines for weaning and discontinuing ventilatory support. A collective task force facilitated by the American College of Chest Physicians; the American Association of Respiratory Care; and the American College of Critical Care Medicine. *Chest* 2001; **120**: 375S–395S.

32. Yang KL, Tobin MJ. A prospective study of indexes predicting the outcome of trials of weaning from mechanical ventilation. *N Engl J Med* 1991; **324**: 1445–50.

33. Smith IE, Shneerson JM. A progressive care programme for prolonged ventilatory failure: analysis of outcome. *Br J Anaesth* 1995; **75**: 399–404.

34. Hill JD, Main FB, Osborn JJ, Gerbode F. Correct use of respirator on cardiac patient after operation. *Arch Surg* 1965; **91**: 775–8.

35. Gottfried SB, Reissman H, Ranieri M. A simple method for the measurement of intrinsic end-expiratory pressure during controlled and assisted modes of mechanical ventilation. *Crit Care Med* 1992; **20**: 621–9.

*36. Conacher ID. Dynamic hyperinflation – the anaesthetist applying a tourniquet to the right heart. *Br J Anaesth* 1998; **81**; 116–17.

37. Vellody VPS, Nassery M, Balasaraswathi K, Goldberg NB, Sharp JT. Compliances of human ribcage and diaphragm-abdomen pathways in relaxed versus paralyzed states. *Am Rev Respir Dis* 1978; **118**: 479–91.

38. Hulands GH, Greene R, Iliff LD, Nunn JF. Influence of anaesthesia on the regional distribution of perfusion and ventilation in the lung. *Clin Sci* 1970; **38**: 451–60.

39. Bindslev LG, Hedenstierna G, Santesson J, Gottlieb I, Carvallhas A. Ventilation–perfusion distribution during inhalational anaesthesia. *Acta Anaesthesiol Scand* 1981; **25**: 360–71.

40. Biondi JW, Schulman DS, Soufer R, *et al.* The effect of incremental positive end-expiratory pressure on right ventricular hemodynamics and ejection fraction. *Anesth Analg* 1988; **67**: 144–51.

*41. Pinsky MR. The hemodynamic consequences of mechanical ventilation: an evolving story. *Intens Care Med* 1997; **23**: 493–503.

*42. Tyberg JV, Grant DA, Kingma I, *et al.* Effects of positive intrathoracic pressure on pulmonary and systemic hemodynamics. *Respir Physiol* 2000; **119**: 163–71.

43. Cournand A, Motley HL, Werko L, Richards DW. Physiological studies of the effects of intermittent positive pressure breathing on cardiac output in man. *Am J Physiol* 1948; **152**: 162–74.

44. Jardin F, Farcot J-C, Boisante L, Curien N, Margairaz A, Bourdarias J-P. Influence of positive end-expiratory pressure on left ventricular performance. *N Engl J Med* 1981; **304**: 387–92.

45. Nunn JF. Positive end-expiratory pressure. *Int Anaesthesiol Clin* 1984; **22**: 149–64.

46. Mitaka C, Nagura T, Sakanishi N, Tsunoda Y, Amaha K. Two-dimensional echocardiographic evaluation of inferior vena cava, right ventricle and left ventricle during positive-pressure ventilation with varying levels of positive end-expiratory pressure. *Crit Care Med* 1989; **17**: 205–10.

47. Cassidy SS, Gaffney FA, Johnson RL. A perspective on PEEP. *N Engl J Med* 1981; **304**: 421–2.

48. Traverse JH, Korvenranta H, Adams EM, Goldthwait DA, Carlo WA. Impairment of hemodynamics with increasing mean airway pressure during high-frequency oscillatory ventilation. *Pediatr Res* 1988; **23**: 628–31.

49. Marquez JM, Douglas ME, Downs JB, *et al.* Renal function and cardiovascular responses during positive airway pressure. *Anesthesiology* 1979; **50**: 393–8.

50. Markos J, Hooper RO, Kavanagh-Gray D, Wiggs BR, Hogg JC. Effect of raised alveolar pressure on leukocyte retention in the human lung. *J Appl Physiol* 1990; **69**: 214–21.

51. Loick HM, Wendt M, Rötker J, Theissen JL. Ventilation with positive end-expiratory airway pressure causes leukocyte retention in human lung. *J Appl Physiol* 1993; **75**: 301–6.

*52. Dreyfuss D, Saumon G. Ventilator-induced lung injury: lessons from experimental studies. *Am J Respir Crit Care Med* 1998; **157**: 294–323.

*53. Slutsky AS. Lung injury caused by mechanical ventilation. *Chest* 1999; **116**(supp): 9S–15S.

54. Fothergill J. Observations on a case published in the last volume of the medical essays, & c. of recovering

a man dead in appearance, by distending the lungs with air. *Philos Trans Roy Soc Lond* 1745; **43**: 275–81.

55. Slutsky AS, Tremblay LN. Multiple system organ failure – is mechanical ventilation a contributing factor? *Am J Respir Crit Care Med* 1998; **157**: 1721–5.

56. Dreyfuss D, Soler P, Basset G, Saumon G. High inflation pressure pulmonary edema. Respective effects of high airway pressure, high tidal volume and positive end-expiratory pressure. *Am Rev Respir Dis* 1988; **137**: 1159–64.

57. Slavin G, Nunn JF, Crow J, Doré CJ. Bronchiolectasis – a complication of artificial ventilation. *Br Med J* 1982; **285**: 931–4.

58. Rouby JJ, Lherm T, de Lassale EM, *et al.* Histologic aspects of pulmonary barotrauma in critically ill patients with acute respiratory failure. *Intens Care Med* 1993; **19**: 383–9.

59. Navaratnarajah M, Nunn JF, Lyons D, Milledge JS. Bronchiolectasis caused by positive end-expiratory pressure. *Crit Care Med* 1984; **12**: 1036–8.

60. Taghizadeh A, Reynolds EOR. Pathogenesis of bronchopulmonary dysplasia following hyaline membrane disease. *Am J Pathol* 1976; **82**: 241–64.

61. Hooper J. Advances in mechanical ventilation. *Can J Anaesth* 1998; **45**: R149–R154.

62. Faridy EE. Effect of ventilation on movement of surfactant in airways. *Respir Physiol* 1976; **27**: 323–34.

63. Pugin J. Molecular mechanisms of lung cell activation induced by cyclical stretch. *Crit Care Med* 2003; **31**(Supp): S200–6.

64. Minnear FL. Vascular endothelial cells actively participate in high inflation pressure-induced permeability and edema. *Am J Physiol Lung Cell Mol Physiol* 2002; **283**: L1200–2.

65. Slutsky AS. Consensus conference on mechanical ventilation – January 28–30, 1993 at Northbrook, Illinois, USA. *Intens Care Med* 1994; **20**: 64–79.

*66. Wenzel V, Idris AH, Dörges V, *et al.* The respiratory system during resuscitation: a review of the history, risk of infection during assisted ventilation, respiratory mechanics and ventilation strategies for patients with an unprotected airway. *Resuscitation* 2001; **49**: 123–34.

67. Herholdt JD, Rafn CG. *Life-saving methods for drowning persons*. Copenhagen: T Tikiob, 1796. Reprinted in 1960; Aarhuus, Denmark: Stiftsbogtrykkerie.

68. Thierbach AR, Wolcke BB, Krummenauer F, Kunde M, Jänig C, Dick WF. Artificial ventilation for basic life support leads to hyperventilation in first aid providers. *Resuscitation* 2003; **57**: 269–77.

69. Idris AH. Reassessing the need for ventilation during CPR. *Ann Emerg Med* 1996; **27**: 569–75.

70. Hallstrom A, Cobb L, Johnson E, Copass M. Cardiopulmonary resuscitation by chest compression alone or with mouth-to-mouth ventilation. *N Engl J Med* 2000; **342**: 1546–53.

71. Jack D. Artificial lungs on the way – but don't hold your breath. *Lancet* 1997; **349**: 260.

72. Zwischenberger JB, Alpard SK. Artificial lungs: a new inspiration. *Perfusion* 2002; **17**: 253–68.

73. Wegner JA. Oxygenator anatomy and function. *J Cardiothorac Vasc Anaesth* 1997; **11**: 275–81.

74. Videm V, Svennevig JL, Fosse E, Semb G, Osterud A, Mollnes TE. Reduced complement activation with heparin-coated oxygenator and tubings in coronary bypass operations. *J Thorac Cardiovasc Surg* 1992; **103**: 806–13.

75. Briegel J, Hummel T, Lenhart A, Heyduck M, Schelling G, Haller M. Complications during long-term extracorporeal lung assist (ECLA). *Acta Anaesthesiol Scand Suppl* 1996; **109**: 121–2.

76. Walker G, Liddell M, Davis C. Extracorporeal life support – state of the art. *Paediatr Respir Rev* 2003; **4**: 147–52.

77. Peek GA, Killer MK, Sosnowski AW, Firmin RK. Extracorporeal membrane oxygenation: potential for adults and children? *Hosp Med* 1998; **59**: 304–8.

78. Lewandowski K. Extracorporeal membrane oxygenation for severe acute respiratory failure. *Crit Care* 2000; **4**: 156–68.

*79. Cook LN. Update on extracorporeal membrane oxygenation. *Paediatr Respir Rev* 2004; **5**(Supp A): S329–37.

80. Rossaint R, Pappert D, Gerlach H, Lewandowski K, Keh D, Falke K. Extracorporeal membrane oxygenation for transport of hypoxaemic patients with severe ARDS. *Br J Anaesth* 1997; **78**: 241–6.

81. Gattinoni L, Pesenti A, Rossi GP, *et al.* Treatment of acute respiratory failure with low-frequency positive-pressure ventilation and extracorporeal removal of CO_2. *Lancet* 1980; **2**: 292–4.

82. Gattinoni L, Pesenti A, Mascheroni D, Marcolin R, Fumagalli R, Rossi F. Low-frequency positive-pressure ventilation with extracorporeal CO_2 removal in severe acute respiratory failure. *JAMA* 1986; **256**: 881–6.

83. Bidani A, Zwischenberger JB, Cardenas V. Intracorporeal gas exchange: current status and future development. *Intens Care Med* 1996; **22**: 91–3.

84. Conrad SA, Eggerstedt JM, Grier LR, Morris VF, Romero MD. Intravenacaval membrane oxygenation and carbon dioxide removal in severe acute respiratory failure. *Chest* 1995; **107**: 1689–97.

85. Mira JP, Brunet F, Belghith M, *et al.* Reduction of ventilator settings allowed by intravenous oxygenator (IVOX) in ARDS patients. *Intens Care Med* 1995; **21**: 11–17.

86. Soll RF. Neonatal extracorporeal membrane oxygenation – a bridging technique. *Lancet* 1996; **348**: 70–1.

87. Mansfield RT, Parker MM. Cerebral autoregulation during venovenous extracorporeal membrane oxygenation. *Crit Care Med* 1996; **24**: 1945–6.

88. Field D, Davis C, Elbourne D, Grant A, Johnson A, Macrea D and UK Collaborative ECMO Trial Group. UK collaborative randomised trial of neonatal extracorporeal membrane oxygenation. *Lancet* 1996; **348**: 75–82.

89. Peek GJ, Firmin RK. Extracorporeal membrane oxygenation, a favourable outcome? *Br J Anaesth* 1997; **78**: 235–6.

90. Zapol WM, Snider MT, Hill JD, *et al*. Extracorporeal membrane oxygenation in severe respiratory failure. *JAMA* 1979; **242**: 2193–6.

91. Lennartz H. Extracorporeal lung assist in ARDS: history and state of the art. *Acta Anaesthesiol Scand Suppl* 1996; **109**: 114–16.

92. Morris AH, Wallace CJ, Menlove RL, *et al*. Randomized clinical trial of pressure-controlled inverse ratio ventilation and extracorporeal CO_2 removal for adult respiratory distress syndrome. *Am J Respir Crit Care Med* 1994; **149**: 295–305.

KEY POINTS

- Lung transplantation is an established technique for treating advanced lung disease, with chronic obstructive pulmonary disease currently being the most common indication.
- The procedure performed may involve a single-lung, bilateral lung or heart–lung transplant, depending on the indication.
- Although there is still a significant mortality soon after the procedure, survivors have substantial improvements in quality of life, lung function tests and exercise tolerance.
- Lung transplant results in completely denervated lungs, which leaves the respiratory pattern unaffected but impairs the cough reflex and so causes chest infections.

Transplantation of a human lung was first performed in 1963,[1] but in the years following this few patients survived for longer than a month. Improved immunosuppression led to a resurgence of interest in the early 1980s and the technique has now become an established form of treatment. The function of a transplanted lung is important for the well-being of the recipient, but also furthers our understanding of certain fundamental issues of pulmonary physiology. The subject has been reviewed recently.[2–6]

CLINICAL ASPECTS

Indications

Patients who are considered for transplant have severe respiratory disease and are receiving optimal therapy, but still have a life expectancy of less than 2–3 years. Uncontrolled respiratory infection, significant disease of other organs, continued smoking or an age in excess of 55–65 years are normally contraindications. Precise selection criteria for recipients vary between transplant centres and with the respiratory disease, but in general patients

referred for transplant have a forced expiratory volume in 1 second (FEV_1) of less than 30% predicted, resting hypoxia, hypercapnia and commonly pulmonary hypertension. The indications for lung transplant are shown in Table 33.1, where it can be seen that chronic obstructive pulmonary disease (COPD) is now by far the most common. Further discussion of the lung diseases shown in Table 33.1 may be found elsewhere (COPD, page 379; α_1-antitrypsin deficiency, page 202; idiopathic pulmonary fibrosis, page 404; cystic fibrosis (CF), page 381; and primary pulmonary hypertension, page 396).

In most countries with transplant programmes the number of patients awaiting transplant exceeds the number of donors. In recent years the number of donor organs available has remained static whereas the number of candidates for lung transplants has risen rapidly. As a result, median waiting time for an organ to become available has increased, as has the number of patients who die while on the waiting list.[8] Cadaveric donor lungs are taken from patients less than 65 years of age with limited smoking history and no evidence of lung disease. Using current selection criteria, only about 20% of organ donors are suitable for lung donation. Strategies to improve the number of lung transplants being performed include increasing numbers of living-related lobar transplants (see below), extending donor selection criteria to include older patients or recent smokers or using non-heart beating donors.[9] This last approach potentially offers unique advantages for lung donation, as oxygenation of the donor lung after cessation of circulation can conserve lung function for up to an hour.

Types of transplant

Donor and recipient chest sizes are matched. With current organ preservation solutions, lung transplants must be performed within 6–8 hours of organ removal.

Single-lung transplant is the simplest procedure. The recipient's pneumonectomy is undertaken via a thoracotomy using one-lung ventilation (page 317), which presents a significant challenge in these patients.[10] The donor lung is implanted, with anastomoses of the main

Table 33.1 Indications for lung transplantation and the type of operation performed

Indication	Total number	Operations performed for each indication		
		Heart–lung (%)	*Bilateral (%)*	*Single (%)*
COPD	3717	0.5	26.9	72.6
α_1-Antitrypsin deficiency	868	0.6	50.0	49.4
Idiopathic pulmonary fibrosis	1600	0.7	25.2	74.1
Cystic fibrosis	1605	6.8	90.2	3.1
Primary pulmonary hypertension	912	13.4	39.6	47.0
Congenital heart disease	354	69.2	28.0	2.8
Retransplantation	172	3.5	48.8	47.7

Bilateral lung transplant includes double-lung and bilateral single-lung procedures.
Data are from the Registry of the International Society for Heart and Lung Transplantation[7] and include transplants performed worldwide between 1995 and June 2002 for the indications shown.

bronchus, the left or right pulmonary artery and a ring of left atrium containing both pulmonary veins of one side. Cardiopulmonary bypass is required in some cases, particularly those patients with preoperative pulmonary hypertension who are at risk of right-sided heart failure during one-lung ventilation. Cardiopulmonary bypass may have a role in preventing lung injury in transplanted lungs and its routine, rather than emergency, use in patients having lung transplants has been suggested.[11] Evidence of beneficial outcome with the use of cardiopulmonary bypass for lung transplantation is lacking and the technique remains controversial.[11,12]

Bilateral lung transplant. Double-lung transplant performed at a single operation is a more complex procedure for which sternotomy and cardiopulmonary bypass are required. The donor lungs are implanted with anastomoses of either the trachea or both bronchi, the main pulmonary artery and the posterior part of the left atrium containing all four pulmonary veins. Tracheal anastomoses have a high complication rate (see below). A simpler alternative is to transplant two lungs sequentially (termed a double single-lung transplant) through bilateral thoracotomies, and this has now almost completely replaced double-lung transplant.

Heart–lung transplant was originally used for patients with primary pulmonary hypertension and Eisenmenger's syndrome and continues to be the operation of choice for the latter (Table 33.1). Total cardiopulmonary bypass is, of course, essential and the anastomoses involve the right atrium, the aorta and the trachea. The complexity and complication rates of heart–lung trans-

plant are high and, wherever possible, alternative procedures are now preferred, leading to a decline in the number of heart–lung transplant procedures being performed.[7]

Choice of operation depends on the indication for the transplant and types of surgery performed are shown in Table 33.1. Single-lung transplantation is favoured, partly because mortality may be lower following this operation but also because each suitable donor can be used to transplant two recipients. Congenital heart disease commonly requires heart–lung transplant, whereas diseases associated with pulmonary hypertension ideally need either heart–lung transplant or bilateral lung transplant to normalise pulmonary arterial pressure. Lung disease alone is satisfactorily treated with single-lung transplant. Patients with cystic fibrosis have widespread pulmonary infection and so are rarely suitable for single-lung transplant if infection of the transplanted lung is to be avoided.

Living-related lung transplants are now being carried out at several centres in the world.[13–15] Left or right lower lobes of the donor relative are transplanted into the whole hemithorax of the recipient, so the technique is only suitable for children or very small adults, such as patients with CF. The same selection criteria apply as for cadaveric transplantation, so CF patients must have bilateral transplants and therefore two related donors. Early results show survival figures at least comparable with other forms of lung transplantation[13] and evidence is emerging of better survival in paediatric lung transplants when living-related, rather than cadaveric, organs are used.[7,9] The technique is in its infancy and offers theoretical benefits in the availability of organs and attenuated organ rejection, but the ethical issues for donors are substantial.

Airway anastomosis. The tracheal or bronchial circulation of the donor lung is usually compromised and the problem of stenosis, leakage or even occasional dehiscence of the airway anastomosis remains in up to 15% of transplanted lungs. This is a particular problem for tracheal anastomoses, which seem to be in a watershed where both tracheal and bronchial blood supply is poor. The earliest approach to this problem was omentopexy, in which omentum was brought up through the diaphragm and wrapped round the anastomosis to provide collateral circulation. Later, 'telescoping' bronchial anastomoses or direct anastomosis of the internal mammary artery to the donor bronchial circulation were advocated. There is no agreement on which, if any, of these techniques is the most useful.[16]

Outcome following transplant

Mortality. The actuarial survival of lung transplant recipients is shown in Figure 33.1. Given the nature of the surgery, it is not surprising that there is significant perioperative and early postoperative mortality. Thereafter, mortality rates are low when consideration is given to the 2-year predicted survival of recipients prior to transplant. Survival following single-lung or bilateral lung transplants is better than after a heart–lung transplant.

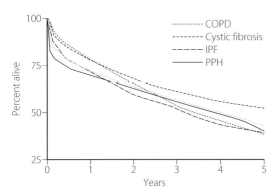

Figure 33.1 Actuarial survival following lung transplantation. The blue line shows results for all lung transplants, whereas the other lines show results for individual diseases as indicated. Data are from the Registry of the International Society for Heart and Lung Transplantation[7] and include transplants performed worldwide between January 1990 and June 2001. COPD, chronic obstructive pulmonary disease; IPF, idiopathic pulmonary fibrosis; PPH, primary pulmonary hypertension.

Ventilatory performance. After lung transplantation FEV_1 is initially poor owing to the effects of the surgery, but then shows a gradual improvement, reaching a peak 3–6 months after surgery. From pretransplant values of 20–30% of predicted normal, recipients of a single-lung transplant achieve values of 50–60% and patients receiving bilateral lung transplant typically have normal values.[2–4] These improvements in ventilatory performance contribute to the huge improvement in quality of life following lung transplant.

Exercise performance. The attainable level of exercise depends on many factors which, in addition to pulmonary function, include circulation, condition of the voluntary muscles, motivation and freedom from pain on exertion. Improvement in performance does occur following lung transplantation but exercise limitation remains common, with maximal oxygen uptake (page 239) of about half normal. There is no evidence that this limitation results from poor pulmonary function and a muscular origin is more likely, possibly related to myopathy induced by immunosuppressant drugs.[2,4]

Rejection[2,4]

Acute rejection occurs following activation of cytotoxic T-lymphocytes by helper T-cells which 'recognise' the foreign tissue. This form of rejection occurs in about 15% of patients and presents as acute lung injury (see Chapter 31) within 72 hours of the transplant operation. Treatment involves escalation of immunosuppressive therapy and supportive management as for other forms of lung injury. Recovery of the transplanted lung may occur, but mortality from acute rejection is substantial.

Chronic rejection in the lung manifests itself as obliterative bronchiolitis syndrome, the origin of which is not clear but which occurs in up to half of patients, normally more than a year after transplantation.

Detection of chronic rejection. There is a major difficulty in detecting the early stages of acute rejection because it is difficult to distinguish rejection from infection on clinical evidence. Both conditions feature arterial hypoxaemia, pyrexia, leucocytosis, dyspnoea and a reduced capacity for exercise. These changes are followed by a decrease in diffusing capacity and FEV_1 and later by perihilar infiltration or graft opacification on the chest radiograph.

Chronic rejection can normally be detected from a deterioration in previously stable lung function. Bronchiolitis obliterans, as the name suggests, causes significant air flow limitation; the FEV_1 is used as a screening test and also to stage the degree of rejection.

None of the symptoms and signs described are truly diagnostic of either acute or chronic threatened rejection. The gold standard is the histopathology of an open-lung biopsy, which shows perivascular lymphocytic infiltration or bronchiolitis obliterans. However, this procedure is unsuitable for routine screening. Transbronchial biopsy is less invasive, but unreliable in comparison with open-lung biopsy and also not entirely free from hazard.

Immunosuppression.[17] Except in the case of identical twins, survival of the transplanted lung depends on immunosuppression. Current therapy involves immunosuppression by three groups of drugs.

1. Steroids to suppress the transcription of numerous proinflammatory cytokines (page 378).
2. Calcineurin inhibitors, such as ciclosporin-A or tacrolimus, which also reduce cytokine production.
3. Cell-cycle inhibitors, such as azathioprine or mycophenolate mofetil, which suppress cellular production of purines and inhibit lymphocyte subset proliferation.

The continued use of immunosuppression greatly reduces resistance to infection and the transplanted lung is particularly vulnerable to cytomegalovirus, herpes simplex and *Pneumocystis carinii*.

PHYSIOLOGICAL EFFECTS OF LUNG TRANSPLANT

Transplantation inevitably disrupts innervation, lymphatics and the bronchial circulation. The condition of the recipient is further compromised by immunosuppressive therapy.

The denervated lung

The transplanted lung has no afferent or efferent innervation and there is, as yet, no evidence that re-innervation occurs in patients.[18] However, in dogs, vagal stimulation has been observed to cause bronchoconstriction 3–6 months after lung reimplantation[19], and sympathetic reinnervation has been demonstrated after 45 months.[20]

Respiratory rhythm. In Chapter 5, attention was paid to the weakness of the Hering–Breuer reflex in humans. It was therefore to be expected that denervation of the lung, with block of pulmonary baroreceptor input to the medulla, would have minimal effect on the respiratory rhythm. This is in contrast to the dog and most other laboratory animals, in whom vagal block is known to cause slow deep breathing. Bilateral vagal block in human volunteers was already known to leave the respiratory rhythm virtually unchanged[21], and it was therefore no great surprise when it was shown that bilateral lung transplant had no significant effect on the respiratory

rate and rhythm in patients, after the early postoperative period.[22] Breathing during sleep is also normal.[23] Chemical control of ventilation (see Chapter 5) does not depend on either afferent or efferent innervation of the lung and there is no evidence of any abnormality after lung transplant.

Bronchial hypersensitivity. Enhanced sensitivity to the bronchoconstrictor effects of inhaled methacholine and histamine can be demonstrated after heart–lung transplantation.[24] This is thought to be due to hypersensitivity of receptors in airway smooth muscle, following denervation of the predominantly constrictor autonomic supply, though not all studies have demonstrated this.[18] In spite of these findings, airway hyperresponsiveness (page 374) is rarely a problem in transplanted patients.[2]

The cough reflex, in response to afferents arising from below the level of the tracheal or bronchial anastomosis, is permanently lost after lung transplantation.[25] Following single-lung transplant, the remaining diseased lung will continue to stimulate coughing, which will facilitate clearance of secretions from the transplanted lung. Similarly, a bilateral single-lung transplant will be preferable to a double-lung transplant, as the former will maintain intact the potent carinal cough reflex. The abnormality in cough reflex is a major contributor to lung infection following transplant, along with altered mucus clearance as described below.

Ventilation/perfusion ($\dot{V}/\dot{Q}$) relationships

Bilateral lung or heart–lung transplants usually result in normal $\dot{V}/\dot{Q}$ relationships, but following single-lung transplant the situation is more complex. For most indications, including COPD, the single transplanted lung receives the majority of pulmonary ventilation (60–80% of the total) and a similar proportion of pulmonary blood flow and so $\dot{V}/\dot{Q}$ relationships are acceptable, though not normal.[26,27] However, following single-lung transplant for primary pulmonary hypertension, ventilation to the two lungs remains approximately equal although the majority of blood flow (often >80%) is to the transplanted lung. This $\dot{V}/\dot{Q}$ mismatch fortunately has little effect on arterial oxygenation at rest. During exercise in patients with a single-lung transplant, the already high blood flow to the transplanted lung seems not to increase further and the normal recruitment of apical pulmonary capillaries (page 96) cannot be demonstrated.[26]

Hypoxic pulmonary vasoconstriction seems to be an entirely local mechanism and, as might be expected, has been shown to persist in the human transplanted lung,[28] though some studies have demonstrated abnormalities, particularly in patients with pulmonary hypertension.[26,27]

Pleural effusion[29]

The hilar lymphatics are severed at pneumonectomy and it is not feasible to anastomose with the lymphatics of the donor lung. In animals, restoration of pulmonary lymphatics occurs spontaneously within a few weeks, but this has not been demonstrated in humans. In the meantime lymph drains from the severed ends of the donor lung into the recipient's pleural cavity and an effusion develops which may need to be drained with a chest tube. Also, there is some degree of increased pulmonary capillary permeability in the first few days after transplantation, probably as a result of ischaemia/reperfusion injury (page 353) of the graft.[2] This will cause a substantial increase in lymph production and further contribute to pleural fluid accumulation. Drainage of pleural fluid is minimal by a few days after the transplant.

Mucociliary clearance

Mucociliary clearance is defective after transplantation.[30] The cause seems to be defective production of mucus, rather than changes in the frequency of cilial beat. This, together with the absent cough reflex below the line of the airway anastomosis, means that the patient is at a disadvantage in clearing secretions. Side effects of immunosuppression compound these changes and lead to enhanced susceptibility to infection of the transplanted lung. Although these factors clearly do not preclude long-term survival of the graft, one-quarter of deaths following lung transplantation result from infection.[2]

REFERENCES

1. Hardy JD, Webb WR, Dalton ML, Walker GR. Lung homotransplantation in man. *JAMA* 1963; **186**: 1065–74.
2. Trulock EP. Lung transplantation. *Am J Respir Crit Care Med* 1997; **155**: 789–818.
*3. Bracken CA, Gurkowski MA, Naples JJ. Lung transplantation: historical perspectives, current concepts and anesthetic considerations. *J Cardiothorac Vasc Anesth* 1997; **11**: 220–41.
4. Arcasoy SM, Kotloff RM. Lung transplantation. *N Engl J Med* 1999; **340**: 1081–91.
*5. DeMeo DL, Ginns LC. Lung transplantation at the turn of the century. *Annu Rev Med* 2001; **52**: 185–201.
*6. Lau CL, Patterson GA. Current status of lung transplantation. *Eur Respir J* 2003; **22**(Supp 47): 57S–64S.
7. International Society for Heart and Lung Transplantation. 20th Official Annual Data Report 2003. www.ishlt.org/registries
8. Keller CA. The donor lung: conservation of a precious resource. *Thorax* 1998; **53**: 506–13.
9. de Perrot M, Weder W, Patterson GA, Keshavjee S. Strategies to increase limited donor resources. *Eur Respir J* 2004; **23**: 477–82.
10. Singh H, Bossard RF. Perioperative anaesthetic considerations for patients undergoing lung translantation. *Can J Anaesth* 1997; **44**: 284–99.
11. Marczin N, Royston D, Yacoub M. Pro: lung transplantation should be routinely performed with cardiopulmonary bypass. *J Cardiothorac Vasc Anesth* 2000; **14**: 739–45.
12. McRae K. Con: lung transplantation should not be routinely performed with cardiopulmonary bypass. *J Cardiothorac Vasc Anesth* 2000; **14**: 746–50.
13. Starnes VA, Barr ML, Cohen RG, *et al*. Living-donor lobar lung transplantation experience: intermediate results. *J Thorac Cardiovasc Surg* 1996; **112**: 1284–91.
14. Quinlan JJ, Gasior T, Firestone S, Firestone LL. Anesthesia for living-related (lobar) lung transplantation. *J Cardiothorac Vasc Anesth* 1996; **10**: 391–6.
15. Dark JH. Lung: living related transplantation. *Br Med Bull* 1997; **53**: 892–903.
16. Patterson GA. Airway revascularization: is it necessary? *Ann Thorac Surg* 1993; **56**: 807–8.
17. Knoop C, Haverich A, Fischer S. Immunosuppressive therapy after human lung transplantation. *Eur Respir J* 2004; **23**: 159–71.
18. Stretton CD, Mak JCW, Belvisi MG, Yacoub MH, Barnes PJ. Cholinergic control of human airways *in vitro* following extrinsic denervation of the human respiratory tract by heart-lung transplantation. *Am Rev Respir Dis* 1990; **142**: 1030–3.
19. Edmunds LH, Graf PD, Nadel JA. Reinnervation of reimplanted canine lung. *J Appl Physiol* 1971; **31**: 722–7.
20. Lall A, Graf PD, Nadel JA, Edmunds LH. Adrenergic reinnervation of the reimplanted dog lung. *J Appl Physiol* 1973; **35**: 439–42.
21. Guz A, Noble MIM, Widdicombe JG, Trenchard D, Mushin WW, Makey AR. The role of the vagal and glossopharyngeal afferent nerves in respiratory sensation, control of breathing and arterial pressure regulation in conscious man. *Clin Sci* 1966; **30**: 161–70.
22. Shaw IH, Kirk AJB, Conacher ID. Anaesthesia for patients with transplanted hearts and lungs undergoing non-cardiac surgery. *Br J Anaesth* 1991; **67**: 772–81.
23. Sanders MH, Costantino JP, Owens GR, *et al*. Breathing during wakefulness and sleep after human heart-lung transplantation. *Am Rev Respir Dis* 1989; **140**: 45–51.
24. Glanville AR, Burke CM, Theodore J, *et al*. Bronchial hyper-responsiveness after human cardiopulmonary transplantation. *Clin Sci* 1987; **73**: 299–303.

25. Higenbottam T, Jackson M, Woolman P, Lowry R, Wallwork J. The cough response to ultrasonically nebulized distilled water in heart-lung transplantation patients. *Am Rev Respir Dis* 1989; **140**: 58–61.

26. Ross DJ, Waters PF, Waxman AD, Koerner SK, Mohsenifar Z. Regional distribution of lung perfusion and ventilation at rest and during steady-state exercise after unilateral lung transplantation. *Chest* 1993; **104**: 130–5.

27. Kuni CC, Ducret RP, Nakhleh RE, Boudreau RJ. Reverse mismatch between perfusion and aerosol ventilation in transplanted lungs. *Clin Nucl Med* 1993; **18**: 313–17.

28. Robin ED, Theodore J, Burke CM, *et al.* Hypoxic pulmonary vasconstriction persists in the human transplanted lung. *Clin Sci* 1987; **72**: 283–7.

29. Judson MA, Handy JR, Sahn SA. Pleural effusions following lung transplantation: time course, characteristics and clinical implications. *Chest* 1996; **109**: 1190–4.

30. Herve P, Silbert D, Cerrina J, Simonneau G, Dartevelle P and the Paris-Sud Lung Transplant Group. Impairment of bronchial mucociliary clearance in long-term survivors of heart/lung and double-lung transplantation. *Chest* 1993; **103**: 59–63.

Appendix

A Physical quantities and units of measurement

SI UNITS

A clean transition from the old to the new metric units failed to occur. The old system was based on the centimetre-gram-second (CGS) and was supplemented with many non-coherent derived units such as the millimetre of mercury for pressure and the calorie for work, which could not be related to the basic units by factors which were powers of ten. The new system, the Système Internationale or SI, is based on the metre-kilogram-second (MKS) and comprises base and derived units which are obtained simply by multiplication or division without the introduction of numbers, not even powers of ten.[1]

Base units are metre (length), kilogram (mass), second (time), ampere (electric current), kelvin (thermodynamic temperature), mole (amount of substance) and candela (luminous intensity).

Derived units include newton (force: kilograms metre second^{-2}), pascal (pressure: newton metre^{-2}), joule (work: newton metre) and hertz (periodic frequency: second^{-1}).

Special non-SI units are recognised as having sufficient practical importance to warrant retention for general or specialised use. These include litre, day, hour, minute and the standard atmosphere.

Non-recommended units include the dyne, bar, calorie, and gravity-dependent units such as the kilogram-force, centimetre of water and millimetre of mercury, the demise of which has been expected for many years.

The introduction of SI units into anaesthesia and respiratory physiology remains incomplete. The kilopascal is replacing the millimetre of mercury for blood gas tensions, the transition being almost complete in most European countries but barely started in the USA, where mmHg had been replaced by the almost identical torr. The introduction of the kilopascal for fluid pressures in the medical field is being delayed for what appears to be an entirely specious attachment to the mercury or water manometer. We appear to be condemned to a further period during which we record arterial pressure in mmHg, venous pressure in cmH$_2$O and cerebrospinal fluid pressure in mmH$_2$O. This absurd situation would be less dangerous if all staff knew the relationship between a millimetre of mercury and a centimetre of water.

As in previous editions of this book, it has proved necessary to make text and figures bilingual, with both SI and CGS units for the benefit of readers who are unfamiliar with one or other of the systems. Some useful conversion factors are listed in Table A.l. There are still some areas of physiology and medicine where non-SI units continue to be extensively used, such as mmHg for most vascular pressures and cmH$_2$O for airway pressure, so these units are retained throughout this book to aid clarity.

Physical quantities relevant to respiratory physiology are defined below, together with their mass/length/time (MLT) units. These units provide a most useful check of the validity of equations and other expressions which are derived in the course of studies of respiratory function. Only quantities with identical MLT units can be added or subtracted, and the units must be the same on both sides of an equation.

VOLUME (DIMENSIONS: L^3)

In this book we are concerned with volumes of blood and gas. Strict SI units would be cubic metres and sub-multiples. However, the litre (l) and millilitre (ml) are recognised as special non-SI units and will remain in use. For practical purposes, we may ignore changes in the volume of liquids which are caused by changes of temperature. However, the changes in volume of gases caused by changes of temperature or pressure are by no means negligible and constitute an important source of error if they are ignored. These are discussed in detail in Appendix C.

Table A.1 Conversion factors for units of measurement

Force

1 N (newton)	$= 10^5$ dyn

Pressure

1 kPa (kilopascal)	= 7.50 mmHg
	= 10.2 cmH_2O
	= 0.009 87 standard atmospheres
	= 10 000 $dyn.cm^{-2}$
1 standard atmosphere	= 101.3 kPa
	= 760 mmHg
	= 1033 cmH_2O
	= 10 m of sea water (SG 1.033)
1 mmHg	= 1.36 cmH_2O
	= 1 torr (approx)

Compliance

1 $l.kPa^{-1}$	= 0.098 $l.cmH_2O^{-1}$

Flow resistance

1 $kPa.l^{-1}.s^{-1}$	= 10.2 $cmH_2O.l^{-1}.s^{-1}$

Work

1 J (joule)	= 0.102 kilopond metres
	= 0.239 calories

Power

1 W (watt)	= 1 $J.s^{-1}$
	= 6.12 $kp.m.min^{-1}$

Surface tension

1 $N.m^{-1}$ (newton metre or pascal metre)	= 1000 $dyn.cm^{-1}$

In the figures, tables and text of this book 1 kPa has been taken to equal 7.5 mmHg or 10 cmH_2O.

FLUID FLOW RATE (DIMENSIONS: L^3/T OR L^3T^{-1})

In the case of liquids, flow rate is the physical quantity of cardiac output, regional blood flow etc. The strict SI units would be $metre^3.second^{-1}$ but litres per minute ($l.min^{-1}$) and millilitres per minute ($ml.min^{-1}$) are special non-SI units which may be retained. For gases, the dimension is applied to minute volume of respiration, alveolar ventilation, peak expiratory flow rate, oxygen consumption etc. The units are the same as those for liquids, except that litres per second are used for the high instantaneous flow rates that occur during the course of inspiration and expiration.

In the case of gas flow rates, just as much attention should be paid to the matter of temperature and pressure as when volumes are being measured (see Appendix C).

FORCE (DIMENSIONS: MLT^{-2})

Force is defined as mass times acceleration. An understanding of the units of force is essential to an understanding of the units of pressure. Force, when applied to a free body, causes it to change either the magnitude or the direction of its velocity.

The units of force are of two types. The first is the force resulting from the action of gravity on a mass and is synonymous with weight. It includes the kilogram-force and the pound-force (as in the pound per square inch). All such units are non-recommended under the SI and have almost disappeared. The second type of unit of force is absolute and does not depend on the magnitude of the gravitational field. In the CGS system, the absolute unit of force was the dyne, and this has been replaced under the MKS system and the SI by the newton (N), which is defined as the force which will give a mass of 1 kilogram an acceleration of 1 metre per second per second.

$$1 \text{ N} = 1 \text{ kg.m.s}^{-2}$$

PRESSURE (DIMENSIONS: MLT^{-2}/L^2 OR $ML^{-1}T^{-2}$)

Pressure is defined as force per unit area. The SI unit is the pascal (Pa), which is 1 newton per square metre.

$$1 \text{ Pa} = 1 \text{ N m}^{-2}$$

The pascal is inconveniently small (one hundred-thousandth of an atmosphere) and the kilopascal (kPa) has been adopted for general use in the medical field. Its introduction is simplified by the fact that the kPa is very close to 1% of an atmosphere. Thus a standard atmosphere is 101.3 kPa and the PO_2 of dry air is very close to 21 kPa. The kilopascal will eventually replace the millimetre of mercury and the centimetre of water, both of which are gravity based.

The standard atmosphere may continue to be used under SI. It is defined as $1.013\ 25 \times 10^5$ pascals.

The torr came into use only shortly before the move towards SI units. This is unfortunate for the memory of Torricelli, as the torr will disappear from use. The torr is defined as exactly equal to 1/760 of a standard atmosphere and it is therefore very close to the millimetre of mercury, the two units being considered identical for practical purposes. The only distinction is that the torr is absolute, whereas the millimetre of mercury is gravity based.

The bar is the absolute unit of pressure in the old CGS system and is defined as 10^6 dyn.cm^{-2}. The unit was convenient because the bar is close to 1 atmosphere (1.013 bars) and a millibar is close to 1 centimetre of water (0.9806 millibars).

COMPLIANCE (DIMENSIONS: $M^{-1}L^4T^2$)

The term 'compliance' is used in respiratory physiology to denote the volume change of the lungs in response to a change of pressure. The dimensions are therefore volume divided by pressure and the commonest units have been litres (or millilitres) per centimetre of water. This continues to slowly change over to litres per kilopascal (l.kPa^{-1}).

RESISTANCE TO FLUID FLOW (DIMENSIONS: $ML^{-4}T^{-1}$)

Under conditions of laminar flow (see Figure 4.2) it is possible to express resistance to gas flow as the ratio of pressure difference to gas flow rate. This is analogous to electrical resistance, which is expressed as the ratio of potential difference to current flow. The dimensions of resistance to gas flow are pressure difference divided by gas flow rate and typical units in the respiratory field have been cmH$_2$O per litre per second (cmH$_2$O.l^{-1}.s^{-1}) or dynes.s.cm^{-5} in absolute units. Appropriate SI units will probably be kPa.l^{-1}.s^{-1}.

WORK (DIMENSIONS: ML^2T^{-2}, DERIVED FROM $MLT^{-2} \times L$ OR $ML^{-1}T^{-2} \times L^3$)

Work is done when a force moves its point of application or gas is moved in response to a pressure gradient. The dimensions are therefore either force times distance or pressure times volume, in each case simplifying to ML^2T^{-2}. The multiplicity of units of work has caused confusion in the past. Under SI, the erg, calorie and kilopond-metre will disappear in favour of the joule, which is defined as the work done when a force of 1 newton moves its point of application 1 metre. It is also the work done when 1 litre of gas moves in response to a pressure gradient of 1 kilopascal. This represents a welcome simplification.

$$1 \text{ joule} = 1 \text{ newton metre} = 1 \text{ litre kilopascal}$$

POWER (DIMENSIONS: ML^2T^{-2}/T OR ML^2T^{-3})

Power is the rate at which work is done and so has the dimensions of work divided by time. The SI unit is the watt, which equals 1 joule per second. Power is the correct dimension for the rate of continuous expenditure of biological energy, although one talks loosely about the 'work of breathing'. This is incorrect and 'power of breathing' is the correct term.

SURFACE TENSION (DIMENSIONS: MLT^{-2}/L OR MT^{-2})

Surface tension has been important to the respiratory physiologist since the realisation of the part it plays in lung recoil (see Chapter 3). The CGS units of surface tension are dynes per centimetre (of interface). The appropriate SI unit would be the newton per metre. This has the following rather curious relationships:

$$1 \text{ N m}^{-1} = 1 \text{ Pa m} = 1 \text{ kg.s}^{-2}$$

The unit for surface tension is likely to be called the pascal metre (Pa m), which is identical to the newton per metre.

REFERENCE

1. Baron DN. *Units, symbols, and abbreviations. A guide for medical and scientific editors and authors*, 5th edn. London: Royal Society of Medicine Press, 1994.

A knowledge of physics is more important to the understanding of the respiratory system than of any other system of the body. Not only gas transfer but also ventilation and perfusion of the lungs occur largely in response to physical forces, with vital processes playing a less conspicuous role than is the case, for example, in brain, heart or kidney.

Certain physical attributes of gases are customarily presented under the general heading of the gas laws. These are of fundamental importance in respiratory physiology.

Boyle's law describes the inverse relationship between the volume and absolute pressure of a perfect gas at constant temperature:

$$PV = K \qquad (1)$$

where P represents pressure and V represents volume. At temperatures near their boiling point, gases deviate from Boyle's law. At room temperature, the deviation is negligible for oxygen and nitrogen and of little practical importance for carbon dioxide or nitrous oxide.

Charles' law describes the direct relationship between the volume and absolute temperature of a perfect gas at constant pressure:

$$V = KT \qquad (2)$$

where T represents the absolute temperature. There are appreciable deviations at temperatures immediately above the boiling point of gases. Equations (1) and (2) may be combined as:

$$PV = RT \qquad (3)$$

where R is the universal gas constant, which is the same for all perfect gases and has the value of 8.1314 joules.degrees kelvin^{-1}.moles^{-1}. From this it may be derived that the mole volume of all perfect gases is 22.4 litres at standard temperature and pressure, dry (STPD). Carbon dioxide and nitrous oxide deviate from the behaviour of perfect gases to the extent of having mole volumes of about 22.2 litres at STPD.

Henry's law describes the solution of gases in liquids with which they do not react. The general principle of Henry's law is simple enough. The number of molecules of gas dissolving in the solvent is directly proportional to the partial pressure of the gas at the surface of the liquid, and the constant of proportionality is an expression of the solubility of the gas in the liquid. This is a constant for a particular gas and a particular liquid at a particular temperature but usually falls with rising temperature.

Unfortunately, confusion often arises from the multiplicity of units that are used. For example, when considering oxygen dissolved in blood, it has been customary to consider the amount of gas dissolved in units of vols% (ml of gas at STPD per 100 ml blood) and the pressure in mmHg. Solubility is then expressed as vols% per mmHg, the value for oxygen in blood at 37°C being about 0.003. However, for carbon dioxide in blood, we tend to use units of mmol.l^{-1} of carbon dioxide per mmHg. The units are then mmol.l^{-1}.mmHg^{-1}, the value for carbon dioxide in blood at 37°C being 0.03. Both vols% and mmol.l^{-1} are valid measurements of the quantity (mass or number of molecules) of the gas in solution and are interchangeable with the appropriate conversion factor.

Physicists are more inclined to express solubility in terms of the *Bunsen coefficient*. For this, the amount of gas in solution is expressed in terms of volume of gas (STPD) per unit volume of solvent (i.e. one-hundredth of the amount expressed as vols%) and the pressure is expressed in atmospheres.

Biologists, on the other hand, prefer to use the *Ostwald coefficient*. This is the volume of gas dissolved, expressed as its volume under the conditions of temperature and pressure at which solution took place. It might be thought that this would vary with the pressure in the gas phase, but this is not so. If the pressure is doubled, according to Henry's law, twice as many molecules of gas dissolve. However, according to Boyle's law, they would occupy half the volume at double the pressure. Therefore, if Henry's and Boyle's laws are obeyed, the Ostwald coefficient will be independent of changes in pressure at which solution occurs. It will differ from the Bunsen coefficient only because the gas volume is expressed as the volume it would occupy at the temperature of the experiment rather than at 0°C. Conversion is thus in accord with Charles' law and the two coefficients will be identical at 0°C. This should not be confused with the fact that, like the Bunsen coefficient, the Ostwald coefficient falls with rising temperature.

The partition coefficient is the ratio of the number of molecules of gas in one phase to the number of molecules of gas in another phase when equilibrium between the two has been attained. If one phase is gas and the other liquid, the liquid/gas partition coefficient will be identical to the Ostwald coefficient. Partition coefficients are also used to describe partitioning between two media (e.g. oil/water, brain/blood etc.).

Graham's law of diffusion governs the influence of molecular weight on the diffusion of a gas through a gas mixture. Diffusion rates through orifices or through porous plates are inversely proportional to the square root of the molecular weight. This factor is only of importance in the gaseous part of the pathway between ambient air and the tissues, and is, in general, only of importance when the molecular weight is greater than that of oxygen or carbon dioxide. Graham's law is not relevant to the process of 'diffusion' through the alveolar/capillary membrane (page 136).

Dalton's law of partial pressure states that, in a mixture of gases, each gas exerts the pressure that it would exert if it occupied the volume alone (see Figure 13.8). This is known as the partial pressure (or tension) and the sum of the partial pressures equals the total pressure of the mixture. Thus, in a mixture of 5% carbon dioxide in oxygen at a total pressure of 101 kPa (760 mmHg), the carbon dioxide exerts a partial pressure of $5/100 \times 101$ = 5.05 kPa (38 mmHg). In general terms:

$$P_{CO_2} = F_{CO_2} \times P_B$$

In the alveolar gas at sea level there is about 6.2% water vapour, which exerts a partial pressure of 6.3 kPa (47 mmHg). The available pressure for other gases is therefore $(P_B - 6.3)$ kPa or $(P_B - 47)$ mmHg. Gas concentrations are usually measured in the dry gas phase and therefore it is necessary to apply this correction for water vapour in the lungs.

Tension is synonymous with partial pressure and is applied particularly to gases dissolved in a liquid such as blood. Molecules of gases dissolved in liquids have a tendency to escape, but net loss may be prevented by exposing the liquid to a gas mixture in which the partial pressure of the gas exactly balances the escape tendency. The two phases are then said to be in equilibrium and *the tension of a gas in a liquid is defined as the tension of the gas in a gas mixture with which the liquid is in equilibrium*. Thus a blood P_{CO_2} of 5.3 kPa (40 mmHg) means that there would be no net exchange of carbon dioxide if the blood were exposed to a gas mixture which had a P_{CO_2} of 5.3 kPa (40 mmHg).

C Conversion factors for gas volumes

Gas volumes are usually measured at ambient (or environmental) temperature and pressure, either dry (e.g. from a cylinder passing through a rotameter) or saturated with water vapour at ambient temperature (e.g. an expired gas sample). Customary abbreviations are ATPD (ambient temperature and pressure, dry) and ATPS (ambient temperature and pressure, saturated).

CONVERSION OF GAS VOLUME – ATPS TO BTPS

Gas volumes measured by spirometry and other methods usually indicate the volume at ambient temperature and pressure, saturated (ATPS). Tidal volume, minute volume, dead space, lung volumes and ventilatory gas flow rates etc. should be converted to the volumes they would occupy in the lungs of the patient at body temperature and pressure, saturated (BTPS).

Conversion from ATPS to BTPS is based on Charles' and Boyle's laws (see Appendix B) and conversion factors are listed in Table C.1.

Derivation of conversion factors

$$\text{Volume}_{(BTPS)} = \text{volume}_{(ATPS)} \left(\frac{273 + 37}{273 + t} \right) \left(\frac{P_B - P_{H_2O}}{P_B - 6.3} \right)$$

P_B is barometric pressure (kPa) and Table C.1 has been prepared for a barometric pressure of 100 kPa (750 mmHg); variations in the range 99–101 kPa (740–760 mmHg) have a negligible effect on the factors.

t is ambient temperature (°C). Table C.1 has been prepared for a body temperature of 37°C; variations in the range 35–39°C are of little importance.

P_{H_2O} is the water vapour pressure of the sample (kPa) at ambient temperature (see Table C.1).

CONVERSION OF GAS VOLUME – ATPS TO STPD

In measurement of absolute amounts of gases such as oxygen uptake, carbon dioxide output and the exchange of 'inert' gases, we need to know the actual quantity (i.e. number of molecules) of gas exchanged and this is most conveniently expressed by stating the gas volume as it would be under standard conditions, i.e. 0°C, 101.3 kPa (760 mmHg) pressure and dry (STPD). Under these conditions, one mole of an ideal gas occupies 22.4 litres.

Conversion from ATPS to STPD is again by application of Charles' and Boyle's laws, as follows:

$$\text{Volume}_{(STPD)} = \text{volume}_{(ATPS)} \left(\frac{273}{273 + t} \right) \left(\frac{P_B - P_{H_2O}}{101} \right)$$

P_B is barometric pressure (kPa).

t is ambient temperature (°C).

P_{H_2O} is the saturated water vapour pressure of the sample (kPa) at ambient temperature

Table C.1 Factors for conversion of gas volumes measured under conditions of ambient temperature and pressure, saturated (ATPS) to volumes that would be occupied under conditions of body temperature and pressure, saturated (BTPS)

Ambient temperature °C	Conversion factor	Saturated water vapour pressure	
		kPa	mmHg
15	1.129	1.71	12.8
16	1.124	1.81	13.6
17	1.119	1.93	14.5
18	1.113	2.07	15.5
19	1.108	2.20	16.5
20	1.103	2.33	17.5
21	1.097	2.48	18.6
22	1.092	2.64	19.8
23	1.086	2.80	21.0
24	1.081	2.99	22.4
25	1.075	3.16	23.7
26	1.069	3.66	25.2

Appendix

D Symbols and abbreviations

Symbols used in this book are in accordance with recommendations for editors of medical and scientific publications in the United Kingdom.[1] There continues to be variation between journals, particularly between Europe and the USA. The use of these symbols is very helpful for an understanding of the quantitative relationships that are so important in respiratory physiology.

Primary symbols (large capitals) denoting physical quantities.

F fractional concentration of gas
P pressure, tension or partial pressure of a gas
V volume of a gas
Q volume of blood
C content of a gas in blood
S saturation of haemoglobin with oxygen
R respiratory exchange ratio (RQ)
D diffusing capacity

˙ denotes a time derivative, e.g. $\dot{V}$ ventilation, $\dot{Q}$ blood flow

Secondary symbols denoting location of quantity.

in gas phase (small capitals)	in blood (lower case)
I inspired gas	a arterial blood
E expired gas	v venous blood
A alveolar gas	c capillary
D dead space	t total
T tidal	s shunt
B barometric (usually pressure)	

⁻ denotes mixed or mean, e.g. v̄ mixed venous blood, Ē mixed expired gas
′ denotes end, e.g. E′ end-expiratory gas, c′ end-capillary blood

Tertiary symbols indicating particular gases.
O_2 oxygen
CO_2 carbon dioxide
N_2O nitrous oxide
etc.
f denotes the respiratory frequency
BTPS, ATPS and STPD: see Appendix C.

Examples of respiratory symbols

$P_{A_{O_2}}$ alveolar oxygen partial pressure
$C\bar{v}_{O_2}$ oxygen content of mixed venous blood
$\dot{V}_{O_2}$ oxygen consumption

REFERENCE

1. Baron DN. *Units, symbols, and abbreviations. A guide for medical and scientific editors and authors*, 5th edn. London: Royal Society of Medicine Press, 1994.

Appendix

E

Nomograms and correction charts

BLOOD GAS CORRECTION NOMOGRAMS FOR TIME

This nomogram (Figure E.1) is designed for the application of corrections for metabolism of blood occurring between sampling and analysis (page 161). The effect of temperature is based on the cooling curve when blood is drawn at 37°C into a 5 ml glass or 2 ml plastic syringe at room temperature, followed by storage at room temperature. Elapsed time between sampling and analysis is shown on the ordinate. Line charts indicate the change in $P\mathrm{CO_2}$ (which rises), pH (which falls) and base excess (which falls). A graph is required for the change in $P\mathrm{O_2}$ (which falls) because the rate of fall depends upon the $P\mathrm{O_2}$. For details, see reference 1.

BLOOD GAS CORRECTION NOMOGRAM FOR PATIENT TEMPERATURE (Figure E.2)

Enter with the patient's temperature on the abscissa. *Multiply* the measured gas tension by the factor shown on the ordinate, using the appropriate curve for $P\mathrm{O_2}$ based on the saturation of the sample. The broken line should be used for $P\mathrm{O_2}$, whatever the level of $P\mathrm{CO_2}$. The line chart at the top of the graph may be used for the pH correction, which should be *added*. For details, see reference 1.

THE SIGAARD-ANDERSEN CURVE NOMOGRAM

The *in vitro* relationship between pH and $P\mathrm{CO_2}$ of oxygenated blood is indicated either by a line joining two points obtained after *in vitro* equilibration or by a line passing through the actual arterial values and with a slope dependent on the haemoglobin concentration. The slope is that of a line joining the normal arterial point (indicated by a small circle in the diagram) and the appropriate point on the haemoglobin scale (i.e. 14 g.dl^{-1} in the example shown). Intersections of the buffer line indicate three indices of metabolic acid–base state: buffer base, standard bicarbonate and base excess, the last of which is the most commonly used. Interpolation of $P\mathrm{CO_2}$ indicates corresponding (*in vitro*) pH values and vice versa.

The example in Figure E.3 is normal arterial blood (*in vitro* changes); other equilibration curves are shown in Figure 10.5.

THE ISO-SHUNT CHART

Figure E.4 is a diagram of the theoretical relationship between arterial $P\mathrm{O_2}$ and inspired oxygen concentration for different values of virtual shunt. It is based on assumed values as follows:

Arterial $P\mathrm{CO_2}$ 5.3 kPa (40 mmHg)
Arterial/mixed venous oxygen content difference 5 ml.dl^{-1}
Haemoglobin concentration 14 g.dl^{-1}

Virtual shunt is defined as the shunt that gives the relationships depicted when the arterial/mixed venous oxygen content difference is 5 ml.dl^{-1}. These curves include a small component for moderate non-uniformity of ventilation/perfusion ratios of the ventilated alveoli.[3,4] For further details, see page 124 *et seq.*

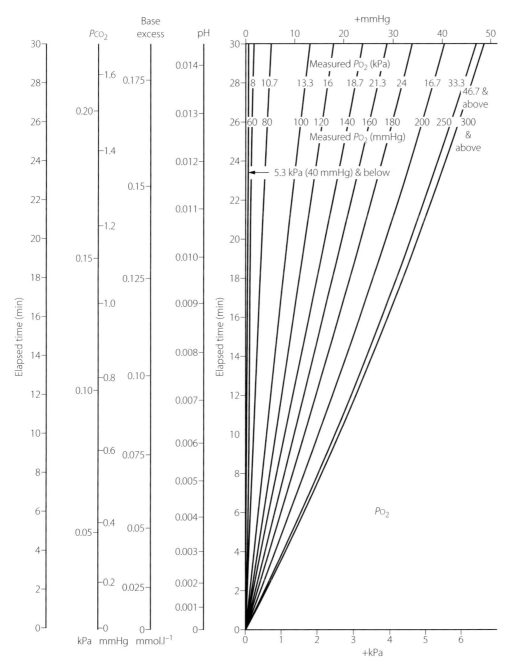

Figure E.1 Nomogram for correcting blood P_{CO_2}, P_{O_2}, pH and base excess for metabolic changes occurring between sampling and analysis. (Reproduced from reference 1 by permission of the Editors of the *Journal of Applied Physiology*.)

461

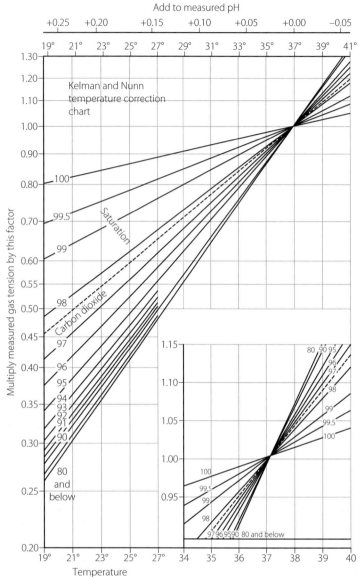

Figure E.2 Nomogram for correction of blood P_{CO_2}, P_{O_2} and pH for differences between temperature of patient and electrode system (assumed to be 37°C). (Reproduced from reference 1 by permission of the Editors of *Journal of Applied Physiology*.)

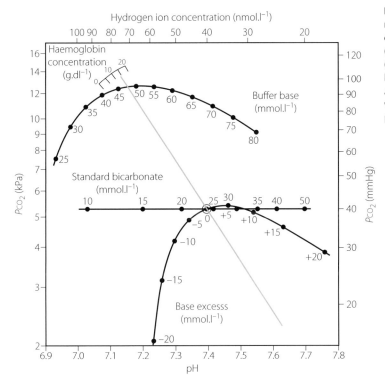

Figure E.3 The Sigaard-Andersen curve nomogram relating pH and P_{CO_2} for oxygenated blood *in vitro*. The example shown (blue line) is for normal arterial blood. (Reprinted from The pH, log P_{CO_2} blood acid–base nomogram revisited by O. Sigaard-Andersen from *Scand J Clin Lab Invest*, www.tandf.no/sjcli, 1962; **14**: 598–604 by permission of Taylor & Francis AS.)

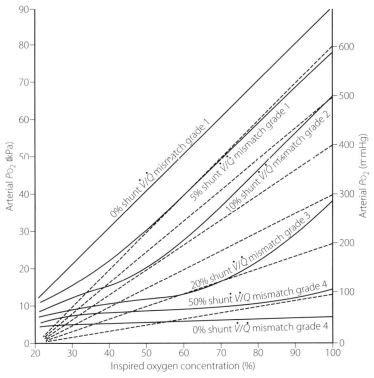

Figure E.4 Arterial P_{O_2} as a function of inspired oxygen concentration on a modified iso-shunt diagram (see Figure 8.11), incorporating a factor for ventilation/perfusion mismatch (see Figure 8.14). Normal values are assumed for P_{CO_2}, haemoglobin concentration and arterial/mixed venous oxygen content difference. Note the reverse curves below an inspired oxygen concentration of 40% with mismatch grades of 2–4. The broken lines indicate arterial P_{O_2} expressed as a ratio of inspired oxygen concentration, as used for example in the calculations of lung injury score (see Table 31.1).

REFERENCES

1. Kelman GR, Nunn JF. Nomograms for correction of blood P_{O_2}, P_{CO_2}, pH and base excess for time and temperature. *J Appl Physiol* 1966; 21: 1484–90.
2. Sigaard-Andersen O. The pH, log P_{CO_2} blood acid-base nomogram revisited. *Scand J Clin Lab Invest* 1962; **14**: 598–604.
3. Benator SR, Hewlett AM, Nunn JF. The use of iso-shunt lines for control of oxygen therapy. *Br J Anaesth* 1973; **45**: 711–18.
4. Petros AJ, Doré CJ, Nunn JF. Modification of the iso-shunt lines for low inspired oxygen concentrations. *Br J Anaesth* 1994; **72**: 515–22.

F Mathematical functions relevant to respiratory physiology

This book contains many examples of mathematical statements, which relate respiratory variables under specified conditions. Appendix F is intended to refresh the memory of those readers whose knowledge of mathematics has been attenuated under the relentless pressure of new information acquired in the course of study of the biological sciences.

The most basic study of respiratory physiology requires familiarity with at least four types of mathematical relationship. These are:

1. the linear function
2. the rectangular hyperbola or inverse function
3. the parabola or squared function
4. exponential functions.

These four types of function will now be considered separately with reference to examples drawn from this book.

THE LINEAR FUNCTION

Examples

1. Pressure gradient against flow rate with laminar flow (page 40). There is no constant factor and the pressure gradient is zero when flow rate is zero.
2. Respiratory minute volume against P_{CO_2} (page 62). In this case there is a constant factor corresponding to a 'negative' respiratory minute volume when P_{CO_2} is zero.
3. Over a limited range, lung volume is proportional to inflating pressure (page 29). The slope of the line is then the compliance.

Mathematical statement. A linear function describes a change in one variable (dependent or y variable) that is directly proportional to another variable (independent or x variable). There may or may not be a constant factor which is equal to y when x is zero. Thus:

$$y = ax + b$$

where a is the slope of the line and b is the constant factor. In any one particular relationship a and b are assumed to be constant, but both may have different values under other circumstances. They are not there-

fore true constants (like π, for example) and are more precisely termed parameters, whereas y and x are variables.

Graphical representation. Figure F.1 shows a plot of a linear function following the convention that the independent variable (x) is plotted on the abscissa and the dependent variable (y) on the ordinate. Note that the relationship is a straight line, and simple regression analysis is based on the assumption that the relationship is of this type. If the slope (a) is positive, the line goes upwards and to the right. If the slope is negative, the line goes upwards and to the left.

THE RECTANGULAR HYPERBOLA OR INVERSE FUNCTION

Examples

1. The ventilatory response to hypoxia (expressed in terms of P_{O_2}) approximates to a rectangular hyperbola, asymptotic on the horizontal axis to the respiratory minute volume at high P_{O_2} and, on the vertical axis, to the P_{O_2} at which it is assumed ventilation increases towards infinity.
2. The relationships of alveolar gas tensions to alveolar ventilation are conveniently described by rectangular hyperbolas (for carbon dioxide see page 157 and for oxygen see page 168). The curves are concave upwards for gases that are eliminated (e.g. carbon dioxide) and concave downwards for gases that are taken up from the lungs (e.g. oxygen). Curvature is governed by gas output (or uptake), and the asymptotes in each case are zero ventilation and partial pressure of the gas under consideration in the inspired gas. The relationship is extremely helpful for understanding the quantitative relationship between ventilation and alveolar gas tensions.
3. Airway resistance approximates to an inverse function of lung volume (page 43).

Mathematical statement. A rectangular hyperbola describes a relationship when the dependent variable y

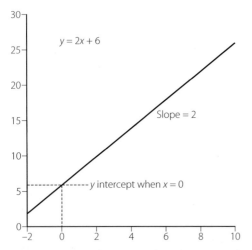

Figure F.1 A linear function plotted on linear coordinates. Examples include pressure/flow rate relationships with laminar flow (see Figure 4.2) and P_{CO_2}/ventilation response curves (see Figure 5.5).

is inversely proportional to the independent variable x thus:

$$y = a/x + b$$

The asymptote of x is its value when y is infinity and the asymptote of y is its value when x is infinity. If b is zero, then the relationship may be simply represented as follows:

$$xy = a$$

Graphical representation. Figure F.2a shows rectangular hyperbolas with and without constant factors. Changes in the value of a alter the curvature but not the asymptotes. Figure F.2b shows the same relationships plotted on logarithmic coordinates. The relationship is now linear but with a negative slope of unity because, if:

$$xy = a$$

then:

$$\log y = -\log x + \log a$$

THE PARABOLA OR SQUARED FUNCTION

Example

With fully turbulent gas flow, pressure gradient changes according to the square of gas flow and the plot is a typical parabola (see Chapter 4).

Mathematical statement. A parabola is described when the dependent variable (y) changes in proportion to the square of the independent variable (x), thus:

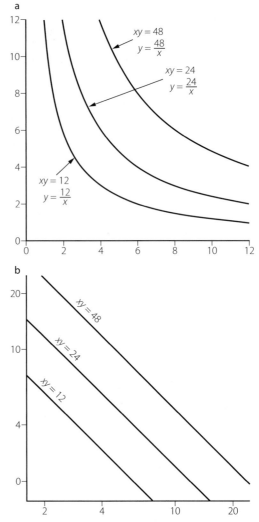

Figure F.2 Rectangular hyperbolas plotted on **(a)** linear coordinates and **(b)** logarithmic coordinates. Examples include the relationships between alveolar gas tensions and alveolar ventilation (see Figures 10.9, 11.2), P_{O_2}/ventilation response curves (see Figure 5.8) and the relationship between airway resistance and lung volume (see Figures 4.5 and 22.13).

$$y = ax^2$$

Graphical representation. On linear coordinates, a parabola, with positive values of the abscissa, shows a steeply rising curve (Figure F.3a), which may be confused with an exponential function (see below) although it is fundamentally different. On logarithmic coordinates for both abscissa and ordinate, a parabola becomes a straight line with a slope of 2 (Figure F.3b) because log $y = \log a + 2 \log x$ (a and log a are parameters).

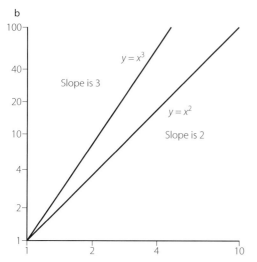

Figure F.3 Parabolas plotted on (a) linear coordinates and (b) logarithmic coordinates. An example is the pressure/volume relationship with turbulent flow (see Figure 4.3b).

EXPONENTIAL FUNCTIONS

General statement

An exponential function describes a change in which the rate of change of the dependent variable is proportional to the magnitude of the independent variable at that time. Thus, the rate of change of y with respect to x (i.e. dy/dx)* varies in proportion to the value of y at that instant. That is to say:

---

*dy/dx is the mathematical shorthand for the rate of change of y with respect to x. The 'd' means 'a very small bit of'; therefore dy/dx means a very small bit of y divided by the corresponding very small bit of x. This is equal to the slope of the graph of y against x at that point. In the case of a curve, it is the slope of a tangent drawn to the curve at that point.

$$\frac{dy}{dx} = ky$$

where k is a constant or a parameter.

This general equation appears with minor modifications in three main forms. To the biological worker they may be conveniently described as the tear-away, the wash-out and the wash-in.

The tear-away exponential function

This must be described first, as it is the simplest form of the exponential function. It is, however, the least important of the three in relation to respiratory function.

Simple statement. In a tear-away exponential function, the quantity under consideration increases at a rate which is in direct proportion to its actual value – the richer one is, the faster one makes money.

Examples. Classic examples are compound interest and the mythical water-lily that doubles its diameter every day (Figure F.4). A typical biological example is the free spread of a bacterial colony in which (for example) each bacterium divides every 20 minutes. The doubling time of this example would be 20 minutes.

Mathematical statement. In the case of exponential functions relevant to respiratory function, the independent

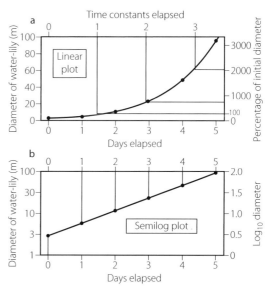

Figure F.4 The growth of a water-lily that doubles its diameter every day – a typical tear-away exponential function. Initial diameter, 3 metres; size doubled every day (i.e. doubling time = 1 day).

variable x almost invariably represents time, and so we shall take the liberty of replacing x with t throughout. The tear-away function may thus be represented as follows:

$$\frac{dy}{dt} = ky$$

A little mathematical processing will convert this equation into a more useful form, which will indicate the instantaneous value of y at any time t.

First multiply both sides by dt/y:

$$\frac{1}{y}dy = kdt$$

Next integrate both sides with respect to t:

$$\log_e y + C_1 = kt + C_2$$

(C_1 and C_2 are constants of integration and may be collected on the right-hand side.)

$$\log_e y = (C_2 - C_1) + kt$$

Finally, take antilogs of each side to the base e:

$$y = e^{(C_2-C_1)} \times e^{kt}$$

At zero time, $t = 0$ and $e^{kt} = 1$. Therefore the constant $e^{(C_2-C_1)}$ equals the initial value of y, which we may call y_0. Our final equation is thus:

$$y = y_0 e^{kt}$$

y_0 is the initial value of the variable y at zero time.
e is the base of natural logarithms. This constant (2.71828 . . .) possesses many remarkable mathematical properties.
k is a constant that defines the speed of the particular function. For example, it will differ by a factor of 2 if our mythical water-lily doubles its size every 12 hours instead of every day. In the case of the wash-out and wash-in, we shall see that k is directly related to certain important physiological quantities, from which we may predict the speed of certain biological changes.

Instead of using e, it is possible to take logs to the more familiar base 10, thus:

$$y = y_0 10^{k_1 t}$$

This is a perfectly valid way of expressing a tear-away exponential function, but you will notice that the constant k has changed to k_1. This new constant does not have the simple relationships of physiological variables mentioned above. It does, however, bear a constant relationship to k, as follows:

$$k_1 = 0.4343k \text{ (approx.)}$$

Graphical representation. On linear graph paper, a tear-away exponential function rapidly disappears off the top

of the paper (see Figure F.4). If plotted on semi-logarithmic paper (time on a linear axis and y on a logarithmic axis), the plot becomes a straight line and this is a most convenient method of presenting such a function. The logarithmic plots in Figures F.4–F.6 are all plotted on semi-log paper.

The wash-out or die-away exponential function

The account of the tear-away exponential function has really been an essential introduction to the wash-out or die-away exponential function, which is of great importance to the biologist in general and the respiratory physiologist in particular.

Simple statement. In a wash-out exponential function, the quantity under consideration falls at a rate which decreases progressively in proportion to the distance it still has to fall. It approaches but, in theory, never reaches zero.

Examples. Familiar examples are cooling curves, radioactive decay and water running out of the bath. In the last example the rate of flow of bath water to waste is proportional to the pressure of water, which is proportional to the depth of water in the bath, which in turn is proportional to the quantity of water in the bath (assuming that the sides are vertical). Therefore, the flow rate of water to waste is proportional to the amount of water left in the bath and decreases as the bath empties. The last molecule of bath water takes an infinitely long time to drain away.

In the field of respiratory physiology, examples include:

1. passive expiration (Figure F.5)
2. the elimination of inhalational anaesthetics
3. the fall of arterial P_{CO_2} to its new level after a step increase in ventilation
4. the fall of arterial P_{O_2} to its new level after a step decrease in ventilation
5. the fall of blood P_{CO_2} towards the alveolar level as it progresses along the pulmonary capillary
6. the fall of blood P_{O_2} towards the tissue level as blood progresses through the tissue capillaries.

Mathematical statement. When a quantity *decreases* with time, the rate of change is *negative*. Therefore, the wash-out exponential function is written thus:

$$\frac{dy}{dt} = -ky$$

from which we may derive the following equations, which give the value of y at any time t:

$$y = y_0 e^{-kt}$$

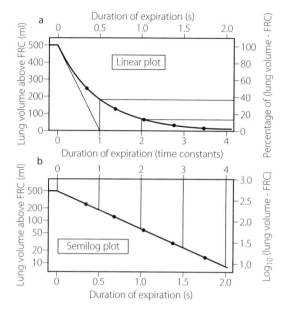

Figure F.5 Passive expiration – a typical wash-out exponential function. Tidal volume, 500 ml; compliance, 0.5 l.kPa^{-1} (50 ml.cmH$_2$O^{-1}); airway resistance, 1 kPa.l^{-1}.s (10 cmH$_2$O.l^{-1}.s); time constant, 0.5 s; half-life, 0.35 s. The points on the curve indicate the passage of successive half-lives. Note that the logarithmic coordinate has no zero. This accords with the lung volume approaching, but never actually equalling, the FRC.

which is simply another way of saying:

$$y = \frac{y_0}{e^{kt}}$$

y_0 is again the initial value of y at zero time. In Figure F.5, y_0 is the initial value of (lung volume – FRC) at the start of expiration; that is to say, the tidal volume inspired.

e is again the base of natural logarithms (2.71828 . . .).

k is the constant that defines the rate of decay and is the reciprocal of a most important quantity known as the *time constant*, represented by the Greek letter tau (τ). Three things should be known about the time constant.

1. Figure F.5 shows a tangent drawn to the first part of the curve. This shows the course events would take if the initial rate were maintained instead of slowing down in the manner characteristic of the wash-out curve. The time that would then be required for completion would be the time constant (τ) or $1/k$. The wash-out exponential function may thus be written:

$$y = y_0 e^{-t/\tau}$$

2. After 1 time constant, y will have fallen to $1/e$ of its initial value or approximately 37% of its initial value.

After 2 time constants, y will have fallen to $1/e^2$ of its initial value or approximately 13.5% of its initial value.

After 3 time constants, y will have fallen to $1/e^3$ of its initial value or approximately 5% of its initial value.

After 5 time constants, y will have fallen to $1/e^5$ of its initial value or approximately 1% of its initial value.

3. The time constant is often determined by physiological factors. When air escapes passively from a distended lung, the time constant is governed by two variables, compliance and resistance (see Chapters 3, 4 and 32).

We may now consider the example of passive expiration. Let V represent the lung volume (above FRC), then $-dV/dt$ is the instantaneous expiratory gas flow rate. Assuming Poiseuille's law is obeyed:

$$-\frac{dV}{dt} = \frac{P}{R}$$

when P is the instantaneous alveolar-to-mouth pressure gradient and R is the airway resistance. However, compliance $(C) = V/P$. Therefore:

$$-\frac{dV}{dt} = \frac{1}{CR}V$$

or:

$$\frac{dV}{dt} = -\frac{1}{CR}V$$

Then by integration and taking antilogs as described above:

$$V = V_0 e^{-(t/CR)}$$

By analogy with the general equation of the wash-out exponential function, it is clear that $CR = 1/k = \tau$ (the time constant). Thus the *time constant equals the product of compliance and resistance.*[†] This is analogous to the discharge of an electrical capacitor through a resistance, when the time constant of discharge equals the product of the capacitance and the resistance.

Half-life. It is often convenient to use the half-life instead of the time constant. This is the time required for y to change to half of its previous value. The special attraction of the half-life is its ease of measurement. The half-

---

[†] It is strange at first sight that two quantities as complex as compliance and resistance should have a product as simple as time. In fact, the MLT units (see Appendix A) check perfectly well:

Compliance × resistance = time

$M^{-1}L^4T^2 \times ML^{-4}T^{-1} = T$

life of a radioactive element may be determined quite simply. First of all, the degree of activity is measured and the time noted. Its activity is then followed and the time noted at which its activity is exactly half the initial value. The difference between the two times is the half-life and is constant at all levels of activity. Half-lives are shown in Figures F.4–F.6 as dots on the curves. For a particular exponential function there is a constant relationship between the time constant and the half-life.

$$\text{Half-life} = 0.69 \times \text{time constant}$$

$$\text{Time constant} = 1.44 \times \text{half-life}$$

Graphical representation. Plotting a wash-out exponential function is similar to the tear-away function (see Figure F.5). A semilog plot is particularly convenient as the curve (being straight) may then be defined by far fewer observations. It is also easy to extrapolate backwards to zero time if the initial value is required but could not be measured directly for some reason. It is, for example, an essential step in the measurement of cardiac output with a dye that is rapidly lost from the circulation (page 107).

The wash-in exponential function

The wash-in function is also of special importance to the respiratory physiologist and is the mirror image of the wash-out function.

Simple statement. In a wash-in exponential function, the quantity under consideration rises towards a limiting value, at a rate that decreases progressively in proportion to the distance it still has to rise.

Examples. A typical example would be a mountaineer who each day manages to climb half the remaining distance between his overnight camp and the summit of the mountain. His rate of ascent declines exponentially and he will never reach the summit. A graph of his altitude plotted against time would resemble a wash-in curve.

Biological examples include the reverse of those listed for the wash-out function.

1. Inflation of the lungs of a paralysed patient by a sustained increase of mouth pressure (Figure F.6).
2. The uptake of inhalational anaesthetics.
3. The rise of arterial $P\text{CO}_2$ to its new level after a step decrease of ventilation.
4. The rise of arterial $P\text{O}_2$ to its new level after a step increase of ventilation.
5. The rise of blood $P\text{O}_2$ to the alveolar level as it progresses along the pulmonary capillary.
6. The rise of blood $P\text{CO}_2$ to the venous level as blood progresses through the tissue capillaries.

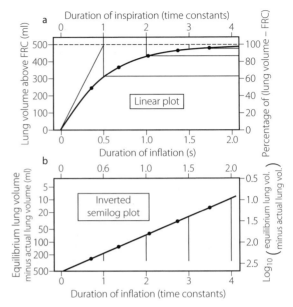

Figure F.6 Passive inflation of the lungs with a sustained mouth pressure – a typical wash-in exponential function. Final tidal volume, 500 ml; compliance, 0.5 l.kPa^{-1} (50 ml.cmH$_2$O^{-1}); airway resistance, 1 kPa.l^{-1}.s (10 cmH$_2$O.l^{-1}.s); time constant, 0.5 s; half-life, 0.35 s. The points on the curves indicate the passage of successive half-lives. Note that, for the semilog plot, the log scale (ordinate) is from above downwards and indicates the difference between the equilibrium lung volume (inflation pressure maintained indefinitely) and the actual lung volume.

Mathematical statement. With a wash-in exponential function, y increases with time and therefore the rate of change is positive. As time advances, the rate of change falls towards zero. The initial value of y is often zero and y approaches a final limiting value that we may designate y_∞; that is, the value of y when time is infinity (∞). A change of this type is indicated thus:

$$\frac{dy}{dt} = k(y_\infty - y)$$

As y approaches y_∞ so the quantity within the parentheses approaches zero and the rate of change slows down. The corresponding equation that indicates the instantaneous value of y is:

$$y = y_\infty(1 - e^{-kt})$$

y_∞ is the limiting value of y (attained only at infinite time).

e is again the base of natural logarithms.

k is a constant defining the rate of build-up and, as is the case of the wash-out function, it is the reciprocal of the *time constant* the significance of which is described above. It is the time that would be required to reach completion, if the initial rate of change were maintained without slowing down.

After 1 time constant, y will have risen to approximately $100 - 37 = 63\%$ of its final value.

After 2 time constants, y will have risen to approximately $100 - 13.5 = 86.5\%$ of its final value.

After 3 time constants, y will have risen to approximately $100 - 5 = 95\%$ of its final value.

After 5 time constants, y will have risen to approximately $100 - 1 = 99\%$ of its final value.

As in the wash-out function representing passive exhalation, the time constant for the corresponding wash-in exponential function (passive inflation of the lungs) equals the product of compliance and resistance. For the wash-in of a substance into an organ, the time constant equals tissue volume divided by blood flow or FRC divided by alveolar ventilation, as the case may be. As above, the time constant is approximately 1.5 times the half-life.

There are many situations in which the same parameters apply to both wash-in and wash-out functions of the same system. The time constant for each function will then be the same. A classic example is the charging of an electrical capacitor through a resistance and then allowing it to discharge to earth through the same resistor. The time constant is the same for each process and equals the product of capacitance and resistance. This is approximately true for passive deflation and inflation of the lungs (see Figures F.5 and F.6), on the assumption that compliance and airway resistance remain the same.

Graphical representation. The wash-in function may be represented on linear paper as for the other types of exponential function. However, for the semi-log plot, the paper must be turned upside down and the plot made as indicated in Figure F.6. The curve will then be a straight line.

Index